T0226697

Pain Management: A Multidisciplinary Approach

Editorial Advisor

JOEL J. HEIDELBAUGH

ELSEVIER

1600 John F. Kennedy Boulevard • Suite 1800 • Philadelphia, Pennsylvania, 19103-2899

http://www.theclinics.com

CLINICS COLLECTIONS
ISSN 2352-7986, ISBN-13: 978-0-323-37073-8

Editor: Patrick Manley (p.manley@elsevier.com)
Developmental Editor: John Vassallo (j.vassallo@elsevier.com)

Clinics Collections (ISSN 2352-7986) is published by Elsevier Inc., 360 Park Avenue South, New York, NY 10010-1710. Business and editorial offices: 1600 John F. Kennedy Boulevard, Suite 1800, Philadelphia, PA 19103-2899. **POSTMASTER:** Send address changes to *Clinics Collections*, Elsevier Health Sciences Division, Subscription Customer Service, 3251 Riverport Lane, Maryland Heights, MO 63043. **Customer Service: Telephone: 1-800-654-2452** (U.S. and Canada); **1-314-447-8871** (outside U.S. and Canada). **Fax: 314-447-8029. E-mail: journalscustomerserviceusa@elsevier.com** (for print support); **journalsonlinesupport-usa@elsevier.com** (for online support).

Reprints. For copies of 100 or more of articles in this publication, please contact the Commercial Reprints Department, Elsevier Inc., 360 Park Avenue South, New York, NY 10010-1710. Tel.: 212-633-3874; Fax: 212-633-3820; E-mail: reprints@elsevier.com.

Contributors

EDITORIAL ADVISOR

JOEL J. HEIDELBAUGH, MD, FAAFP, FACG
Clinical Associate Professor, Departments of Family Medicine and Urology; Clerkship Director, Department of Family Medicine, University of Michigan Medical School, Ann Arbor, Michigan; Ypsilanti Health Center, Ypsilanti, Michigan

AUTHORS

PENNE ALLISON, RN, BSN, MSOM, NE-BC
Director of Emergency Services, University of Kentucky HealthCare, Lexington, Kentucky

KEVIN N. ALSCHULER, PhD
Acting Assistant Professor, Department of Rehabilitation Medicine, University of Washington School of Medicine, Seattle, Washington

AMBA AYLOO, MD
Chief Resident, Family Medicine Residency Program, Department of Family Medicine, Mount Sinai Hospital, Chicago, Illinois

JONATHAN A. BECKER, MD
Program Director, Primary Care Sports Medicine Fellowship, Jewish Hospital and University of Louisville; Associate Professor, Department of Family and Geriatric Medicine, University of Louisville, Louisville, Kentucky

JOANNE BORG-STEIN, MD
Associate Professor, Department of Physical Medicine and Rehabilitation, Harvard Medical School, Boston, Massachusetts

SARAH BOURNE, MD
Resident, Department of Neurosurgery, Cleveland Clinic, Cleveland, Ohio

LUIS F. BUENAVER, PhD
Assistant Professor, Department of Psychiatry and Behavioral Sciences, Johns Hopkins University School of Medicine, Baltimore, Maryland

IAN CARROLL, MD, MS
Assistant Professor, Department of Anesthesia, Stanford University, Palo Alto, California

GRACE CHEN, MD
Assistant Professor, Department of Anesthesiology and Perioperative Medicine, Oregon Health and Science University, Portland, Oregon

MICHAEL C. CHEN, PhD
Galderma Laboratories, LP, Fort Worth, Texas

CATHERINE M. CURTIN, MD
Staff Physician, Palo Alto VA; Assistant Professor, Division of Plastic Surgery, Stanford University, Palo Alto, California

TERESA CVENGROS, MD, CAQSM
Attending Physician, Family Medicine Residency Program, Department of Family Medicine, Mount Sinai Hospital, Chicago, Illinois

LAURA J. DAVILA, DDS
Chief Resident, General Practice, Division of Dentistry and Oral & Maxillofacial Surgery, Weill-Cornell Medical College, New York Presbyterian Hospital, Cornell University, New York, New York

ARTHUR JASON De LUIGI, DO
Department of Rehabilitation Medicine, Georgetown University School of Medicine, Washington, DC

SCOTT S. De ROSSI, DMD
Chair, Department of Oral Health and Diagnostic Sciences, College of Dental Medicine; Associate Professor, Departments of Dermatology and Otolaryngology/Head and Neck Surgery, Medical College of Georgia, Georgia Regents University, Augusta, Georgia

DAVID M. DICKERSON, MD
Assistant Professor, Department of Anesthesia and Critical Care, University of Chicago Medicine, Chicago, Illinois

JOHN A. DiPRETA, MD
Clinical Associate Professor, Division of Orthopaedic Surgery, Capital Region Orthopaedic Group, Albany Medical Center, Albany Medical College, Albany, New York

DAWN M. EHDE, PhD
Professor, Department of Rehabilitation Medicine, University of Washington School of Medicine, Seattle, Washington

ERIC EMANSKI, MD
Department of Orthopaedic Surgery, Penn State–Milton S. Hershey Medical Center, Hershey, Pennsylvania

GINGER EVANS, MD
Acting Instructor, Department of Medicine, VA Puget Sound Health Care System, University of Washington, Seattle, Washington

PATRICK H. FINAN, PhD
Assistant Professor, Department of Psychiatry and Behavioral Sciences, Johns Hopkins University School of Medicine, Baltimore, Maryland

JENNIFER FORMAN, RN, BSN
Patient Care Manager, Critical Care Services, Good Samaritan Hospital, University of Kentucky HealthCare, Lexington, Kentucky

MITCHELL FREEDMAN, DO
Associate Professor and Clinical Instructor of Rehabilitation Medicine, Jefferson Medical College, Thomas Jefferson University; Director of Physical Medicine and Rehabilitation, Rothman Institute, Philadelphia, Pennsylvania

DEBORAH L. GREENBERG, MD
Associate Professor of Medicine; University of Washington School of Medicine, Seattle, Washington

ARI C. GREIS, DO
Clinical Instructor of Rehabilitation Medicine, Jefferson Medical College, Thomas Jefferson University; Rothman Institute, Philadelphia, Pennsylvania

SALIM M. HAYEK, MD, PhD
Chief, Division of Pain Medicine; Professor, Department of Anesthesiology, University Hospitals of Cleveland, Case Western Reserve University, Cleveland, Ohio

JEFFREY HENSTENBURG
Rochester Institute of Technology College Student Volunteer, Rothman Institute, Philadelphia, Pennsylvania

LAURIE ANNE HIEMSTRA, MD, PhD, FRCSC
Banff Sport Medicine, Banff, Alberta, Canada; Department of Surgery, University of Calgary, Calgary, Alberta, Canada

M. BRIGID HOLLORAN-SCHWARTZ, MD
Professor, Saint Louis University School of Medicine, St Louis, Missouri

ULA HWANG, MD, MPH
Associate Professor, Department of Emergency Medicine; Brookdale Department of Geriatrics and Palliative Medicine, Mount Sinai School of Medicine, New York; Geriatric Research, Education and Clinical Center, James J. Peters Veterans Affairs Medical Center, Bronx, New York

MARY ALEXIS IACCARINO, MD
Department of Physical Medicine and Rehabilitation, Harvard Medical School, Boston, Massachusetts

CHRISTOPHER IRVING, MD
Banff Sport Medicine, Banff, Alberta, Canada

HOWARD A. ISRAEL, DDS
Professor of Clinical Surgery, Division of Dentistry and Oral & Maxillofacial Surgery, Weill-Cornell Medical College, New York Presbyterian Hospital, Cornell University; Adjunct Professor of Clinical Dentistry, Columbia University College of Dental Medicine, New York, New York

MARK P. JENSEN, PhD
Professor, Department of Rehabilitation Medicine, University of Washington School of Medicine, Seattle, Washington

BRIAN KAHAN, DO, FAAPMR, DAOCRM, DABIPP, DABPM, FIPP
Founder, The Kahan Center for Pain Management, Annapolis, Maryland

CHRISTOPHER KARRASCH, MD
Department of Orthopaedic Surgery, Penn State–Milton S. Hershey Medical Center, Pennsylvania State University College of Medicine, Hershey, Pennsylvania

SARAH KERSLAKE, BPhty(Hons)
Banff Sport Medicine, Banff, Alberta, Canada; Department of Physical Therapy, University of Alberta, Edmonton, Alberta, Canada

MARK A. KNAUB, MD
Assistant Professor, Department of Orthopaedic Surgery; Chief of Adult Spine Service, Penn State–Milton S. Hershey Medical Center, Hershey, Pennsylvania

PATRICIA KUNZ HOWARD, PhD, RN, CEN, CPEN, NE-BC, FAEN, FAAN
Operations Manager, Emergency Services, University of Kentucky Chandler Medical Center, Lexington, Kentucky

FAH CHE LEONG, MS, MD
Professor, Obstetrics, Gynecology, and Women's Health; Professor, Surgery, Saint Louis University School of Medicine, St Louis, Missouri

SCOTT LYNCH, MD
Associate Professor, Department of Orthopaedic Surgery, Penn State–Milton S. Hershey Medical Center, Hershey, Pennsylvania

ANDRE G. MACHADO, MD, PhD
Staff Neurosurgeon, Department of Neurosurgery, Center for Neurological Restoration; Associate Professor, Cleveland Clinic Lerner College of Medicine, Cleveland Clinic, Cleveland, Ohio

SRIMANNARAYANA MARELLA, MD
Resident, Family Medicine Residency Program, Department of Family Medicine, Mount Sinai Hospital, Chicago, Illinois

LISA MARINO, DO
Associate Physician, Rothman Institute, Philadelphia, Pennsylvania

MATTHEW H. MECKFESSEL, PhD
Galderma Laboratories, LP, Fort Worth, Texas

DAVID MISENER, BSc (HK), CPO, MBA
Clinical Prosthetics and Orthotics, Albany, New York

SEAN J. NAGEL, MD
Staff Neurosurgeon, Department of Neurosurgery, Center for Neurological Restoration; Assistant Professor, Cleveland Clinic Lerner College of Medicine, Cleveland Clinic, Cleveland, Ohio

JOEL J. NAPEÑAS, DDS
Assistant Professor, Division of Oral Medicine and Radiology, Schulich School of Medicine and Dentistry, Western University, London, Ontario, Canada; Department of Oral Medicine, Carolinas Medical Center, Charlotte, North Carolina

NATHAN PATRICK, MD
Department of Orthopaedic Surgery, Penn State–Milton S. Hershey Medical Center, Hershey, Pennsylvania

TIMOTHY F. PLATTS-MILLS, MD
Assistant Professor, Department of Emergency Medicine; Department of Anesthesiology, University of North Carolina at Chapel Hill, Chapel Hill, North Carolina

MATTHEW PROUD, BSN, RN, CEN
Patient Care Manager, Emergency Services, University of Kentucky Chandler Medical Center, Lexington, Kentucky

ANDREW J. ROSENBAUM, MD
Resident, Division of Orthopaedic Surgery, Albany Medical Center, Albany Medical College, Albany, New York

VIRGINIA T. RUNKO, PhD
Clinical Associate, Department of Psychiatry and Behavioral Sciences, Johns Hopkins University School of Medicine, Baltimore, Maryland

JOSEPH SALAMA-HANNA, MBBS
Department of Anesthesiology and Perioperative Medicine, Henry Ford Hospital, Detroit, Michigan

MICHAEL SAULINO, MD, PhD
Physiatrist, MossRehab, Elkins Park; Assistant Professor, Department of Rehabilitation Medicine, Jefferson Medical College, Thomas Jefferson University, Philadelphia, Pennsylvania

ATIT SHAH, MD
Pain Management Fellow, Department of Anesthesiology, Case Western University, Chicago, Illinois

ANUPAM N. SINHA, DO
Associate Physician, Rothman Institute, Philadelphia, Pennsylvania

MICHAEL T. SMITH, PhD
Professor, Department of Psychiatry and Behavioral Sciences, Johns Hopkins University School of Medicine, Baltimore, Maryland

ANDREW STEELE, MD
Professor, Obstetrics, Gynecology, and Women's Health; Professor, Surgery, Saint Louis University School of Medicine, St Louis, Missouri

SHARON L. STEIN, MD
Associate Professor, Division of Colorectal Surgery, Department of Surgery, University Hospitals Case Medical Center, Cleveland, Ohio

JESSICA R. STUMBO, MD
Associate Program Director, Primary Care Sports Medicine Fellowship, Jewish Hospital and University of Louisville; Assistant Professor, Department of Family and Geriatric Medicine, University of Louisville; Centers for Primary Care, Louisville, Kentucky

Contents

including sympathetic blocks, sympathectomy, and spinal cord stimulation are also reviewed.

This article discusses current trends in managing cancer pain, with specific regard to opioid transmission, descending pathway inhabitation, and ways to facilitate the endogenous antinociceptive chemicals in the human body. Various techniques for opioid and nonopioid control of potential pain situations of patients with cancer are discussed. The benefits of using pharmacogenetics to assess the appropriate medications are addressed. Finally, specific treatment of abdominal cancer pain using radiofrequency lesioning is discussed.

Musculoskeletal

Head and Neck

Chronic neck pain is a common and often disabling problem. It can describe pain in the neck region alone or include related disorders of radiculopathy or myelopathy. This review of the literature is aimed at the practicing primary care provider, who is diagnosing and managing nontraumatic neck pain in the clinic. It includes an anatomic review, definition of related disorders, differential diagnosis, and discussion of common diagnostic uncertainty for mechanical neck pain. Important history and physical examination techniques, the role of imaging, and the available literature on conservative and invasive treatment options are reviewed.

This article clarifies the current state of knowledge of chronic oral, head, and facial pain (COHFP) conditions with the inclusion of temporomandibular joint disorders as just one component of the variety of conditions that can cause head and facial pain. Obtaining an accurate diagnosis in a timely manner is extremely important because COHFP symptoms can be caused by a variety of pathologic conditions that can be inflammatory, degenerative, neurologic, neoplastic, or systemic in origin. The essential role of the specialty of otolaryngology in the diagnosis and management of patients with these complex COHFP conditions is emphasized.

Orofacial pain refers to pain associated with the soft and hard tissues of the head, face, and neck. It is a common experience in the population that has profound sociologic effects and impact on quality of life. New scientific evidence is constantly providing insight into the cause and pathophysiology of orofacial pain including temporomandibular disorders, cranial neuralgias, persistent idiopathic facial pains, headache, and dental pain. An evidence-based approach to the management of orofacial pain is imperative for the general clinician. This article reviews the basics of pain epidemiology and neurophysiology and sets the stage for in-depth discussions of various painful conditions of the head and neck.

Dental and oral diseases are common findings in the general population. Pain associated with dental or periodontal disease is the primary reason why most patients seek treatment from providers. Thus, it is essential that all complaints of pain in the mouth and face include ruling out pain of dental origin. However, intraoral pain is not exclusively a result of dental disorders. This review outlines common somatic intraoral pain disorders, which can originate from disease involving one or more broad anatomic areas: the teeth, the surrounding soft tissues (mucogingival, tongue, and salivary glands), and bone.

Back

Low back pain is an extremely common presenting complaint that occurs in upward of 80% of persons. Treatment of an acute episode of back pain includes relative rest, activity modification, nonsteroidal anti-inflammatories, and physical therapy. Patient education is also imperative, as these patients are at risk for further future episodes of back pain. Chronic back pain (>6 months' duration) develops in a small percentage of patients. Clinicians' ability to diagnose the exact pathologic source of these symptoms is severely limited, making a cure unlikely. Treatment of these patients should be supportive, the goal being to improve pain and function.

This article provides a summary of the many causes of back pain in adults. There is an overview of the history and physical examination with attention paid to red flags that alert the clinician to more worrisome causes of low back pain. An extensive differential diagnosis for back pain in adults is provided along with key historical and physical examination findings. The various therapeutic options are summarized with an emphasis on evidence-based findings. These reviewed treatments include medication, physical therapy, topical treatments, injections, and complementary and alternative medicine. The indications for surgery and specialty referral are also discussed.

Clinicians must have knowledge of the growth and development of the adolescent spine and the subsequent injury patterns and other spinal conditions common in the adolescent athlete. The management and treatment of spinal injuries in adolescent athletes require a coordinated effort between the clinician, patients, parents/guardians, coaches, therapists, and athletic trainers. Treatment should not only help alleviate the current symptoms but also address flexibility and muscle imbalances to prevent future injuries by recognizing and addressing risk factors. Return to sport should be a gradual process once the pain has resolved and the athlete has regained full strength.

Neurologic

of this information across disciplines is slow. This article synthesizes some of this literature and provides a systematic presentation of the evidence on pain associated with peripheral nerve injury. It highlights the use of perioperative and early intervention to decrease this debilitating problem.

Obstetric and Gynecologic

should be avoided. If patients present for evaluation of disease states such as endometriosis or interstitial cystitis already using regular narcotics, physicians should be aware of ways to mediate misuse and diversion. Women with chronic pain should be screened for depression as well as a history of prior sexual abuse, and treatment or referral initiated when indicated.

Psychologic

Pain is the number 1 reason patients seek care in an emergency department (ED). A limiting factor for effective pain management may be clinical staff attitudes about pain and pain management. Analysis of data from an investigation into pain, perceptions, and perceived conflicts of ED staff pain management revealed a need for change. Operation Pain and ED pain champions created an environment that promoted enhanced pain management resulting in measurable outcomes. Emergency nurses participating in Operation Pain placed a higher priority on pain management for their patients.

This article summarizes the literature on cognitive-behavioral therapy for insomnia (CBT-I) in patients with comorbid insomnia and chronic pain. An empiric rationale for the development of CBT-I in chronic pain is provided. The 6 randomized controlled trials in this area are described and contrasted. The data suggest that CBT-I for patients with comorbid insomnia and chronic pain produces clinically meaningful improvements in sleep symptoms. Effects on pain are inconsistent, but tend to favor functional measures over pain severity. Hybrid interventions for insomnia and pain have demonstrated feasibility, but additional trials must be conducted to determine the efficacy relative to CBT-I alone.

Depression and pain are highly prevalent among individuals with multiple sclerosis, and they often co-occur. The purpose of this article is to summarize the literature and theory related to the comorbidity of pain and depression and describe how their presence can impact individuals with multiple sclerosis. Additionally, the article discusses how existing treatments of pain and depression could be adapted to address shared mechanisms and overcome barriers to treatment utilization.

Special Considerations

Myofascial pain syndrome (MPS) is a regional pain disorder caused by taut bands of muscle fibers in skeletal muscles called myofascial trigger points. MPS is a common disorder, often diagnosed and treated by physiatrists. Treatment strategies for MPS include exercises, patient education, and trigger point injection. Pharmacologic interventions are also common, and a variety of analgesics, antiinflammatories, antidepressants, and other medications are used in clinical practice. This review explores the various treatment options for MPS, including those therapies that target myofascial trigger points and common secondary symptoms.

Autoinflammatory disorders are disorders of the innate immune system that are distinct from autoimmune disorders. Dysregulation of the innate immune system, specifically an increase in interleukin-1 beta (IL-1β), gives rise to a spectrum of symptoms marked by inflammation and pain. Identification of causative gene mutations led to the discovery of the inflammasome. Many autoinflammatory disorders also have a strong pain component. The contribution of IL-1β to pain and neural involvement is underappreciated. This article provides an overview of the current autoinflammatory disorders and highlights the contribution IL-1β makes to pain in these disorders.

Effective treatment of acute pain in older patients is a common challenge faced by emergency providers. Because older adults are at increased risk for adverse events associated with systemic analgesics, pain treatment must proceed cautiously. Essential elements to quality acute pain care include an early initial assessment for the presence of pain, selection of an analgesic based on patient-specific risks and preferences, and frequent reassessments and retreatments as needed. This article describes current knowledge regarding the assessment and treatment of acute pain in older adults.

Preface

Clinics Review Articles have been a part of the physician's, nurse's, and resident's library for nearly 100 years. This trusted resource covers over 50 medical disciplines every year, producing thousands of articles focused on the most current concepts and techniques in medicine. This collection of articles, devoted to pain management, draws from this *Clinics* database to provide multidisciplinary teams with practical, clinical advice on comorbidities and complications of this highly prevalent condition.

A multidisciplinary perspective is key to effective team-based pain management. Featured articles from the *Medical Clinics of North America, Nursing Clinics of North America, Physical Medicine and Rehabilitation Clinics of North America, Gastroenterology Clinics of North America, Obstetrics and Gynecology Clinics of North America,* and *Hand Clinics,* reflect the wide range of clinicians who manage patients with pain-related disorders.

I encourage you to share this volume with your colleagues in hopes that it may promote more collaboration, new perspectives, and informed, effective care for your patients.

Joel J. Heidelbaugh, MD, FAAFP, FACG
Ypsilanti, Michigan
November 2014

http://dx.doi.org/10.1016/j.ccol.2014.10.001
2352-7986/14/$ – see front matter © 2014 Published by Elsevier Inc.

Basic Anatomy and Physiology of Pain Pathways

Sarah Bourne, MD[a], Andre G. Machado, MD, PhD[b],
Sean J. Nagel, MD[b],*

KEYWORDS

- Hyperalgesia • Allodynia • Peripheral sensitization • Spino-thalamic tract
- Gait control theory • Descending systems

KEY POINTS

- Pain signals are transmitted along Aδ and C nociceptive nerve fibers to the central nervous system.
- Most peripheral nerve fibers will synapse in the Rexed lamina and then ascend in the contralateral spinothalamic tract before terminating in the ventral posterior nuclei and central nuclei of the thalamus.
- The receptive fields of the thalamus may reorganize following injury.
- The primary and secondary somatosensory cortex receive the bulk of direct projections from the thalamus; the insula, orbitofrontal cortex, dorsolateral prefrontal cortex, amygdala and cingulate are additional early relay sites important in pain processing.
- The rostral ventromedial medulla, the dorsolateral pontomesencephalic tegmentum, and the periaquaductal gray region are important structures in the descending regulation of noxious stimuli at the dorsal horn.
- The neuromatrix theory of pain incorporates the gate control theory of pain that focused on pain regulation at the spinal cord with more recent evidence that expands the role of the cortex.

INTRODUCTION

The pain pathways form a complex, dynamic, sensory, cognitive, and behavioral system that evolved to detect, integrate, and coordinate a protective response to incoming noxious stimuli that threatens tissue injury or organism survival.[1] This defense system includes both the primitive spinal reflexes that are the only protection

This article originally appeared in Neurosurgery Clinics of North America, Volume 25, Issue 4, October 2014.

[a] Department of Neurosurgery, Cleveland Clinic, 9500 Euclid Avenue, S4, Cleveland, OH 44195, USA; [b] Department of Neurosurgery, Center for Neurological Restoration, Cleveland Clinic Lerner College of Medicine, Cleveland Clinic, 9500 Euclid Avenue, S31, Cleveland, OH 44195, USA

* Corresponding author.

E-mail address: nagels@ccf.org

for simple organisms all the way up to the complex emotional responses humans consciously and subconsciously experience as pain. The mental representation of pain is stored as both short-term and long-term memory and serves as an early warning avoidance system for future threats.[1] When severe, mental anguish may be projected with a physical complaint or symptom. Although many of the basic structures of the pain pathways have been defined, a more complete understanding of the interactions that would enable the development of targeted therapies remains elusive.

PERIPHERAL SENSORY SYSTEM AND MECHANISMS OF SENSITIZATION

The location, intensity, and temporal pattern of noxious stimuli are transduced into a recognizable signal through unmyelinated nociceptors at the terminal end of sensory neurons. Through physical deformation or molecular binding, membrane permeability and, consequently, the membrane potential fluctuate.[2] If depolarization reaches a critical threshold, an action potential is propagated along the length of a sensory nerve toward the spinal cord.

Most sensory receptors respond to a single stimulus modality. Nociceptors, designed to detect tissue injury, are excited by three noxious stimuli: mechanical, thermal, and chemical. Mechanical stimuli deform the receptor to augment receptor ion permeability,[3] whereas chemicals such as bradykinin, serotonin, histamine, potassium ions, acids, acetylcholine, and proteolytic enzymes[2] bind directly to receptors to influence membrane permeability. Prostaglandins and substance P (SP) do not directly activate pain receptors but indirectly influence membrane permeability.

Nociceptive receptors sit at the ends of pseudounipolar sensory neurons with cell bodies in the dorsal root, trigeminal, or nodose ganglia (**Fig. 1**).[4] Pain receptors are unencapsulated free nerve endings. Sensory nerve fibers range from 0.5 to 20 μm in diameter and can conduct impulses at speeds ranging from 0.5 to 120 m/sec. Larger diameter neurons conduct information at a faster speed.[2] Nerve fibers are divided up into two main categories: type A, which are medium to large diameter myelinated neurons, and type C, small diameter unmyelinated neurons.[2] Pain transmission is divided into two categories, fast and slow. A-delta fibers detect and transmit pain quickly. These fibers are relatively small (1–6 m), thinly myelinated neurons that can conduct at speeds of 6 to 30 m/sec.[3] C fibers are small (<1.5 m) and unmyelinated, conducting pain at 0.5 to 2 m/sec.[2] A-beta are large (6–12 m) myelinated fibers that are high speed (30–70 m/sec).[2] They have encapsulated receptors and transmit information about touch, pressure, and vibration.[3] Most A-delta fibers are associated with thermo or mechanoreceptors. C fibers can be associated with polymodal receptors, suggesting a role in monitoring the overall tissue condition.[3]

Innocuous stimuli may elicit excitation of neurons in the peripheral nociceptive system following repeated injury or inflammation. These pathologic changes contribute to phenomena such as sensitization, allodynia, or hyperalgesia. In peripheral sensitization, neurons fire at a lower threshold and have greater response magnitude to a given stimuli,[5] may fire spontaneously, or may even have altered receptive field areas.[6,7] This occurs via inflammatory mediators, including bradykinin, prostaglandins, serotonin, tumor necrosis factor alpha, and histamine.[8] After integration in the brainstem, descending pronociceptive and antinociceptive pathways contribute to peripheral sensitization. When the function of these pathways becomes abnormal, chronic pain may occur.

The expression of molecules, including GABA, histamine, serotonin, and opiate receptors in nociceptive neurons, may be modulated by inflammation or injury.[8] Near the receptor there is a high concentration of sodium channels. Increased channel

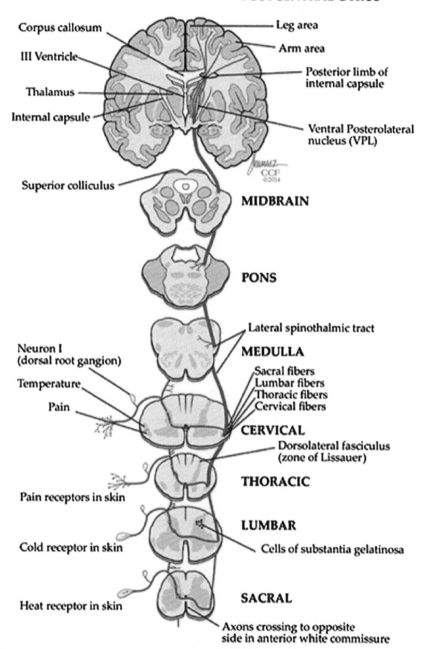

POSTCENTRAL GYRUS

Corpus callosum

III Ventricle

Thalamus

Internal capsule

Leg area

Arm area

Posterior limb of internal capsule

Ventral Posterolateral nucleus (VPL)

Superior colliculus

MIDBRAIN

PONS

Lateral spinothalmic tract

Neuron I (dorsal root gangion)

Temperature

Pain

MEDULLA

Sacral fibers
Lumbar fibers
Thoracic fibers
Cervical fibers

CERVICAL

Dorsolateral fasciculus (zone of Lissauer)

THORACIC

Pain receptors in skin

LUMBAR

Cold receptor in skin

Cells of substantia gelatinosa

Heat receptor in skin

SACRAL

Axons crossing to opposite side in anterior white commissure

Fig. 1. Pain and temperature transmission from receptors in the skin ascend in the spinal cord to the postcentral gyrus via the lateral spinothalamic tract. First-order neurons transmit this sensory information via pseudounipolar neurons that enter the spinal cord in the Lissauer tract where they synapse in the Rexed lamina. Second-order neurons from the dorsal horn then decussate at the ventral commissure and ascend in the lateral spinothalamic tract before ending in the ventral posterolateral nuclei of the thalamus. Third-order neurons then project to the postcentral gyrus. (*Courtesy of* the Cleveland Clinic Foundation, Cleveland, Ohio.)

expression can alter sensitivity of nerve endings to noxious stimuli by modulating integration of stimuli and threshold potential for action potential generation.[3] Increased sodium channel expression has been reported after nerve injury and may contribute to hyperexcitability and associated abnormal sensation.[9] C fibers have long response times and are slow to adapt. Because of this, they show summation of response to noxious stimuli in the presence of tissue injury,[10] perhaps contributing to sensitization and hyperalgesia.

Inflammation results in an upregulation of SP, including in A-beta fibers.[11] In this setting, A fibers may play a role in central sensitivity, perhaps contributing to hypersensitivity.[11,12] A-beta fibers terminate in lamina III of the spinal cord where SP receptors are present. They may contribute to ongoing activation of SP expressing nociceptive neurons in chronic pain states.[12]

DORSAL ROOT GANGLIA

Sensory neuron cell bodies are located in the dorsal root ganglia (DRG). DRG neurons are classically pseudounipolar; one process extends into the peripheral nerve and the other process extends centrally, transmitting information through the dorsal root into the spinal cord. Each DRG contains thousands of unique sensory neuron cell bodies that are capable of encoding and then transmitting specific information gathered from external stimuli.[13] Cells in the DRG are subclassified into peptidergic neurons and nonpeptidergic neurons. Peptidergic neurons contain peptides such as SP, calcitonin gene–related peptide (CGRP), and somatostatin.[14] Each DRG neuron is surrounded by glial cell cytoplasm. The surface of the DRG neuron cell bodies are covered with perikaryal projections that are invested in the surrounding glial cytoplasm, increasing the surface area.[15]

The soma of DRG neurons synthesizes and transports the substances needed for neuron functioning to the far reaches of the axon terminals, including receptors, ion channels, as well as molecules essential for synaptic transmission.[13] The most common neurotransmitter that is synthesized by DRG cells is glutamate; however, many DRG cells also express SP, which facilitates pain transmission.[3] There are no direct synaptic connections between DRG neurons but their activity is indirectly modulated.[16] After injury, DRG neurons may become innervated by postganglionic axons in a neurotrophin-mediated process.[8] C fibers may also modulate DRG sensitivity by altering intracellular calcium concentration affecting N-methyl-d-aspartate receptor configuration and sensitivity.[11] Therefore, plastic reorganization of the DRG is one of the many mechanisms involved in pain sensitization and chronification.

SPINAL CORD

Most sensory fibers project from the DRG through the dorsal root and into the dorsal root entry zone (DREZ). There is evidence that the ventral roots also receive projections from unmyelinated fibers originating from DRG cells that are involved in sensation, including nociception, violating the Bell-Magendie law.[17–20] At the DREZ, most unmyelinated and small myelinated axons project laterally to enter. Lissauer tract (see **Fig. 1**)[21] fibers then extend vertically in this tract for several spinal segments before synapsing. Second-order neurons then cross to the opposite side, in the ventral decussation of the central canal of the spinal cord.[22] The Lissauer tract contains both unmyelinated C fibers and myelinated A-delta fibers. A-delta fibers may ascend 3 to 4 segments in the Lissauer tract before finally terminating in lamina of Rexed I, II_o, or V. C fibers typically ascend one segment before terminating, most often in Rexed lamina II.[21]

Rexed lamina I, or the marginal layer, is composed of two main types of cells, nociceptive-specific neurons, and wide dynamic range neurons (WDRs). Nociceptive-specific neurons respond to noxious stimuli and express neuropeptides such as SP, CGRP, enkephalin, and serotonin.[3] WDRs dynamic range neurons transmit both noxious and nonnoxious information.[10] WDR display graded responses, proportional to the input stimulus by firing at a higher frequency.[3] WDR neurons have a large receptive field, including a center that responds to both noxious and nonnoxious stimuli and surrounding area responds to noxious stimuli only.[4] The large receptive fields of WDR neurons reflect its proposed integrative function that may contribute to allodynia through increased and disproportionate responsiveness to nonnoxious stimuli.[8]

Lamina II (substantia gelatinous) may play a role modulating spinothalamic and spinobulbar projection neurons via its numerous inhibitory interneurons that primarily release GABA. C fibers and A-delta fibers are the primary afferent inputs of lamina II. Lamina II inhibitory neurons then arborize locally to other lamina, including I, II, III, and IV.[3,23] There are very few projection neurons in lamina II. It has been hypothesized that disinhibition related to the functional loss of lamina II inhibitory neurons facilitates chronic neuropathic pain.

A-beta fibers project to lamina III and IV. Layer III also receives A-delta fiber mechanoreceptive input and may have sprouting of A-category neurons to lamina I and II after injury, possibly contributing to chronic pain and allodynia.[10,24] Some layer IV neurons project to layer I, which contributes to integration of sensation.[3] Lamina V receives input from A-delta and C fibers and neurons project to the spinothalamic tract (STT). Lamina V also contains a large number of WDR neurons with projections to reticular formation, periaqueductal gray, and medial thalamic nuclei, forming part of the mesial pathways that mediate the emotional characteristics of pain.[3,8] Lamina X surrounds the spinal cord central canal. The function of this region is less well defined but likely is involved in visceral pain. It receives some direct input from A-delta fibers and may play a role in integration of nociception.[3]

Dorsal horn (DH) nociceptive neurons form glutamatergic synapses that may also release neuropeptides, including SP, CGRP, vasoactive intestinal peptide (VIP), and somatostatin. Expression of these substances may be altered in the setting of injury,[8] leading to sensitization, allodynia, and secondary hyperalgesia. WDR neurons have also been implicated in the development of these phenomena. Secondary hyperalgesia may occur due to central sensitization which is, in turn, mediated by abnormal connections between nonnociceptive neurons and centrally transmitting nociceptive pathways, as well as receptive field plasticity of DH neurons.[25]

SPINOTHALAMIC PATHWAYS

The STT is oriented vertically along the ventrolateral portion of the spinal cord (see **Fig. 1**). It serves as the main conduit from the peripheral nerves to the brain by transmitting pain, temperature and deep touch signals to the thalamus. It receives projections from contralateral lamina I and IV-VI[26] and is composed of two tracts: one dorsolateral, carrying axons from the superficial lamina, and the other ventrolateral, carrying axons from deeper lamina.[27] Most projections are contralateral, although there is also an ipsilateral contribution.[8] There is somatotopic organization of the STT with the lower limbs dorsolaterally and upper body and limbs positioned ventromedially. Cells projecting to ventral posterolateral nuclei originate from laminae I and V. Lateral STT neurons have small contralateral receptive fields and are most likely involved in sensory-discriminative aspects of pain signaling.[8] Cells projecting to the medial thalamic nuclei originate from the deep dorsal laminae (ie, layer V; see above discussion) and ventral horn. The medial STT relays the motivational and affective components of noxious stimuli.[28] These neurons have large receptive fields to support this purpose.

The paleospinothalamic tract projects to brainstem reticular formation, hypothalamus, and thalamic nuclei.[3] Neurons in lamina VI, VII, and VIII have direct projections to reticular formation nuclei, some of which are bilateral.[29] Neurons in lamina I, VII, and VIII project to pons.[29] Neurons in the marginal zone, nucleus proprius, and lateral reticulated area project both to thalamus and hypothalamus. These neurons include both WDR neurons and nociceptive-specific neurons.[30] They project to reticular formation, periaquaductal gray (PAG), and medial thalamic nuclei, and may also be involved in motivational-affective component of pain.

Most of the projections to the reticular formation arise from A fibers, although A and C fiber innervation has been described.[29] Reticular formation response is proportional to noxious characteristics of the stimulus.[29] The spinoreticular tract travels with STT in ventrolateral spinal cord. Fibers largely terminate in ventral medial portion of the medulla reticular formation, medullae oblongatae centralis, pars ventralis, and nucleus gigantocellularis.[29,31] These cells have large receptive fields and exhibit heterotopic convergence. This tract functions to activate homeostatic mechanisms in brainstem autonomic centers as well as to provide input to antinociceptive systems and motivational-affective systems.

The spinomesencephalic tract originates in laminae I and IV-VI, with some contribution from lamina X and ventral horn. It projects to areas including periaqueductal gray, pretectal nuclei, red nucleus, Edinger-Westphal nucleus, and interstitial nucleus of Cajal. Neurons in this tract are nociceptive, and generally have large, complex receptive fields.[8] They are involved in aversive behavior and orientation responses, and may activate descending antinociceptive systems.

The 1965 gate control theory of pain by Melzack and Wall[32] proposed that there were three spinal cord systems involved in pain transmission: the substantia gelatinosa, dorsal column fibers, and central transmission cells in the DH (**Fig. 2**). The substantia gelatinosa functions as a gate that modulates signals before they reach the brain. Large diameter fibers have inhibitory effects to "shut the gate" whereas small diameter fibers carrying noxious stimuli open the gate to pain transmission. In a simplistic view of this model, rubbing of the injured area promotes proprioceptive (ie, large diameter) fiber input and reduces pain perception.[32] The gate-control theory has been criticized and revisited because it is inherently incomplete in its view of the nervous system. Nevertheless, it needs to be recognized for its key role in advancing the understanding of pain perception five decades ago and promoting the development of modern neurostimulation for pain management.

THALAMUS

The sensory thalamus is divided into nuclei that roughly maintain the segmentation of the noxious and innocuous divisions from the periphery. The ventral caudal (Hassler's nomenclature) or ventroposterior (VP) nucleus thalamic nuclei are the most direct subcortical relay site for the STT and the trigeminal thalami ctract (TTT)[27,33] before relaying pain signals to the primary sensory cortex and other cortical regions.[34] Glutaminergic projections from the dorsal column nuclei and from the DH via the STT synapse on neurons in the VP.[33] The VP is somatotopically organized with neurons excited by face stimulation medially (VPM) and arm and leg laterally (VPL). Cutaneous sensation from the distal extremities is located ventrally and truncal representation dorsally in the VP.[8] The VP can be further subdivided into a core that responds to

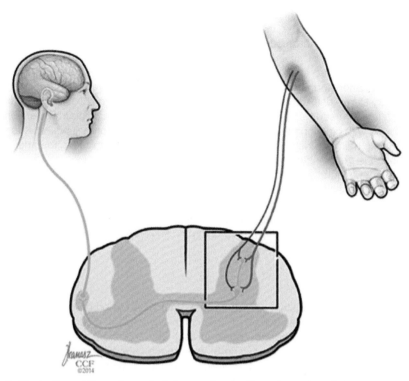

Fig. 2. Illustration of the gate control theory of pain. The substantia gelatinosa (SG) serves as a gate in the spinal cord that closes in response to large fiber (L) inputs, suppressing pain transmission. Alternatively, small fiber inputs open the gate or facilitate pain transmission. The summated pain signal then ascends in a projection neuron (P) via the spinothalamic (S) tract. This theory has since been revised to include the role of higher cortical processing to explain pain perception. (*Courtesy of* the Cleveland Clinic Foundation, Cleveland, Ohio.)

mechanical, nonnoxious stimuli and a posterior inferior region that transmits nociceptive signals.[35] Deep brain stimulation (DBS) of VP (Vc [Ventralis caudalis]) has been studied as a target to treat intractable, chronic pain.[35]

VP also receives WDR nociceptive neurons with large receptive fields and responses proportional to stimulus intensity.[26] Some of these neurons project to areas 3b and 1.

The ventralis posterior inferior (VPI) nucleus, which lies inferior to VPL and lateral to VPM, has larger receptive fields than VPL but retains somatotopic organization. It projects to SII.[26] The ventromedial posterior (VMpo) nucleus plays an important role in pain processing.[33] It receives projections from lamina I STT neurons and is composed of nociceptive-specific neurons with small, contralateral, receptive fields.[26] VMpo neurons project to the insula and area 3a.

The central nuclei of the thalamus are also involved in pain transmission. Neurons from the STT terminate in the intralaminar nuclei, including the central medial nuclei, parafasicularis, medial dorsal nucleus, and in the centralis laterals.[27] These midline intralaminar thalamic nuclei also receive indirect projections important in pain processing from the parabrachial nucleus and brainstem reticular nuclei. Neurons in these thalamic nuclei have large and nonspecific receptive fields that integrate pain signals and initiate protective responses such as arousal in response to noxious stimuli.[36]

The receptive fields of the specific nuclei of the thalamus have been shown to reorganize following injury. This thalamic reorganization subsequently influences downstream cortical reorganization.[35] Thalamic neurons with receptive fields adjacent to the receptive fields of an injured area gain a larger representation in the homunculus.[35,37] Decreased excitatory input or increased inhibitory input leads to neuronal hyperpolarization and aberrant bursting.[26] For example, membrane hyperpolarization secondary to loss of excitatory STT input following spinal cord injury contributes to cell bursting interspersed with periods of low firing between bursts.[35] This irregular firing is associated with development of central pain following spinal cord injury. Patients with neuropathic pain also demonstrate detrimental thalamic reorganization that may lead to innocuous thermal stimuli encoded as nociceptive signals.[37]

In some patients with chronic pain, the surface encephalographic recordings demonstrate a recognizable shift from normal alpha rhythms to low-frequency theta rhythms.[38] This cortical dysrhythmia is best observed between the medial thalamic nuclei and the insular, parietal opercular, and cingulate cortices.[38] Simultaneous thalamic recordings in patients with chronic pain show an increase in low frequency, coherent thalamocortical activity.[38]

CORTICAL AREAS

Painful stimuli activate distant cortical regions, including the primary somatosensory cortex (SI; Brodmann areas 3a/b, 2, 1, postcentral gyrus), secondary somatosensory cortex (SII), insula, orbitofrontal cortex, dorsal-lateral prefrontal cortex, extended amygdala, and cingulate cortex.[27] The SI is arranged with somatotopic organization of nociceptive signals that follows Penfield's homuncular pattern.[39] Projections from the VPM and VPL nuclei synapse directly in the SI. These neurons in SI demonstrate a graded response according to intensity of noxious stimulus.[27] This suggests that SI is involved in the discriminative quality of pain. The SII (parietal operculum) receives projections from ventrobasal thalamus, the VPM-VPL, and from the SI, as well as contralateral input.[27] Neurons in both the SII and Broadmann's area 7 also show responses proportional to magnitude of noxious stimuli.[27]

C fibers stimulation is associated with activation of the contralateral SI, in particular area 3a, the SII, and ipsilateral SII.[34] Similarly, activation of A-group fibers causes activation of the contralateral SI followed by SII.[34] This nociceptive input mainly projects to cortical layers III and IV.[3] The insula receives input from SI, SII, VPI, pulvinar, central median and parafascicular nuclei, medial dorsal nucleus, and Vmpo.[27] It demonstrates a graded response proportional to intensity of noxious stimulus and is likely involved in the sensory-discriminative processing of pain.[27] The insula projects to limbic structures such as amygdala and perirhinal cortex.[27] These widespread connections of the insula are involved in higher order pain processing and require consciousness for activation with painful stimuli.[3] Insula lesions have been associated with altered motivational-affective responses to pain.

The anterior cingulate cortex (ACC) and middle cingulate cortex receive projections from the medial and intralaminar thalamic nuclei and the VPI. These areas are activated with noxious stimuli that elicit an affective or motivational response to pain. Lesioning of the cingulate cortex attenuates these motivational-affective characteristics of pain, particularly in patients with chronic cancer pain.[27] Increased ACC activity may be seen in those with chronic pain.[39]

In the late 1990s, Melzack[1] revisited the original gate control theory and proposed the neuromatrix theory, adding higher cortical functions as key elements of pain transmission and interpretation. It postulates that individuals possess a genetically determined neural matrix that is shaped and modulated by sensory input. The neuromatrix contains parallel and interacting thalamocortical and limbic loops. Nodes in the sensory signaling circuitry are predetermined pattern generators and contribute to abnormal nociception. The structure and output of the neuromatrix is also controlled by cognitive and affective spheres. Thus, the final pain experience is determined not only by sensory input but also by behavioral and cognitive interpretation of pain, which includes prior experiences, injuries, and cultural background.

DESCENDING SYSTEMS

Descending pathways originating in the brain regulate incoming signals from noxious stimuli primarily through synapses on DH neurons (**Fig. 3**). Facilitative regulation amplifies the response as observed in sensitization. Alternatively, inhibitory regulation suppresses ascending pain signals during life-threatening events and other periods of extraordinary stress. These descending pathways include several relevant supraspinal structures: the rostral ventromedial medulla (RVM), the dorsolateral pontomesencephalic tegmentum, and the PAG region. The descending systems exert their effect predominantly in lamina I and II in the DH through the release of the monamine-serotonin, norepinephrine, and dopamine.[40] The monoamine released and receptor subtype will dictate an antinociceptive or pronociceptive effect. Dysregulation of these descending systems are believed to play a major role in chronic pain states.

The PAG-RVM-DH pathway is a descending pain modulatory system that has been well characterized. Stimulation of the PAG, first reported in the 1960s, induces analgesia and blocks the response of lamina V interneurons to noxious stimuli.[41,42] This net analgesic effect of PAG stimulation depends, in part, on the release of serotonin from neurons activated in the RVM.[43] Functional depletion of 5-hydroxytryptamine (5-HT) from RVM neurons has been shown to inhibit persistent pain in a rat model.[44] In addition to these serotonergic neurons, three additional neuron subtypes found in the RVM regulate pain transmission. Unlike the 5-HT neurons, the bulk of these neurons are GABA-ergic. ON-cells are inhibited by opioids and excite DH neurons to facilitate nociceptive pain. OFF-cells are excited by opioids and inhibit DH neurons to attenuate nociceptive pain. The function of the third population of neurons, NEUTRAL-cells, is not known. These three neuron types project to the spine and branch locally within the RVM.

The PAG also has direct projections to the spinal cord and additional indirect projections via the reticular formation and the parabrachial nuclei. Furthermore, the PAG has widespread connections with structures in rostral midbrain, diencephalon, and telencephalon.[28] The PAG projects to central nuclei of the thalamus, including centrolateral, paraventricular, parafascicular, and central medial areas, along with several dopaminergic areas, including ventral tegmental area and substantia nigra pars compacta. The PAG is likely also involved in the ascending modulation of nociception and integration of behavioral responses.[28]

Descending noradrenergic systems originating from the pontine A7 cell group (subcoerulus) and A5, A6 (locus coerulus) also show bidirectional pain control.[45] This pontine noradrenergic system is at least partly influenced by direct projections from neurons that release SP located in the RVM.[46] The regulation of pain signals transiting through the DH of the spinal cord is also under the control of dopaminergic descending neurons from the periventricular region of the hypothalamus (A11).[47] The dopamine receptor subtype expressed by primary afferents or DH neurons in lamina I dictate an antinociceptive or pronociceptive effect.[47] Dysfunction of this descending

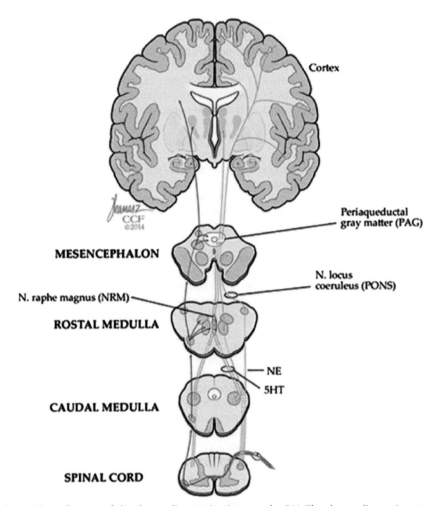

Fig. 3. The influence of the descending projections on the DH. The descending pain system regulates incoming pain signals at the DH. Input into the descending pain system is encoded at several sites in the brainstem including the PAG, dorsolateral pontine tegmentum (DLPT) and the RVM. The PAG exerts both direct and indirect descending control at the DH. The indirect pathway induces the release of 5-HT from neurons in the nucleus raphe magnus (NRM) located in the RVM. The descending noradrenergic system includes the nucleus locus coeruleus in the DLPT. (*Courtesy of* the Cleveland Clinic Foundation, Cleveland, Ohio.)

pain system may lead to chronic pain conditions; however, this descending dopaminergic system is another potential target for treatment.[47]

The descending endogenous opioid pain modulation system also augments pain processing. Activation of opioid receptors in the brain, specifically the mu receptor, blocks pain transmission centrally in the brain but also will activate descending systems. Opioid receptor binding alters membrane conductance and protein phosphorylation states.[3] Dynorphin is found in laminae I and V as well as PAG and midbrain reticular formation. It hypothesized that dynorphin contributes to pain centralization.

The interactions of the descending systems are still being defined although several hypothesis have been proposed to explain certain abnormal pain states. For example, central sensitization is believed to involve an increase in the activity of the ascending pain pathway coupled with a decrease in activity in the descending inhibitory pathway. Similarly, the release of tonic inhibition at the DH is associated with chronic pain.

SUMMARY

Although the details underpinning the pain systems are debatable, the evolutionary advantage to having an integrative pain system culminating in the conscious recognition of pain is not. When studied using modern neuroimaging or electrophysiological studies, the nature of the perceptual experience of pain still remains fragmented. This has unfortunately delayed the development of novel neurosurgical approaches to treat chronic noncancer pain. Nevertheless, the surgical treatments represented in this issue have taken advantage of what is known currently and represent an important step forward for those patients with chronic pain.

REFERENCES

1. Melzack R. From the gate to the neuromatrix. Pain 1999;(Suppl 6):S121–6.
2. Hall JE, Guyton AC. Guyton and Hall textbook of medical physiology. 12th edition. Philadelphia: Saunders/Elsevier; 2011.
3. Rosenow JM, Henderson JM. Anatomy and physiology of chronic pain. Neurosurg Clin N Am 2003;14(3):445–62, vii.
4. Fishman S, Ballantyne J, Rathmell JP, et al. Bonica's management of pain. 4th edition. Baltimore (MD): Lippincott, Williams & Wilkins; 2010.
5. Cooper B, Ahlquist M, Friedman RM, et al. Properties of high-threshold mechanoreceptors in the goat oral mucosa. II. Dynamic and static reactivity in carrageenan-inflamed mucosa. J Neurophysiol 1991;66(4):1280–90.
6. Handwerker HO, Anton F, Reeh PW. Discharge patterns of afferent cutaneous nerve fibers from the rat's tail during prolonged noxious mechanical stimulation. Exp Brain Res 1987;65(3):493–504.
7. Thalhammer JG, LaMotte RH. Spatial properties of nociceptor sensitization following heat injury of the skin. Brain Res 1982;231(2):257–65.
8. Willis WD, Westlund KN. Neuroanatomy of the pain system and of the pathways that modulate pain. J Clin Neurophysiol 1997;14(1):2–31.
9. England JD, Happel LT, Kline DG, et al. Sodium channel accumulation in humans with painful neuromas. Neurology 1996;47(1):272–6.
10. Benzel EC, Francis TB. Spine surgery: techniques, complication avoidance, and management. 3rd edition. Philadelphia: Elsevier/Saunders; 2012.
11. Neumann S, Doubell TP, Leslie T, et al. Inflammatory pain hypersensitivity mediated by phenotypic switch in myelinated primary sensory neurons. Nature 1996; 384(6607):360–4.
12. Pitcher GM, Henry JL. Nociceptive response to innocuous mechanical stimulation is mediated via myelinated afferents and NK-1 receptor activation in a rat model of neuropathic pain. Exp Neurol 2004;186(2):173–97.
13. Devor M. Unexplained peculiarities of the dorsal root ganglion. Pain 1999;(Suppl 6):S27–35.
14. McMahon SB. Wall and Melzack's textbook of pain. 6th edition. Philadelphia: Elsevier/Saunders; 2013.
15. Pannese E, Ledda M, Conte V, et al. The perikaryal projections of rabbit spinal ganglion neurons. A comparison of thin section reconstructions and scanning microscopy views. Anat Embryol (Berl) 1990;181(5):427–32.

16. Amir R, Devor M. Chemically mediated cross-excitation in rat dorsal root ganglia. J Neurosci 1996;16(15):4733–41.
17. Applebaum ML, Clifton GL, Coggeshall RE, et al. Unmyelinated fibres in the sacral 3 and caudal 1 ventral roots of the cat. J Physiol 1976;256(3):557–72.
18. Coggeshall RE, Applebaum ML, Fazen M, et al. Unmyelinated axons in human ventral roots, a possible explanation for the failure of dorsal rhizotomy to relieve pain. Brain 1975;98(1):157–66.
19. Coggeshall RE, Maynard CW, Langford LA. Unmyelinated sensory and preganglionic fibers in rat L6 and S1 ventral spinal roots. J Comp Neurol 1980;193(1): 41–7.
20. Sykes MT, Coggeshall RE. Unmyelinated fibers in the human L4 and L5 ventral roots. Brain Res 1973;63:490–5.
21. Traub RJ, Mendell LM. The spinal projection of individual identified A-delta- and C-fibers. J Neurophysiol 1988;59(1):41–55.
22. Earle KM. The tract of Lissauer and its possible relation to the pain pathway. J Comp Neurol 1952;96(1):93–111.
23. Gobel S. Golgi studies of the neurons in layer II of the dorsal horn of the medulla (trigeminal nucleus caudalis). J Comp Neurol 1978;180(2):395–413.
24. Mannion RJ, Doubell TP, Gill H, et al. Deafferentation is insufficient to induce sprouting of A-fibre central terminals in the rat dorsal horn. J Comp Neurol 1998;393(2):135–44.
25. Treede RD, Meyer RA, Raja SN, et al. Peripheral and central mechanisms of cutaneous hyperalgesia. Prog Neurobiol 1992;38(4):397–421.
26. Dostrovsky JO. Role of thalamus in pain. Prog Brain Res 2000;129:245–57.
27. Lenz FA, Weiss N, Ohara S, et al. The role of the thalamus in pain. Suppl Clin Neurophysiol 2004;57:50–61.
28. Cameron AA, Khan IA, Westlund KN, et al. The efferent projections of the periaqueductal gray in the rat: a Phaseolus vulgaris-leucoagglutinin study. I. Ascending projections. J Comp Neurol 1995;351(4):568–84.
29. Bowsher D. Role of the reticular formation in responses to noxious stimulation. Pain 1976;2(4):361–78.
30. Dado RJ, Katter JT, Giesler GJ Jr. Spinothalamic and spinohypothalamic tract neurons in the cervical enlargement of rats. II. Responses to innocuous and noxious mechanical and thermal stimuli. J Neurophysiol 1994;71(3):981–1002.
31. Bowsher D, Mallart A, Petit D, et al. A bulbar relay to the centre median. J Neurophysiol 1968;31(2):288–300.
32. Melzack R, Wall PD. Pain mechanisms: a new theory. Science 1965;150(3699): 971–9.
33. Ralston HJ 3rd. Pain and the primate thalamus. Prog Brain Res 2005;149:1–10.
34. Tran TD, Inui K, Hoshiyama M, et al. Cerebral activation by the signals ascending through unmyelinated C-fibers in humans: a magnetoencephalographic study. Neuroscience 2002;113(2):375–86.
35. Anderson WS, O'Hara S, Lawson HC, et al. Plasticity of pain-related neuronal activity in the human thalamus. Prog Brain Res 2006;157:353–64.
36. Krout KE, Belzer RE, Loewy AD. Brainstem projections to midline and intralaminar thalamic nuclei of the rat. J Comp Neurol 2002;448(1):53–101.
37. Lenz FA, Lee JI, Garonzik IM, et al. Plasticity of pain-related neuronal activity in the human thalamus. Prog Brain Res 2000;129:259–73.
38. Llinas RR, Ribary U, Jeanmonod D, et al. Thalamocortical dysrhythmia: a neurological and neuropsychiatric syndrome characterized by magnetoencephalography. Proc Natl Acad Sci U S A 1999;96(26):15222–7.

39. Jones AK, Kulkarni B, Derbyshire SW. Pain mechanisms and their disorders. Br Med Bull 2003;65:83–93.
40. Møller AR. Textbook of tinnitus. New York: Springer; 2011.
41. Oliveras JL, Woda A, Guilbaud G, et al. Inhibition of the jaw opening reflex by electrical stimulation of the periaqueductal gray matter in the awake, unrestrained cat. Brain Res 1974;72(2):328–31.
42. Reynolds DV. Surgery in the rat during electrical analgesia induced by focal brain stimulation. Science 1969;164(3878):444–5.
43. Mayer DJ, Liebeskind JC. Pain reduction by focal electrical stimulation of the brain: an anatomical and behavioral analysis. Brain Res 1974;68(1):73–93.
44. Wei F, Dubner R, Zou S, et al. Molecular depletion of descending serotonin unmasks its novel facilitatory role in the development of persistent pain. J Neurosci 2010;30(25):8624–36.
45. Yeomans DC, Proudfit HK. Antinociception induced by microinjection of substance P into the A7 catecholamine cell group in the rat. Neuroscience 1992; 49(3):681–91.
46. Yeomans DC, Clark FM, Paice JA, et al. Antinociception induced by electrical stimulation of spinally projecting noradrenergic neurons in the A7 catecholamine cell group of the rat. Pain 1992;48(3):449–61.
47. Kwon M, Altin M, Duenas H, et al. The role of descending inhibitory pathways on chronic pain modulation and clinical implications. Pain Pract 2013. [Epub ahead of print].

Acute Pain Management

David M. Dickerson, MD

KEYWORDS

- Acute pain management • Multimodal analgesia • Multimodal pain management
- Ambulatory surgery • Outpatient surgery

KEY POINTS

- The cost to the patient and society of uncontrolled postoperative pain and chronic post-surgical pain requires a focus on prevention and effective multimodal intervention.
- The ambulatory anesthesiologist should be skilled at regional anesthesia and the application of continuous peripheral nerve catheters.
- The ambulatory surgical setting should make these techniques and their implementation possible.
- Effective communication in the perioperative period among the patient, nursing staff, and providers is necessary for rapid assessment and treatment of a patient's pain.
- The cost of maintaining a formulary with multiple analgesic drug classes and supplies and equipment for regional anesthesia may be offset by revenue in an outcomes-based reimbursement model.

INTRODUCTION

Acute postsurgical pain poses treatment challenges for the anesthesiologist, challenges augmented by the ambulatory surgical setting. The "fifth vital sign," pain, has become a focal point and continues to be a primary determinant of delayed discharge, unanticipated admission, and quality of recovery.[1–5] Although the prevalence of uncontrolled postoperative pain, frequently moderate to severe, has been characterized, the continued cost of uncontrolled pain has led to publication of practice guidelines for its control.[6] Most recently, the American Society of Anesthesiologists practice guidelines for acute pain management establish a paradigm for the more frequent and specific use of multimodal analgesia (MMA) (**Table 1**).[7]

This article updates acute pain management in ambulatory surgery and proposes a practical three-step approach, the "three I's" (**Box 1**), for reducing the impact and incidence of uncontrolled surgical pain. By identifying at-risk patients, implementing MMA, and intervening promptly with rescue therapies, the anesthesiologist may

This article originally appeared in Anesthesiology Clinics, Volume 32, Issue 2, June 2014.
Disclosure: No conflicts or relationships to disclose.
Department of Anesthesia and Critical Care, University of Chicago Medicine, 5841 South Maryland Avenue MC4028, Office O-416, Chicago, IL 60637, USA
E-mail address: ddickerson@dacc.uchicago.edu

Table 1
American Society of Anesthesiologists practice guidelines for acute pain management in the perioperative setting

	Recommendations

Institutional policies	• Anesthesiologists should provide ongoing, up-to-date education and training on the safe and effective use of available treatment options within the institution. Including:
	  ○ Basic bedside pain assessment
	  ○ Nonpharmacologic techniques
	  ○ Sophisticated pain management techniques (eg, regional anesthesia)
	• Providers should use standardized, validated instruments for the regular evaluation and documentation of pain intensity, therapeutic response, and side effects.
	• Anesthesiologists responsible for perioperative analgesia should be available at all times to assist in the evaluation and treatment of perioperative pain.
	• Standardized, institutional policies and procedures should be developed and an integrated approach used for pain management by an anesthesiologist-led acute pain service.

Preoperative preparation of the patient	• A directed pain history, directed physical examination, and pain control plan should be included in the anesthetic preoperative evaluation.
Perioperative techniques	• Anesthesiologists who manage perioperative pain should use therapeutic options, such as central regional opioids, systemic opioid PCA, or peripheral regional techniques after an analysis of the risk/benefit ratio for the individual patient. • The therapy implemented should reflect the individual anesthesiologist's expertise and a respect for the capacity for safe application of the modality in the specific practice setting. This includes the ability to recognize and treat adverse effects from the therapy.
Multimodal techniques for pain management	• Whenever possible, anesthesiologists should use multimodal pain management therapy, regional block should be considered. • Unless contraindicated, patients should receive an around-the-clock regimen of COXIBs, NSAIDS, or acetaminophen. • Dosing regimens should optimize efficacy and minimize adverse events. • Specific medication, dose, route, and duration of therapy should be individualized.

Abbreviations: COXIB, cyclooxygenase-2 inhibitor; NSAID, nonsteroidal anti-inflammatory drugs; PCA, Patient-Controlled Analgesia.

Adapted from American Society of Anesthesiologists Task Force on Acute Pain Management. Practice guidelines for acute pain management in the perioperative setting. Anesthesiology 2012;116:255–6; with permission.

Box 1
Planning for pain: the three "I's"

Identify patients at risk for uncontrolled postoperative pain

Implement effective preventative multimodal analgesia

Intervene with rescue regional analgesia, additional opioids, or nonopioid agents improve outcomes, reduce cost, and optimize the patient's experience and quality of recovery.

IDENTIFY: RISK STRATIFICATION, PREPROCEDURAL PLANNING

The preanesthetic assessment identifies a history of uncontrolled postsurgical pain, intolerance or contraindications to analgesics, contraindications to regional anesthesia, and presence of preoperative pain or anxiety.[7] Several patient and surgical characteristics predispose to moderate or severe postoperative pain (**Box 2**).[8–12] Identifying a high-risk cohort preoperatively warrants prompt initiation of MMA. Comprehensive MMA may impact the patient's quality of recovery, prevent discharge delay or unanticipated admission, and reduce the risk of chronic postsurgical pain (**Box 3**).[13–22]

Katz[23] suggested controlling pain throughout all phases of the perioperative period and not just the period of surgical intervention.[24] Uncontrolled postdischarge pain can lead to unanticipated admission, defined as readmission within 24 hours of surgery, and greater risk for chronic postsurgical pain. For these reasons, the anesthesiologist should assist the surgical team in planning postdischarge multimodal analgesic regimens for the most immediate and intense period of surgical pain. Appreciation of the multitude of neural pathways involved in nociceptive afferent neurotransmission is the foundation for a targeted, comprehensive multimodal approach (**Table 2**). Preoperative blocking of the afferent injury barrage during and after surgery prevents the induction of central sensitization, lowering postoperative pain and analgesic requirements.

IMPLEMENT: MMA, REGIONAL ANESTHESIA

Multiple days of effective analgesia minimizing adverse effects can be accomplished with continuous peripheral neural blockade (cPNB). A single-shot PNB reduces opioid exposure, improves patient comfort and circulation to the anesthetized extremity, reduces time in recovery, increases patient satisfaction, and lowers rates of adverse events.[25] Catheter-based continuous techniques have similar benefit.[4,26] Compared with single-shot PNBs, cPNBs are associated with better pain control and the need for decreased opioid analgesics, resulting in less nausea. Chronic pain after surgery

---

Box 2
Preoperative predictors of moderate-to-severe postoperative pain

- Increased preoperative pain
- Increased preoperative anxiety
- Younger patients
- Female gender
- Surgery type
  - Appendectomy
  - Cholecystectomy
  - Hemorrhoidectomy
  - Tonsillectomy
- Duration of surgery

Box 3
Preoperative predictors of the development of chronic postsurgical pain

- Increased preoperative pain
- Increased preoperative anxiety
- Increased postoperative pain
- Female gender
- Surgical type

---

also is decreased and patient satisfaction is augmented.[27,28] cPNBs can be safely placed at multiple sites with proved analgesic efficacy for a multitude of ambulatory surgeries (**Table 3**).[29] The cost and risks of these techniques must be weighed in the context of the benefit to the patient during the first postoperative days. Some

Table 2
Pathway approach to multimodal analgesia

	Peripheral vs Central Nervous Site of Action	Analgesic Agent	Receptor Target
Peripheral afferent blockade, inhibition of central hyperexcitability	Peripheral +/− central	Local anesthetic (wound infiltration)	Sodium channel (free nerve endings of peripheral)
		Local anesthetic (peripheral nerve block)	Sodium channel (peripheral afferent neuron)
		Local anesthetic systemic infusion	Sodium channel (central and peripheral)
Inflammation reduction (reduction in proinflammatory mediators, decreased afferent neurotransmission)	Peripheral and central	Acetaminophen, paracetamol	Cox-II, cannabinoid
		NSAIDs	Cox-I, Cox-II
		Dexamethasone	Cox-II
Afferent slowing	Peripheral and central	Gabapentanoids (Lyrica, gabapentin)	Calcium-channel
Spinal and supraspinal modulation	Central	Opioids	Opioid receptors
Antinociceptive interneuron activation	Membrane stabilization	Benzodiazepines SNRI/TCA (chronic use)	GABAa Norepinephrine reuptake, serotonin reuptake
Pronociceptive interneuron blockade	Central (dorsal horn of spinal cord)	Ketamine, dextromethorphan, levorphanol, methadone	NMDA receptor
Descending inhibition	Central	Tizanidine, clonidine, dexmedetomidine	Alpha-2 in locus ceruleus

Abbreviations: Cox, cyclooxygenase; GABA, γ-aminobutyric acid; NMDA, N-methyl-D-aspartate; NSAID, nonsteroidal anti-inflammatory drugs; SNRI, selective norepinephrine reuptake inhibitor; TCA, tricyclic antidepressant.

Table 3
Indications for continuous nerve blocks in orthopedic procedures and trauma

Surgical Procedure or Site of Injury	Continuous Block	Doses for Initial Bolus Followed by Continuous Infusion
Total shoulder arthroplasty, shoulder hemiarthroplasty, rotator cuff repair, shoulder arthrodesis, "frozen" shoulder physical therapy, biceps surgery, proximal humerus fractures	Interscalene	20 mL ropivacaine 0.5% 5–10 mL·h^{-1} ropivacaine 0.2%
Distal humerus fractures, elbow arthroplasty, elbow arthrodesis, radius fractures and surgery, ulna fractures and surgery, wrist arthrodesis, reimplantation surgery	Supraclavicular, infraclavicular, axillary	20 mL ropivacaine 0.5% 5–10 mL·h^{-1} ropivacaine 0.2%
Breast surgery	Thoracic paravertebral (T4-5)	15 mL ropivacaine 0.5% via catheter 5–10 mL·h^{-1} ropivacaine 0.2% via catheter
Total knee arthroplasty, anterior cruciate ligament reconstruction, patella repair, knee active and passive physical therapy	Femoral nerve	20 mL ropivacaine 0.5% 5–10 mL·h^{-1} ropivacaine 0.2%
Total knee arthroplasty, posterior cruciate ligament reconstruction	Femoral + sciatic	6–12 mL ropivacaine 0.2%–0.5% 3–8 mL·h^{-1} ropivacaine 0.1%–0.2%
Tibia fracture and repair, fibular fracture and repair, ankle fusion, subtalar fusion, total knee arthroplasty, hallux valgus repair	Sciatic or popliteal	5–10 mL ropivacaine 0.2%–0.5% 3–8 mL·h^{-1} ropivacaine 0.1%–0.2%
Ankle fusion, total ankle arthroplasty	Femoral or saphenous + sciatic	20 mL ropivacaine 0.2% 5–10 mL·h^{-1} ropivacaine 0.1%

Adapted from Chelly JE, Ghisi D, Fanelli A. Continuous peripheral nerve blocks in acute pain management. Br J Anaesth 2010;105(Suppl 1):i88; with permission.

procedures and patients, however, are not suitable for regional anesthesia because of contraindication or surgical site. These patients should still receive local anesthetic infiltration at incision sites.

IMPLEMENT: MMA, PHARMACOTHERAPY

Much emphasis has been placed on MMA to improve the quality of recovery, decrease length of postanesthesia care unit stay, and potentially reduce the opioid requirement.[1–3,30–33] Opioid-sparing methods help to reduce delayed discharge, prevent unanticipated admission, and potentially alter the rates of cancer recurrence or metastasis.[34–36] The American Society of Anesthesiologists practice guidelines provide a framework for incorporating nonopioid medications perioperatively.[7] The selection of the type and number of specific nonopioid agents should be evidence-based and directed toward minimizing risk and maximizing benefit.

Several studies support preoperative initiation of nonsteroidal anti-inflammatory drugs (NSAIDs), yet the necessary dose, route, frequency, and duration are unclear. The potent inhibition of prostaglandin synthesis by NSAID therapy may have analgesic benefits that must be weighed against the potential renal, cardiovascular, gastrointestinal, and bleeding risks.[37–39] Whether or not NSAIDs impair bone healing is controversial.[40]

Among its potent antiemetic effects, dexamethasone also may contribute to postoperative pain relief and reduce opioid consumption.[41,42] α_2-Agonists, ketamine, β-blockers, local anesthetics, and acetaminophen can improve postoperative pain management (see **Table 1**).[43–50] When acetaminophen and an NSAID were combined, the benefit was synergistic. When not contraindicated, these agents should be administered concurrently for maximal benefit.[51]

The efficacy of preoperative gabapentinoids in reducing postoperative pain has been evaluated in randomized controlled trials and meta-analyses. Most studies demonstrated a reduction in postoperative pain scores, but there was discrepancy in the reduction of opioid consumption; postoperative nausea and vomiting; and other adverse effects, such as sedation, dizziness, or visual disturbances.[52–55]

Because preoperative anxiety correlates with severe postoperative pain, anxiolysis may be another target for intervention. A 1200-mg dose of gabapentin significantly reduced preoperative anxiety and pain catastrophization in highly anxious patients compared with placebo.[56] In a recent, randomized, double-blind study, preoperative coadministration of midazolam and diclofenac resulted in significant reduction of pain scores and postoperative nausea and vomiting compared with diclofenac alone for hernia repair surgery performed with general anesthesia.[57]

IMPLEMENT: NONPHARMACOLOGIC TECHNIQUES

Nonpharmacologic techniques may influence patient stress, anxiety, and pain. Intraoperative music has been shown to reduce opioid consumption and increase patient comfort after gynecologic surgery.[58] Transcutaneous electrical nerve stimulation and other complementary therapies offer additional patient comfort.[59]

INTERVENE: RECOVERY ROOM RESCUE

If preoperative and intraoperative interventions fail to produce patient comfort, the anesthesiologist must first rule out superimposed medical issues in a timely fashion (eg, anginal chest pain, pneumoperitoneum-related shoulder or abdominal pain). Assuming surgical pain, the anesthesiologist must implement a treatment algorithm to promptly intervene in hopes of improving the patient's comfort and preventing potential discharge delay or admission. Application of other classes or doses of nonopioid analgesics and additional opioids should be initiated while the possible need for a neuraxial block is evaluated.

SUMMARY

The cost to the patient and society of uncontrolled postoperative pain and chronic postsurgical pain requires a focus on prevention and effective intervention. The ambulatory anesthesiologist should be skilled at regional anesthesia and the application of continuous peripheral nerve catheters.

The ambulatory surgical setting should make these techniques and their implementation possible. For rapid assessment and treatment of a patient's pain, communication in the perioperative period among the patient, nursing staff, and providers is necessary. The cost of maintaining a formulary with multiple analgesic drug classes and supplies and equipment for regional anesthesia may be offset by revenue in an outcomes-based reimbursement model.

REFERENCES

1. Pavlin DJ. Pain as a factor complicating recovery and discharge after ambulatory surgery. Anesth Analg 2002;95:627–34.
2. Pavlin DJ. A survey of pain and other symptoms that affect recovery process after discharge from an ambulatory surgical unit. J Clin Anesth 2004;16:200–6.
3. Pavlin DJ. Factors affecting discharge time in adult outpatients. Anesth Analg 1998;89:1352–9.
4. Coley KC, Williams BA, DaPos SV, et al. Retrospective evaluation of unanticipated admissions and readmissions after same day surgery and associated costs. J Clin Anesth 2002;14(5):349–53.
5. Mezei G, Chung F. Return hospital visits and hospital readmissions after ambulatory surgery. Ann Surg 1999;230:721–7.
6. Apfelbaum JL, Chen C, Mehta SS, et al. Postoperative pain experience results: results from a national survey suggest postoperative pain continues to be undermanaged. Anesth Analg 2003;97:534–40.
7. American Society of Anesthesiologists Task Force on Acute Pain Management. Practice guidelines for acute pain management in the perioperative setting. Anesthesiology 2012;116:248–73.
8. Ip HY, Abrishami A, Peng PW, et al. Predictors of postoperative pain and analgesic consumption: a qualitative systematic review. Anesthesiology 2009;111: 657–77.
9. Herbershagen HJ, Aduckathil A, Van Wijck AJ, et al. Pain intensity on the first day after surgery. Anesthesiology 2013;118:934–44.
10. Kalkman CJ, Visser K, Moen J, et al. Preoperative prediction of severe postoperative pain. Pain 2004;105:415–23.
11. Caumo W, Schmidt AP, Schneider CN, et al. Preoperative predictors of moderate to intense acute postoperative pain in patients undergoing abdominal surgery. Acta Anaesthesiol Scand 2002;46:1265–71.
12. Singh JA, Gabriel S, Lewallen D. The impact of gender, age, and preoperative pain severity on pain after TKA. Clin Orthop Relat Res 2008;466(11):2717–23.
13. Kehlet H, Jensen TS, Woolf CJ. Persistent postsurgical pain risk factors and prevention. Lancet 2006;267(9522):1618–25.
14. Macrae WA, Davies HT. Chronic postsurgical pain. In: Crombie IK, editor. Epidemiology of pain. Seattle (WA): IASP Press; 1999. p. 125–42.
15. Macrae WA, Bruce J. Chronic pain after surgery. In: Wilson PR, Watson PJ, Haythornthwaite JA, et al, editors. Clinical pain management: chronic pain. London: Hodder Arnold; 2008. p. 405–14.
16. Singh JA, Lewallen D. Predictors of pain and use of pain medications following primary total hip arthroplasty (THA): 5,707 THAs at 2-years and 3,289 THAs at 5-years. BMC Muscloskelet Disord 2010;11:90.
17. Perkins FM, Kehlet H. Chronic pain as an outcome of surgery: a review of predictive factors. Anesthesiology 2000;93(4):1123–33.
18. Forsythe MD, Dunbar MJ, Hennigar AW, et al. Prospective relation between catastrophizing and residual pain following knee arthroplasty: two year follow-up. Pain Res Manag 2008;13:335–41.
19. Katz J, Seltzer Z. Transition from acute to chronic postsurgical pain: risk factors and protective factors. Expert Rev Neurother 2009;9(5):723–44.
20. Jung BF, Ahrendt GM, Oaklander AL, et al. Neuropathic pain following breast cancer surgery: proposed classification and research update. Pain 2003; 204(102):1–13.

21. Granot M, Ferber SG. The roles of catastrophising and anxiety in the prediction of postoperative pain intensity: a prospective study. Clin J Pain 2005;21: 429–45.
22. Katz J, Poleshuck EL, Andrus CH, et al. Risk factors for acute pain and its persistence following breast cancer surgery. Pain 2005;119(1–3):16–25.
23. Katz J, Clark H, Seltzer Z. Preventive analgesia: quo vadimus? Anesth Analg 2011;24:545–50.
24. Diatchenko L, Slade GD, Nackley AG, et al. Genetic basis for individual variations in pain perception and the development of a chronic pain condition. Hum Mol Genet 2005;14(1):135–43.
25. Carli F, Kehlet H, Baldini G, et al. Evidence basis for regional anesthesia in multidisciplinary fast-track surgical care pathways. Reg Anesth Pain Med 2011;36: 63–72.
26. Lenart MJ, Wong K, Gupta RK, et al. The impact of peripheral nerve techniques on hospital stay following major orthopedic surgery. Pain Med 2012;13(6): 828–34.
27. Borghi B, D'Addabbo M, White PF, et al. The use of prolonged peripheral neural blockade after lower extremity amputation: the effect on symptoms associated with phantom limb syndrome. Anesth Analg 2010;111:1308–15.
28. Ilfeld BM. Continuous peripheral nerve blocks: a review of the published evidence. Anesth Analg 2011;113(4):904–25.
29. Chelly JE, Ghisi D, Fanelli A. Continuous peripheral nerve blocks in acute pain management. Br J Anaesth 2010;105(Suppl 1):i86–96.
30. White PF, Kehlet H. Improving postoperative pain management: what are the unresolved issues? Anesthesiology 2010;112:220–5.
31. Elvir-Lazo O, White PF. The role of multimodal analgesia in pain management after ambulatory surgery. Curr Opin Anesthesiol 2010;23:697–703.
32. Joshi GP. Multimodal analgesia techniques for ambulatory surgery. Int Anesthsiol Clin 2005;43:197–204.
33. Bisgaard T. Analgesic treatment after laparoscopic cholecystectomy: a critical assessment of the evidence. Anesthesiology 2006;104:835–46.
34. Exadaktylos AK, Buggy DJ, Moriary DC, et al. Can anesthetic technique for primary breast cancer surgery affect recurrence or metastasis? Anesthesiology 2006;105(4):660–4.
35. Singleton PA, Moreno-Vinaco L, Sammani S, et al. Attenuation of vascular permeability by methylnaltrexone: role of mOP-R and S1P3 transactivation. Am J Respir Cell Mol Biol 2007;37(2):222–31.
36. De Oliveira GS, Ahmad S, Schink JC, et al. Intraoperative neuraxial anesthesia but not postoperative neuraxial analgesia is associated with increased relapse-free survival in ovarian cancer patients after primary cytoreductive surgery. Reg Anesth Pain Med 2011;36(3):271–7.
37. White PF, Sacan O, Tufanogullari B, et al. Effect of short-term postoperative celecoxib administration on patient outcome after outpatient laparoscopic surgery. Can J Anaesth 2007;54:342–8.
38. Gan TJ, Joshi GP, Viscusi E, et al. Preoperative parenteral paracoxib and follow-up oral valdecoxib reduce length of stay and improve quality of patient recovery after laparoscopic cholecystectomy surgery. Anesth Analg 2004;98: 1665–73.
39. De Oliviera GS, Agarwal D, Benzon HT. Perioperative single dose ketorolac to prevent postoperative pain: a meta-analysis of randomized trials. Anesth Analg 2012;114:424–33.

40. Pountos I, Georgouli T, Calori GM, et al. Do nonsteroidal anti-inflammatory drugs affect bone healing? A critical analysis. Scientific World Journal 2012;2012: 606404.
41. Mattila K, Kontinen VK, Kalso E, et al. Dexamethasone decreases oxycodone consumption following osteotomy of the first metatarsal bone: a randomized controlled trial in day surgery. Acta Anaesthesiol Scand 2010;54:268–76.
42. De Oliviera GS, Almeida MD, Benzon HT, et al. Perioperative single dose systemic dexamethasone for postoperative pain. Anesthesiology 2011;115: 575–88.
43. Salman N, Uzun S, Coskun F, et al. Dexmedetomidine as a substitute for remifentanil in ambulatory gynecologic laparoscopic surgery. Saudi Med J 2009;102: 117–22.
44. Viscomi CM, Friend A, Parker C, et al. Ketamine as an adjuvant in lidocaine intravenous regional anesthesia: a randomized, double-blind, systematic control trial. Reg Anesth Pain Med 2009;34:130–3.
45. Suzuki M. Role of N-methyl-D-aspartate receptor antagonists in postoperative pain management. Curr Opin Anesthesiol 2009;22:618–22.
46. Laskowski K, Stirling A, McKay WP, et al. A systematic review of intravenous ketamine for postoperative analgesia. Can J Anesth 2011;58:911–23.
47. Collard V, Mistraletti G, Taq A, et al. Intraoperative esmolol infusion in the absence of opioids spares postoperative fentanyl in patients undergoing ambulatory laparoscopic cholecystectomy. Anesth Analg 2007;105:1255–62.
48. McCarthy GC, Megalla SA, Habib AS. Impact of intravenous lidocaine infusion on postoperative analgesia and recovery from surgery: a systematic review of randomized controlled trials. Drugs 2010;70:1149–63.
49. Wininger SJ, Miller H, Minkowitz HS, et al. A randomized, double-blind, placebo-controlled, multicenter, repeat-dose study of two intravenous acetaminophen dosing regimens for the treatment of pain after abdominal laparoscopic surgery. Clin Ther 2010;32(14):2348–69.
50. Api O, Unal O, Ugurel V, et al. Analgesic efficacy of intravenous paracetamol for outpatient fractional curettage: a randomized controlled trial. Int J Clin Pract 2009;63(1):105–11.
51. Ong CK, Seymour RA, Lirk P, et al. Combining paracetamol (acetaminophen) with nonsteroidal anti-inflammatory drugs: a qualitative systematic review of analgesic efficacy for acute postoperative pan. Anesth Analg 2010;110:1170–9.
52. Moore A, Costello J, Wieczorek P, et al. Gabapentin improves postcesarean delivery pain management: a randomized, placebo-controlled trial. Anesth Analg 2011;112:167–73.
53. McQuay HJ, Poon KH, Derry S, et al. Acute pain: combination treatments and how we measure their efficacy. Br J Anaesth 2008;101:69–76.
54. Kim SY, Song JW, Park B, et al. Pregabalin reduces postoperative pain after mastectomy: a double blind, randomized, placebo-controlled study. Acta Anaesthesiol Scand 2011;55:290–6.
55. Engleman E, Cateloy F. Efficacy and safety of perioperative pregabalin for postoperative pain: a meta-analysis of randomized-controlled trials. Acta Anaesthesiol Scand 2011;55:290–6.
56. Clarke H, Kirkham KR, Orser BA, et al. Gabapentin reduces preoperative anxiety and pain catastrophizing in highly anxious patients prior to major surgery: a blinded randomized placebo-controlled trial. Can J Anesth 2013;60:432–43.
57. Hasani A, Maloku H, Sallahu F, et al. Preemptive analgesia with midazolam and diclofenac for hernia repair pain. Hernia 2011;15:267–72.

58. Angioli R, Cicco Nardone CD, Plotti F, et al. The use of music to reduce anxiety during office hysteroscopy: a prospective randomized trial. J Minim Invasiv Gynecol 2013. http://dx.doi.org/10.1016/j.jmig.2013.07.020.

59. Chen L, Tang J, White PF, et al. The effect of location of transcutaneous electrical nerve stimulation on postoperative opioid analgesic requirement: acupoint versus nonacupoint stimulation. Anesth Analg 1998;87:1129–34.

Patients with Chronic Pain

Joseph Salama-Hanna, MBBS[1], Grace Chen, MD*

KEYWORDS

- Preoperative evaluation • Opioid tolerance • Postoperative pain
- Multimodal analgesia • Multidisciplinary pain treatment • Preoperative opioid abuse
- Buprenorphine

KEY POINTS

- Preoperative assessment and treatment of chronic pain and its comorbidities are essential to assure a positive operative outcome and smooth recovery.
- Multimodal analgesia can decrease postoperative pain, increase patient satisfaction, and reduce opioid requirements and may help avoid the development of chronic pain.
- If there is adequate preoperative time, multidisciplinary treatment of chronic pain to minimize catastrophizing, anxiety, deconditioning, and medication tolerance can improve perioperative outcomes in chronic pain patients.
- Special situations, such as patients with intrathecal drug delivery systems and patients who are on buprenorphine, may warrant coordination of care with subspecialists.

OVERVIEW

Chronic pain afflicts more than 100 million Americans,[1] making it approximately 4 times more common than diabetes and 10 times more common than cancer. The Institute of Medicine recognizes ongoing pain as a disease, with far-reaching physiologic, psychological, and emotional implications that are frequently inadequately assessed and treated. These issues are often in the forefront when a chronic pain patient presents for surgery, requiring individualized assessment and preparation to assure effective postoperative pain control and a seamless recovery. Surgical patient satisfaction and pain control have been shown to correlate closely. One study, by Hanna and colleagues,[2] of 4349 patients found that surgical patient satisfaction was significantly improved when their pain was well treated.

Chronic pain patients undergoing surgery often experience more postoperative pain and consume more opioids than patients without chronic pain.[3,4] Possible

This article originally appeared in Medical Clinics of North America, Volume 97, Issue 6, November 2013.

Disclosures: None.

Department of Anesthesiology and Perioperative Medicine, Oregon Health & Science University, 3303 Southwest Bond Avenue, Portland, OR 97239, USA

[1] Present address: Henry Ford Hospital, 2799 West Grand Boulevard, Detroit, MI 48202, USA.

* Corresponding author.

E-mail address: cheng@ohsu.edu

Clinics Collections 4 (2014) 25–39

http://dx.doi.org/10.1016/j.ccol.2014.10.004

factors contributing to increased postoperative pain include increased preoperative pain, anxiety, age, and type of surgery. The type of surgery, age, and psychological distress are significant predictors for analgesic consumption.[5] Psychological variables, including anxiety, depression, and patients overwhelmed by out-of-proportion fear—all predictors of increased postoperative pain, are more common in chronic pain patients.[6,7] Effectively managing these issues requires a multidisciplinary approach incorporating multimodal analgesic approaches initiated prior to incision, thus emphasizing the importance of effective preoperative evaluation and planning.

IMPORTANT CONCEPTS

Acute pain accompanies trauma and injury (such as surgery) and typically resolves as tissues heal. In contrast, chronic pain can be defined as ongoing pain that extends beyond the typical period of healing and adversely affects the function and well being of the individual.[8] Chronic pain is a complex biopsychosocial disease process with accompanying changes in physiology that promote ongoing pain. Chronic pain is associated with depression, anxiety, deconditioning, poor sleep, increased medication use, and increased use of health services. Chronic pain and its comorbidities are associated with poor postoperative pain control, and patients who come into surgery without chronic pain are more likely to develop chronic postsurgical pain when perioperative pain is not well controlled. Chronic pain is a national problem, having an impact on more than 100 million Americans and costing the US economy more than $600 million per year.[1]

Out of the approximately 40 million surgical procedures performed each year in North America, 10% to 15% of patients continue to have ongoing pain 1 year later because they develop chronic postsurgical pain. This process of transition from acute pain to chronic pain is complex and poorly understood. In a given individual, there is likely interplay between genetic, biologic, psychological, and social-environmental factors that leads to ongoing pain.[9,10]

Demographically, younger female patients seem an increased risk group for developing chronic postsurgical pain.[11] Patients with anxiety, depression, or other chronic pain; those with longer preoperative opioid requirements[12]; or those who have out-of-proportion fear[13] or are less optimistic about their postoperative pain and outcomes have more postoperative pain and may be at increased risk for developing chronic pain.[14–16] Although not routinely performed clinically, preoperative assessment of pain perception by assessing sensitivity to pressure or other stimuli that reflect physiologic and processing changes is associated with more postoperative pain.[17–19] Patients with poor pain control in the hours and days after surgery are more likely to have ongoing chronic pain.[20]

Another quantifiable factor associated with a more challenging postoperative pain experience is the use of long-term opioids to treat chronic pain. Patients with opioid prescription for preoperative pain are likely to have more pain and increased opioid requirements. Given these identifiable factors associated with both increased acute pain and chronic postsurgical pain, it is clear that preoperative evaluation is helpful in identifying patients at increased risk for this complication of surgery. This is particularly true for chronic pain patients who often manifest many of these risk factors as part of their pain syndrome. For example, patients with neuropathic pain associated with diabetes have increased anxiety, depression, and sleep disturbance.[21] Additionally, many chronic pain syndromes are treated with opioids, which pose special challenges in the perioperative period.

In the forefront of perioperative pain control is the concept of multimodal analgesia—the practice of implementing together several pharmaceutical and nonmedication treatments to reduce postoperative pain and enhance recovery. Multimodal analgesia shifts the focus away from opioids to a host of treatments that can reduce pain by complementary mechanisms of action. The common theme of these treatments is that by reducing the physiologic response to the intense nociceptive (pain) stimulus of surgery, pain is reduced. Related concepts include pre-emptive analgesia (initiating treatment before the surgery to reduce pain after surgery) and preventive analgesia (a broader time frame for intervention including the entire perioperative period). Overwhelming evidence shows that multimodal strategies improve clinical outcomes. For chronic pain patients, this is of increased importance, and the therapy likely has enhanced benefit if doses and strategies are individualized.[22,23] This multimodal analgesia review suggests a 5-step approach to optimize the preoperative care of patients who suffer from chronic pain.

Step One: Preoperative Evaluation of Chronic Pain Patients

According to the International Association for the Study of Pain, pain is defined as an unpleasant subjective physical and emotional experience.[24] Acute pain tends to be adaptive and signals impending or ongoing tissue damage.

Chronic pain (excluding cancer pain) persists beyond the expected period of recovery. The exact pathway of transformation is the focus of intensive study. The process seems to begin in the periphery with up-regulation of cyclooxygenase-2 and interleukin 1β–sensitizing first-order neurons, which eventually sensitize second-order spinal neurons, a process that requires activating N-methyl-D-aspartic acid (NMDA) receptor-channel activity. Prostaglandins, endocannabinoids, a variety of ion channels, microglia, and scavenger cells have all been implicated in the transformation of acute to chronic pain.[25] Clinically, intense uncontrolled pain seems to be a risk factor for the development of postoperative chronic pain, making pre-emptive analgesia important for chronic pain prevention.[26,27]

In the United States, pain is termed, *the fifth vital sign*, emphasizing its importance in patient care, and is often recorded on a numeric rating scale.[28] More sophisticated and function-focused instruments, such as the Brief Pain Inventory, are also used. To optimize postoperative recovery and patient satisfaction, physicians and midlevel providers who evaluate patients for surgery should inquire about pain and document pain intensity, location, functional impairment, and concomitant medication use for treatment. Like cardiopulmonary disease, patients' chronic pain can significantly affect surgical outcome and patient satisfaction. One European study found that of factors of nociception, depression and anxiety, and activities of daily living, only pain caused dissatisfaction with surgical care.[29] Patients who have their chronic pain, anxiety, and depression under reasonable control are in the best position to cope effectively with the additional stress of acute postoperative pain and have a lower risk of developing new chronic pain.

If depression or anxiety is not well controlled, it is reasonable to consider either additional pharmacotherapy or appropriate psychotherapy. Beyond the medical preparations for surgery, patient education is an important aspect of optimizing surgical recovery, with patients who participate in preoperative education experiencing less pain and anxiety along with better recovery.[30,31] Patients who have realistic expectations, understand how to report their pain, and understand their options for treatment have less anxiety and are able to play a more active role in their recovery. The earlier this education process starts, the more likely they are to effectively implement it during the stresses of the perioperative period. Providers seeing patient pre-operatively should discuss a patient's fears and concerns, explain perioperative routines, and provide education for optimal use of patient-controlled analgesia (PCA) and other analgesic methods, such as regional analgesia. Patients may receive additional information during the preanesthetic evaluation, including educational materials they can take home with them for review. A clear evaluation of chronic pain risk factors and concise patient preparation are fundamentally important to optimize surgical outcome and patient satisfaction.

Step Two: Pain Specialist Preoperative Evaluation of the Patient on Opioids

Millions of people are prescribed long-term opioid therapy for the treatment of chronic pain and opioid abuse had been rising steadily over the decade, with unintentional opioid overdose deaths rising from 1/100,000 in 1970 to 10/100,000 in 2007.[32,33] The majority of these patients use their medications as prescribed by their health care providers. Some patients, however, have issues of abuse and addiction. For all patients on any type of opioid therapy, the main goals of opioid therapy are the same: avoid withdrawal, account for tolerance, avoid unnecessary dose escalation, provide reasonable postoperative pain control, and avoid opioid overdose. If patients understand these opioid goals, they are more likely to actively participate and fear may be allayed.[34]

Chronic opioid use alters physiology and the body's future response to the ongoing use of opioids. Long-term opioid use has been linked to endocrine derangements, such as sex hormone deficiency and cortisol deficiency.[35] Some studies suggest that patients exposed to opioids may have increased sensitivity for pain, thus exhibiting opioid-induced hyperalgesia.[7,36] Patients who suffer from substance abuse may benefit from psychiatric treatment and stabilization of their psychological state before elective surgery.

In addition to simply tallying preoperative opioid use, it is appropriate for a preoperative pain consultation to assess for opioid misuse and addiction to improve the care of patients in the vulnerable preoperative time period. If opioid addiction is suspected, a team approach involving the primary care provider, anesthesiologist, surgeon, pain specialist, and addiction specialist (psychiatry) facilitates achieving successful pain management without unintended long-term complications of addiction relapse (**Table 1**).

Many addiction-screening tools are available, including the Screening Tool for Addiction Risk, to identify opioid abuse potential in chronic pain patients. Patients who have an opioid abuse problem often display an overwhelming focus on opioid issues during preoperative pain clinic visits and clinicians should have a high index of suspicion for opioid abuse in those who exhibit such behavior. Patients with opioid abuse or misuse, those who often request early refills or escalate drug use in the absence of an acute change in medical condition, and young white male patients tend to be the most susceptible population for prescription opioid abuse.[37] In addition, an addictionologist should be consulted for patients who are identified as opioid abusers and have self-insight and a sincere desire to stop abusing.

If surgery needs to proceed without delay, multimodal analgesia, including acetaminophen, nonsteroidal anti-inflammatory drugs (NSAIDs), regional blocks, antidepressants, anticonvulsants, muscle relaxants, α-adrenergic agonists, or benzodiazepines, should be considered.[38] Patients should be monitored for opioid withdrawal if not offered opioids. If patients receive opioids in the acute postoperative setting, tapering the opioids should be implemented when a patient's acute pain is expected to subside. The most important factor in the perioperative care of a patient who suffers from opioid addiction is to establish a support structure for the patient to cope with the

Table 1
Substance use disorders and their definitions

Substance Use Disorder	Related Definitions
Addiction	Commonly used term meaning the aberrant use of a specific psychoactive substance in a manner characterized by loss of control, compulsive use, preoccupation, and continued use despite harm; pejorative term, replaced in the *DSM-IV11* in a nonpejorative way by the term, *substance use disorder*, with psychological and physical dependence
Dependence	1. Psychological dependence: need for a specific psychoactive substance either for its positive effects or to avoid negative psychological or physical effects associated with its withdrawal 2. Physical dependence: a physiologic state of adaptation to a specific psychoactive substance characterized by the emergence of a withdrawal syndrome during abstinence, which may be relieved in total or in part by readministration 3. One category of psychoactive substance use disorder
Chemical dependence	A generic term relating to psychological and/or physical dependence on one or more psychoactive substances
Substance use disorders	Term of *DSM-IV13* comprising 2 main groups: 1. Substance dependence disorder and substance abuse disorder 2. Substance-induced disorders (eg, intoxication, withdrawal, delirium, and psychotic disorders)
Tolerance	A state in which an increased dosage of a psychoactive substance is needed to produce a desired effect. Cross-tolerance: induced by repeated administration of one psychoactive substance that is manifested toward another substance to which an individual has not been recently exposed.
Withdrawal syndrome	The onset of a predictable constellation of signs and symptoms after the abrupt cessation of the drug
Polydrug dependence	Discontinuation of, or a rapid decrease in, dosage of a psychoactive substance
Recovery	A process of overcoming both physical and psychological dependence on a psychoactive substance with a commitment to sobriety
Abstinence	Nonuse of any psychoactive substance
Maintenance	Prevention of craving behavior and withdrawal symptoms of opioids by long-acting opioids (eg, methadone, buprenorphine)
Substance abuse	Use of a psychoactive substance in a manner outside of sociocultural conventions

Abbreviation: DSM-IV, Diagnostic and Statistical Manual of Mental Disorders (Fourth Edition).

stresses of the disease that necessitated the surgery, the preexisting addiction challenge, and the new stress of postoperative pain with exposure to the substance of abuse.

Step Three: Formulating a Perioperative Analgesic Plan

Formulating and communicating the plan for multidisciplinary preoperative treatment and multimodal perioperative pain control[39] to patients and care teams help alleviate patient anxiety and improve care.[32] Initiating treatment before surgical incision requires planning and is associated with the best outcomes (**Fig. 1**).

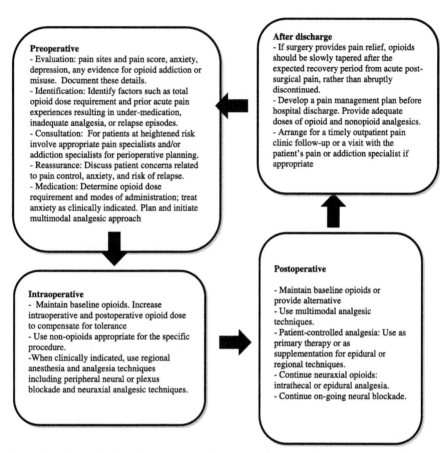

Preoperative
- Evaluation: pain sites and pain score, anxiety, depression, any evidence for opioid addiction or misuse. Document these details.
- Identification: Identify factors such as total opioid dose requirement and prior acute pain experiences resulting in under-medication, inadequate analgesia, or relapse episodes.
- Consultation: For patients at heightened risk involve appropriate pain specialists and/or addiction specialists for perioperative planning.
- Reassurance: Discuss patient concerns related to pain control, anxiety, and risk of relapse.
- Medication: Determine opioid dose requirement and modes of administration; treat anxiety as clinically indicated. Plan and initiate multimodal analgesic approach

After discharge
- If surgery provides pain relief, opioids should be slowly tapered after the expected recovery period from acute post-surgical pain, rather than abruptly discontinued.
- Develop a pain management plan before hospital discharge. Provide adequate doses of opioid and nonopioid analgesics.
- Arrange for a timely outpatient pain clinic follow-up or a visit with the patient's pain or addiction specialist if appropriate

Intraoperative
- Maintain baseline opioids. Increase intraoperative and postoperative opioid dose to compensate for tolerance
- Use non-opioids appropriate for the specific procedure.
- When clinically indicated, use regional anesthesia and analgesia techniques including peripheral neural or plexus blockade and neuraxial analgesic techniques.

Postoperative
- Maintain baseline opioids or provide alternative
- Use multimodal analgesic techniques.
- Patient-controlled analgesia: Use as primary therapy or as supplementation for epidural or regional techniques.
- Continue neuraxial opioids: intrathecal or epidural analgesia.
- Continue on-going neural blockade.

Fig. 1. Plan for multidisciplinary preoperative treatment and multimodal perioperative pain control.

Step Four: Specifics to Execute the Plan; the Key is Multimodal Analgesia

Multimodal analgesia optimizes analgesia and minimizes functionally limiting side effects. In the perioperative period, the use of steroids, such as dexamethasone; anticonvulsants, such as gabapentin; acetaminaphen; NSAIDs, such as celecoxib; and ketamine has been shown to be opioid sparing. A recent study of multilevel spine surgery patients demonstrated that, compared with a historic group of patients receiving usual care, multimodal analgesia significantly reduced opioid consumption, improved postoperative mobilization, and was associated with concomitant low levels of nausea, sedation, and dizziness.[40] Many other studies show multimodal analgesia has opioid-sparing properties concomitant with reduction of opioid side effects.[41]

The orally administered medications with the best evidence for reducing postoperative pain and opioid requirements are the NSAIDs, acetaminophen, and gabapentin/pregabalin.[42–44] Despite the desire to have patients nothing by mouth prior to transport to the operating room, it is common to administer a combination of oral medications (eg, acetaminophen, NSAID, and pregabalin) in the preoperative holding area. Initiating treatment with these medications the night before surgery is also an option that can provide adequate pre-emptive analgesia. In addition to the analgesic effects, gabapentin is an anxiolytic, with demonstrated efficacy in anxious patients undergoing surgery.[45] Standard preoperative doses for gabapentin are typically 600 mg to 1200 mg and, for acetaminophen, 650 mg to 1000 mg.

The nonopioid intravenous (IV) analgesic with the most impact seems to be ketamine, an anesthetic agent that is an NMDA receptor antagonist.[46,47] Ketamine reduces pain and opioid requirements and is particularly helpful in opioid-tolerant patients.[48] Ketamine is often given as a bolus dose prior to incision and may be continued through the operation and at times into the postoperative period.

Regional and neuraxial blocks with local anesthetics and opioids are key components of effective multimodal analgesia. Options include a field block or wound infiltration[49] (before or after incision), neuraxial analgesia (epidural or intrathecal often combined with an opioid), and peripheral nerve/plexus blockade (divisions of brachial plexus, lumbar plexus, and femoral nerve). Simple use of local anesthetic at the surgical site may reduce pain and opioid requirements, and contraindications or adverse effects are rare, making this option widely applicable.[50,51] For patients who are not candidates for neuraxial or peripheral nerve analgesic techniques, IV lidocaine infusion may reduce pain and opioid requirements while enhancing recovery.[52–55]

Neuraxial analgesia

Neuraxial analgesia (intrathecal or epidural) involves the delivery of local anesthetic and/or opioid to the spinal cord and surrounding nerve tissues to decrease pain at the spinal level.[56] Epidural analgesia with local anesthetic and opioid combination delivered via an indwelling catheter and continued into the postoperative period is the best-studied neuraxial technique. Particularly in high-risk patients, epidural analgesia can reduce pain and improve patient outcomes and is often used for many surgical procedures.[57–59] For opioid-tolerant patients, special attention is required for success, including a multimodal analgesia plan. One of the rare but potentially devastating complications of neuraxial analgesia is hematoma formation in the spinal canal. Anticoagulation and coagulation abnormalities are major risk factors for this complication. Readers are encouraged to refer to the American Society of Regional Anesthesia and Pain Medicine[60] guidelines if neuraxial therapy is expected in an anticoagulated patient. Consensus guidelines are recommendations and specific decisions on nerve blocks in patients on anticoagulants should be made on an individual basis. Optimal monitoring, adequate follow-up, and timely treatment should be practiced for patients taking anticoagulants and who had neuraxial or peripheral nerve blocks.

Patients should be educated regarding IV-PCA prior to surgery. The PCA is a programmable delivery system by which patients self-administer predetermined doses of analgesic medication, via the IV route, at the push of a button. The PCA can optimize drug delivery and improve satisfaction by enabling patients to titrate analgesia. Safe use of the PCA requires patients to control analgesic delivery. Increasing plasma concentrations of opioid usually causes sedation prior to causing clinically significant respiratory depression, but sedation usually impairs the ability of the patient to activate the PCA. Thus, it is important that patients are instructed to not allow family members or friends to activate the PCA while they are resting. In addition, each PCA pump is programmed to limit the amount of drug delivered. Thus, repeatedly pressing the activation button does not deliver an amount that exceeds the preset limit. This upper set limit may be enough, however, to cause apnea in an individual patient, if a family member or friend takes control of the control button while a patient is sleeping. Because the dose can be varied to accommodate patient needs, the IV-PCA is a reasonable choice for opioid-tolerant chronic pain patients. **Table 2** provides

Table 2
Sample bolus doses and lockout intervals for opioid IV

Drug	Bolus (mg)	Lockout Interval (min)
Fentanyl	0.015–0.05	3–10
Hydromorphone	0.1–0.5	5–15
Meperidine	5–15	5–15
Morphine	0.5–3	5–20
Oxymorphone	0.2–0.8	5–15
Remifentanil (labor)	0.5 µg/kg	2
Sufentanil	0.003–0.015	3–10

Data from Kong B, Ya Deau JT. Patient-controlled analgesia. In: Benzon HT, Fishman SM, Raja RT, et al, eds. Essentials of Pain Medicine, 3rd edition. Philadelphia: Saunders, 2011; with permission.

examples of guideline boluses and lockout intervals (time between the next dose of medication even if the PCA is activated) for different IV-PCA opioids.

Preoperative placement of a peripheral nerve block can be helpful in preventing postoperative pain. In adult patients, it is standard to place the nerve block under mild or moderate sedation. This practice allows patients to provide direct feedback to the provider placing the block, in the event that the block needle comes in contact with the target nerve. In addition, for patients who are thought to require several days of strong analgesia, local anesthetic can be continuously infused through a catheter positioned (usually with ultrasound) alongside the target nerve (referred to as continuous peripheral nerve block [CPNB]). Examples include femoral nerve catheters for knee surgery, paravertebral catheters for thoracotomy, and brachial plexus catheters for upper extremity orthopedic procedures. CPNB can reduce baseline pain, improve pain control with movement, facilitate recovery, and reduce opioid requirements.[61,62] For appropriate surgical procedures, CPNB is an important option for chronic pain patients undergoing surgery.[63,64]

Nonpharmacologic approaches

There are several approaches and techniques that have gained popularity in the chronic pain management field that may be helpful in perioperative pain management.[65] Physical modalities, including cooling, acupuncture, heat, and massage, are low-risk approaches that offer potential benefit. Among these, the best evidence is for transcutaneous electrical nerve stimulation (TENS). The TENS units are small portable devices that deliver electrical energy through the skin. There are more than 20 controlled trials of TENS for postoperative pain control with reasonable evidence to suggest an opioid-sparing effect.[66] Several cognitive techniques that offer the possibility of reducing anxiety and pain have been studied for postoperative pain control, including relaxation techniques, guided imagery, hypnosis, music, and positive suggestions. Given the low risk of these techniques, they are reasonable to suggest for chronic pain patients undergoing surgery.

Step Five: Special Situations that May Benefit from Acute Pain Specialist Referral for Preoperative Pain Optimization

Patients who suffer from special chronic pain conditions, especially those who are on multiple psychotropic medications, may benefit from a preoperative consult by a rheumatologist, psychiatrist, neurologist, or pain specialist. Special consideration should be given to the following patient situations.

Patients with intrathecal drug delivery systems
Intrathecal drug delivery systems (IDDSs)[67] should be interrogated preoperatively to assess proper functioning of the system and identify medication and dose. Cross tolerance of different opioids is unpredictable, even though there are approximate opioid conversion tables available. For example, patients may have improved response to fentanyl if the intrathecal pump is infusing hydromorphone. At the time of surgery, care should be taken to prevent surgical or regional anesthetic disruption of the intrathecal infusion. Electrocautery does not interfere with the device but there are case reports of the device being deactivated in patients undergoing an MRI. Intrathecal therapy should be continued (recognizing that abrupt cessation of baclofen as a baseline analgesic requirement is dangerous). Supplementation of appropriate doses of opioids, either orally or by using PCA for breakthrough pain as needed, is warranted. Because many patients with IDDS therapy are opioid tolerant, a multimodal analgesic approach is advisable.

Patients with arthritis
Osteoarthritis is usually treated with exercise, NSAIDs, and, in rare cases, opioids and surgery. Rheumatoid arthritis is treated with disease-modifying agents, biologic response modifiers, and steroids. If patients have recently been taking steroids, stress-dose steroids should be given perioperatively. Methotrexate is commonly prescribed to this group of patients. Because this drug can cause severe liver damage,[68] the status of liver function should be documented in the preoperative period. Multinational recommendations on pain management by pharmacotherapy should be followed in all patients with inflammatory arthritis in the preoperative period. For patients with arthritis, a multimodal analgesic technique is appropriate with continuation of their preoperative anti-inflammatory or disease-modifying agents as dictated by the specific surgical situation.

Patients with central pain syndrome
Central pain syndrome is a neurologic condition caused by damage to, or dysfunction of, the central nervous system, which includes the brain, brainstem, and spinal cord. Stroke, multiple sclerosis, tumors, epilepsy, brain/spinal cord trauma, or Parkinson disease may cause this syndrome.[69] If a patient presents with a diagnosis of central pain syndrome, investigating the underlying cause is recommended because this may have anesthetic implications. These patients may have a component of pain that is resistant to opioid therapy so management can be challenging. Multimodal analgesia is important, and often these patients are already taking gabapentin or pregabalin because these agents are considered first-line treatments.

Complex regional pain syndrome
The complex regional pain syndrome (CRPS) is a painful condition of a limb associated with physiologic changes and sensitivity to normally nonpainful stimuli. Because of this sensitivity to pain and because the inciting factor for CRPS is often trauma or surgery, it is important to provide aggressive multimodal analgesia to patients who already have the condition. Vitamin C (ascorbic acid) has potential to prevent CRPS, with specific evidence in wrist and foot/ankle surgery.[70,71] It is reasonable to suggest 500 mg of vitamin C for approximately 6 to 8 weeks for patients undergoing such procedures and for CRPS patients undergoing any surgical procedure.[72]

Fibromyalgia
Diagnostic criteria for fibromyalgia[73] include wide spread pain that lasts for at least 3 months; it is usually a diagnosis of exclusion. Treatment options include

antidepressants, such as amitriptyline (a tricyclic antidepressant), venlafaxine in high doses (serotonin-norepinephrine reuptake inhibitors), duloxetine, and milnacipran (nonselective serotonin reuptake inhibitor). Anticonvulsants, mainly α-2-β ligands (gabapentin and pregabalin), are also used to effectively help with fibromyalgia pain. It should be emphasized that the current Food and Drug Administration–approved medications for fibromyalgia are pregabalin, duloxetinem, and milnacipran. Fibromyalgia patients have impaired diffuse noxious inhibitory control, a measurement of endogenous analgesia efficacy, which is predictive of more postoperative pain. Because these patients also have heightened responses to painful stimuli, postoperative pain control can be challenging. **Fig. 2** demonstrates different forms of soft tissue pain syndrome. It is important to differentiate among the different forms, because the clinical picture is sometimes confusing.

Preoperative evaluation of patients on buprenorphine

Buprenorphine is a partial μ-opioid receptor agonist and a κ-opioid receptor antagonist that has been used to treat pain and opioid addiction. To counteract potential abuse by injection, Subutex and Suboxone were formulated with the strategy of having buprenorphine in combination with the opioid receptor antagonist, naloxone, in a ratio of 4 to 1, for sublingual administration. Naloxone has poor bioavailability in the sublingual form and has high bioavailability if injected IV.[74] Suboxone and Subutex are the only Food and Drug Administration–approved office-based medications to treat opioid abuse. Patients are sometimes put on buprenorphine/naloxone formulations for chronic pain if they do not have previous addiction history. This is an off-label use. At the opioid receptor, buprenorphine has low intrinsic activity and

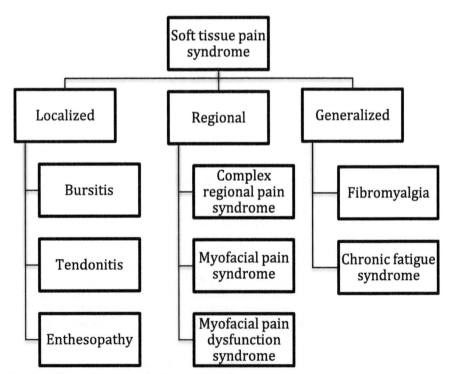

Fig. 2. Different forms of soft tissue pain syndrome.

high binding affinity and can induce withdrawal in opioid-dependent patients who are using full agonists.[75] Ceiling effect and poor bioavailability make buprenorphine safer for overdose potential than are opioid receptor full agonists. The maximal effects of buprenorphine seem to occur in the 16-mg to 32-mg dose range for sublingual tablets.[76] Preoperative pain, addiction history, and last dose of buprenorphine/naloxone should be reviewed before surgery. Previous experience with surgery and buprenorphine/naloxone should also be checked because it can help with opioid dosing. If buprenorphine/naloxone had been stopped for greater than 5 days and switched to pure agonists, patients likely need increased doses of opioids preoperatively and perioperatively for adequate pain control. If buprenorphine/naloxone was not stopped preoperatively, increased doses can be used perioperatively for pain control. Patients may need to convert to methadone, a stronger, longer-acting opioid, if the surgery is painful and not likely treated by partial agonists. Intraoperatively, fentanyl may be an optimal choice due to its high opioid receptor affinity and ability to displace the partial agonist. If a pure opioid agonist was used intraoperatively and postoperatively, an addiction specialist may transition patients back onto a partial agonist when the acute postoperative period is over and pain subsided.

SUMMARY

Patients with chronic pain face many challenges in maintaining function and pain control in their day-to-day lives. The stresses of surgery, the accompanying postoperative pain, and altered physiology add to this challenge. Appropriate planning for surgery and implementation of an individualized multimodal analgesia strategy can reduce the pain and suffering after surgery for these patients and help speed their recovery.

REFERENCES

1. Institute of Medicine Report from the Committee on Advancing Pain Research, Care, and Education. Relieving pain in America, a blueprint for transforming prevention, care, education and research. Washington (DC): The National Academies Press; 2011.
2. Hanna MN, et al. Does patient perception of pain control affect patient satisfaction across surgical units in a tertiary teaching hospital. Am J Med Qual 2012; 27(5):411–6.
3. Bruce J, Thornton AJ, et al. Chronic preoperative pain and psychological robustness predict acute postoperative pain outcomes after surgery for breast cancer. Br J Cancer 2012;107(6):937–46.
4. Althaus A, Hinrichs-Rocker A, et al. Development of a risk index for the prediction of chronic post-surgical pain. Eur J Pain 2012;16(6):901–10.
5. Ip HY, et al. Predictors of postoperative pain and analgesic consumption: a qualitative systematic review. Anesthesiology 2009;111(3):657–77.
6. Angst MS, Clark JD. Opioid-induced hyperalgesia. A qualitative systematic review. Anesthesiology 2006;104(3):570–87.
7. Chu LF, Angst MS, Clark D. Opioid-induced hyperalgesia in humans. Molecular mechanisms and clinical considerations. Clin J Pain 2008;24(6):479–96.
8. American Society of Anesthesiologists Task Force on Chronic Pain Management, American Society of Regional Anesthesia and Pain Medicine. Practice guidelines for chronic pain management: an updated report by the American Society of Anesthesiologists Task Force on Chronic Pain Management and the American Society of Regional Anesthesia and Pain Medicine. Anesthesiology 2010;112: 810–33.

9. Katz J, Seltzer Z. Transition from acute to chronic postsurgical pain: risk factors and protective factors. Expert Rev Neurother 2009;9(5):723–44.
10. Tammimaki A, Mannisto PT. Catechol-O-methyltransferase gene polymorphism and chronic human pain: a systematic review and meta-analysis. Pharmacogenet Genomics 2012;22(9):673–91.
11. Katz J, Poleshuck EL, Andrus CL, et al. Risk factors for acute pain and its persistence following breast cancer surgery. Pain 2005;119:16–25.
12. Zywiel MG, Stroh DA, Lee SY, et al. Chronic opioid use prior to total knee arthroplasty. J Bone Joint Surg Am 2011;93(21):1988–93.
13. Cohen L, Fouladi RT, Katz J. Preoperative coping strategies and distress predict postoperative pain and morphine consumption in women undergoing abdominal gynecologic surgery. J Psychosom Res 2005;58(2):201–9.
14. Caumo W, Schmidt AP, Schneider CN, et al. Preoperative predictors of moderate to intense acute postoperative pain in patients undergoing abdominal surgery. Acta Anaesthesiol Scand 2002;46(10):1265–71.
15. Theunissen M, Peters ML, et al. Preoperative anxiety and catastrophizing: a systematic review and meta-analysis of the association with chronic postsurgical pain. Clin J Pain 2012;28(9):819–41.
16. Powell R, Johnston M, Smith WC, et al. Psychological risk factors for chronic postsurgical pain after inguinal hernia repair surgery: a prospective cohort study. Eur J Pain 2012;16(4):600–10.
17. Werner MU, Mjobo HN, et al. Prediction of postoperative pain: a systematic review of predictive experimental pain studies. Anesthesiology 2010;112(6):1494–502.
18. Brandsborg B, Dueholm M, Kehlet H, et al. Mechanosensitivity before and after hysterectomy: a prospective study on the prediction of acute and chronic postoperative pain. Br J Anaesth 2011;107(6):940–7.
19. Werner MU, Duun P, Kehlet H. Prediction of postoperative pain by preoperative nociceptive responses to heat stimulation. Anesthesiology 2004;100(1):115–9.
20. van Gulik L, Janssen LI, Ahlers SJ, et al. Risk factors for chronic thoracic pain after cardiac surgery via sternotomy. Eur J Cardiothorac Surg 2011;40(6):1309–13.
21. Gore M, Brandenburg NA, Dukes E, et al. Pain severity in diabetic peripheral neuropathy (DPN) is associated with patient functioning, symptom levels of anxiety and depression, and sleep. J Pain Symptom Manage 2005;30(4):374–85.
22. Woolf CJ, Salter MW. Neuronal plasticity: increasing the gain in pain. Science 2000;288:1765–9.
23. Watkins LR, Milligan ED, Maier SF. Spinal cord glia: new players in pain. Pain 2001;93:201–5.
24. Loeser JD, Treede RD. The Kyoto protocol of IASP basic pain terminology. Pain 2008;137(3):473–7.
25. Voscopoulos C, Lema M. When does acute pain become chronic? Br J Anaesth 2010;105(Suppl 1):i69–85.
26. Katz J, McCartney CJ. Current status of preemptive analgesia. Curr Opin Anaesthesiol 2002;15:435–41.
27. Pogatzki-Zahn EM, Zahn PK. From preemptive to preventive analgesia. Curr Opin Anaesthesiol 2006;19:551–5.
28. Lorenz KA, et al. How reliable is pain as the fifth vital sign? J Am Board Fam Med 2009;22(3):291–8.
29. Royse CF, et al. Predictors of patient satisfaction with anaesthesia and surgery care: a cohort study using the Postoperative Quality of Recovery Scale. Eur J Anaesthesiol 2013;30(3):106–10.

30. Crabtree TD, Puri V, Bell JM, et al. Outcomes and perception of lung surgery with implementation of a patient video education module: a prospective cohort study. J Am Coll Surg 2012;214(5):816–21.
31. Livbjerg AE, Froekjaer S, Simonsen O, et al. Pre-operative patient education is associated with decreased risk of arthrofibrosis after total knee arthroplasty: a case control study. J Arthroplasty 2013. [Epub ahead of print].
32. Mitra S, Sinatra RS. Perioperative management of acut pain in the opioid depnedant patient. Anesthesiology 2004;101:212–27.
33. Okie S. A flood of opioids, a rising tide of deaths. N Engl J Med 2010;363(21):1981–5.
34. Kearney M, et al. Effects of preoperative education on patient outcomes after joint replacement surgery. Orthop Nurs 2011;30(6):391–6.
35. Rhodin A, Stridsberg M, Gordh T. Opioid endocrinopathy: a clinical problem in patients with chronic pain and long-term oral opioid treatment. Clin J Pain 2010;26(5):374–80.
36. Célèrier E, Rivat C, Jun Y, et al. Long-lasting hyperalgesia induced by fentanyl in rats: preventive effect of ketamine. Anesthesiology 2000;92:465–72.
37. Sehgal N, Manchikanti L, Smith HS. Prescription opioid abuse in chronic pain: a review of opioid abuse predictors and strategies to curb opioid abuse. Pain Physician 2012;15(3):ES67–92.
38. Lewis M, Souki F. "The anesthetic implications of opioid addiction." Perioperative addiction. New York: Springer; 2012. p. 73–93.
39. Costantini R, et al. Controlling pain in the post-operative setting. Int J Clin Pharmacol Ther 2011;49(2):116.
40. Mathiesen O, et al. A comprehensive multimodal pain treatment reduces opioid consumption after multilevel spine surgery. Eur Spine J 2013;1–8.
41. Rasmussen ML, et al. Multimodal analgesia with gabapentin, ketamine and dexamethasone in combination with paracetamol and ketorolac after hip arthroplasty: a preliminary study. Eur J Anaesthesiol 2010;27(4):324–30.
42. Maund E, McDaid C, et al. Paracetamol and selective and non-selective non-steroidal anti-inflammatory drugs for the reduction in morphine-related side-effects after major surgery: a systematic review. Br J Anaesth 2011;106(3):292–7.
43. Zhang J, Ho KY, et al. Efficacy of pregabalin in acute postoperative pain: a meta-analysis. Br J Anaesth 2011;106(4):454–62.
44. Clarke H, Bonin RP, et al. The prevention of chronic postsurgical pain using gabapentin and pregabalin: a combined systematic review and meta-analysis. Anesth Analg 2012;115(2):428–42.
45. Clarke H, Kirkham KR, Orser BA, et al. Gabapentin reduces preoperative anxiety and pain catastrophizing in highly anxious patients prior to major surgery: a blinded randomized placebo-controlled trial. Can J Anaesth 2013;60(5):432–43.
46. Laskowski K, Stirling A, et al. A systematic review of intravenous ketamine for postoperative analgesia. Can J Anaesth 2011;58(10):911–23.
47. Suzuki M. Role of N-methyl-D-aspartate receptor antagonists in postoperative pain management. Curr Opin Anaesthesiol 2009;22(5):618–22.
48. Gharaei B, Jafari A, et al. Opioid-sparing effect of preemptive bolus low-dose ketamine for moderate sedation in opioid abusers undergoing extracorporeal shock wave lithotripsy: a randomized clinical trial. Anesth Analg 2013;116(1):75–80.
49. Ganapathy S, Brookes J, Bourne R. Local infiltration analgesia. Anesthesiol Clin 2011;29(2):329–42.
50. Scott NB. Wound infiltration for surgery. Anaesthesia 2010;65(Suppl 1):67–75.
51. Gupta A. Wound infiltration with local anaesthetics in ambulatory surgery. Curr Opin Anaesthesiol 2010;23(6):708–13.

52. Sun Y, Li T, et al. Perioperative systemic lidocaine for postoperative analgesia and recovery after abdominal surgery: a meta-analysis of randomized controlled trials. Dis Colon Rectum 2012;55(11):1183–94.
53. Kang JG, Kim MH, et al. Intraoperative intravenous lidocaine reduces hospital length of stay following open gastrectomy for stomach cancer in men. J Clin Anesth 2012;24(6):465–70.
54. Grigoras A, Lee P, et al. Perioperative intravenous lidocaine decreases the incidence of persistent pain after breast surgery. Clin J Pain 2012;28(7):567–72.
55. Vigneault L, Turgeon AF, et al. Perioperative intravenous lidocaine infusion for postoperative pain control: a meta-analysis of randomized controlled trials. Can J Anaesth 2011;58(1):22–37.
56. de Leon-Casasola OA, Lema MJ. Epidural bupivacaine/sufentanil therapy for postoperative pain control in patients tolerant to opioid and unresponsive to epidural bupivacaine/morphine. Anesthesiology 1994;80(2):303–9.
57. Manion SC, Brennan TJ. Thoracic epidural analgesia and acute pain management. Anesthesiology 2011;115(1):181–8.
58. Pottecher J, Falcoz PE, et al. Does thoracic epidural analgesia improve outcome after lung transplantation? Interact Cardiovasc Thorac Surg 2011;12(1):51–3.
59. Nishimori M, Low JH, et al. Epidural pain relief versus systemic opioid-based pain relief for abdominal aortic surgery. Cochrane Database Syst Rev 2012;(7):CD005059.
60. Horlocker TT, Wedel DJ, Rowlingson JC, et al. Regional anesthesia in the patient receiving antithrombotic or thrombolytic therapy. American Society of Regional Anesthesia and Pain Medicine evidence-basedguidelines. 3rd edition. Reg Anesth Pain Med 2010;35(2):226.
61. Bingham AE, Fu R, et al. Continuous peripheral nerve block compared with single-injection peripheral nerve block: a systematic review and meta-analysis of randomized controlled trials. Reg Anesth Pain Med 2012;37(6):583–94.
62. Ilfeld BM. Continuous peripheral nerve blocks: a review of the published evidence. Anesth Analg 2011;113(4):904–25.
63. Hurley RW, Cohen SP, Williams KA, et al. The analgesic effects of perioperative gabapentin on postoperative pain. A meta-analysis. Reg Anesth Pain Med 2006;31:237–47.
64. Gilron I. Gabapentin and pregabalin for chronic neuropathic and early postsurgical pain. Current evidence and future directions. Curr Opin Anaesthesiol 2007;20:456–72.
65. Srinivas P, Gan TJ. Perioperative pain management. Durham (NC): Department of Anesthesiology, Duke university Medical Center. CNS drugs 2007:185–211.
66. Bjordal JM, Johnson MI, et al. Transcutaneous electrical nerve stimulation (TENS) can reduce postoperative analgesic consumption. A meta-analysis with assessment of optimal treatment parameters for postoperative pain. Eur J Pain 2003;7(2):181–8.
67. Grider JS, Brown RE, Colclough GW. Perioperative management of patients with intrathecal durg delivery system for chronic pain. Anesth Analg 2008;107:1393–6.
68. Lindsay K, Gough A. Psoriatic arthritis, methotrexate and the liver. Rheumatology (Oxford) 2008;47:939–41.
69. Klit H, Nanna BF, Troels SJ. Central post-stroke pain: clinical characteristics, pathophysiology, and management. The Lancet Neurology 2009;857–68.
70. Besse JL, Gadeyne S, et al. Effect of vitamin C on prevention of complex regional pain syndrome type I in foot and ankle surgery. Foot Ankle Surg 2009;15(4):179–82.

71. Zollinger PE, Tuinebreijer WE, et al. Can vitamin C prevent complex regional pain syndrome in patients with wrist fractures? A randomized, controlled, multicenter dose-response study. J Bone Joint Surg Am 2007;89(7):1424–31.
72. Harden RN, Bruehl S. Proposed new diagnostic criteria for complex regional pain syndrome. Pain Med 2007;8(4):326–31.
73. Wolfe F, Häuser W. Fibromyalgia diagnosis and diagnostic criteria. Ann Med 2011;43(7):495–502. http://dx.doi.org/10.3109/07853890.2011.595734.
74. Bezchlibnyk-Butler KZ, Jeffries J, Virani A. Clinical handbook of psychotropic drugs. 17th edition. Cambridge (MA): Hogrefe & Huber Publishers; 2007.
75. Rosado J, Walsh SL, Bigelow GE, et al. Sublingual buprenorphine/naloxone precipitated withdrawal in subjects maintained on 100 mg of daily methadone. Drug Alcohol Depend 2007;90:261–9.
76. Ducharme S, Ronald F, Kathryn G. Update on the clinical use of buprenorphine In opioid-related disorders. Canadian Family Physician 2012;37–41.

Complex Regional Pain Syndrome
Diagnosis and Treatment

Mitchell Freedman, DO[a,b,]*, Ari C. Greis, DO[a,b], Lisa Marino, DO[b],
Anupam N. Sinha, DO[b], Jeffrey Henstenburg[b]

KEYWORDS

- Complex regional pain syndrome • Neuropathic pain syndromes
- Reflex sympathetic dystrophy sympathetic nerve block • Spinal cord stimulation

KEY POINTS

- Complex regional pain syndrome (CRPS) is characterized by pain out of proportion to the usual time or degree of a specific lesion.
- The diagnosis of CRPS is based on 4 distinct subgroups of signs and symptoms: sensory, vasomotor, sudomotor, and motor/trophic changes.
- Treatment should be multidisciplinary, consisting of medications, physical/occupational therapy, psychotherapy, and sympathetic blocks targeted toward pain relief and functional restoration.
- More aggressive treatment, such as sympathectomy and spinal cord stimulation, have a low level of evidence but may be considered for therapy-resistant CRPS type I.

INTRODUCTION

Complex regional pain syndrome (CRPS) is characterized by pain that is out of proportion to the usual time or degree of a specific lesion. It does not present within the distribution of one peripheral nerve or nerve root, and has a distal predominance of abnormal sensory, motor, sudomotor, vasomotor, and/or trophic findings. Progression is variable.[1] CRPS has been known by many other names including reflex sympathetic dystrophy (RSD) and causalgia. These terms date back to Claude Bernard, who in 1851 referred to a pain syndrome that was accompanied by changes in the sympathetic nervous system. During the American Civil War, Silas Weir Mitchell described cases of soldiers suffering from ongoing burning pain after recovering from gunshot wounds, and coined the term Causalgia.[2,3] Evans first used the term reflex sympathetic dystrophy in the 1940s to emphasize that the sympathetic nervous system

This article originally appeared in Physical Medicine and Rehabilitation Clinics of North America, Volume 25, Issue 2, May 2014.
Disclosures: None.
[a] Department of Rehabilitation Medicine, Jefferson Medical College, Thomas Jefferson University, 9th and Chestnut Street, Philadelphia, PA 19107, USA; [b] Rothman Institute, 925 Chestnut Street, Philadelphia, PA 19107, USA
* Corresponding author. Rothman Institute, 925 Chestnut Street, Philadelphia, PA 19107.
E-mail address: mitchell.freedman@rothmaninstitute.com

http://dx.doi.org/10.1016/j.ccol.2014.10.005
2352-7986/14/$ – see front matter

was involved in the pathophysiology of the disease.[4] CRPS replaced the term RSD for several reasons. Sympathetic changes and dystrophy may not be present throughout the disease course.[5,6] Furthermore, there is no specific reflex arc that is responsible for the CRPS; pain is secondary to multisynaptic pathologic changes involving the brain, spinal cord, and peripheral nerves.

EPIDEMIOLOGY

CRPS has a female to male ratio of 2:1 to 4:1, which is more common with increasing age. There are 50,000 new cases of CRPS in the United States annually. The most common initiating events of the syndrome include fractures, sprains, and trauma such as crush injuries and surgery. Immobilization after injury is a contributing factor in more than half of patients.[7,8]

DIAGNOSIS

The Budapest Consensus Workshop introduced criteria to identify patients with CRPS and exclude other neuropathic conditions. More stringent criteria are used for research purposes to eliminate false-positive inclusions. Less stringent criteria are used in the clinical setting to avoid missing the diagnosis. A patient must report symptoms of, and display signs on physical examination, in the following categories: sensory, vasomotor, sudomotor/edema, and motor/trophic (**Figs. 1** and **2**). For both clinical and research purposes, a patient with CRPS should have physical examination evidence of at least 1 sign in 2 or more of the categories. The symptom criteria are different when assessing patients in a clinical rather than a research setting. In a clinical setting, patients must report 1 symptom in 3 out of the 4 categories, whereas in the research setting the patient must report 1 symptom in each of the 4 categories (**Box 1**). This minor adjustment in data collection creates a sensitivity of 0.85 and a specificity of 0.69 for the research group, compared with the clinical criteria that have a sensitivity of 0.94 and a specificity of 0.36.[1,9]

There are 2 subgroupings of CRPS. CRPS I is CRPS without major nerve damage (formerly known as RSD) while CRPS II is CRPS with major nerve damage (formerly known as causalgia). A third subtype is CRPS NOS (not otherwise specified), which captures patients who only partially meet the current criteria but were diagnosed with CRPS under previous criteria.[1,6,9]

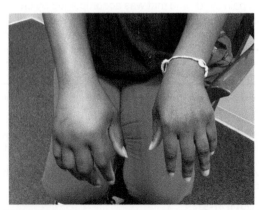

Fig. 1. A patient with 3 months of pain following brachial plexus injury has significant fusiform edema and color changes in the right upper extremity.

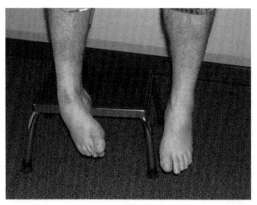

Fig. 2. A patient with chronic complex regional pain syndrome exhibits dystonic posture of the right ankle along with trophic skin changes.

Accurate diagnosis of CRPS is challenging despite the standardization of diagnostic criteria. There is no one definitive objective test that confirms the clinical diagnosis. Physical findings may not be present at all times, but the diagnostic criteria for signs require that the findings be present at the time of the diagnosis. At present, the diagnosis is made primarily on the basis of physical examination, but there are objective tests that may help verify the physical examination findings. Functional imaging, visual

---

Box 1
Budapest clinical diagnostic criteria for CRPS

1. Continuing pain that is disproportionate to any inciting event

2. Patient must report 1 symptom in 3 of the 4 following categories:

   a. Sensory: Reports of hyperesthesia and/or allodynia

   b. Vasomotor: Reports of temperature asymmetry and/or skin color changes and/or skin color asymmetry

   c. Sudomotor/edema: Reports of edema and/or sweating changes and/or sweating asymmetry

   d. Motor/trophic: Reports of decreased range of motion and/or motor dysfunction (weakness, tremor, dystonia) and/or trophic changes (hair, nail, and/or skin)

3. Patient must have 1 sign at the time of evaluation in 2 or more of the following categories:

   a. Sensory: Evidence of hyperalgesia to pin prick and/or allodynia to light touch and/or deep somatic pressure and/or joint movement

   b. Vasomotor: Evidence of temperature asymmetry and/or skin color changes and/or asymmetry

   c. Sudomotor/edema: Evidence of edema and/or sweating changes and/or sweating asymmetry

   d. Motor/trophic: Evidence of decreased range of motion and/or motor dysfunction (weakness, tremor, dystonia) and/or trophic changes (hair, nail and/or skin)

4. There is no other diagnosis that better explains the signs and symptoms

From Harden RN, Bruehl S, Perez RS, et al. Validation of proposed diagnostic criteria (the "Budapest Criteria") for complex regional pain syndrome. Pain 2010;150(2):274; with permission.

analog scales, and devices to quantify temperature and mechanical allodynia are available. Vasomotor findings are supported with a thermometer and Doppler measurement of vasomotor tone. Edema is quantitated with volumetry. Sudomotor function can be measured directly with quantitative sudomotor axon response testing, and indirectly with biopedance and skin potential fluctuations. Weakness and range of motion are measured by clinicians. Bone density testing is available. Small-fiber dropout via skin biopsy can be measured to validate a decrease in small nerve density.[10] Most of these technologies are not readily available in the office.

Diagnostic testing may include rheumatologic workup to assess for inflammatory arthritis. Electrodiagnostic testing serves to evaluate the peripheral nervous system, which can help in the diagnosis of CRPS II. Plain films may reveal advanced osteoporosis or fracture in the symptomatic limb with CRPS. Magnetic resonance imaging evaluates soft-tissue injuries and bone edema. A triple-phase bone scan is generally not diagnostic of CRPS.

Pain may or may not be mediated by the sympathetic nervous system. A fluoroscopic guided lumbar paravertebral block for the lower extremity and a stellate ganglion block for the upper extremity may be useful in determining how much sympathetic input contributes to a patient's symptoms. Because CRPS may or may not have a sympathetic component, a positive or negative response to a sympathetic block does not substantiate the diagnosis of CRPS.

PROGRESSION AND COURSE OF DISEASE

Schwartzman and colleagues[7] report that after 1 year most of the signs and symptoms are well developed. Most patients have abnormalities of pain processing such as allodynia, which is present in 90% of patients at 5 years and in 98% of patients by 15 years. Swelling is noted in 75% of patients at 5 years and 90% by 15 years. Loss of strength and difficult movement is seen in 90% of patients at 5 years. Spread of the pain occurs in 92% of patients.[7,11]

In a study of 27 patients with CRPS I, Maleki and colleagues[12] reported contiguous spread in all patients, 70% of whom had independent spread to another site, 15% mirror-image spread to the initial site, and 19% contiguous spread alone. Van Rijn and colleagues[13] reported that CRPS usually affects one limb but can spread to the contralateral or ipsilateral limb in 53% and 30% of cases, respectively. A diagonal spread was seen the least in 14% of cases. Aberrant regulation of neurogenic inflammation, maladaptive neuroplasticity, and genetic predisposition are theorized as the pathophysiology behind the spread of CRPS. Spontaneous spread is at the level of the spinal cord, as opposed to a systemic etiology.[13]

The CRPS Severity Score (CSS) was developed in an attempt to assess the severity of CRPS. The concept of staging CRPS has been abandoned owing to the lack of empirical statistical evidence to suggest the existence of the stages.[1,14] The CSS is based on the presence or absence of 17 clinically assessed signs and symptoms. Patients with higher CSS scores had greater reported pain intensity, distress, and functional impairments. Greater temperature asymmetry and abnormalities in thermal perception were seen more frequently.[14,15]

PSYCHIATRIC ISSUES

There is a debate as to whether patients who have CRPS are predisposed to develop the condition based on their psychiatric profile. Harden and colleagues[16] found that preoperative anxiety and severity of pain predicted the development of CRPS signs and symptoms following total knee arthroplasty. However, most studies do not find a unique relationship between CRPS and psychiatric factors. Shiri and colleagues[17] compared psychological profiles of patients with CRPS with those of patients suffering from conversion disorders. High somatization and depression and low anxiety scores were seen in both groups. Reedijk and colleagues[18] compared patients with CRPS I–related dystonia with those with conversion disorders and affective disorders. Although the CRPS patients did exhibit elevated scores for somatoform dissociation, traumatic experiences, general psychopathology, and lower quality of life compared with the general population, they also had lower total scores for personality traits, recent life events, and general psychopathology relative to the patients with conversion disorder and affective disorder. The investigators concluded that patients with CRPS I–related dystonia did not have a uniquely disturbed psychological profile as a group. Puchalski and Zyluk[19] reported that 62 patients who underwent distal radius fractures and developed CRPS did not exhibit significant differences in personality or depression scales relative to patients who did not develop CRPS. Monti and colleagues[20] compared 25 CRPS I patients with a control group with chronic back pain. Both groups exhibited similar findings of major depressive and personality disorders. It was concluded that the abnormal findings are a result of severe chronic pain and are not uniquely secondary to CRPS.

Beerthuizen and colleagues[21] conducted a systematic review of the literature since 1980, and concluded that there was no relationship between psychological factors and CRPS; they concluded that CRPS was associated only with patients who experienced more life events (divorce, death of spouse, vacation, and so forth). Geertzen and colleagues[22] also reported that a difficult time in life or a painful affective loss (stressful life event) is more common during the onset of CRPS when a group of patients with subacute CRPS were compared with a group of patients preparing for hand surgery over the next 24 hours.

TREATMENT

In 1997, consensus guidelines were generated for the functional restoration of CRPS. Medication, psychological counseling, and interventional options were reserved for patients who were failing to progress with physical and occupational therapy.[23] Current literature supports the use of medication, modalities, interventions, and psychological treatment more acutely.[24] Multiple articles support the use of physical therapy to treat CRPS.[25,26] Interdisciplinary treatment of CRPS is supported without high-level evidence by the aforementioned consensus-building conferences.[23,24] Interdisciplinary treatment of the more general category of chronic pain has been used for decades. The objectives of physical and occupational therapy in patients with CRPS are to minimize edema, desensitize a painful limb and normalize sensation, promote normal positioning, decrease muscle guarding, and increase functional use of the extremity. Edema management consists of specialized compressive garments along with manual edema mobilization techniques. Aquatic therapy has also been shown to aid in edema control and to facilitate early weight bearing.[27]

Desensitization can be achieved through a stress-loading program consisting of scrubbing and carrying techniques. Scrubbing involves using the affected limb to move a brush against a surface. Carrying involves a gradual weight-loading program whereby the patient carries objects and weights either in the hand or in a handled bag.[28] For the lower extremities, weight-shifting and balancing techniques are used to gradually stress the affected leg. Contrast baths can also be beneficial in mild cases of CRPS. Desensitization and improved circulation may be accomplished in the affected extremity by alternating vasodilation (heat) with vasoconstriction (cold).

Patient education involves explaining fear-avoidance models using the symptoms, beliefs, and behaviors of the individual patients. Patients are taught to view their various autonomic and vasomotor disturbances as a condition that can be self-managed, rather than a disease whereby the affected limb needs careful protection. Under therapist supervision, the patient identifies dangerous and threatening situations and gradually increases exposure to these activities as much as possible until anxiety levels have decreased.[29]

Mirror therapy, or mirror visual feedback, is conducted with the patient seated before a mirror that is oriented parallel to the midline. View of the affected limb is blocked behind the mirror. The patient first closes his or her eyes and describes both the affected and unaffected limb, followed by imagined movements of both extremities. When looking into the mirror, the patient sees the reflection of the unaffected limb positioned as the affected limb. The patient is then asked to look at the mirrored limb without movement. Finally, the patient moves the unaffected extremity through different planes of movement. Movement of or touch to the intact limb may be perceived as affecting the painful limb.[30]

Graded motor imagery (GMI) acts on the reorganization of cortical networks presumed to be involved in chronic pain and CRPS. GMI consists of a sequential set of brain exercises comprising laterality training, imagined hand movements, and mirror feedback therapy. The patient looks at a photograph of a hand or foot, then imagines moving the painful limb into the position in the photograph. This action is progressed to moving both limbs into the position while observing the unaffected limb in a mirror that obscures the affected limb.[30]

Alternative therapeutic techniques include acupuncture, Qigong therapy, and relaxation training. However, there is very low-quality evidence that any of these methods are effective in reducing CRPS I–related pain.[31] Hyperbaric oxygen therapy has been reported to reduce pain and edema in a placebo-controlled, randomized study of 71 CRPS patients.[32]

PHARMACOTHERAPY

There are many medication options for the treatment of CRPS. Unfortunately, there is a paucity of evidence to support their use in treating CRPS specifically. CRPS affects the vascular, neurologic, osseous, integumentary, and immunologic systems. In most cases, polypharmacy is required to manage the various symptoms of CRPS. The use of medications from complementary drug classes minimizes side effects from any one medication by lessening individual dosage requirements. As in any syndrome, it is important to analyze the efficacy and side effects of all drugs that are added to the treatment regimen.

Nonsteroidal anti-inflammatory drugs (NSAIDs) are used in a variety of pain conditions to manage inflammation. It is unclear whether the inflammatory component of CRPS follows the traditional cyclooxygenase (COX) pathway or is more neurogenic in nature (mediated by afferent nociceptors). NSAIDs inhibit COX, which is responsible for the production of prostaglandins that mediate inflammation and hyperalgesia. Their use may help block spinal nociceptive processing as well.[33] Small clinical trials looking at NSAID use in neuropathic pain have shown mixed results, and one study showed no benefit in the treatment of CRPS I.[33] The use of COX-2 selective inhibitors has not been formally studied in the treatment of CRPS, but there is some anecdotal mention in the literature.[34]

Clinical evidence supports the use of oral corticosteroids in cases of CRPS.[35] Improvements in symptoms of acute patients were seen in randomized controlled studies that used approximately 30 mg of corticosteroids per day for 2 to 12 weeks followed by a taper.[36,37] Their role in chronic CRPS in comparison with more acute cases is uncertain. Long-term use of steroids has not proved to be effective. Given the significant complications of steroids, it is not recommended that steroids be prescribed for long-term use.

Neuropathic pain is often related to increased excitability of neurons. Gabapentin and pregabalin work by blocking voltage-dependent calcium channels, and are effective in treating post-herpetic neuralgia and diabetic neuropathy. There are limited data addressing the effect of gabapentin on CRPS, and no studies are available to evaluate whether CRPS patients benefit from pregabalin.[1] Carbamazepine (Tegretol) is approved by the Food and Drug Administration (FDA) for the treatment of trigeminal neuralgia.[38] One randomized controlled trial showed pain reduction in CRPS symptoms after 8 days of carbamazepine when compared with placebo.[39] Oxcarbazepine (Trileptal), phenytoin (Dilantin), and lamotrigine (Lamictal) are alternative anticonvulsants.

Norepinephrine and, possibly, serotonin have been shown to mediate inhibition of the dorsal horn and block peripheral sodium channels. The tricyclic and heterocyclic drugs, such as amitriptyline, augment descending inhibition by blocking presynaptic reuptake.[40] These agents are considered a first-line option for neuropathic conditions but have not been formally studied in CRPS. Their antidepressant and sedative effects provide additional benefit to patients in chronic pain. Combined serotonin and norepinephrine reuptake inhibitors, such as venlafaxine, milnacipran, and duloxetine, are FDA-approved for several chronic pain conditions but have not been studied in CRPS.

Several studies document the safety and benefit of opioids in treating neuropathic pain.[41] However, neuropathic pain does not seem to respond as well to opioids as acute nociceptive pain. Opioids are considered second-line or third-line agents that should be used cautiously in conjunction with other medications. It is possible that tramadol and tapentadol may be more efficacious in treating neuropathic pain related to CRPS, owing to their ability to block the reuptake of serotonin and norepinephrine. Opioids for chronic benign pain syndromes remain controversial secondary to potential for abuse, misuse, diversion, and overdoses leading to death.

N-Methyl-D-aspartate receptor antagonists are a class of anesthetics that have been used in the treatment of neuropathic pain and CRPS. Ketamine, amantadine, and dextromethorphan have been studied, but toxicity at effective doses has generally been too high.[42,43] These agents are popular as recreational drugs because of their dissociative, hallucinogenic, and euphoric effects.

An outpatient subanesthetic course of intravenous ketamine over 5 days provided significant relief of pain for up to 3 months.[44] Quality of life did not change. Side effects included nausea, headache, tiredness, and dysphoria. Pain relief was obtained in 16 of 20 patients in an open-label phase II study of anesthetic-dose intravenous ketamine in patients with refractory CRPS,[45] with treatment lasting 5 days. Quality of life, associated movement disorder, and ability to work significantly improved in most patients at 6 months after the study. Anxiety, nightmares, and difficulties with sleep were observed in most patients. Epidural ketamine administration for CRPS[46] and topical ketamine gel for neuropathic pain[47] have also been evaluated.

Clonidine has been used orally, transdermally, and epidurally to treat sympathetically maintained pain in CRPS.[48] A systematic review found no convincing support for clonidine in the treatment of CRPS.[35] Two uncontrolled case series showed nifedipine, a calcium-channel blocker, to be effective in managing vasoconstriction in patients with CRPS.[49,50]

Phenoxybenzamine is an irreversible α-antagonist that has antiadrenergic effects and has been shown to be beneficial in treating CRPS. It is considered a third-line agent and works best in cases lasting less than 3 months.[49,51] At higher doses, side effects include orthostatic hypotension and inhibition of ejaculation.

CRPS is frequently associated with localized osteopenia/osteoporosis. Active bone resorption and remodeling may be seen on triple-phase bone scan, and results in nociceptive bone pain. In addition, disuse of the affected limb in CRPS can cause reduction in bone mineral density. Calcitonin reduces blood calcium levels and is usually administered nasally. Calcitonin can help to preserve bone mass and also has antinociceptive effects that have been found to be useful in treating both acute and chronic pain. A meta-analysis of a limited number of controlled studies supported the use of intranasal doses of 100 to 300 U per day for 3 to 4 weeks.[52] Other clinical trials have revealed equivocal evidence regarding the efficacy of calcitonin in treating CRPS.[53,54]

Bisphosphonates, such as alendronate, improve bone density by slowing the resorption of bone. Multiple high-quality studies support the benefits of some older short-acting bisphosphonates in treating CRPS-related pain.

Baclofen administration via intrathecal pump is effective for pain and dystonia while minimizing sedation. The long-term use of other muscle relaxants such as benzodiazepines and cyclobenzaprine are usually not effective or recommended.[1] Injection of botulinum toxin can be considered in focal areas of spasticity. Intradermal injections of botulinum toxin extended the duration of pain relief in a subset of patients with CRPS who received a sympathetic chain block with bupivacaine.[55]

Intravenous immunoglobulin (IVIG) is a potent anti-inflammatory and immune modulator. In CRPS, peripheral and central glial-mediated neuroimmune activation sustains chronic pain. A randomized, double-blind, placebo-controlled trial of 13 patients with chronic CRPS compared low-dose IVIG with treatment with intravenous normal saline. The 12 patients who completed the trial described some pain relief in the IVIG group at 6 to 19 days after treatment. Further research is needed to determine whether IVIG, which is relatively costly, has a role in treating CRPS.[56]

Topical medications for the treatment of local symptoms are an attractive option when treating limb pain. EMLA cream and Lidoderm patches are local anesthetics used to treat CRPS. Capsaicin is a compound found in chili peppers. Topical application overstimulates nociceptive nerve endings and causes a "dying-back" phenomenon that can decrease neuropathic pain locally. It is not well tolerated by patients secondary to burning pain. DMSO is a cream that acts as a scavenger of free radicals. A 2-month trial of 50% DMSO cream decreased pain in CRPS in comparison with placebo.[57]

INTERVENTIONAL AND SURGICAL TREATMENTS

Sympathetic blockade may be particularly beneficial if pain and swelling is limiting participation in therapy despite medication. These blocks involve the injection of local anesthetics along the lumbar sympathetic chain (for lower limbs) or stellate ganglion (for upper limbs) under fluoroscopic guidance. A good response includes an increase in temperature in the affected extremity, without a motor or sensory block, reduced pain, decreased allodynia, and improved range of motion.[58] Blocks may be repeated if there is short-term benefit. These blocks are most beneficial in patients who demonstrate sympathetically mediated symptoms. Response duration and efficacy is variable. Success would be expected to be greater in the patient who has a sympathetically maintained pain than in a patient who has sympathetic independent pain.

Cepeda and colleagues[59] conducted a systematic review on the role of sympathetic blockade in CRPS, and found 2 small randomized, double-blind, crossover studies that evaluated 23 subjects. The combined effect of the 2 trials produced a relative risk of 1.17 to achieve at least 50% of pain relief 30 minutes to 2 hours after the sympathetic blockade (95% confidence interval 0.80–1.72). It was not possible to determine the effect of sympathetic blockade on long-term pain relief because the investigators evaluated different outcomes in the 2 studies. No conclusion concerning the effectiveness of this procedure could be drawn.

Chemical or surgical sympathectomies may be performed for sympathetically maintained pain from CRPS in patients who have had good but transient relief from sympathetic blocks. Chemical sympathectomy is a procedure whereby alcohol or phenol injections serve as agents to destroy the sympathetic chain. Outcomes are variable, and the procedure has uncertain efficacy.[58] Surgical ablation can be performed by open removal or electrocoagulation of the sympathetic chain, or minimally invasive procedures using stereotactic thermal or laser interruption of the sympathetic chain. The effects may be longer lasting, up to 1 year, with radiofrequency ablation.[58] Nerve regeneration commonly occurs following both surgical and chemical ablation, but may take longer with surgical ablation.

Manjunath and colleagues[60] randomized 20 patients with lower limb CRPS I to either radiofrequency or phenol lumbar sympathectomy. There were statistically significant reductions from baseline in all the pain scores used in both treatment groups. A 2012 Cochrane review found that lower-quality evidence seems to suggest that sympathectomy for neuropathic pain can be effective. Complications of sympathectomy are common, including postsympathectomy neuralgia, hyperhidrosis, and Horner syndrome (in cases of upper limb CRPS). Because there is poor evidence for the long-term effectiveness of sympathectomy, it should be used with great caution and only after failure of other treatment options.[61]

Intravenous regional anesthesia (IVRA) involves injection of medication directly into the involved extremity. Numerous IVRA trials have been conducted using atropine, guanethidine, lidocaine, bretylium, clonidine, droperidol, ketanserin, and reserpine. Bretylium and ketanserin IVRA been proved to have some efficacy, although there is a high risk of false-positive results.[62] All other trials have proved to be ineffective.

Spinal cord stimulation (SCS) involves surgical placement of electrodes within the epidural space at the level of the cervical or lower thoracic spinal cord. Kemler and colleagues[63] performed a randomized study to compare SCS combined with physical therapy (SCT/PT) with physical therapy (PT) alone in 54 chronic CRPS I patients (pain of at least 6 months' duration) who had failed conventional treatment. Patients in the SCT/PT group underwent 1 week of test stimulation. The SCS system was implanted if they had a 50% reduction in their visual analog score or if they reported that they were "much improved" or "best ever" on the global perceived effect scale; 24 patients proceeded to permanent lead placement. Detection thresholds and pain thresholds for pressure, warmth and cold, and the extent of dynamic and static hyperalgesia were evaluated at baseline, and at 1, 3, 6, and 12 months after implantation. At 2 years, the SCS/PT group had statistically better results.[64] However, in the last follow-up at 5 years there were no statistical differences in any of the measured variables. Complications include pulse-generator failure, lead displacement, and pulse-generator pocket revision. Despite the diminishing effectiveness of SCS, 95% of patients responded that they would repeat the treatment for the same result.[65]

Successful results of SCS include significant reductions in pain perception, allodynia, and muscle dysfunction, and improvement in blood flow. When applied early in the course of the disease, SCS can greatly increase the functionality of the affected limb.[66]

CRPS as an indication for amputation remains controversial. The predominant reasons for amputation have been pain, dysfunctional limb, gangrene, infection, or ulcers. Recurrence of CRPS I in the residual limb following the amputation was reported in 48% of the patients in 14 studies. Phantom pain was reported in 41% of patients in 15 studies.[67] In a recent retrospective study, 21 patients with long-standing therapy-resistant CRPS I underwent amputation of the affected limb. Pain reduction and improvements in mobility and sleep were seen in most patients. Only 4 patients (14%) had recurrence of CRPS I in the residual limb.[68]

Amputation should be considered for therapy-resistant CRPS only when the patient has no major psychopathology and has a realistic point of view about the possible beneficial and adverse effects of an amputation. Further research is necessary.[67,68]

SUMMARY

CRPS is a formidable disease to diagnose and treat. It is important to apply the current diagnostic criteria in making the diagnosis. Treatment should be aggressive early in the disease, and a multidisciplinary approach is often required. Medication, sympathetic blocks, and SCS may also be beneficial.

REFERENCES

1. Harden RN, Oaklander AL, Burton AW, et al. Complex regional pain syndrome: practical diagnostic and treatment guidelines, 4th edition. Pain Med 2013; 14(2):180–229.
2. Dommerholt J. Complex regional pain syndrome—1: history, diagnostic criteria and etiology. J Bodyw Mov Ther 2004;8(3):167–77.
3. Mitchell SW, Morehouse GR, Keen WW. Gunshot wounds and other injuries of nerves. 1864. Clin Orthop Relat Res 2007;458:35–9.
4. Evans JA. Reflex sympathetic dystrophy. Surg Clin North Am 1946;8:260–3.
5. Harden RN, Bruehl SP. Diagnosis of complex regional pain syndrome: signs, symptoms, and new empirically derived diagnostic criteria. Clin J Pain 2006; 22(5):415–9.
6. Harden R, Bruehl S. Introduction and diagnostic considerations. Milford (CT): Reflex Sympathetic Dystrophy Syndrome Association; 2006.
7. Schwartzman RJ, Erwin KL, Alexander GM. The natural history of complex regional pain syndrome. Clin J Pain 2009;25(4):273–80.
8. Bruehl S. An update on the pathophysiology of complex regional pain syndrome. Anesthesiology 2010;113(3):713–25.
9. Harden RN, Bruehl S, Perez RS, et al. Validation of proposed diagnostic criteria (the "Budapest Criteria") for complex regional pain syndrome. Pain 2010;150(2): 268–74.
10. Harden RN. Objectification of the diagnostic criteria for CRPS. Pain Med 2010; 11(8):1212–5.
11. Sandroni P, Benrud-Larson LM, McClelland RL, et al. Complex regional pain syndrome type I: incidence and prevalence in Olmsted county, a population-based study. Pain 2003;103(1–2):199–207.
12. Maleki J, LeBel AA, Bennett GJ, et al. Patterns of spread in complex regional pain syndrome, type I (reflex sympathetic dystrophy). Pain 2000;88(3):259–66.
13. van Rijn MA, Marinus J, Putter H, et al. Spreading of complex regional pain syndrome: not a random process. J Neural Transm 2011;118(9):1301–9.

14. Bruehl S, Harden RN, Galer BS, et al. Complex regional pain syndrome: are there distinct subtypes and sequential stages of the syndrome? Pain 2002;95(1–2): 119–24.
15. Harden RN, Bruehl S, Perez RS, et al. Development of a severity score for CRPS. Pain 2010;151(3):870–6.
16. Harden RN, Bruehl S, Stanos S, et al. Prospective examination of pain-related and psychological predictors of CRPS-like phenomena following total knee arthroplasty: a preliminary study. Pain 2003;106(3):393–400.
17. Shiri S, Tsenter J, Livai R, et al. Similarities between the psychological profiles of complex regional pain syndrome and conversion disorder patients. J Clin Psychol Med Settings 2003;10(3):193–9.
18. Reedijk WB, van Rijn MA, Roelofs K, et al. Psychological features of patients with complex regional pain syndrome type I related dystonia. Mov Disord 2008; 23(11):1551–9.
19. Puchalski P, Zyluk A. Complex regional pain syndrome type 1 after fractures of the distal radius: a prospective study of the role of psychological factors. J Hand Surg Br 2005;30(6):574–80.
20. Monti DA, Herring CL, Schwartzman RJ, et al. Personality assessment of patients with complex regional pain syndrome type I. Clin J Pain 1998;14(4):295–302.
21. Beerthuizen A, van 't Spijker A, Huygen FJ, et al. Is there an association between psychological factors and the complex regional pain syndrome type 1 (CRPS1) in adults? A systematic review. Pain 2009;145(1–2):52–9.
22. Geertzen JH, de Bruijn-Kofman AT, de Bruijn HP, et al. Stressful life events and psychological dysfunction in complex regional pain syndrome type I. Clin J Pain 1998;14(2):143–7.
23. Stanton-Hicks MM, Baron RD, Boas RM, et al. Complex regional pain syndromes: guidelines for therapy. Clin J Pain 1998;14(2):155–66.
24. Stanton-Hicks MD, Burton AW, Bruehl SP, et al. An updated interdisciplinary clinical pathway for CRPS: report of an expert panel. Pain Pract 2002;2(1):1–16.
25. Perez RS, Zollinger PE, Dijkstra PU, et al. Evidence based guidelines for complex regional pain syndrome type 1. BMC Neurol 2010;10:20.
26. Baron R, Wasner G. Complex regional pain syndromes. Curr Pain Headache Rep 2001;5(2):114–23.
27. Sherry DD, Wallace CA, Kelley C, et al. Short- and long-term outcomes of children with complex regional pain syndrome type I treated with exercise therapy. Clin J Pain 1999;15(3):218–23.
28. Carlson LK, Watson HK. Treatment of reflex sympathetic dystrophy using the stress-loading program. J Hand Ther 1988;1(4):149–54.
29. de Jong JR, Vlaeyen JW, Onghena P, et al. Reduction of pain-related fear in complex regional pain syndrome type I: the application of graded exposure in vivo. Pain 2005;116(3):264–75.
30. Moseley GL. Graded motor imagery for pathologic pain: a randomized controlled trial. Neurology 2006;67(12):2129–34.
31. O'Connell NE, Wand BM, McAuley J, et al. Interventions for treating pain and disability in adults with complex regional pain syndrome. Cochrane Database Syst Rev 2013;(4):CD009416.
32. Yildiz S, Uzun G, Kiralp MZ. Hyperbaric oxygen therapy in chronic pain management. Curr Pain Headache Rep 2006;10(2):95–100.
33. Geisslinger G, Muth-Selbach U, Coste O, et al. Inhibition of noxious stimulus-induced spinal prostaglandin E2 release by flurbiprofen enantiomers: a microdialysis study. J Neurochem 2000;74(5):2094–100.

34. Pappagallo M, Rosenberg AD. Epidemiology, pathophysiology, and management of complex regional pain syndrome. Pain Pract 2001;1(1):11–20.
35. Kingery WS. A critical review of controlled clinical trials for peripheral neuropathic pain and complex regional pain syndromes. Pain 1997;73(2):123–39.
36. Christensen K, Jensen EM, Noer I. The reflex dystrophy syndrome response to treatment with systemic corticosteroids. Acta Chir Scand 1982;148(8): 653–5.
37. Braus DF, Krauss JK, Strobel J. The shoulder-hand syndrome after stroke: a prospective clinical trial. Ann Neurol 1994;36(5):728–33.
38. Rull JA, Quibrera R, Gonzalez-Millan H, et al. Symptomatic treatment of peripheral diabetic neuropathy with carbamazepine (Tegretol): double blind crossover trial. Diabetologia 1969;5(4):215–8.
39. Harke H, Gretenkort P, Ladleif HU, et al. The response of neuropathic pain and pain in complex regional pain syndrome I to carbamazepine and sustained-release morphine in patients pretreated with spinal cord stimulation: a double-blinded randomized study. Anesth Analg 2001;92(2):488–95.
40. Sindrup SH, Jensen TS. Pharmacologic treatment of pain in polyneuropathy. Neurology 2000;55(7):915–20.
41. Dellemijn PL, van Duijn H, Vanneste JA. Prolonged treatment with transdermal fentanyl in neuropathic pain. J Pain Symptom Manage 1998;16(4):220–9.
42. Eide PK, Jorum E, Stubhaug A, et al. Relief of post-herpetic neuralgia with the N-methyl-D-aspartic acid receptor antagonist ketamine: a double-blind, cross-over comparison with morphine and placebo. Pain 1994;58(3):347–54.
43. Nelson KA, Park KM, Robinovitz E, et al. High-dose oral dextromethorphan versus placebo in painful diabetic neuropathy and postherpetic neuralgia. Neurology 1997;48(5):1212–8.
44. Schwartzman RJ, Alexander GM, Grothusen JR, et al. Outpatient intravenous ketamine for the treatment of complex regional pain syndrome: a double-blind placebo controlled study. Pain 2009;147(1–3):107–15.
45. Kiefer RT, Rohr P, Ploppa A, et al. Efficacy of ketamine in anesthetic dosage for the treatment of refractory complex regional pain syndrome: an open-label phase II study. Pain Med 2008;9(8):1173–201.
46. Takahashi H, Miyazaki M, Nanbu T, et al. The NMDA-receptor antagonist ketamine abolishes neuropathic pain after epidural administration in a clinical case. Pain 1998;75(2–3):391–4.
47. Gammaitoni A, Gallagher RM, Welz-Bosna M. Topical ketamine gel: possible role in treating neuropathic pain. Pain Med 2000;1(1):97–100.
48. Rauck RL, Eisenach JC, Jackson K, et al. Epidural clonidine treatment for refractory reflex sympathetic dystrophy. Anesthesiology 1993;79(6):1163–9 [discussion: 27A].
49. Muizelaar JP, Kleyer M, Hertogs IA, et al. Complex regional pain syndrome (reflex sympathetic dystrophy and causalgia): management with the calcium channel blocker nifedipine and/or the alpha-sympathetic blocker phenoxybenzamine in 59 patients. Clin Neurol Neurosurg 1997;99(1):26–30.
50. Prough DS, McLeskey CH, Poehling GG, et al. Efficacy of oral nifedipine in the treatment of reflex sympathetic dystrophy. Anesthesiology 1985;62(6):796–9.
51. Ghostine SY, Comair YG, Turner DM, et al. Phenoxybenzamine in the treatment of causalgia. Report of 40 cases. J Neurosurg 1984;60(6):1263–8.
52. Perez RS, Kwakkel G, Zuurmond WW, et al. Treatment of reflex sympathetic dystrophy (CRPS type 1): a research synthesis of 21 randomized clinical trials. J Pain Symptom Manage 2001;21(6):511–26.

53. Bickerstaff DR, Kanis JA. The use of nasal calcitonin in the treatment of post-traumatic algodystrophy. Br J Rheumatol 1991;30(4):291–4.
54. Gobelet C, Waldburger M, Meier JL. The effect of adding calcitonin to physical treatment on reflex sympathetic dystrophy. Pain 1992;48(2):171–5.
55. Carroll I, Clark JD, Mackey S. Sympathetic block with botulinum toxin to treat complex regional pain syndrome. Ann Neurol 2009;65(3):348–51.
56. Goebel A, Baranowski A, Maurer K, et al. Intravenous immunoglobulin treatment of the complex regional pain syndrome: a randomized trial. Ann Intern Med 2010; 152(3):152–8.
57. Zuurmond WW, Langendijk PN, Bezemer PD, et al. Treatment of acute reflex sympathetic dystrophy with DMSO 50% in a fatty cream. Acta Anaesthesiol Scand 1996;40(3):364–7.
58. Nelson DV, Stacey BR. Interventional therapies in the management of complex regional pain syndrome. Clin J Pain 2006;22(5):438–42.
59. Cepeda MS, Carr DB, Lau J. Local anesthetic sympathetic blockade for complex regional pain syndrome. Cochrane Database Syst Rev 2005;(4):CD004598.
60. Manjunath PS, Jayalakshimi TS, Dureja GP, et al. Management of lower limb complex regional pain syndrome type 1: an evaluation of percutaneous radiofrequency thermal lumbar sympathectomy versus phenol lumbar sympathetic neurolysis—a pilot study. Anesth Analg 2008;106(2):647–9.
61. Straube S, Derry S, Moore RA, et al. Cervico-thoracic or lumbar sympathectomy for neuropathic pain and complex regional pain syndrome. Cochrane Database Syst Rev 2010;(7):CD002918.
62. Jadad AR, Carroll D, Glynn CJ, et al. Intravenous regional sympathetic blockade for pain relief in reflex sympathetic dystrophy: a systematic review and a randomized, double-blind crossover study. J Pain Symptom Manage 1995;10(1):13–20.
63. Kemler MA, Barendse GA, van Kleef M, et al. Spinal cord stimulation in patients with chronic reflex sympathetic dystrophy. N Engl J Med 2000;343(9):618–24.
64. Kemler MA, De Vet HC, Barendse GA, et al. The effect of spinal cord stimulation in patients with chronic reflex sympathetic dystrophy: two years' follow-up of the randomized controlled trial. Ann Neurol 2004;55(1):13–8.
65. Kemler MA, de Vet HC, Barendse GA, et al. Effect of spinal cord stimulation for chronic complex regional pain syndrome Type I: five-year final follow-up of patients in a randomized controlled trial. J Neurosurg 2008;108(2):292–8.
66. Stanton-Hicks M. Complex regional pain syndrome: manifestations and the role of neurostimulation in its management. J Pain Symptom Manage 2006;31(Suppl 4): S20–4.
67. Bodde MI, Dijkstra PU, den Dunnen WF, et al. Therapy-resistant complex regional pain syndrome type I: to amputate or not? J Bone Joint Surg Am 2011;93(19): 1799–805.
68. Krans-Schreuder HK, Bodde MI, Schrier E, et al. Amputation for long-standing, therapy-resistant type-I complex regional pain syndrome. J Bone Joint Surg Am 2012;94(24):2263–8.

Cancer Pain and Current Theory for Pain Control

Brian Kahan, DO, DAOCRM, DABIPP, DABPM, FIPP

KEYWORDS

- Cancer pain • Opioid therapy • NMDA antagonists
- Splanchnic nerve blocks opioid pharmacogenetic testing

KEY POINTS

- Although the diagnosis of cancer has been stereotyped as a disease to end all, treatment of pain in cancer is showing hopeful prospects.
- A strong background in anatomy and physiology is the foundation on which to approach pain in cancer patients, with multiple options accessible.
- Use of new medications geared at enhancing the descending inhibitory pathways in combination with classic pharmacologic treatment can improve a patient's quality of life and reduce side effects.
- Reducing pain has been reported to enhance patients' quality of life and has been associated with longer survival rates.
- Being diligent in the reassessment of treatment is the answer to effectively managing complicated cases of cancer pain.
- Pain is always changing and, therefore, an astute physician will know how to address the treatment of patients at any time by understanding how pain works.

INTRODUCTION

Cancer is a disease that many people prefer not to talk about. Patients with a diagnosis of cancer are met with fear and thoughts of a life-ending illness. During their treatment they suffer significant pain. Various studies have looked at the prevalence of cancer pain, with one study reporting that 50% to 60% of all patients with cancer will experience pain, and other studies reporting a range of anywhere from 19% to 95% of patients with cancer have had or are still having pain. Although studies vary in the reported prevalence of pain in patients with cancer, approximately 70% of patients who die from cancer experience unrelieved pain. Despite national efforts by

This article originally appeared in Physical Medicine and Rehabilitation Clinics of North America, Volume 25, Issue 2, May 2014.

The author has nothing to disclose.

The Kahan Center for Pain Management, 2002 Medical Parkway, Suite 150, Annapolis, MD 21401, USA

E-mail address: bkahan@thekahancenter.com

http://dx.doi.org/10.1016/j.ccol.2014.10.006

the Joint Commission on Accreditation of Hospitals and health organizations in the Agency for Healthcare Research and Quality, World Health Organization, and the International Association for the Study of Pain, pain continues to be a significant problem in patients with cancer.

In a European study, the prevalence of pain based on the type of cancer has been well documented (**Fig. 1**). The most painful cancers appear to be pancreatic, bone, and lung.

In 2011, Marcus and colleagues[1] reported the prevalence of cancer pain to be consistent, with 56% of patients in their study suffering from pain. Thirty-three percent had pain after they underwent treatment, 59% had pain during treatment, and 64% had pain secondary to metastatic disease. All patients suffered functional limitations related to their cancer pain. Patients with head and neck cancer, gynecologic cancer, gastrointestinal cancer, and breast cancer appeared to suffer the most pain. The most consistent barriers to effective treatment of pain were concerns about addiction, cost of therapy, or lack of endorsement by health care providers.[2]

This article discusses pharmacologic management, interventional treatment, and specific cancers that seem to have the highest prevalence of pain, and how interventional treatment and medications can help.

PAIN IN CANCER

Treating cancer pain needs to be systematically evaluated. The etiology of cancer pain is related to either direct neoplasm involvement, side effects of chemotherapeutic agents, or radiation-induced plexopathies. The clinician must determine whether the cause of pain is neuropathic, nociceptive, or a combination of both, after which effective treatment can be decided upon.

The OPQRSTU mnemonic will help assess a patient's pain (**Table 1**).[3]

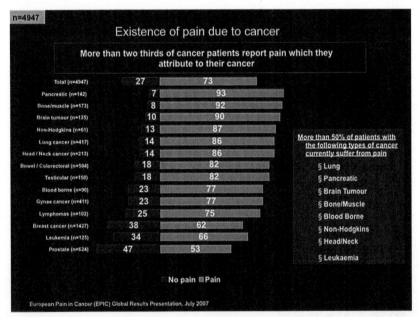

Fig. 1. Existence of pain due to cancer, reported by patients when asked "have you suffered any pain due to cancer?"

Table 1		
Cancer pain assessment mnemonic		
O	Onset	When did it start? Acute or gradual? Pattern since onset?
P	Provoking/ palliating	What brings it on? What makes it better or worse (eg, rest, medication)?
Q	Quality	Identifying neuropathic pain (burning, tingling, numb, itchy, etc)
R	Region/radiation	Primary location(s) of pain, radiation pattern(s)
S	Severity	Use verbal description and/or 1–10 scale
T	Treatment	Current and past treatment; side effects
U	Understanding	Meaning of the pain to the sufferer, "total pain"
V	Values	Goals and expectations of management for this symptom

PHARMACOLOGIC MANAGEMENT OF CANCER PAIN
Opioid Therapy

The most common medication used to treat cancer pain is opioids. Although opioids have been used for many years, their efficacy in alleviating cancer pain is questioned.[4] When opioids were discovered, medical knowledge was extremely limited with regard to how pain was transmitted. Early theories attributed pain to only an afferent pathway generating a tissue-injuring message to the spinal dorsal horn. Thus treatment of this pathway for pain consisted of pharmacologic management specific to modulation of components of this sensory message to higher centers.[5] Management consisted of opioid receptor blockers and sodium/potassium channel blockers. Although opioids demonstrated antinociception to the brainstem, forebrain, spinal cord, and the periphery, binding occurred heterogeneously, leading to inadequate treatment of pain.

Descending Pathway Inhibitors

In 1985 Fields and Heinricher[6] demonstrated the presence of a dual-projection system to be highly effective in treating pain through use of the descending pathway.

The interrelationship of major neuroanatomic components exerting descending nociceptive control is shown in **Fig. 2**. The periaqueductal gray and rostral ventral medulla are strategically located to integrate input from cerebral structures and relay processed information to the spinal dorsal horn. Noradrenergic pontine and medullary nuclei constitute a second important structure directly projecting to the dorsal horn. Presynaptic and postsynaptic mechanisms modulate nociceptive information that is transmitted from primary afferents to spinal projection neurons. Alternatively, indirect actions are exerted via inhibition or excitation of spinal interneurons. Cortical areas, the amygdala and the hypothalamus, are among the cerebral structures exerting top-down control. These structures are relevant for the modulation of pain by stress, emotion, and cognition.[7]

The discovery of a descending inhibitory pathway for pain led to the discovery of various nociceptive neurotransmitters (**Box 1**). In addition to finding more pain regulators, scientists have also determined how and where these neurotransmitters exert their affect (**Fig. 3**).

Fig. 3 illustrates that descending control of spinal nociceptive processes is exerted by multiple neurotransmitters. Transmitters contributing to inhibition of nociceptive signaling are depicted on the left while transmitters enhancing nociceptive signaling are depicted on the right. This physical separation serves didactic reasons and has no anatomic foundation. Transmitters are contained in descending pathways, in inhibitory or excitatory interneurons, and in primary afferent terminals. Only principal transmitter locations are shown, with subtypes indicated in parentheses.[7]

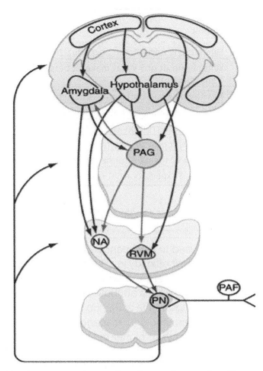

Fig. 2. Major structural components exerting descending nociceptive control. NA, noradren-ergic pontine and medullary nuclei; PAF, primary afferents; PAG, periaqueductal gray; PN, spinal projection neurons; RVM, rostral ventral medulla. (*From* Ottestad E, Angst MS. Nocicep-tive Physiology. In: Hemmings HC, Egan TD, eds. Pharmacology and physiology for anesthesia: foundations and clinical application. Philadelphia: Saunders/Elsevier, 2013; with permission. *Modified from* Millan MJ. Descending control of pain. Prog Neurobiol 2002;66:355–474.)

Neuropathic pain does not respond well to opioid therapy and tends to be more problematic. The focus of treating neuropathic pain should be blocking the ascending pathways or increasing the inhibition provided by the descending pathways.

It is theorized that an initiation phase of neuropathic pain is driven by activity from primary afferents, whereas the maintenance phase is mediated by central neuroplastic adaptations.[8] Treatment focused on blocking transmission to the rostral ventromedial medulla (see **Fig. 2**) through lesions or pharmacologic addition of medications that prevent upregulation of spinal dynorphin will help reduce neuropathic pain and neuropathic pain states. Newer medications attempt to work on these descending pathways, on the periphery by modulating GABAergic receptors and centrally by increasing serotonin and norepinephrine. Selective norepinephrine medications such as duloxetine (Cymbalta) are showing promise in treating various forms of pain by enhancing the descending pathways and working centrally on norepinephrine and serotonin receptors and voltage gated calcium-channel blockers such as gabapentin (Neurontin) and pregabalin (Lyrica). Today research is focusing not on opioids but on ways to block these neuropeptides.

NMDA Antagonists

Pharmacology assays in animal behavioral models of neuropathic pain suggest that the *N*-methyl-D-aspartate (NMDA) receptor is at least partially responsible for

---

Box 1
Nociceptive neurotransmitters

Peripheral neurotransmitters

Hydrogen ions

Norepinephrine

Bradykinin

Histamine

Potassium ions

Prostanoids

Purines

Cytokines (interleukin, tumor necrosis factor)

Serotonin (5-HT)

Neuropeptides

  Substance P, calcitonin gene-related peptide, neurokinin A

Leukotrienes

Central neurotransmitters

Glutamate

Neurokinin 1

Substance P

G protein

Neurokinin A

γ-Aminobutyric acid

Calcitonin gene-related peptide

Calcium

Nitric oxide

---

facilitated processing, augmentation of painful responses, and subsequent stimuli, but not normal pain sensation.[9] Using NMDA-receptor antagonists such as methadone and buprenorphine can allow titration of analgesic therapy while preventing respiratory depression. Opioid tolerance results in a requirement for increasing doses to achieve a given degree of analgesia. It is thought that continued doses of an opioid will enhance levels of cyclic adenosine monophosphate, protein phosphorylation, and subsequent upregulation of the NMDA-receptor mechanisms within the dorsal horn and supraspinal sites. In addition, accumulation of morphine metabolites may antagonize the analgesic action normally produced by opioid receptor activation. Animal studies indicate that the administration of NMDA antagonists can prevent both the development of tolerance to morphine and the withdrawal syndrome in morphine-dependent rats. Therefore, coadministration of NMDA antagonists such as methadone, buprenorphine, and ketamine with opioids may attenuate the development of opioid tolerance and potentiate opioid analgesic mechanisms.[10] However, the therapeutic window needs to be improved by the use of drug combinations and more selective administration of systemic NMDA-receptor antagonists, and physicians must understand the benefits of NMDA antagonists in comparison with their current

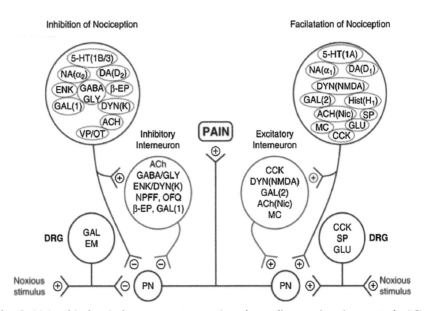

Fig. 3. Major biochemical components exerting descending nociceptive control. ACH, acetylcholine; β-EP, β-endorphin; CCK, cholecystokinin; DA, dopamine; DRG, dorsal root ganglion; DYN, dynorphin; EM, endomorphin; ENK, enkephalin; GABA, γ-hydroxybutyric acid; GAL, galanin; GLU, glutamate; GLY, glycine; Hist, histamine; MC, melanocortin; NA, noradrenaline; NMDA, N-methyl-D-aspartate; NPFF, neuropeptide FF; OFQ, orphanin FQ; OT, oxytocin; PN, projection neuron; SP, substance P; VP, vasopressin; 5-HT, serotonin. (*From* Ottestad E, Angst MS. Nociceptive Physiology. In: Hemmings HC, Egan TD, eds. Pharmacology and physiology for anesthesia: foundations and clinical application. Philadelphia: Saunders/Elsevier, 2013; with permission. *Modified from* Millan MJ. Descending control of pain. Prog Neurobiol 2002;66:355–474.)

use as adjunctive medications. It is hoped that more education on the transmission of pain in medical school, residency, fellowship, and continuing medical education will lead to elimination of the stereotyping of NMDA antagonists.

Cannabis

Various societies are debating the efficacy of cannabinoids in treating pain. Cannabinoid receptors are found throughout the central and peripheral nervous system, and even in the immune system. CB1 receptor tends to predominate in the central nervous system, and CB2 receptors are more extensive in the peripheral and immune systems.[11] Endogenous cannabinoid compounds such as anandamide, 2-arachidonyl-glycerol, and palmitoylethanolamide act on the CB1 and CB2 receptors to help modulate inflammatory pain and possibly provide analgesic effects. *Cannabis sativa* L. contains 60 or more cannabinoids; the most prevalent are δ9-tetrahydrocannabinol (THC) and cannabidiol (CB). These 2 cannabinoids seem to mimic the action of endogenous cannabinoid compounds. THC seems to be a partial CB1 and CB2 receptor agonist, thus acting centrally and peripherally, and may produce more psychoactive side effects, whereas cannabidiol seems to act more centrally and produce analgesic and anti-inflammatory effects.

A systemic review of single-dose studies of dronabinol, nabilone, and levonantradol found them to be as effective as 5 to 120 mg of oral codeine.[12] There are also suggestions that cannabis can augment opioid analgesia.[13] Although there is public interest in the utilization of cannabis, more controlled, sizable studies demonstrating true effectiveness are required.

Intrathecal Administration

Intrathecal administration offers an advanced way of delivering opioid therapy with a more direct effect on supraspinal pathways. Although relatively uncommon in patients with cancer, it has some advantages. Patients undergoing intrathecal administration of opioids via an implantable pump (**Figs. 4** and **5**) will have fewer side effects than those taking oral medications. Owing to the direct effects on the supraspinal pathways, lower doses are required than if used orally. It is generally thought that the concentration ratio from oral to intrathecal is 300:1. A comprehensive review of intrathecal drug-delivery systems is beyond the scope of this article, but certain aspects are highlighted.

Using a dosage 300 times less will reduce systemic absorption and reduce the incidence of gastrointestinal and cognitive side effects. Another advantage over oral medication is once on a stable dosage of intrathecal medication, a patient will require fewer visits to a clinician. In general, patients receiving intrathecal medication will be refilled every 90 days as an outpatient procedure. In addition to supplying a continuous flow of medication, patient dosage adjustments for breakthrough pain or pain increased at night can be programmed into the pump either through flexible dosing schedules or with a patient hand-held device that communicates through telemetry to give the patient a programmed bolus based on the physician-adjusted settings. This procedure is identical to patient-controlled administration in the hospital.

Complications of intrathecal medication tend to be more technical, such as catheter dislodgment and kinking, rather than infection, granulomas, and overdosing. Pump complications tend to involve premature battery failure. However, there are reports that compounded medication can potentially cause corrosion attributable to pH levels.

Intrathecal drug-delivery systems can be used in about 10% to 20% of patients suffering from cancer pain who have failed other therapeutic measures and are eligible

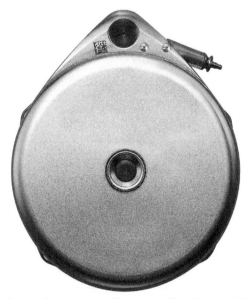

Fig. 4. Implantable drug-delivery system. (*Courtesy of* Medtronic, Minneapolis, MN; with permission.)

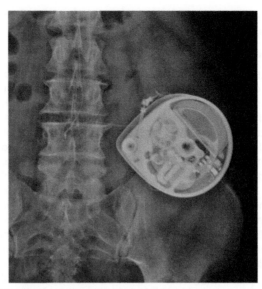

Fig. 5. Radiographic view of implantable drug-delivery system.

for an intrathecal trial. Patient selection can be subjective, but there are some definitive contraindications. **Table 2** lists some of the relevant indications and contraindications for intrathecal drug-delivery systems.

Once the appropriate patient is selected, he or she undergoes an intrathecal trial performed with single boluses, epidural continuous trials, or intrathecal continuous trials. Based on patients' response as measured by 50% reduction in pain, improved functional capability, or reduced side effects, the patient can proceed with an implant. Medications currently approved for intrathecal use are morphine, ziconotide, and baclofen. **Table 3** lists the various combinations of intrathecal medications.[14]

Table 2
Patient selection for intrathecal drug-delivery systems

Relative Indications	Relative Contraindications
Inability to tolerate oral medications	Anticoagulation therapy
Fear of side effects or addiction	Leukopenia <2 × 10⁹/L Neutropenia <1000 μL Thrombocytopenia <20 × 10³/μL
Receiving aggressive chemotherapy regimens with high toxicity profile	Active infections or methicillin-resistant *Staphylococcus aureus*
Pain refractory	Spinal cord tumors
Visceral tumors that affects other forms of absorption of medications	Body size not sufficient to accept pump bulk
Pathologic fractures or diffuse bone metastasis	
Neuropathic pain states due to surgery, chemotherapy, or radiation	
Minimum life expectancy >3 mo	
Pelvic tumors or tumors with high rate of metastatic spread to bone[14]	

Table 3
Lists the cancer pain best practices algorithm

	Nociceptive	Mixed Pain	Neuropathic Pain
First line	Morphine or hydromorphone	Morphine/ hydromorphone with bupivacaine	Bupivacaine
Second line	First-line drugs or fentanyl/sufentanil with bupivacaine and clonidine	First-line drugs or fentanyl/sufentanil with bupivacaine and clonidine	First-line drugs or fentanyl/sufentanil with bupivacaine
Third line	Second-line drugs with either baclofen or other lipophilic or hydrophilic opioid	—	—
Fourth line	Second-line drugs with anesthetic, antineuropathic medication, and NMDA antagonist	—	—

Abbreviation: NMDA, *N*-methyl-ᴅ-aspartate.

INTERVENTIONAL TREATMENT FOR CANCER PAIN

Various nociceptive pathways can be blocked by using local anesthetics in the nervous system to alleviate cancer pain on a temporary or long-term basis, allowing them to undergo treatment that might be needed to alleviate the cancer. An example concerns a patient with mesothelioma and metastatic disease to the rib cage. He required a series of 8 radiation treatments to suppress the expansion of his tumor. Unfortunately he was unable to lie still for 45 minutes to undergo these treatments. The patient therefore underwent intercostal blockade with 0.5% marcaine 45 minutes before radiation therapy, which provided pain relief to undergo the radiation treatment required. Neurolytic blockade can also assist the oncologist and radiation oncologist to facilitate cancer treatment. Another example is anesthetizing the lumbar plexus and its roots for patients undergoing treatment of sacral malignancies caused by direct invasion of bladder or rectal cancer, to facilitate temporary pain relief while undergoing treatment. There have also been case reports of physicians inserting lumbosacral plexus catheters for continuous infusions of anesthetic for palliative care (**Figs. 6** and **7**).[15]

Neurolysis and Chemotactic Agents

Neurolysis with chemotaxic agents has also been described over the years to be effective in treating refractory cancer pain for periods of time, but in certain anatomic regions there is risk of motor deficit or paralysis if there is too much diffusion of medication. Radiofrequency ablation is another option for destroying or denaturing nerves. Pancreatic and abdominal cancers are extremely painful, as shown in **Fig. 1**. If pancreatic cancer is diagnosed early enough, some patients will undergo surgical resection. However, those who have advancing stages of pancreatic cancer will suffer from direct invasion into the celiac plexus. There are multiple ways of blocking the celiac plexus, but these techniques carry risk owing to the close proximity of the aorta. Even if blockade is obtained for short-term relief, performing neurolytic blockade with phenol has been associated with spinal cord infarction and paralysis. Therefore, other approaches to the pancreas include lesser and greater splanchnic nerve supply

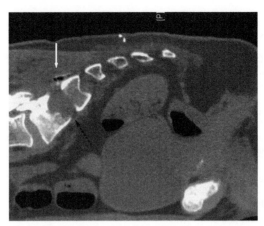

Fig. 6. A patient with metastatic lung cancer to S1 with continuous pain. Dashed arrow indicates tumor. White arrow indicates catheter tip and continuous infusion of ropivacaine over tumor.

branches to the celiac plexus (**Fig. 8**). Various techniques have been described for blocking the splanchnic nerves. In the author's practice, patients receiving a greater than 50% reduction in pain after splanchnic nerve blocks are considered for radiofrequency lesioning. The splanchnic nerve blocks are performed under fluoroscopic guidance with a combination of 2 mL of 2% xylocaine, 3 mL of 0.5% marcaine, and 40 mg dexamethasone phosphate (**Figs. 9** and **10**). The patient is evaluated with a pain diagram for the first 24 hours and the efficacy of the procedure recorded via a follow-up call. The patient is then followed up after 1 week. Should the procedure be effective, the patient is considered as a candidate for rhizotomy.

SPLANCHNIC NERVE RHIZOTOMY FOR PANCREATIC PAIN RELIEF

Treating pain derived from pancreatic cancer can be extremely difficult. Pancreatic cancer is one of the most deadly, and is associated with a high degree of pain. Aside

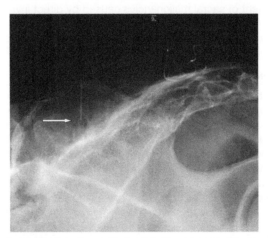

Fig. 7. Lateral radiograph showing catheter placement over S1 neuroforamen (*white arrow*). Personal files.

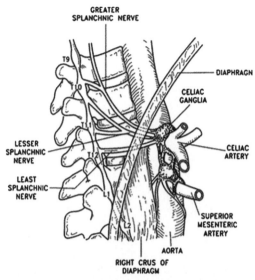

Fig. 8. Anatomy of splanchnic chain. (*From* Carachi R, Currie JM. New Tools in the treatment of motility disorders in children. Semin Pediatr Surg 2009;18:274–7; with permission.)

from medications, interventional techniques such as celiac plexus blocks and neurolysis have been associated with severe complications. An alternative is to use radiofrequency lesioning of the splanchnic nerves to provide a safe and longer-term treatment for the pancreatic pain.

Raj and colleagues[16] described rhizotomy as an effective technique for the treatment of pancreatic pain, with minimal side effects. The author uses a technique similar to that described by Gauci,[17] performed on an outpatient basis with local anesthetic. Sedation is not used for this procedure because it tends not to be painful with local

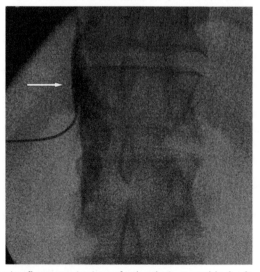

Fig. 9. Anteroposterior fluoroscopic view of splanchnic nerve block after 2 mL of Omnipaque, 180 mg/mL. White arrow indicates lateral dye spread.

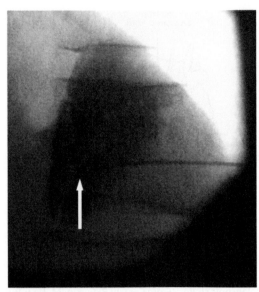

Fig. 10. Lateral fluoroscopic view of splanchnic nerve block after 2 mL of Omnipaque, 180 mg/mL. White arrow indicates needle of T12 anterior part of vertebral body.

anesthetic and a blunt-needle technique. The procedure takes less than 15 minutes, so patient does not have to fast. Should patients have problems with anxiety or pain, lorazepam (Ativan) is prescribed if they do not already have it, with the recommendation that that they take their pain medications 30 minutes before the procedure.

- The patient is placed in a prone position on the fluoroscopy table, and the T11 and T12 vertebral body is identified. The image is then rotated obliquely so that the supra-articular process is under the anterior third of the superior vertebral body. One must pay close attention to the silhouette of the pleura to avoid pneumothorax.
- Under intermittent fluoroscopy, the skin is locally anesthetized with 1 to 2 mL of 2% lidocaine without epinephrine with a 25-gauge needle.
- A 3.5-inch 25 gauge spinal needle is advanced under intermittent fluoroscopy to anesthetize the deep muscle structures with lidocaine without epinephrine.
- A 16-gauge intravenous angiocatheter is guided under intermittent fluoroscopy in the direction of the anterior vertebral body of T12 with a slight superior tilt. The stylet is then removed. A 100- or 145-mm blunt radiofrequency cannula with a 10-mm active tip is then advanced under intermittent fluoroscopy until contact with vertebral body. Once the vertebral body is contacted, the fluoroscope is angled to a lateral position.
- With a lateral projection, the needle tip is advanced to the anterior one-third of the vertebral body. Confirmation is obtained with lateral and anteroposterior pictures (**Fig. 11**; lateral view only).
- Confirm position by stimulating at 50 Hz at 0.6 mV. In general, patients will feel no sensation at all but sometimes patients will complain of tightness in their stomach. Position is further confirmed with 2 Hz at a voltage of 3.0 mV to make sure there is no motor stimulation. If placement is not proper, one can contact the diaphragmatic nerves and discern stimulation of the diaphragm.
- Use of Omnipaque to demonstrate spread along the lateral vertebral bodies and avoidance of intravascular uptake may be beneficial.

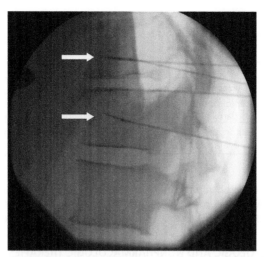

Fig. 11. Placement of radiofrequency needles for splanchnic lateral view. White arrows over the anterior third of T11 and T12 vertebral body.

- The splanchnic nerve is anesthetized with 3 mL of 2% xylocaine without epinephrine, and lesioning is carried out at 80°C for 75 seconds, after which the cannulas are rotated 180° and lesioning is repeated.
- This procedure is performed on both sides of the patient.
- The cannulas are removed and a sterile dressing is applied.

POSTOPERATIVE CARE

- The patient is monitored for 15 minutes to make sure vital signs are stable, and discharged home.
- Unlike with typical rhizotomy of the medial branch nerves, the author has not seen a postinjection flare. In general any soreness can be managed with patients' current pain medications. If they are sore at the injection site, ice is applied. Patients should experience about 6 to 9 months of pain relief, and the procedure may be repeated.

COMPLICATIONS AND MANAGEMENT

- Complications from the procedure consist of:
  1. Infection
  2. Bleeding
  3. Pneumothorax from improper placement
- To help minimize the risk of pneumothorax, use of blunt needles in addition to understanding of proper fluoroscopic guidance is necessary.

OUTCOMES AND FUTURE CONSIDERATIONS

The success rate of splanchnic nerve radiofrequency is sparse in the literature. Papadopoulos and colleagues[18] demonstrated in patients with malignant pain a significant improvement in quality of life and reduction in pain during the first 5 months after the procedure. Raj and colleagues[16] looked at 107 patients with both malignant and nonmalignant abdominal pain, and found that 40% of patients who had both splanchnic nerve blocks and radiofrequency lesioning had excellent results at

Table 4
Genetic markers and their association with pharmacologic metabolism

Genetic Marker	Pharmacologic Implications
CYP2C9, VKORC1	NSAID therapy, phenytoin, warfarin metabolism
CYP2C19	Diazepam, citalopram, sertraline
CYP2D6	Opioids, tapentadol, amphetamines, tramadol, duloxetine, fluoxetine, paroxetine, venlafaxine, cyclobenzaprine, bupropion
CYP3A4, CYP3A5	Buprenorphine, methadone, buprenorphine and naloxone, meperidine, fentanyl

6 months. Future research into utilization of splanchnic nerve rhizotomy for pancreatic pain should involve more prospective studies and look at bipolar radiofrequency lesioning to provide a bigger lesion and potentially longer duration of efficacy.

FUTURE PHARMACOLOGIC AND NONPHARMACOLOGIC THERAPIES
Genetic Testing

Over the past decade there has been increasing concern about the cost of health care. Often, inefficiency is due to using a trial-and-error approach to determine the appropriate medications, because of lack of evidence. Recent advances in pharmacogenetic testing have enabled physicians to obtain a drug-metabolism profile of their patients by obtaining a swab from the inside of the buccal mucosa. In opioid therapy one will examine the CYP450 system, primarily at the CYP2D6, CYP2C9, CYP2C19, CYP3A4, CYP3A5, and VKORC1. These genetic markers evaluate the patient's ability to metabolize certain drugs (**Table 4**). Test results assess a person's ability to metabolize medications. The analysis of the cytochrome P450 system is broken down into accelerated, broad/normal, compromised, and deficient. To interpret these grades one must know the outcomes of each grade (**Table 5**).

Case Example

A 58 year old female with metastatic pancreatic cancer to bone presents for treatment. She is unable to take nonsteroidal anti-inflammatory therapy because she is being treated with anticoagulants. Before starting treatment, genetic testing is obtained and reveals the following:

CYP2C9/VKORC1	Grade B normal/broad/extensive metabolizer
CYP2C19	Grade B normal/broad/extensive metabolizer
CYP2D6	Grade C compromised/intermediate metabolizer
CYP3A4	Grade B normal/broad/extensive metabolizer
COMT	Grade B normal/broad/extensive metabolizer
CYP1A2	Grade B normal/broad/extensive metabolizer

These results demonstrate that she is compromised to opioids or other medications that primarily use the CYP2D6 system to become active in the body. Therefore, normal dosages of a medication using this genetic marker to break down into an active metabolite might cause inadvertent overdose of adverse reactions if this test was not performed before initiating therapy. **Table 4** lists some of the medications that are metabolized by the CY2D6 as well as the other enzymes.

Table 5
List of enzymes and associated pharmacological metabolism

CYP2C19 Enzymes Metabolize	CYP2D6 Enzymes Metabolize		CYP2C9 Enzymes Metabolize
Tricyclics	AHDH	Opioids	Hypoglycemics
Amitriptyline	Modafinil	Hydrocodone	Glipzide
Imipramine	Amphetamine	Codeine	Glimepiride
SSRI's	Atomoxetine	Tramadol	Tolbutamide
Citalopram	Methyphenidate	Beta blockers	Glyburide
Escitalopram	Psychotropics	Carvedilol	Anticoagulants
Sertaline	Aripiprazole	Metoprolol	S-warfarin
Anticonvulsant	Risperidone	Timolol	Diuretic
Diazepam	Haloperidol	Propanolol	Torsemide
Oncology	Thioridazine	Antiarrythmics	ARB's
Cyclophosphamide	Clozipine	Flecainide	Losartan
Proton Pump	Donepezil	Propafenone	Irbesartan
Omeprazole	Tricyclics	Quinadine	
Lansoprazole	Nortriptyline	Mexilitine	Statins
Pantoprazole	Clomipramine	Oncology	Fluvastatin
ETC.	Deipramine	Tamoxifen	Rosuvastatin
Antiplatelet	SSRI's	Doxorubicine	NSAID's
Clopidogrel	Fluoxetine	SNRI's	Celecoxib
Other	Paroxetine	Duloxetine	Diclofenac
Proquanil	Sertaline	Venlafaxine	Meloxicam
Atovaquone			Naproxen
Melfinavir			Ibuprofen
Tolbutamide			Indomethacin
Carisoprodol			Anticonvulsant
			Valproic acid
			Phenytoin
			Other:
			Sildenafil

(continued on next page)

Table 5
(continued)

CYP3A4 Enzymes Metabolize		CYP1A2 Enzymes Metabolize		COMT Enzymes Metabolize	
Psychotropics	Statins	Psychotropics	Muscle relaxers	Catecholamines	Cardiac inotropic
Carbamazepine	Atorvastatin	Clomipramine	Cyclobenzaprine	Epinephrine	Dobutamine
Aripiprazole	Lovastatin	Imipramine	Tizanidine	Norepinephrine	Isoproterenol
Quetiapine	Simvastatin	Fluvoxamine	Cardiovascular	Dopamine	Methyldopa
Mirtazapine	Sex hormones	Antipsychotics	Mexiletine	Parkinsons	Catechol estrogens
Trazodone	Finasteride	Haloperidol	Other	Carbidopa/levodopa	2-hydroxyestrodial
Sertaline	Estradiol	Clozipine	Theophylline		4-hydroxyestrodial
Oncology	Progesterone	Olanzapine	Caffeine		
Vincristine	Ethinylestradiol		Zolmitriptan		
Vinblastine	Testosterone		Acetaminophen		
Imatinib	HIV				
Erlotinib	Amprenavir				
Doxorubicin	Efavirenz				
Cardiovascular	Atripla				
Amilodipine	Atazanavir				
Diltiazem	Ritonavir				
Felodipine	Opioids				
Nifedipine	Buprenorphine				
Verapamil	Fentanyl				
Antiarrythmic	Methadone				
Amiodarone	Oxycodone				
Other	Tranquilizers				
Tacrolimus	Alprazolam				
Cyclosporine	Midazolam				
Hydrocortisone	Sedative				
Dexamethasone	Zolpidem				
Donepezil	Eszoplidone				
Erythromycin					
Clarithromycin					

TRANSCRANIAL MAGNETIC STIMULATION

A nonpharmacologic technique that is proving interesting in the management of pain is transcranial magnetic stimulation. This treatment is based on enhancing the descending inhibitory pathways through magnetic stimulation of the prefrontal cortex. Studies have demonstrated that repetitive transcranial magnetic stimulation of the prefrontal cortex can enhance production of serotonin and norepinephrine. This method has obtained approval from the Food and Drug Administration for major depression refractory to oral medication. Transcranial magnetic stimulation consists of repetitive stimulation over the prefrontal cortex at an intensity of 120% of motor threshold. Repetitive impulses are provided to the patient at a rate of more than 5 seconds with a 25-second rest. The sessions take 37.5 minutes to complete and are performed daily for a total of 30 treatments. Studies evaluating functional magnetic resonance imaging (MRI) have demonstrated in patients without pain that one treatment of transcranial magnetic stimulation can increase the thermal threshold in almost 13% of patients treated. This finding correlates with those of functional MRI demonstrating increased activity in the right superior frontal gyrus and insula, and anterior and posterior cingulate gyri. Increased superior frontal activity was significantly associated with decreased pain-intensity ratings.[19] Various clinical trials studying the effects of transcranial magnetic stimulation on fibromyalgia and other areas of pain are currently under way.

SUMMARY

Although the diagnosis of cancer has been stereotyped as a disease to end all, pain treatment in cancer is showing hopeful prospects. A strong background in anatomy and physiology is the foundation on which to approach pain in a patient with cancer, with multiple options accessible. Using new medications geared at enhancing the descending inhibitory pathways in combination with classic pharmacologic treatment can improve a patient's quality of life and reduce side effects. Interventional therapy to inhibit various peripheral structures improves a patient's quality of life. Clinicians must look not only at the disease but also how it is affecting the patient. Reducing pain has been reported to enhance the quality of life of patients with cancer and has been associated with longer survival rates. Being diligent to always reassess treatment is the answer to effectively managing complicated cases of cancer pain. It is hoped that this article will give the reader pause for thought as to how patients suffering from pain can be helped, rather than being merely instructive. Pain is always changing and, therefore, an astute physician will know how to address the treatment at any time by understanding how pain works.

REFERENCES

1. Marcus DA. Epidemiology of cancer pain. Current Pain Headache Rep Aug 2011; 15(4):231–4.
2. Simone C. Cancer patient attitudes toward analgesic usage and pain intervention. Clin J Pain 2012;28(2):157–62.
3. Medical Services Commission. Palliative care for the patient with incurable cancer or advanced disease. Part 2. Pain and symptom management. Victoria (Canada): British Columbia Medical Services Commission; 2011. p. 44.
4. Moulin DE. Opioid treatment for cancer pain and chronic noncancer pain. In: Merskey H, Loeser JD, Dubner R, editors. The paths of pain 1975-2005. Seattle (WA): IASP Press; 2005. p. 469–82.

5. Yaksh TL. Opioid analgesia: the last 30 years. In: Merskey H, Loeser JD, Dubner R, editors. The paths of pain 1975-2005. Seattle (WA): IASP Press; 2005. p. 209–28.
6. Fields HL, Heinricher MM. Anantomy and physiology of a nocioceptive modulatory system. Philos Trans R Soc Lond B Biol Sci 1985;308(1136):361–74.
7. Millan MJ. Descending control of pain. Prog Neurobiol 2002;66:355–474.
8. Burgess SE, Gardell LR, Ossipov MH, et al. Time dependent descending facilitation from the rostral ventromedial medulla maintains, but does not initiate, neuropathic pain. J Neurosci 2002;22:5129–36.
9. Sang CN. NMDA-receptor antagonists in neuropathic pain: experimental methods of clinical trials. J Pain Symptom Manage 2000;19(Suppl 1):S21–5.
10. Hemmings H, Egan T. Pharmacology and physiology for anesthesia: foundations and clinical application. Chapter 14. 2013. p. 235–52.
11. Dray A. Pharmacology of inflammatory pain. In: Merskey H, Loeser JD, Dubner R, editors. The paths of pain 1975-2005. Seattle (WA): IASP Press; p. 177–90.
12. Campbell FA, Tramer MR, Carroll D, et al. Are cannabinoids an effective and safe treatment option in the management of pain? A quality systematic review. BMJ 2001;323:13–6.
13. Johnson JR, Burnell-Nugent M, Lossignol D, et al. Multicenter, double-blind, randomized, placebo-controlled, parallel group study of the efficacy, safety, and tolerability of THC: CBD extract and THC extracts in patients with intractable cancer related pain. J Pain Symptom Manage 2010;39:169–79.
14. Stearns L, Boortz-Marx R, Du Pen S, et al. Intrathecal drug delivery for management of cancer pain: a multidisciplinary consensus of best clinical practices. J Support Oncol 2005;3(6):399–408.
15. Zaporowska-Stachowiak I, Kotlinska-Lemieszek A, Kowalski G, et al. Lumbar paravertebral blockade as intractable management method in palliative care. Onco Targets Ther 2013;6:1187–96.
16. Raj PP, Sahinler B, Lowe M. Radiofrequency lesioning of the splanchnic nerves. Pain Pract 2002;2(3):241–7.
17. Gauci CA. Sympathetic nervous system radiofrequency and pulsed radiofrequency. In: Manual of RF techniques. Meggen (Switzerland): Flivo Press SA; 2004. p. 95–100.
18. Papadopoulos D, Kostopanagiotou G, Batistaki C. Bilateral thoracic splanchnic nerve radiofrequency thermocoagulation for the management of end stage pancreatic abdominal cancer pain. Pain Physician 2013;16:125–33.
19. Martin L, Borckardt J, Reeves S, et al. A pilot functional MRI study of the effects of prefrontal rTMS on pain perception. Pain Med 2011;14:999–1009.

Identifying and Treating the Causes of Neck Pain

Ginger Evans, MD

KEYWORDS

- Neck pain • Cervical spondylosis • Radiculopathy • Myelopathy • Chronic pain

KEY POINTS

- The first step in evaluating neck pain is to look for red flags to suggest serious underlying disease, analogous to the evaluation of low back pain.
- It is important to distinguish mechanical neck pain from radiculopathy or myelopathy based on history and physical examination; techniques are reviewed herein.
- The role of magnetic resonance imaging in mechanical neck pain is dubious.
- Many conservative treatment options are available. Those options with the best support in the literature include educational videos, select exercise interventions, mobilization accompanied by exercise, some medications, and possibly, acupuncture.
- There is no role for surgery in mechanical neck pain.
- Patients with severe or progressive radiculopathy or myelopathy are appropriately referred for surgery; those with mild to moderate radiculomyelopathy have short-term benefits from surgery, but long-term outcomes may be similar to conservative treatment.

INTRODUCTION

Neck pain is a common condition, with approximately 15% to 20% of people reporting neck pain each year and 1.5% to 1.8% of adults seeking ambulatory health care for this complaint annually.[1] Despite the frequency of this presenting complaint, a clear understanding of the cause and the best treatment course is often elusive. This review is aimed at primary care providers evaluating patients in clinic with the complaint of neck pain. Workup of neck pain in trauma victims is outside the scope of this review.

Anatomy

A brief review of the anatomy of the neck sets the stage for a better appreciation of potential causes of pain in the region. There are 7 cervical vertebrae. C1 and C2, atlas

This article originally appeared in Medical Clinics of North America, Volume 98, Issue 3, May 2014.

The author has no conflicts of interest to disclose.

Department of Medicine, VA Puget Sound Health Care System, University of Washington, 1660 South Columbia Way, S-123-PCC, Seattle, WA 98108, USA

E-mail address: gingere@u.washington.edu

Clinics Collections 4 (2014) 73–89

http://dx.doi.org/10.1016/j.ccol.2014.10.007

2352-7986/14/$ – see front matter Published by Elsevier Inc.

and axis, have no intervertebral disk between them. The remaining C3-7 vertebrae are connected superiorly and inferiorly to intervertebral disks, and articulate with adjacent vertebrae through 2 important joints:

- Uncovertebral joints (also called the joints of Luschka)
- Zygapophyseal joints (also called z-joints or facet joints)

To help envision the important structures in the vertebrae, we can begin at C4 and imagine moving posterolaterally from the vertebral body as it arches around toward the spinous process. First, a protuberance called the uncinate process is encountered (which abuts the C3-4 intervertebral disk and C3 vertebral body, forming the uncovertebral joints and comprising the anterior wall of the intervertebral foramen for the exiting C4 spinal nerve). Second, the uncinate process is followed by a depression (which forms the inferior wall of the intervertebral foramen). Third, there is another protuberance, called the articular facet (which connects, through a true synovial joint, to the C3 vertebra to form the zygapophyseal joint and the posterior wall of the intervertebral foramen). Therefore, (1) the anteromedial wall of the intervertebral foramen is the uncovertebral joint, which is not a true synovial joint and is a frequent site of bony overgrowth, and (2) the posterolateral wall of the intervertebral foramen is composed of the zygapophyseal joint, which is a true synovial joint and provides stability to the spine.[2–4]

There are 8 cervical spinal nerves; C1-7 exit superiorly to their named vertebra. C8 exits between C7 and T1.

- Motor efferent fibers have cell bodies in the anterior horn of the ventral spinal cord, exiting the cord to the ventral root, and then merging with sensory afferents to become the spinal nerve (a short nerve located inside the intervertebral foramen).
- Sensory afferents ascend from the periphery. The cell bodies form the dorsal root ganglion, which is located within the intervertebral foramen, just before merging with the spinal nerve (also inside the foramen). Sensory afferents enter the spinal cord through the dorsal root.[2,4,5]

Other surrounding structures to highlight include:

- The vertebral artery, which ascends adjacent laterally to the intervertebral foramina
- The intervertebral disks, comprising a gelatinous nucleus pulposis surrounded by an annulus fibrosis, and protected in the midline from herniating into the spinal cord by the posterior longitudinal ligament
- Cervical muscles and soft tissue

Diagnostic Uncertainty

Significant uncertainty still surrounds the pathophysiology of chronic neck pain, and in many cases, the chance of a clinician accurately identifying a specific cause is low.[1,6] A more critical task is to evaluate patients with neck pain for the following: cervical radiculopathy, cervical myelopathy, and dangerous underlying causes of pain (eg, cancer, fractures, osteomyelitis).[6,7]

Categorization of Neck Pain and Associated Cervical Spine Disorders

Radiculopathy

Radiculopathy is the constellation of symptoms caused by dysfunction of 1 or more cervical spinal nerve roots. It is less common than mechanical neck pain, with 1 population-based study[8] showing an average annual age-adjusted incidence of 83.2 per 100,000 people. Although noncompressive causes should be considered (eg, diabetes, herpes zoster, root avulsion), most (approximately 90%) radiculopathies result from compressive causes. In a large retrospective review at Mayo Clinic,[8] 21.9% of all radiculopathy cases were believed to have a probable cause of disk herniation (based on radiologic or surgical findings). Spondylosis is the major contributor to the remaining cases. Spondylosis usually refers to progressive, age-associated, degenerative changes of the vertebrae and intervertebral disks. These changes can lead to radiculopathy through bony hypertrophy of the uncovertebral joints and, less commonly, the zygapophyseal joints, both of which may cause narrowing of the intervertebral foramen and consequent compression of the spinal nerve.

Myelopathy
Myelopathy is related to narrowing of the spinal canal, most often from spondylosis (including osteophytes of the uncovertebral or zygapophyseal joints, or degenerative hypertrophy of the ligamentum flavum or posterior longitudinal ligaments). Pathophysiology may involve direct spinal cord or nerve root compression or ischemia from compression of arterial or venous supplies to the cord.[9]

Neck pain
Neck pain in the absence of radiculopathy, myelopathy, or clear serious underlying disease is also called mechanical neck pain, and has less well-understood pathophysiology. Among other things, this type of pain may be labeled as cervical muscle strain, myofascial pain, cervical spondylosis, cervical facet joint pain, and diskogenic pain. Because these structures are innervated, all of the muscles, synovial joints, intervertebral disks, dura mater, and vertebral arteries may theoretically generate pain.[2,7] Some studies attempting to more specifically delineate which of these features to implicate have focused on zygapophyseal joints and intervertebral disks. Examples of methods used include delivery of noxious stimuli (eg, saline or contrast injection) to specified structures in asymptomatic volunteers,[10,11] delivery of noxious stimuli to symptomatic volunteers (eg, provocation diskography),[12] and delivery of localized anesthesia in symptomatic volunteers (eg, anesthetic block to zygapophyseal joint either directly or through medial branch blocks).[13]

Some general conclusions from this research include[7,14,15]:

1. Zygapophyseal joints may be a source of pain in some subsets of patients with chronic neck pain caused by minor trauma or degenerative changes. The zygapophyseal joints may also produce referred pain to the head and upper extremities (referred pain is believed to stem from nociceptive afferents from facet joints that converge in the spinal cord with nociceptive afferents from other distal sites).[7,14,15] Attempts to map typical locations of pain derived from each zygapophyseal joint have been created and revised.[14] The prevalence of zygapophyseal pain in a primary care clinic population has not been determined. One estimate from a small population of specialty clinic patients (based on serial positive local anesthetic blocks) was reported at 36%.[16]
2. Although possible, there is no strong evidence that intervertebral disks (through degenerative or other changes) are a source of pain (diskogenic pain). This area remains controversial.[17–19]
3. Other potential sources of pain (eg, soft tissue, muscles, arteries) have not been rigorously studied.

These diagnostic techniques and the conclusions drawn from their use remain controversial.[20,21] Some systematic reviews find adequate evidence to support them,[15,22] but a recent systematic review and guidelines from the Bone and Joint

2000–2010 Task Force on Neck Pain do not endorse these injection techniques as a diagnostic maneuver.[1,19] Furthermore, per the literature review of this task force, there is no "evidence [that was deemed scientifically admissible] demonstrating that disk degeneration is a risk factor for neck pain."[23] Coauthors of related guidelines concur that there is "no evidence that common degenerative changes on cervical magnetic resonance imaging (MRI) are strongly correlated with neck pain symptoms."[19]

Summary

Recent guidelines state, "in most settings a simple descriptive clinical diagnosis might be preferable to a speculative tissue diagnosis as the origin of pain."[1] These guidelines propose a clinically practical grading system to guide workup and therapy by categorizing patients as follows:

Grade I: neck pain with no signs of major disease and no or little interference with daily activities

Grade II: neck pain with no signs of major disease, but interference with daily activities

Grade III: neck pain with neurologic signs of nerve compression

Grade IV: neck pain with signs of major disease

SYMPTOMS
Radiculopathy

The hallmark of radicular pain is some combination of diminished motor strength (described by about 15% of patients at presentation), reflexes, or sensation (paresthesias described by about 90% of patients at presentation) in a nerve root distribution. Lower cervical nerve roots (C5-8) are the most commonly involved in compressive radiculopathies. C7 is involved more than half the time; C6 is involved about 35% of the time.[8] Only a few patients describe trauma or physical exertion preceding their pain.[8] **Table 1** gives a description of history and examination findings for each nerve root. This table represents a compilation of several sources of information; the most distinguishing and consistently reported findings are in bold type.[2,3,6,7]

Pain is not a universal symptom of radiculopathy. Pain associated with radiculopathy may occur directly if the dorsal root ganglion is compressed.[24] Herniated disks, themselves, may also release inflammatory mediators, which may incite pain.[4] Although sensory symptoms like tingling may be felt in a dermatomal distribution, pain does not readily follow this same distribution. Instead, it is often deep feeling and is described as extending through the shoulder, arm, forearm, and hand (the hand being more common in C6-8 involvement).[4,7,8,25]

Myelopathy

Onset of symptoms of cervical myelopathy is often subtle and gradual; years may go by before the patient presents for medical care.[9,26] However, patients can present with sudden or episodic worsening, especially associated with trauma such as sudden hyperextension. If symptoms are mild at onset, the most common clinical course is to remain stable. Less frequently, a steady progression in symptoms is seen.[27,28]

Symptoms are variable and may include[9,29]:

1. Significant pain in the neck, shoulders, or arms (although not present in most patients)[30]
2. Gait spasticity
3. Upper extremity numbness, which is often in a nonspecific distribution but can be dermatomal, especially with a coexisting radiculopathy

Table 1 Signs and symptoms of cervical radiculopathy by involved nerve root			
	C5	**C6**	**C7**	**C8**

	C5	C6	C7	C8
Pain	Neck Scapula Shoulder	Neck Scapula Shoulder Radial forearm	Neck Scapula Chest Hand	Neck Medial forearm Hand
Sensation	**Clavicle, lateral shoulder** (Anterior forearm)	(Lateral arm, forearm) **Thumb** (Index finger)	(Thumb) **Index finger Middle finger** (Ring finger) (Palm)	(Medial forearm, arm) **Ring finger Little finger** (Medial hand)
Muscles innervated	Deltoid Biceps brachii Brachialis	Biceps brachii Brachialis Extensor carpi radialis longus and brevus	Extensor carpi radialis longus, brevus Triceps brachii Flexor digitorum superficialis, profundus	Triceps brachii
Motor	**Shoulder abduction Elbow flexion**	(Shoulder abduction) **Elbow flexion** (Forearm supination) (Forearm pronation) **Wrist extension**	Elbow extension Forearm pronation **Wrist extension** Finger extension	Elbow extension Wrist flexion **Finger, thumb extension** Finger, thumb flexion Finger, thumb abduction Finger, thumb adduction
Reflexes	(Biceps) (Brachioradialis)	Biceps Brachioradialis	Triceps	

This table represents a compilation of several sources of information[2,3,6,7]; the most distinguishing and consistently reported findings are in bold type.

4. Loss of fine motor control in the hands
5. Lower extremity weakness
6. Bowel or bladder dysfunction, including urgency, frequency, retention

Mechanical Neck Pain

As discussed earlier, in the absence of these nerve dysfunction syndromes, the cause of neck pain is not well understood. The prevalence of neck pain increases with age, declining again in late life, and it frequently coexists with other comorbidities such as low back pain, headache, and poor self-rated health.[23] These same comorbidities also portend a worse prognosis. Workers' compensation payments and work-related stress are also reported predictors of persistent pain.[6] Most people who present to primary care clinic with neck pain experience recurrent or persistent problems.[31] In one population-based study of primary care patients with neck pain,[32] only one-third of patients reported resolution of symptoms at 1-year follow-up. Other studies suggest that between 15% and 50% of people in the general population report resolution at one year.[1]

DIAGNOSTIC TESTS/IMAGING STUDIES

Ordering imaging studies for neck pain is tricky. Although neck pain may be causing significant disability, imaging studies are often unhelpful and potentially misleading. A strong correlation between physical examination and imaging studies is paramount.

As most investigators on this subject have advocated, the clinician's first task is to ascertain any symptoms that might suggest serious underlying disease (such as trauma/fracture, osteomyelitis, cancer, inflammatory arthritides, or spinal cord compromise). These red flags,[6,19] as outlined in **Box 1**, should be similar to those

---

Box 1
Red flags for serious underlying disease

Cancer or infection

  Fever, chills, weight loss

  History of cancer

  Age >50 years or <20 years

  Intravenous drug use

  Immunosuppression (steroids, human immunodeficiency virus, transplant)

  Recent infection, especially with bacteremia

  Pain that is worse when supine

  Severe night time pain

  Fail to improve >6 weeks

  Tenderness over vertebral body

Fracture

  Significant trauma

  Osteoporosis

Systemic disease

  History of ankylosing spondylitis or inflammatory arthritis

Myelopathy

  Lower extremity spasticity

  Bowel or bladder changes

  Upper motor neuron signs (eg, Babinski, Hoffman)

reported in patients with low back pain.[33] Such symptoms warrant appropriate, expedited evaluation.

The second and related task is to discern any potential for spinal cord or nerve root compression. This task may be accomplished via the history and physical examination, as described in the next section (see section on symptoms also).

Radiculopathy, History, and Physical Examination

Findings of radiculopathy on examination might include decreased sensation as well as lower motor neuron signs (weakness, hyporeflexia, and less commonly, atrophy or hypotonia). Classically, sensory findings follow a dermatomal distribution, but in clinical practice, sensory findings on examination only follow this distribution in a few patients,[3,8] probably because of significant overlap in dermatomes. Pain into the arm rarely follows a dermatomal pattern, but may run more similar to a myotomal pattern.[4,7,8,25] **Table 1** compiles commonly reported associated findings depending on spinal nerve involved.[2,3,6,8,34] In practice, the experience of pain is variable, and dermatomal/myotomal boundaries overlap significantly. Lower cervical nerve roots are more commonly affected; C7 is the most frequent.[8]

Several provocative maneuvers have been reported for cervical radiculopathy.[19,35,36]

The upper limb tension test (ULTT), also called the brachial plexus tension test or test of Elvey, has been reported as the straight leg raise of the upper extremities; Rubinstein and colleagues[35] reviewed the literature and concurred that it has high sensitivity (97%), with a reasonable negative likelihood ratio (reported at 0.12, but with a large confidence interval). However, it has low specificity (22%–90%).[19,36,37] The ULTT is performed with the patient in a supine position. Provide (1) scapular depression with one hand, while (2) abducting the shoulder to 90°, with the elbow in 90° of flexion. (3) Supinate the forearms and wrist. Extend the wrist and fingers. (4) Push forward on the hand to laterally rotate the shoulder. (5) Extend the elbow. (6) Provocation of pain into the arm can also be further elicited in the final position by having the patient bend their head contralaterally (which should elicit or exacerbate pain)[36,38]; an ipsilateral head bend should diminish pain (**Fig. 1**).[36]

Neck distraction is performed by grasping under the patient's chin while they are supine and applying a modest upward distracting force, which should relieve symptoms. Wainner and colleagues[36] reported low sensitivity (44%) but reasonably high specificity (90%), with a reasonable positive likelihood ratio of 4.4 (although again with a large confidence interval).

Likewise, a positive Spurling sign (**Fig. 2**), Valsalva (pain with 3 seconds of breath holding/bearing down), or abduction relief sign (resolution of pain with placing hand on the patient's head) also have reasonably high specificity (86%–93%, 94%, and 75%–92%, respectively). Their sensitivity is low. They could support a diagnosis of radiculopathy in the context of corroborating history and other examination findings, but their absence does not rule out the disease.[35,36,39–41]

Myelopathy, History, and Physical Examination

In contrast to radiculopathy, the physical examination hallmarks of myelopathy are primarily upper motor neuron findings in a distribution below the level of compression. These findings may include upper or lower extremity weakness, spastic gait, and hyperreflexia. The plantar reflex (Babinski sign) and Hoffman reflex are important to perform, and their presence should alert the clinician to possible myelopathy.[6] The Hoffman reflex is performed by applying a quick pressure (flicking) to the middle finger and then looking for reflexive flexion of the thumb. Please note, this response can be

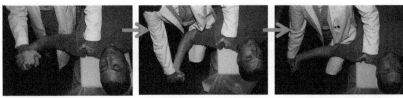

(1) Depress scapula,   (3) Extend wrist and fingers,   (5) Extend elbow
(2) Abduct shoulder   (4) Laterally rotate shoulder

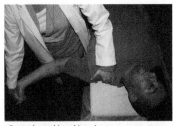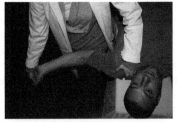

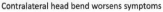

Contralateral head bend worsens symptoms   Ipsilateral head bend improves symptoms

Fig. 1. ULTT. (*Data from* Wainner RS, Fritz JM, Irrgang JJ, et al. Reliability and diagnostic accuracy of the clinical examination and patient self-report measures for cervical radiculopathy. Spine (Phila Pa 1976) 2003;28(1):52–62.)

nonpathologic in naturally hyperreflexic patients. There can be coexisting lower motor neuron findings in myelopathy because of simultaneous nerve root compression; these are classically at the level of involvement, not lower.

Laboratory Tests and Imaging

Blood work is rarely useful in the evaluation of neck pain, except perhaps in the evaluation of someone with red flag symptoms that suggest infection, cancer, and so forth (see **Box 1**).

Plain radiographs for the evaluation of nontraumatic neck pain in primary care clinic, are rarely, if ever, useful. They should be considered only in cases in which the history and examination have yielded red flags for serious disease (in which case the need for more advanced imaging might supersede radiographs, depending on the situation).

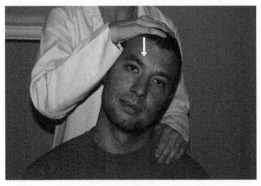

Fig. 2. Spurling maneuver: pain with axial pressure while head is bent ipsilaterally.

Abnormal curvature does not predict muscle spasm as sometimes believed.[42] In one series of 85 patients referred for radiographs based on neck pain,[43] there were no unexpected findings of malignancy or infection. In another series of 848 patients referred for radiographs,[44] there were no unexpected serious diagnoses.

MRI is clearly the test of choice if serious underlying disease, such as infection or cancer, is being considered. However, MRI findings of spinal cord or nerve root compression must be interpreted with caution and always correlated with the patient's history and examination. Degenerative changes, herniated disks, and compression of neural structures on MRI are common, age-related findings.[19] Review of cervical spine MRI scans performed in 100 asymptomatic patients showed herniated disks in 57% of patients older than 64 years, with spinal cord impingement in 26%. Asymptomatic spinal cord compression was observed in 7% of all the patients.[45] MRI can reliably show compression of neural structures, but these findings should then be correlated with any myelopathic or radicular symptoms.[19] Showing degenerative changes in the absence of nerve or cord compression usually does not change management.

Electromyography should be used in conjunction with the physical examination and MRI to evaluate a suspected radiculopathy. It has little role in evaluation of suspected myelopathy, except to rule out alternative explanations of symptoms/findings.[46]

Diskography and diagnostic (anesthetic) injections are controversial, and, although advocated by some investigators, they are generally not recommended based on current evidence for mechanical neck pain.[1,19]

DIFFERENTIAL DIAGNOSIS

A specific cause for neck pain is frequently not found. Rare causes should be considered, especially if red flags are present in the history or physical examination to suggest these. **Table 2** gives a list of common and rare causes.[6,7,19,47-49]

TREATMENT

Because neck pain is a common and sometimes disabling problem, it is not surprising that numerous methods of treatment are routinely used to mitigate symptoms. The scientific literature on treatment is often sparse, conflicting or mired in methodological flaws, making it difficult for the practicing clinician to feel confident about what course of action to recommend. It is not even clear what the benefits and harms of giving a diagnostic label (such as degenerative joint disease) may be for a patient.

Multiple challenges exist in both treating and studying the treatment of patients with neck pain. Lack of clarity on the basic understanding of the cause of neck pain without radiculopathy or myelopathy makes targeted interventions challenging. Gold standards for diagnosis of purported causes are murky. Patients with neck pain are probably a heterogeneous group of patients who respond differently to various interventions. For example, response to treatment may vary depending on (1) presence of radiculopathy, myelopathy or neither, (2) comorbid psychiatric disease or personality,[50] or (3) other premorbid musculoskeletal pains,[23] to name a few. With the inherently subjective nature of pain reporting, it can be hypothesized that a patient's preference for certain treatments (eg, if a friend had a good experience with one type of treatment) may influence a patient's perception or reporting of pain after treatment.

As mentioned earlier, distinctions should be drawn between mechanical neck pain, neck pain with radiculopathy or myelopathy, and neck pain with serious underlying disease (eg, fracture, cancer, infection). Treatment of patients in this final category (serious underlying disease) is often appropriately more aggressive, with excellent

Table 2
Common and rare causes of neck pain, radiculomyelopathy or both

	Neck Pain Alone	Neck Pain with Radiculopathy/ Myelopathy	Radiculopathy/ Myelopathy Symptoms Alone	
Common				
Disk herniation	x	x	x	
Neuroforaminal stenosis (from spondylosis, disk herniation, or both)		x	x	
Spinal canal stenosis (from spondylosis, large central disk herniation, ligament calcification, or combination)		x	x	
Nonspecific pain (also known as mechanical pain) from unknown cause; sometimes, this is labeled as cervical muscle strain, facet joint pain, and so forth	x			
Rare				
Tumor	x	x	x	
Benign tumors (hemangioma, osteoid osteoma, osteoblastoma, osteochondroma, giant cell tumor)		x	x	
Serious infections (diskitis, osteomyelitis, epidural abscess, septic arthritis, meningitis)	x	x	x	
Vascular causes (eg, vertebral artery, internal carotid or aortic dissection)	x	x	x	
Nerve root infarction (vasculitis)		x	x	
Trauma: fracture, root avulsion, spinal cord injuries	x	x	x	
Polymyalgia rheumatica/ temporal arteritis	x			Stiffness should be primary
Inflammatory arthropathies (rheumatoid arthritis, crystal arthropathy, ankylosing spondylitis)	x			Typically multiple joint involvement and systemic inflammatory symptoms

(continued on next page)

Table 2 (continued)	Neck Pain Alone	Neck Pain with Radiculopathy/ Myelopathy	Radiculopathy/ Myelopathy Symptoms Alone	
Fibromyalgia	x			Should not be isolated neck pain
Synovial cyst			x	
Torticollis	x			Not necessarily painful
Diffuse idiopathic skeletal hyperostosis			x	Classically painless, except at risk for cervical fractures from minimal trauma. Stiffness and dysphagia more common symptoms
Paget disease			x	Cervical spine lesions only seen in 11% of patients. In a series of 180 patients, none reported neck pain and only 2 patients had spinal cord compression[48]
Thoracic outlet syndrome		x	x	
Shoulder diseases	x			
Multiple sclerosis			x	
Amyotrophic lateral sclerosis, Guillain-Barré syndrome, normal pressure hydrocephalus			x	
Noncompressive radiculopathies (rare)				
Diabetic monoradiculopathy			x	
Herpes zoster			x	
Lyme disease			x	
Tuberculosis	x		x	
Syphilis			x	
Brucellosis			x	
Cytomegalovirus			x	
Lyme disease			x	
Histiocytosis X			x	
Sarcoidosis			x	
Human immunodeficiency virus–related neuropathy			x	

support in the literature. This subject is outside the scope of this discussion and we focus instead on the first two categories.[1]

Multiple helpful systematic reviews have been published for individual treatment methods, combinations of treatment methods, and overall surgical versus conservative treatment courses.[51–65]

Conservative Treatments

A panoply of conservative treatments are available. Typically, in the absence of severe myelopathic or radicular motor weakness, these treatments are the first attempted courses of action. Of the available options, those believed to have the weight of evidence in support include educational videos after whiplash injury; select exercise interventions; mobilization when used with exercise; some medications; and possibly, acupuncture.

Although reassurance and education are often given at initial consultations, there is no evidence that such counseling is superior to any other noninvasive treatments for mechanical neck pain.[53] Specifically, after whiplash injury, an educational video was shown to predict lower pain ratings at 24 weeks.[66] There is low-quality to moderate-quality evidence for the use of specific cervical and scapular stretching and strengthening exercises for chronic neck pain,[55,67,68] but not upper extremity stretching and strengthening or a general exercise program. The improvement from these stretching and strengthening exercises is often limited to immediately after treatment and decreases after the intermediate-term.

Manual therapies encompass a range of hands-on interventions, which might typically be used by a physical therapist, occupational therapist, chiropractor, or doctor of osteopathic medicine. One type of manual therapy is joint mobilization. Joint mobilizations are a type of passive movement of a skeletal joint, graded and distinguished by positioning of the joint and velocity and amplitude of the movement. Within the spectrum of mobilizations, a high-velocity, low-amplitude thrust has several synonymous terms: manipulation, a grade V mobilization, or an adjustment. Multiple systematic reviews have looked at the evidence for joint mobilization, manipulation, or other manual therapies as a treatment of mechanical neck pain and come to slightly different conclusions. Mior[69] concluded that evidence is limited and that these therapies may or may not be effective. Gross and colleagues[56] in their Cochrane review concluded that mobilization or manipulation when used with exercise is beneficial, but when performed alone is not. The Bone and Joint Task Force[53] concluded that mobilization or exercise sessions alone or in combination with medications are beneficial in the short-term (6–13 weeks).

Several classes of oral medications are frequently used for chronic, mechanical neck pain, including nonsteroidal antiinflammatory drugs, muscle relaxants, opiates, antidepressants, and other analgesics. They all have limited evidence and unclear benefits.[57]

Two systematic reviews of acupuncture[53,58] reported moderate-quality or inconsistent evidence of benefit compared with sham controls.

Because of limited evidence, conclusions cannot be drawn about the effectiveness of massage,[59] and multiple investigators have concluded that passive modalities (transcutaneous electrical nerve stimulation, ultrasonography, diathermy, electrotherapy) are not associated with short-term or long-term pain or functional improvements.[53,60]

Specifically for radiculopathy, traction has been advocated; it is intuitively believed to decrease pressure on the exiting spinal nerve. It is contraindicated in patients with significant or severe spondylosis, who have myelopathy, a positive Lhermitte sign, or rheumatoid arthritis with atlantoaxial subluxation.[70] A recent Cochrane review[61] found only one study deemed to have a low risk of bias and concluded that there was no evidence of benefit. Graham and colleagues[62] also found few high-quality trials and concluded that there was no evidence of benefit to continuous traction and low-quality evidence for intermittent traction. Others have determined that poor methodological quality precludes any conclusions.[4,63]

In a practice environment with a dearth of high-quality evidence, perhaps patient preference should strongly influence choice of therapy. Future research is critical.

Invasive Treatments

Steroid injections may be considered for radiculopathy, with evidence supporting short-term symptom improvement.[54,71] For more significant manifestations of radiculopathy, steroid injections do not seem to decrease the rate of open surgery.[54] Zygapophyseal injections are a controversial therapy for mechanical neck pain (without radiculopathy) and are not endorsed by the Bone and Joint Task Force.[54]

Surgery

For a detailed discussion of surgical outcomes, the reader is referred to the surgical literature. There is not convincing evidence to support the role of surgery in mechanical neck pain,[54] and there is wide variation in current practice with regards to who is referred for surgery.[72]

For patients with severe or progressive radiculomyelopathy, surgery is appropriately considered.[9]

In the presence of mild to moderate radiculopathy, short-term outcomes of pain relief, decreased numbness, and weakness are better with surgery compared with conservative management, but that difference disappears with longer-term (1–2 year) follow-up.[64] In the presence of mild to moderate myelopathy, short-term benefits have been reported, but long-term follow-up (3 years) does not delineate benefits over conservative treatment.[28,54,64]

MANAGEMENT

Mechanical neck pain is frequently a chronic or recurrent problem for individual patients. Regular follow-up with a provider should focus on vigilance for clues to underlying serious disease and monitoring for the onset or progression of radiculopathy or myelopathy. Conservative management is usually the recommended course, and various options were discussed earlier. Given the lack of evidence that one conservative management tool is superior to another,[73] patient preference and availability can figure prominently in the decision. Other pillars of chronic pain management also apply here, such as validating the patient's experience of pain, managing expectations of treatments, refocusing goals of treatment toward functionality, and treating comorbidities such as depression. Although it has not yet been validated in the literature,[65] considering a multidisciplinary approach seems reasonable.

SUMMARY/FUTURE CONSIDERATIONS

Future studies are needed to further understand the pathophysiology of mechanical neck pain. Robust scientific evidence is sparse on which noninvasive treatments are the most beneficial and how to better select patients for particular noninvasive or invasive treatments.

REFERENCES

1. Guzman J, Haldeman S, Carroll L, et al. Clinical practice implications of the Bone and Joint Decade 2000-2010 Task Force on Neck Pain and its associated disorders: from concepts and findings to recommendations. Spine 2008;33(4S): S199–213.
2. Netter FH. Atlas of human anatomy. 3rd edition. Teterboro (NJ): Icon Learning Systems; 2003.
3. Robinson J, Kothari M. Clinical features and diagnosis of cervical radiculopathy. Available at: http://www.uptodate.com/. Accessed September 28, 2013.
4. Carette S, Fehlings MG. Cervical radiculopathy. N Engl J Med 2005;353: 392–9.
5. Zhang J, Tsuzuki N, Hirabayashi S, et al. Surgical anatomy of the nerves and muscles in the posterior cervical spine: a guide for avoiding inadvertent nerve injuries during the posterior approach. Spine 2003;28(13):1379–84.
6. Honet JC, Ellenberg MR. What you always wanted to know about the history and physical exam of neck pain but were afraid to ask. Phys Med Rehabil Clin N Am 2003;14:473–91.
7. Bogduk N. The anatomy and pathophysiology of neck pain. Phys Med Rehabil Clin N Am 2011;22:367–82.
8. Radhakrishnan K, Litchy WJ, O'Fallon WM, et al. Epidemiology of cervical radiculopathy. A population based study from Rochester, Minnesota 1876 through 1990. Brain 1994;117:325–35.
9. McCormick WE, Steinmetz MP, Benzel EC. Cervical spondylotic myelopathy: make a difficult diagnosis, then refer for surgery. Cleve Clin J Med 2003; 70(10):899–904.
10. Dreyfuss P, Michaelsen M, Fletcher D. Atlanto-occipital and lateral atlanto-axial joint pain patterns. Spine 1994;19(10):1125–31.
11. Dwyer A, Aprill C, Bogduk N. Cervical zygapophyseal joint pain patterns. I: a study in normal volunteers. Spine 1990;15(6):453–7.
12. Fukui S, Ohetso K, Shiotani M, et al. Referred pain distribution of the cervical zygapophyseal joints and cervical dorsal rami. Pain 1996;68:79–83.
13. Aprill C, Dwyer A, Bogduk N. Cervical zygapophyseal joint pain patterns. II: a clinical evaluation. Spine 1990;15(6):458–61.
14. Cooper G, Bailey B, Bogduk N. Cervical zygapophysial joint pain maps. Pain Med 2007;8(4):344–53.
15. Sehgal N, Dunbar EE, Shah RV, et al. Systematic review of diagnostic utility of facet (zygapophysial) joint injections in chronic spinal pain: an update. Pain Physician 2007;10:213–8.
16. Speldewinde GC, Bashford GM, Davidson IR. Diagnostic cervical zygapophyseal joint blocks for chronic cervical pain. Med J Aust 2001;174(4): 174–6.
17. Schellhas KP, Smith MD, Gundry CR, et al. Cervical discogenic pain. Prospective correlation of magnetic resonance imaging and discography in asymptomatic subjects and pain sufferers. Spine 1996;21(3):311–2.
18. Slipman CW, Plastaras C, Patel R, et al. Provocative cervical discography symptom mapping. Spine 2005;5(4):381–8.
19. Nordin M, Carragee EJ, Hogg-Johnson S, et al. Assessment of neck pain and its associated disorders. Results of the Bone And Joint Decade 2000– 2010 Task Force on Neck Pain and its Associated Disorders. Spine 2008;33(Suppl): S101–22.

20. Hogan QH, Abram SE. Neural blockade for diagnosis and prognosis. Anesthesiology 1997;86(1):216–41.
21. Ackerman WE, Munir MA, Zhang JM, et al. Are diagnostic lumbar facet injections influenced by pain of muscular origin? Pain Pract 2004;4(4):286–91.
22. Falco FJ, Erhart S, Wargo BW, et al. Systematic review of diagnostic utility and therapeutic effectiveness of cervical facet joint interventions. Pain Physician 2009;12(2):323–44.
23. Hogg-Johnson S, van der Velde G, Carroll LJ, et al. The burden and determinants of neck pain in the general population: results of the Bone and Joint Decade 2000-2010 Task Force on Neck Pain and its Associated Disorders. Spine 2008; 33(4S):S39–51.
24. Song XJ, Hu SJ, Greenquist KW, et al. Mechanical and thermal hyperalgesia and ectopic neuronal discharge after chronic compression of dorsal root ganglia. J Neurophysiol 1999;82(6):3347–58.
25. Slipman CW, Plastaras CT, Palmitier RA, et al. Symptom provocation of fluoroscopically guided cervical nerve root stimulation: are dynatomal maps identical to dermatomal maps? Spine 1998;23(20):2235–42.
26. Brain WR, Northfield D, Wilkinson M. Neurological manifestations of cervical spondylosis. Brain 1952;75(2):187–225.
27. Kadanka Z, Mares M, Bednarıka J, et al. Predictive factors for mild forms of spondylotic cervical myelopathy treated conservatively or surgically. Eur J Neurol 2005;12(1):16–24.
28. Kadanka Z, Mares M, Bednarık J, et al. Approaches to spondylotic cervical myelopathy: conservative versus surgical results in a 3-year follow-up study. Spine 2002;27(20):2205–10.
29. Tracy JA, Bartleson JD. Cervical spondylotic myelopathy. Neurologist 2010;16(3): 176–87.
30. Lunsford LD, Bissonette DJ, Zorub DS. Anterior surgery for cervical disc disease. Part 2: treatment of cervical spondylotic myelopathy in 32 cases. J Neurosurg 1980;53(1):12–9.
31. Carroll L, Hogg-Johnson S, van der Velde G, et al. Course and prognostic factors for neck pain in the general population. Results of the Bone and Joint Decade 2000-2010 Task Force on Neck Pain and its Associated Disorders. Spine 2008; 33(4S):S75–82.
32. Cote P, Cassidy JD, Carroll LJ, et al. The annual incidence and course of neck pain in the general population: a population-based cohort study. Pain 2004; 112(3):267–73.
33. Chou R, Qaseem A, Snow V, et al. Diagnosis and Treatment of Low Back Pain: A Joint Clinical Practice Guideline from the American College of Physicians and the American Pain Society. Ann Intern Med 2007;147(7):478–91.
34. Yoss RE, Corbin KB, MacCarlty CS, et al. Significance of symptoms and signs in localization of involved root in cervical disk protrusion. Neurology 1957;7(10): 673–83.
35. Rubinstein S, Pool JJ, van Tulder MW. A systematic review of the diagnostic accuracy of provocative tests of the neck for diagnosing cervical radiculopathy. Eur Spine J 2007;16(3):307–19.
36. Wainner RS, Fritz JM, Irrgang JJ, et al. Reliability and diagnostic accuracy of the clinical examination and patient self-report measures for cervical radiculopathy. Spine 2003;28(1):52–62.
37. Sandmark H, Nisell R. Validity of five common manual neck pain provoking tests. Scand J Rehabil Med 1995;27(3):131–6.

38. Elvey RL. The investigation of arm pain: signs of adverse responses to the physical examination of the brachial plexus and related tissues. In: Boyling JD, Palastanga N, editors. Grieve's modern manual therapy. 2nd edition. New York: Churchill Livingstone; 1994. p. 577–85.

39. Tong HC, Haig AJ, Yamakawa K. The Spurling test and cervical radiculopathy. Spine 2002;27(2):156–9.

40. Davidson RI, Dunn EJ, Metzmaker JN. The shoulder abduction test in the diagnosis of radicular pain in cervical extradural compressive monoradiculopathies. Spine 1981;6(5):441–6.

41. Viikari-Juntura E, Porras M, Laasonen EM. Validity of clinical tests in the diagnosis of root compression in cervical disc disease. Spine 1989;14(3):253–7.

42. Matsumoto M, Fujimura Y, Suzuki N, et al. Cervical curvature in acute whiplash injuries: prospective comparative study with asymptomatic subjects. Injury 1998;29(10):775–8.

43. Heller CA, Stanley P, Lewis-Jones B, et al. Value of x ray examinations of the cervical spine. Br Med J (Clin Res Ed) 1983;287(6401):1276–8.

44. Johnson MJ, Lucas GL. Value of cervical spine radiographs as a screening tool. Clin Orthop Relat Res 1997;340:102–8.

45. Teresi LM, Lufkin RB, Reicher MA, et al. Asymptomatic degenerative disk disease and spondylosis of the cervical spine: MR imaging. Radiology 1987;164(1):83–8.

46. So YT, Weber CF, Campbell WW. Practice parameter for needle electromyographic evaluation of patients with suspected cervical radiculopathy: summary statement. American Association of Electrodiagnostic Medicine. American Academy of Physical Medicine and Rehabilitation. Muscle Nerve 1999;22(S8):S209–11.

47. Shelerud RA, Paynter KS. Rarer causes of radiculopathy: spinal tumors, infections, and other unusual causes. Phys Med Rehabil Clin N Am 2002;13:645–96.

48. Harinck HI, Bijvoet OL, Vellenga CJ, et al. Relation between signs and symptoms in Paget's disease of bone. Q J Med 1986;58(226):133–51.

49. Mazières B. Diffuse idiopathic skeletal hyperostosis (Forestier-Rotes-Querol disease): what's new? Joint Bone Spine 2013;80(5):466–70. http://dx.doi.org/10.1016/j.jbspin.2013.02.011.

50. Van der Donk J, Shouten J, Passchier J, et al. The associations of neck pain with radiological abnormalities of the cervical spine and personality traits in a general population. J Rheumatol 1991;18(12):1884–9.

51. Nikolaidis I, Fouyas IP, Sandercock PA, et al. Surgery for cervical radiculopathy or myelopathy. Cochrane Database Syst Rev 2010;(1):CD001466. http://dx.doi.org/10.1002/14651858.CD001466.pub3.

52. Vernon H, McDermaid CS, Hagino C. Systematic review of randomized clinical trials of complementary/alternative therapies in the treatment of tension-type and cervicogenic headache. Complement Ther Med 1999;7(3):142–55.

53. Hurwitz EL, Carragee EJ, van der Velde G, et al. Treatment of neck pain. Noninvasive interventions: results of the bone and Joint Decade 2000-2010 Task Force on Neck Pain and its Associated Disorders. Spine 2008;33(4S):S123–52.

54. Carragee EJ, Hurwitz EL, Cheng I, et al. Treatment of neck pain. Injections and surgical interventions: results of the Bone and Joint Decade 2000-2010 Task Force on Neck Pain and its Associated Disorders. Spine 2008;33(4S):S153–69.

55. Kay TM, Gross A, Goldsmith CH, et al. Exercises for mechanical neck disorders. Cochrane Database Syst Rev 2012;(8):CD004250. http://dx.doi.org/10.1002/14651858.CD004250.pub4.

56. Gross A, Hoving JL, Haines TA, et al. A Cochrane review of manipulation and mobilization for mechanical neck disorders. Spine 2004;29(14):1541–8.
57. Peloso PM, Gross A, Haines T, et al, Cervical Overview Group. Medicinal and injection therapies for mechanical neck disorders. Cochrane Database Syst Rev 2007;(3):CD000319. http://dx.doi.org/10.1002/14651858.CD000319.pub4.
58. Trinh K, Graham N, Gross A, et al. Acupuncture for neck disorders. Spine 2007; 32(2):236–43.
59. Patel KC, Gross A, Graham N, et al. Massage for mechanical neck disorders. Cochrane Database Syst Rev 2012;(9):CD004871. http://dx.doi.org/10.1002/14651858.CD004871.pub4.
60. Kroeling P, Gross AR, Goldsmith CH. A Cochrane review of electrotherapy for mechanical neck disorders. Spine 2005;30(21):E641–8.
61. Graham N, Gross A, Goldsmith CH, et al. Mechanical traction for neck pain with or without radiculopathy. Cochrane Database Syst Rev 2008;(3):CD006408. http://dx.doi.org/10.1002/14651858.CD006408.pub2.
62. Graham N, Gross A, Goldsmith C. Mechanical traction for mechanical neck disorders: a systematic review. J Rehabil Med 2006;38(3):145–52.
63. van der Heijden GJ, Beurskens AJ, Koes BW, et al. The efficacy of traction for back and neck pain: a systematic, blinded review of randomized clinical trial methods. Phys Ther 1995;75(2):93–104.
64. Fouyas I, Statham P, Sandercock PA. Cochrane review of the role of surgery in cervical spondylotic radiculomyelopathy. Spine 2002;27(7):736–47.
65. Karjalainen KA, Malmivaara A, van Tulder MW, et al. Multidisciplinary biopsychosocial rehabilitation for neck and shoulder pain among working age adults. Cochrane Database Syst Rev 2003;(2):CD002194. http://dx.doi.org/10.1002/14651858CD002194.
66. Brison RJ, Hartling L, Dostaler S, et al. A randomized controlled trial of an educational intervention to prevent the chronic pain of whiplash associated disorders following rear-end motor vehicle collisions. Spine 2005;30(16):1799–807.
67. Sarig-Bahat H. Evidence for exercise therapy in mechanical neck disorders. Man Ther 2003;8(1):10–20.
68. Mior S. Exercise in the treatment of chronic pain. Clin J Pain 2001;17(4S):S77–85.
69. Mior S. Manipulation and mobilization in the treatment of chronic pain. Clin J Pain 2001;17(4S):S70–6.
70. Ellenberg MR, Honet JC, Treanor WJ. Cervical radiculopathy. Arch Phys Med Rehabil 1994;75:342–52.
71. Stav A, Ovadia L, Sternberg A, et al. Cervical epidural steroid injection for cervicobrachialgia. Acta Anaesthesiol Scand 1993;37(6):562–6.
72. Harland SP, Laing RJ. A survey of the perioperative management of patients undergoing anterior cervical decompression in the UK and Eire. Br J Neurosurg 1998;12(2):113–7.
73. Van der Velde G, Hogg-Johnson S, Bayoumi AM, et al. Identifying the best treatment among common nonsurgical neck pain treatments. Spine 2008;33(4S): S184–91.

The Essential Role of the Otolaryngologist in the Diagnosis and Management of Temporomandibular Joint and Chronic Oral, Head, and Facial Pain Disorders

Howard A. Israel, DDS[a,b],*, Laura J. Davila, DDS[a]

KEYWORDS

- Temporomandibular joint • Chronic oral, facial and head pain • Otalgia
- TMJ arthroscopy • TMJ exercise • Passive motion jaw rehabilitation
- Temporomandibular disorders

KEY POINTS

- Chronic oral, head, and facial pain (COHFP) disorders are frequently misdiagnosed, therefore a constant reevaluation of the diagnosis and response to treatment is required.
- Otologic symptoms are often caused by temporomandibular disorders (TMDs), and a careful history and clinical examination are the most important factors in making an accurate diagnosis and appropriate referral.
- Joint overload and lack of motion lead to pathologic changes resulting in inflammatory and degenerative temporomandibular joint disease.
- Principles for treating inflammatory and degenerative temporomandibular joint disorders are to reduce load, increase mobility with passive motion, reduce inflammation and muscle spasm, and manage pain.
- For patients with severe temporomandibular joint disorders that fail to improve with appropriate treatment, the least invasive procedure to treat the pathologic condition and improve function is indicated.

This article originally appeared in Otolaryngologic Clinics of North America, Volume 47, Issue 2, April 2014.

Portions of this review were updated from: Israel H. The essential role of the oral and maxillofacial surgeon in the diagnosis, management, causation and prevention of chronic orofacial pain: clinical perspectives. In: Fonseca RJ, editor. Oral and maxillofacial surgery. 2nd edition. St. Louis, Missouri: Elsevier Health Sciences; 2009. p. 132–55.

[a] Division of Dentistry Oral & Maxillofacial Surgery, Weill-Cornell Medical College, New York Presbyterian Hospital, Cornell University, 525 East 68th Street, New York, NY 10065, USA; [b] Columbia University College of Dental Medicine, 630 West 168th Street, New York, NY 10032, USA
* Corresponding author. 12 Bond Street, Great Neck, NY 11021.
E-mail address: drhowardisrael@yahoo.com

INTRODUCTION

In 1934, Costen[1] published a paper in the *Annals of Otology, Rhinology and Laryngology* on "A Syndrome of Ear and Sinus Symptoms Dependent on Disturbed Function of the Temporomandibular Joint." Costen observed patients with ear, jaw, and sinus pain and theorized that an altered occlusion resulted in temporomandibular joint disease as the major etiologic factor. Furthermore, he recommended correction of the occlusion to relieve pressure on the temporomandibular joint and surrounding structures, ultimately leading to resolution of the symptoms. Thus, the importance of the specialty of otolaryngology in the diagnosis and treatment of oral, head, and face pain was reinforced 80 years ago and continues to this day. Although Costen's proposal that an altered occlusion was the main cause of head and facial pain has been refuted by evidence-based research, to his credit, he did understand that the site and source of complex head and facial pain are often not the same. Today, 8 decades after the introduction of Costen syndrome, there are many clinicians who still treat patients according to the observations of Dr Costen in 1934.

The diagnosis and management of COHFP has been a subject of great controversy over the years and continues to this day. This situation is unfortunate, because there have been great advances in our understanding of these conditions based on solid research over the past 25 years.

Common clinical scenarios that the otolaryngologist is presented with include the following:

1. Patients with severe persistent ear pain with negative otologic findings who have inflammatory temporomandibular joint disease.
2. Patients with COHFP and masticatory dysfunction who are ultimately diagnosed with neoplasia or other serious disorders (eg, trigeminal neuralgia, temporal arteritis).
3. Patients with oropharyngeal cancers treated with surgery and radiation leading to trismus because of radiation fibrosis, making early detection of recurrent or second primary cancers extremely difficult if not impossible for the clinician.
4. Patients with persistent maxillary dental pain, undergoing multiple dental procedures that fail to reduce symptoms (eg. extractions, root canal therapy) who eventually are diagnosed with acute or chronic maxillary sinusitis.
5. Patients with tinnitus symptoms, resistant to treatment, and coexisting TMDs.

This article clarifies the current state of knowledge of COHFP conditions with the inclusion of temporomandibular joint disorders as just one component of the variety of conditions that can cause head and facial pain. Obtaining an accurate diagnosis in a timely manner is extremely important because COHFP symptoms can be caused by a variety of pathologic conditions that can be inflammatory, degenerative, neurologic, neoplastic, or systemic in origin. The essential role of the specialty of otolaryngology in the diagnosis and management of patients with these complex COHFP conditions is emphasized.

PITFALLS LEADING TO MISDIAGNOSIS OF COHFP

The reasons for the difficulty in properly diagnosing COHFP and TMDs are multifactorial. The following factors that can lead to misdiagnosis are important for the clinician to be aware:

1. Complex regional anatomy of the head and neck, often resulting in disparity between the site and the source of pain.

2. Symptoms of pain, limitation of mandibular movement, joint noise, tinnitus, and altered occlusion are not specific for the pathologic condition. Thus, these symptoms can be caused by local otologic and temporomandibular joint disorders or infectious, neoplastic, neurologic, and systemic conditions.
3. Chronic tissue damage from trauma and/or multiple surgical procedures can lead to central sensitization of sensory nerve pathways, leading to neuropathic pain, allodynia (pain response to nonpainful stimuli), and hyperalgesia (excessive pain response to mildly painful stimuli). The presence of neuropathic pain can make accurate diagnosis extremely difficult because the clinician can easily be misled into believing that the source of the pain is localized, when in fact, there is a central-nervous-system-mediated component.

The following case scenarios are provided to demonstrate common clinical situations that can potentially lead to misdiagnosis of COHFP and TMDs.

Inflammatory/Degenerative Temporomandibular Joint Disorders Initially Presenting with Symptoms of Otalgia

A major factor contributing to confusion between otologic pathology and temporomandibular joint pathology is close anatomic proximity and common sensory innervation via the auriculotemporal nerve. Patients often cannot differentiate ear pain from temporomandibular joint pain, and thus, otologic pathology may cause temporomandibular joint pain and temporomandibular joint pathology may cause otologic pain.

CASE REPORT #1: TEMPOROMANDIBULAR JOINT SYNOVITIS AND OTALGIA

A 26-year-old woman presented to the otolaryngologist with severe right-sided ear pain for the past 9 months. The patient reported having an upper respiratory tract infection 9 months ago and after the resolution of the respiratory infection, developed persistent right-sided ear pain. She also noticed that chewing made her symptoms worse and that there was limitation in her jaw opening. The otologic examination and audiometric findings were normal. Palpation of the anterior aspect of the right external auditory canal revealed significant tenderness, compared to the right. The maximum interincisal mandibular opening distance was measured at 20 mm with deviation to the right and produced severe pain in the right ear (**Fig. 1A**). The patient was unable to shift her jaw to the left because of severe pain in the right ear. The patient was given a tongue blade to bite on, and this produced severe pain in the right ear. The otolaryngologist concluded that the diagnosis was a temporomandibular joint disorder. The recommended course of action was ibuprofen, 600 mg, thrice daily and for the patient to be evaluated by an oral and maxillofacial surgeon with expertise in the diagnosis and management of temporomandibular joint disorders.

The patient was evaluated by an oral and maxillofacial surgeon who diagnosed her with right temporomandibular joint synovitis, masticatory muscle spasm with a clenching habit, as a major etiologic factor. A night guard oral appliance was fabricated to attempt to reduce the forces of nocturnal clenching. The patient was instructed to perform passive jaw motion exercises thrice daily. She was continued on ibuprofen, 600 mg, thrice daily and prescribed diazepam, 5 mg, to be taken at bedtime to help to reduce stress and act as a muscle relaxant. After using the oral appliance for 1 week, the patient's symptoms increased, with further exacerbation of the right-sided ear pain. The patient returned to the otolaryngologist who noted severe pain on palpation over the right temporomandibular joint as well as in the external auditory canal. Although examination of the middle ear with an otoscope did cause pain, the tympanic membrane and middle ear examination was unremarkable. The maximum interincisal opening distance was now 15 mm, and the patient was unable to occlude her teeth properly on the right side because the upper and lower posterior teeth were not meeting. The otolaryngologist and the oral and maxillofacial surgeon conferred, and the patient was diagnosed with an acute temporomandibular joint synovitis. The patient was placed on a 1-week oral steroid medication with a tapering dose and was referred back to the oral and maxillofacial surgeon for further management.

The clinical findings were essentially unchanged when the patient was seen by the oral and maxillofacial surgeon. The pain level was rated as 9 on the visual analog scale (0, no pain; 10, the most severe pain); the maximum interincisal opening distance was measured at 18 mm with deviation to the right and causing severe pain localized to the right ear and temporomandibular joint region. The left lateral excursion of the mandible was severely limited to 3 mm and caused pain in the right temporomandibular joint. The right lateral excursion was 10 mm and did not exacerbate pain. The occlusion was class I with a 1-mm right-sided posterior open bite. Mild manipulation of the mandible to attempt to position the right posterior teeth to occlude caused severe right-sided temporomandibular joint and ear pain. The left temporomandibular joint was nonpainful and had normal rotational and translational movement. A panoramic radiograph was obtained, which was unremarkable. Temporomandibular joint magnetic resonance imaging (MRI) was performed, which revealed anterior disk displacement without reduction of both the right and left temporomandibular joints. A significant finding was a large effusion in the right temporomandibular joint superior joint space as demonstrated by enhanced white signal intensity on the T2 images (see **Fig. 1**B). The clinical examination and MRI findings were consistent with a right temporomandibular joint synovitis. The patient was frustrated having had this problem for 9 months without any significant resolution in spite of a full course of nonsurgical management.

The oral and maxillofacial surgeon recommended right temporomandibular joint arthroscopic surgery, which was performed under sedation and local anesthesia. This surgery revealed a severe grade 4 synovitis of the posterior synovial tissues as well as adhesions in the superior joint space (see **Fig. 1**C). Operative arthroscopy was performed, which involved lysis of adhesions and removal with a motorized minishaver and a 2.0 mm full radius blade. Areas of significant synovitis were localized, and under direct vision, betamethasone (6 mg/mL) was injected with a #25 gauge spinal needle. The disk was mobilized with a graded probe instrument. After the arthroscopic surgery, the patient was placed on nonsteroidal antiinflammatory drugs, muscle relaxants, and a nonchew diet for 3 weeks. Most importantly, passive motion exercises to gradually stretch the mandible open to restore normal range of motion were started immediately. The passive motion exercise sessions were performed for 15 minutes thrice daily. Three weeks after the arthroscopic surgery, the maximum interincisal opening distance was 38 mm and the pain level was reduced to 3 with maximum opening. At rest, without jaw movement, there was no ear or temporomandibular joint pain. The diet was gradually advanced, and at 3 months postoperatively, the maximum interincisal opening distance was 41 mm, the pain level on the visual analog scale was 1, and the patient was able to chew on soft foods. She continued performing her passive motion exercises twice daily. At 1 year postoperatively, the patient has no pain at rest and occasional pain levels of up to 2 with maximum opening. The patient is able to chew on almost all foods, although she avoids very chewy foods such as bagels and hero sandwiches.

Discussion Case #1

A common scenario is a patient who seeks consultation with an otolaryngologist regarding the onset of acute ear pain or the persistence of chronic ear pain. When the clinical findings do not support an otologic cause, the patient is often referred for evaluation of a temporomandibular joint disorder. The patient may seek multiple opinions from otolaryngologists, neurologists, dentists, and oral and maxillofacial surgeons in a quest for appropriate diagnosis and treatment. The importance of establishing an accurate diagnosis cannot be over emphasized because it is essential for proper treatment. Thus, failure to establish the diagnosis will often result in persistent symptoms or inappropriate treatments. In spite of this, the astute clinician can use the following guidelines to help differentiate pathologic conditions of the ear versus those of the temporomandibular joint:

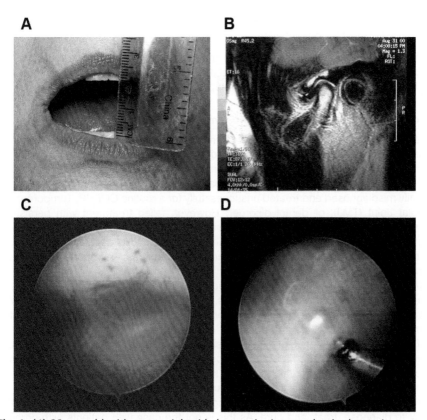

Fig. 1. (*A*) 26-year-old with severe right-sided ear pain, increased pain due to jaw movement, limited jaw opening of 20 mm with deviation to the painful side. (*B*) MRI of the right temporomandibular joint demonstrates a synovial effusion on the T2 images with fluid in the superior joint space. Anterior disk position is also present. (*C, D*) Arthroscopy of the right temporomandibular joint demonstrated grade 4 synovitis and adhesions of the posterior recess. Inflammation of the synovial membrane with associated adhesions area significant tissue changes that cause pain and limitation in joint mobility.

1. Temporomandibular joint pathology is generally increased by mandibular movement and function.
2. If the pain is increased significantly because of chewing (or biting firmly on a tongue blade during the initial examination), it often indicates a temporomandibular joint or masticatory muscle disorder.
3. Temporomandibular joint pathology will often cause a restriction in the range of motion of the affected joint. Thus, a right temporomandibular joint disorder often causes the mandible to deviate to the right with attempts at maximum opening. Furthermore, when a patient attempts an opposite lateral excursion (for example, sliding the lower jaw to the left in the aforementioned scenario) there will be restricted movement and increased pain.
4. Temporomandibular joint noise (clicking or crepitus) does not necessarily indicate temporomandibular joint disease as the cause of the pain.
5. If the patient points directly to the temporomandibular joint as the location of the source of pain during attempts at maximum jaw opening, it usually indicates a temporomandibular joint disorder.

6. Patients who have excessive clenching habits will often have tender temporalis and masseter muscles on palpation.

Although none of the above guidelines are absolute, because there are always exceptions to the rule, these simple observations can give the clinician an important clue as to which direction the diagnostic workup should follow.

Neoplasia Misdiagnosed as COHFP and Temporomandibular Joint Disorders

The specialty of otolaryngology plays a vital role in educating other health professionals about the consequences of misdiagnosing serious neoplastic conditions with symptoms that mimic COFHP and temporomandibular joint disorders. Unfortunately, there are numerous examples of patients with COFHP symptoms who were initially misdiagnosed and treated unsuccessfully for a routine COFHP, Temporomandibular Joint (TMJ), or dental disorder. However, failed treatment with persistent symptoms must alert the clinician that the diagnosis may be faulty. There are serious consequences of continued failed treatment and misdiagnosis because this may lead to delayed diagnosis and treatment of a neoplastic process. An important rule for all clinicians to follow is as follows:

If the patient does not respond as expected to treatment based on the most likely diagnosis in one's differential diagnosis, then the clinician must reevaluate the diagnosis and rule out other conditions that may be causing the patient's symptoms.

The constant reevaluation of the diagnosis based on the patient's response to treatment is referred to as the Flexible Diagnoses-Management Concept. It is common, even for the experienced clinician, to be uncertain of the diagnosis and treatment of a patient with chronic orofacial pain, which is unlike the more common situation in which a patient with acute pain and swelling presents with an abscess that is generally easy to diagnose, treat, and cure. As this is not the case with patients with chronic pain, it is important for the clinician to have a different mind-set with the development of differential diagnoses that remain flexible. The concept here is that the clinician develops an initial differential diagnoses and treats the patient according to the most likely condition or conditions causing the chronic pain. Based on the response to treatment, there is a continual reevaluation of the diagnoses and treatment. Failure to constantly reevaluate the response to treatment and diagnosis can lead to serious consequences with misdiagnosis of lethal pathologic conditions that mimic COFHP and temporomandibular joint disorders.

Most importantly, the clinical presentation needs to be looked at carefully. Patients with jaw pain, limitation of mobility, and deviation of the mandible to one side on opening often have an intra-articular temporomandibular joint pathology. However, there are other pathologic conditions that can lead to deviation of the mandible. The motor branches of the fifth cranial nerve provide innervation to the muscles of mastication, including the masseter, temporalis, lateral, and medial pterygoid muscles. As the lateral pterygoid muscle attaches to the mandibular condyle and anterior capsule of the temporomandibular joint, it is responsible for translation of the temporomandibular joint. Lack of motor function of the lateral pterygoid muscle will cause failure of translation of the mandibular condyle during jaw opening movements, resulting in deviation of the mandible to the affected side because of the unopposed action of the lateral pterygoid muscle on the unaffected side. The clinician must be thorough and check for normal motor function of the muscles of mastication. Lack of muscle tone of the masseter, temporalis and lateral pterygoid muscles must alert the clinician to a fifth cranial nerve deficit as the cause of the mandibular deviation with opening.

Furthermore, once there is clear evidence of a cranial nerve deficit, the clinician must assume a diagnosis of neoplasia until proven otherwise.

Central lesions affecting the trigeminal ganglion often cause symptoms that are located in the peripheral distribution of the fifth cranial nerve (**Fig. 2**). Therefore, dental pain in the absence of objective evidence of local pathologic condition must be viewed with suspicion. Complicating the clinical picture is the fact that there are many painful dental conditions that do not manifest with clear objective clinical findings.

For example, a painful inflammation of the dental pulp caused by decay may not demonstrate any pathologic condition seen on radiographs, particularly if the patient has a metal crown on the tooth. Masticatory muscle pain from clenching also has negative radiographic findings. Therefore, once treatment of these conditions is initiated, it is extremely important to evaluate the patient's response to treatment. If the symptoms persist, it is necessary to reevaluate the diagnosis, and the clinician must consider the possibility of the local pain being caused by a central pathology.

Dental pain does not necessarily originate from the oral cavity. Central nervous system pathology can cause pain in the oral and maxillofacial region. There are numerous examples of dental pain treated by numerous clinicians without any relief because the pain was caused by a central nervous system lesion. A common condition that often presents with a history of numerous failed dental treatments is trigeminal neuralgia. A careful history reveals that the character of the pain is shocklike, usually unilateral and so severe that it stops the patient in the middle of a sentence. Although the pain is of high intensity, it is often short in duration (usually seconds) and there is often a trigger point that will suddenly bring on the severe pain with an innocuous stimulus. A light touch to the face, wind on the face, or brushing teeth is often the triggering stimulus for the severe pain from trigeminal neuralgia. Once the diagnosis is established, initial treatment is usually a course of anticonvulsant medication (eg. gabapentin, carbamazepine). It is extremely important for trigeminal neuralgia to be viewed as a symptom, and thus, a brain scan is necessary to determine if there is a central nervous system lesion compressing the trigeminal nerve. If medications fail to control the severe symptoms, the patient should be referred to a neurologic surgeon.

Another common scenario for the otolaryngologist is the patient with persist dental pain and failed dental treatment in the presence of maxillary sinusitis. Infection of the

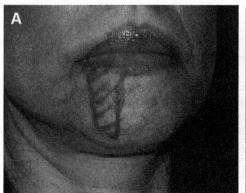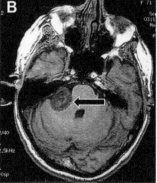

Fig. 2. (*A*) Patient with chronic right mandibular pain treated for 2 years with multiple failed dental treatments. The patient had paresthesia involving the right lower lip and chin. (*B*) MRI demonstrating an acoustic neuroma (*arrow*).

maxillary sinus will cause pain because of nociceptive stimulation of the posterior, middle, and anterior superior divisions of the maxillary nerve (V2). These sensory nerves are also stimulated when there is dental pathology of the maxillary posterior teeth, and therefore, patients with maxillary sinusitis often complain of severe tooth pain with dental interventions failing to resolve symptoms (**Fig. 3**).

The clinician must be aware of systemic pathologic conditions that can cause temporomandibular and oral, facial, and head pain. Conditions such as fibromyalgia, rheumatoid arthritis, psoriasis, and osteoarthritis can affect the temporomandibular joint and the surrounding muscles of mastication causing severe symptoms. Patients with multiple sclerosis are more prone to trigeminal neuralgia. If there is a history of herpes zoster, facial pain can occur because of postherpetic neuralgia. Cardiac ischemia is also a common cause of facial pain. The pain may occur in the throat, mandible, temporomandibular joint, and teeth. Approximately 32% of patients with cardiac ischemia had craniofacial pain along with other cardiac symptoms. One study revealed that craniofacial pain was the only complaint in 6% of individuals with cardiac ischemia.[2] As cardiac ischemia and acute myocardial infarction require immediate referral and management, the implications for the treating clinician are significant.

TEMPOROMANDIBULAR JOINT AND MASTICATORY MUSCLE DISORDERS: CURRENT CONCEPTS OF DIAGNOSIS AND MANAGEMENT

Perhaps one of the most common of the COHFP disorders that causes otologic symptoms without otologic pathology is the group of disorders encompassing inflammatory/degenerative temporomandibular joint disease as well as disorders of the muscles of mastication. TMD is an extremely broad and nonspecific diagnostic term, encompassing both joint and muscle disorders of the masticatory system. To specify whether a diagnosis is primarily intra-articular (coming directly from the temporomandibular joint) or primarily extra-articular (coming from structures outside the temporomandibular joint) is far more useful in patient management.

Other extra-articular conditions beyond the common masticatory muscle disorders can mimic temporomandibular joint disease, for example, coronoid hyperplasia, neoplasia, deep space infections, and myositis ossificans. Here the authors focus on the most common temporomandibular joint and masticatory muscle conditions that the clinician is likely to encounter. The abbreviation TMJ should be avoided and, when used, should refer solely to the anatomic structure. The term TMJ is often inappropriately used by patients and some health professionals to include the variety of disorders of the musculoskeletal component of the head and neck affecting the temporomandibular joint and surrounding masticatory muscles.

Temporomandibular joint disorders are relatively common in the general population. Acute TMD symptoms such as pain, limitation of mandibular opening and impaired masticatory function are experienced in approximately 40% of the US population.[3] LeResche[4] reported that pain in the temporomandibular region occurs in 10% of the adult US population, involves mostly young and middle-aged adults, and has a female predilection. Another study reported that over a 6-month period, 10.8 million adults (6.0% of the US adult civilian population) experienced jaw joint and facial pain.[5] Women reported these symptoms 2.1 times more frequently than men. TMD symptoms have a peak occurrence between ages 20 and 40 years and are reported to be more prevalent in women than in men.[6] Studies show that approximately 5% of people with symptoms seek treatment.

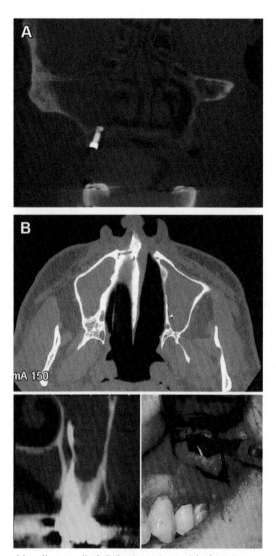

Fig. 3. (*A*) 60-year-old well-controlled diabetic patient with chronic congestion and discomfort of the right side of the face after dental implant placement. This cone beam scan demonstrates a completely opacified right maxillary sinus and an implant that has entered the maxillary sinus. Removal of the implant along with a Caldwell-Luc maxillary antrotomy and debridement revealed aspergillosis as the cause of the maxillary sinusitis. The removal of the pathology along with a 2-month course of antifungal medication resulted in complete resolution of the maxillary sinusitis. (*B*) Image of a 51-year-old man with onset of severe left-sided dental pain 2 days after endodontic therapy on a maxillary left first molar tooth. The diagnosis was acute maxillary sinusitis caused by reaction to endodontic material placed beyond the apex of the palatal root of the maxillary left first molar. Removal of the foreign body material, debridement, and evacuation of infected material from the maxillary sinus along with a course of antibiotics resulted in complete resolution of this infection.

Pathogenesis of Inflammatory/Degenerative Temporomandibular Joint Disorders

Internal derangement theory: a flawed approach to temporomandibular joint disorders

Internal derangement refers to a displaced position of the articular disk (usually anteriorly) of the temporomandibular joint. This condition was once considered to be central in the pathogenesis of temporomandibular joint disorders.[7] Anterior disk displacement was believed to be the major cause of intra-articular symptoms. The progression from anterior disk displacement to osteoarthritis and disk perforation was erroneously believed to be inevitable; therefore, conservative and surgical treatments were designed to reposition a displaced disk. Acceptance of the internal derangement theory led to flawed treatments without a valid research basis. As disk displacement is extremely common in asymptomatic individuals, our current understanding of temporomandibular joint pathogenesis does not support therapeutic interventions designed to reposition or replace a diseased disk.[8]

Current research has presented overwhelming evidence that temporomandibular joint disk displacement is the end result of changes in biochemistry and tissues caused by external factors such as overload and lack of movement. Ultimately, these external factors lead to tissue failure and altered joint biomechanics.

Patients with disk displacement presenting as a clicking joint, without significant symptoms of pain or altered range of motion, do not require surgical treatment. The clinician should view disk displacement as a flaw in joint biomechanics, which has occurred as a result of joint overloading. Disk displacement may be totally asymptomatic without any pain or limitation of function. Much research has been performed on temporomandibular joint pathology over the past 2 decades. The results of findings from clinical studies, magnetic resonance imaging (MRI) studies and synovial fluid analyses have provided compelling evidence that internal derangement theory as a major pathologic entity is flawed.[8–19] Research performed by Stegenga and colleagues[20,21] has furthered our understanding of temporomandibular joint pathogenesis, resulting in cartilage degradation. These studies concluded that abnormal disk position is the end result of degenerative changes that occur within the articular tissues.

Synovial fluid analysis research has provided great insight into the pathogenesis of inflammatory and degenerative conditions involving the temporomandibular joint. Studies involving obtaining synovial fluid samples and correlating the biochemical changes in the fluid with the morphologic alterations seen with arthroscopy have been extremely valuable. Biochemical changes and alteration in the structure and function of the synovial joint tissues occur in response to joint overloading and immobilization. Elevations in levels of inflammatory mediators[12,13,22] and proteoglycan degradation products[15,16,23,24] occur in the synovial fluids of pathologic temporomandibular joints. These biochemical abnormalities result in morphologic changes in the tissues including synovial inflammation and cartilage degradation (fibrillation). Osteoarthritis results in breakdown of the articular cartilage, which also impairs the sliding ability of opposing articular surfaces. Synovial inflammation causes pain and impaired lubrication leading to reduction in joint mobility. The combination of synovial inflammation and immobilization leads to temporomandibular joint adhesions, resulting in a further decrease in mobility.[25] Orthopedic studies[26,27] have shown that joint immobilization leads to adhesions, impaired cartilage nutrition, and cartilage degradation. Therefore, in patients with painful limitation of mandibular opening due to synovitis and osteoarthritis, there is a cycle of joint overloading leading to synovitis and osteoarthritis and reduced joint mobility. This condition leads to further adhesions, decreases in joint motion, pain, and more cartilage degradation (**Fig. 4**).

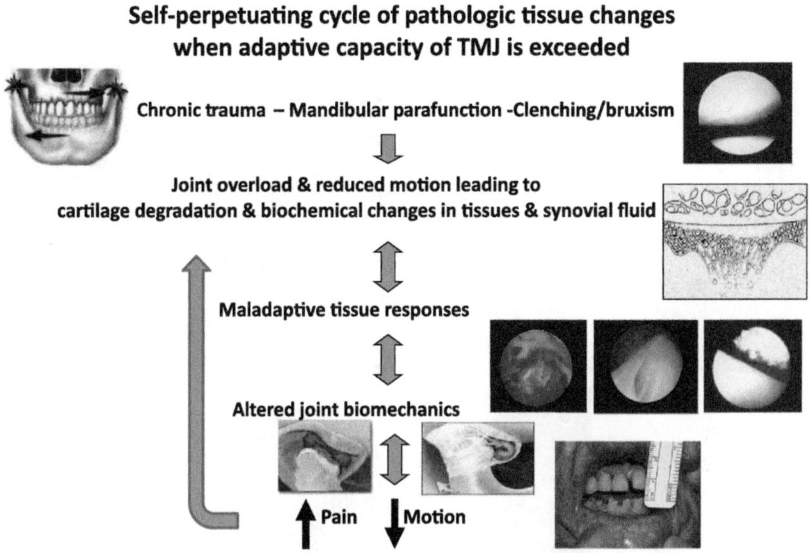

Fig. 4. Excessive loading of a synovial joint leads to biochemical alterations causing mal-adaptive tissue responses, including synovitis, osteoarthritis, and adhesions. Pathologic fail-ure of these tissues lead to pain and altered mobility, which then lead to a cycle of further limitation of mobility, pain, and progression of tissue damage.

Maladaptive changes in synovial joints

Successful management of temporomandibular joint pathology must be based on reducing the external factors that lead to the underlying tissue abnormalities. The 2 major factors that contribute to the loss of structure and function of the temporomandibular joint are joint overloading and joint immobilization. Joint overloading, is usually caused by parafunctional masticatory habits such as clenching or bruxism. When excessive joint loading exceeds the adaptive capacity of the tissue, cartilage degradation occurs. Cartilage degradation products in the synovial fluid lead to synovitis.

Decreased joint mobility also leads to maladaptive tissue responses. Because movement is necessary for the diffusion of synovial fluid through cartilage to provide nutrition of chondrocytes, failure of this movement leads to chondrocyte death, leading to a failure of matrix production and a further breakdown of the articular cartilage. Reduced mobility, as well as the pain from synovial inflammation, leads to the formation of intra-articular adhesions, which further reduces mobility. These factors ultimately lead to a self-perpetuating cycle of reduced range of motion, synovitis, adhesions, and osteoarthritis (see **Fig. 4**).

Maladaptive changes in the tissues can be seen arthroscopically. Osteoarthritis (**Fig. 5**A), synovitis (see **Fig. 5**B), and adhesions (see **Fig. 5**C) are the major tissue pathologies that lead to altered joint biomechanics, pain, and limitation of function. These maladaptive tissue changes are not independent of each other and often coexist within the same damaged joint.

The clinical evaluation

A complete history and clinical examination are the most important diagnostic tools to establish a correct diagnosis. Having the patient point directly to the perceived location of the pain is extremely helpful. Pain due to intra-articular pathology is often well localized to the temporomandibular joint, tends to be more acute in nature, and is

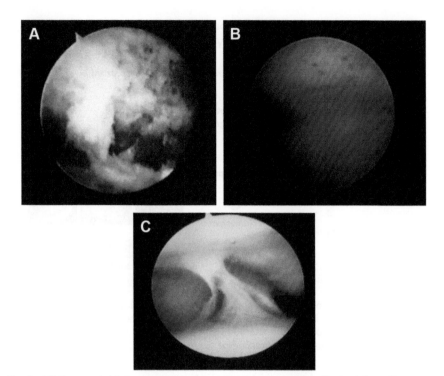

Fig. 5. (*A*) Osteoarthritis is common in symptomatic temporomandibular joints. The process of cartilage degradation because of joint overload leads to the appearance of fibrillation of the articular tissues. (*B*) Arthroscopic view of a temporomandibular joint with a grade 3 synovitis. The inflamed synovial tissues cause pain and swelling, leading to decreased joint movement and adhesions. The temporomandibular joint is constantly being loaded to permit the functions of eating, speaking, and swallowing. The presence of synovial inflammation and swelling along with further function and joint loading leads to further exacerbation and perpetuation of the inflammatory process. (*C*) Adhesions occur in the presence of continued synovitis and limited joint motion, which leads to a further decrease in mobility.

often associated with mandibular movement. Masticatory muscle pain is more diffuse in location and tends to be of a dull aching quality. The chronologic history should include when and how the symptoms began as well as assessment of past treatments and their effectiveness. A positive history of mandibular parafunction (clenching and bruxism) is an important finding. However, a negative history does not necessarily mean that there is an absence of the habit. Patients are often unaware of parafunctional habits, and they should be informed to become more aware of this habit.

Systemic conditions may manifest themselves in the temporomandibular joint and surrounding structures, creating symptoms that may initially seem to be due to local pathology. Therefore, a thorough medical history is required to determine if there are any systemic conditions, such as multiple sclerosis, rheumatoid arthritis, or other connective tissue disorders, that may be the cause of the symptoms.

The clinical examination should include the neck, extraoral structures, and intraoral structures. Examination of the dentition can reveal significant wear patterns on the occlusal surfaces of the teeth, providing secondary evidence of mandibular parafunction. Because the normal rest position of the mandible is with the teeth apart, a good clue to persistent clenching is to ask patients if they are aware of their upper and lower teeth touching during the day, when they are not eating. Once informed of this, patients often indicate that their teeth are together most of the day while they encounter the stresses of their daily life. The occlusion should also be evaluated; however, current research concerning an etiologic relationship between a malocclusion and TMD has failed to establish a definitive relationship.[28,29] An important symptom is an occlusion that is changing and getting worse. The patient often states that "my bite feels off and it is getting worse." Although tumors of the condyle and temporomandibular joint structures are not common, a progressive opening of the occlusion on one side is often the major symptom associated with a slowly expanding neoplasm in this region. An osteochondroma of the condyle is the most common tumor involving the temporomandibular joint (**Fig. 6A–H**).

The extraoral examination should include palpation of the temporomandibular joints including the lateral and posterior capsules (endaurally) to determine if there is tenderness. Pain due to palpation of the capsule is often a sign of synovial inflammation. Mandibular range of motion measurements should be obtained vertically as well as laterally. Maximum vertical opening is measured with a ruler from the incisal edge of the upper and lower central incisors (see **Fig. 1**, normal interincisal opening distance ranges from 35 to 55 mm). Deviation of the mandibular midline to one side during opening movements should be noted and usually represents a failure of translatory movement (sliding forward of the condyle along the articular eminence) on the side to which the mandible is deviating. Lateral excursion distances to the right and left are measured from the midline of the maxillary central incisor teeth to the midline of the mandibular central incisor teeth. Normal lateral excursions usually range from 8 to 15 mm and should not be painful. Protrusive (forward) mandibular movements should be performed, and any deviation should be noted.

Palpation of the muscles of mastication and the presence of tenderness is often a sign of myalgia or muscle spasm. The masseters, temporalis, as well as lateral and medial pterygoid muscles should be palpated bilaterally. Some patients have masseteric or temporalis hypertrophy, with extensive thickening of the muscles that can be seen simply by examining the face. Hypertrophied, firm, and enlarged muscles are usually signs of a mandibular parafunction.

Auscultation of the temporomandibular joints with a stethoscope should be performed to determine if there is clicking and/or crepitus. As TMJ sounds are common in the general population, the clinical significance of joint noise is questionable. Crepitus is often associated with degenerative joint conditions such as osteoarthritis. Clicking noises are associated with internal derangements (disk displacement) of the temporomandibular joint. Joint noise, in general, represents a biomechanical change in the joint as a response to joint overload.

The cranial nerve examination is an essential part of any thorough head and neck. For patients with chronic orofacial pain conditions, a thorough cranial nerve examination is essential and should be performed frequently at follow-up visits. When checking the facial nerve, it is important to determine if the weakness involves the entire side of the face or a portion of the face:

- A complete paralysis of one side of the face is usually an indication of a lower motor neuron lesion.
- If just the lower branches of the facial nerve are involved, this is more likely to be an upper motor neuron lesion.

The distinction between these 2 types of facial nerve dysfunction is important. The temporal branches of the facial nerve on one side receive input from upper motor

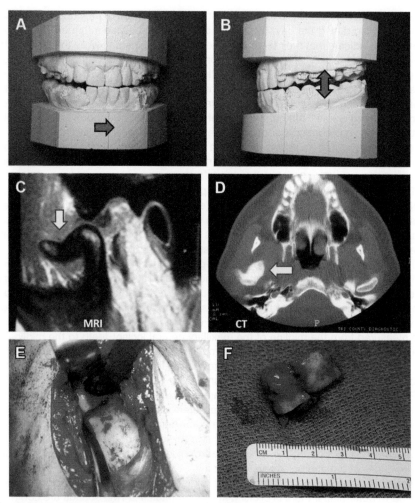

Fig. 6. (*A, B*) A 50-year-old woman presented with complaints of pain in the right temporo-mandibular joint and progressive shifting of her jaw to the left (*arrow*) causing an altered occlusion and facial asymmetry. The patient was treated for 2 years for a temporomandibular disorder with a night guard appliance; however, the symptoms progressed. Study models were obtained that demonstrated shifting of the mandible to the left and a posterior open bite (*arrows*). (*C, D*) MRI and computed tomography reveal a mass emanating from the right condyle (*arrows*). A tentative diagnosis of osteochondroma of the right mandibular condyle was made since this is the most common tumor involving the temporomandibular joint. (*E, F*) The osteochondroma was removed and an autogenous reconstruction was performed which restored the patient to a normal occlusion and total resolution of symptoms. (*G, H*) Postoperative radiograph following condylectomy and autogenous reconstruction resulting in a stable occlusion and correction of the facial asymmetry. The patient is currently 6 years postoperatively without any evidence of recurrence of the tumor or symptoms.

neurons bilaterally, because of decussation of these nerve fibers in the brain. The lower peripheral branches of the facial nerve receive upper motor neuron input from the ipsilateral side only. Thus, a centrally located lesion that affects the facial nerve will cause paralysis of only the lower half of the face. A peripherally located lesion

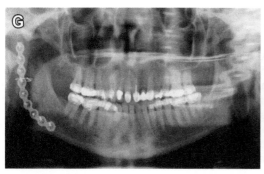
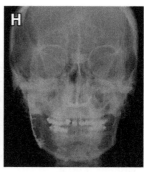

Fig. 6. (*continued*).

that affects the facial nerve, such as a parotid tumor, is likely to cause paralysis of all branches of the facial nerve on the side of the tumor.

Individuals who complain of sensory disturbances require a careful sensory examination. The simplest form of this examination is to map the area of altered sensation. A photograph will serve as a reference point to determine if the area of altered sensation is changing. If the map of the area of altered sensation follows the distribution of one of the sensory nerves, then it is highly suggestive of a pathologic condition or trauma that is altering normal sensory activity. Further investigation of both peripheral and central causes of altered sensory activity is required. Local pathology can often be diagnosed with radiographs and diagnostic images (computed tomography [CT] or MRI). Pathologic condition of the central nervous system that alters sensation requires an MRI and/or CT of the brain. Demyelinating diseases, such as multiple sclerosis, and intracranial tumors, such as acoustic neuroma, are common central causes of altered sensation involving the orofacial structures. Patients with masticatory muscle spasm often have intermittent areas of altered sensation that do not follow an anatomic distribution, which is most likely because of the effect of increased muscle activity causing intermittent impingement of terminal sensory fibers.

Radiographic evaluation of the maxilla, mandible, and temporomandibular joints is often necessary for completion of the examination. A panoramic radiograph is a tomogram of the maxilla and mandible and is nonspecific but useful as a screening tool for gross hard tissue pathology that may be present. The panoramic examination can reveal dental pathology, infections, maxillary sinusitis, facial fractures, and significant bony pathologies of the temporomandibular joint (**Fig. 7**). Bilateral temporomandibular

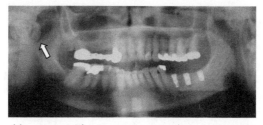

Fig. 7. An 80-year-old woman with no symptoms undergoes a routine panoramic radiographic examination for evaluation for implants. The panoramic radiograph demonstrates severe osteoarthritis of the right temporomandibular joint with heterotopic bone formation (*arrow*). No temporomandibular joint treatment is necessary because the patient is asymptomatic. This case demonstrates that diagnostic images do not necessarily correlate with the clinical examination or the presence of symptoms.

joint radiographs in the open and closed positions can be obtained from most panoramic equipment and are helpful in the assessment of temporomandibular joint structure and function. Panoramic radiographs are readily available in most oral and maxillofacial surgery offices. However, a limitation of the panoramic radiograph is that it will only demonstrate significant bony pathology, and therefore, it is not a sensitive technique for diagnosing intra-articular temporomandibular joint pathology. Cone beam scans are now readily available in many oral and maxillofacial surgery offices, which provide a low-cost, low-radiation option for obtaining a CT scan of the temporomandibular joints in the axial, coronal, and sagittal planes, as well as 3-dimensional reconstruction. A cone beam or CT scan of the temporomandibular joints is most useful for seeing bony pathology such as tumors, bony/fibrous ankylosis, and osteoarthritis (**Fig. 8**).

MRI has been extremely helpful in more recent years in the diagnosis of soft tissue pathology. Synovial joint effusion, osteoarthritis, and disk displacements can be detected with MRIs of the TMJ (**Fig. 9**). Recent studies have demonstrated a high incidence of disk displacement in asymptomatic subjects[9,30,31]; therefore, the clinician must use diagnostic imaging as an adjunct to the overall evaluation of the patient. Advanced diagnostic imaging should be performed when patients do not respond to conservative treatment or when there is clinical and radiographic evidence that significant pathologic condition, such as neoplasia, exists.

Principles of Nonsurgical Management of Inflammatory/Degenerative Temporomandibular Joint Disorders

The most common symptoms that are associated with temporomandibular joint disease are intra-articular pain, limitation of mandibular range of motion, and joint noises (clicking and/or crepitus). As these symptoms are nonspecific, they can reflect common temporomandibular joint pathologies, such as synovitis, adhesions, and osteoarthritis, or they may reflect more serious conditions such as neoplasia (osteochondroma and chondrosarcoma), fibrous/bony ankylosis, or systemic conditions (rheumatoid arthritis, psoriatic arthritis). The principles of treatment are also based on an accurate diagnosis and a thorough understanding of the pathogenesis of the

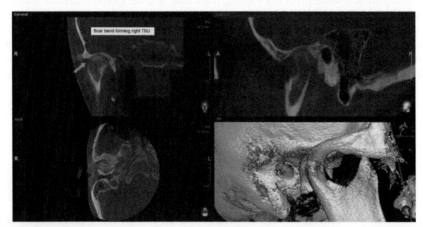

Fig. 8. Cone beam scan of the right temporomandibular joint in a patient with significant restriction in mandibular opening due to intra-articular pathology. The cone beam demonstrates early osteoarthritic changes as well as the development of scar tissue that is beginning to calcify (*arrow*). This patient has a fibrous ankylosis, which will lead to a bony ankylosis without further treatment.

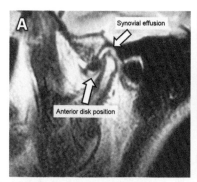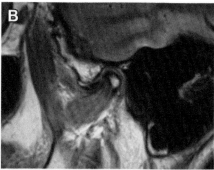

Fig. 9. (*A*) MRI T2 images demonstrating a significant synovial effusion and anterior disk position. (*B*) MRI demonstrating significant osteoarthritic changes. A disk perforation was present when the patient underwent arthroscopic surgery.

disease process. The following concepts are essential in the nonsurgical treatment of patients:

Reduction of joint loading

As joint overload leads to cartilage degradation, the clinician must be aware of parafunctional masticatory activities and control their deleterious effects. A soft nonchew diet for a specified period is necessary to reduce loading of the temporomandibular joint and associated muscles.

Patients' education involves informing them of the deleterious effects of clenching and making them aware of episodes in which their teeth come together during times of stress. Occlusal splint appliances are sometimes fabricated by the patient's dentist to distribute the forces equally between the maxillary and mandibular teeth during mandibular parafunction. These appliances work best in individuals with chronic pain from masticatory muscles. It is important to understand that these appliances do not prevent clenching and bruxism. The clinician must carefully evaluate the patient's response to these appliances because some individuals tend to clench more when there is an appliance in their mouth.

Maximize joint mobility

Orthopedic research has shown that joint immobilization has deleterious effects. Immobilization leads to joint adhesion and muscle atrophy. Passive motion exercises are an important part of synovial joint rehabilitation. Passive motion occurs when joint movement does not involve the use of the muscle groups that normally move the joint.

Passive motion exercises performed as a daily routine at home are essential for the restoration of normal joint mobility. Passive motion therapy for the temporomandibular joint can be achieved with a variety of devices designed to move the mandible by squeezing the device by hand (**Fig. 10**). Patients are generally instructed to perform these exercises for 5 minutes 3 to 4 times daily, after massage or moist heat applications. Frequent moist heat applications, massage, and ice applications are important adjuncts to passive motion exercises and help to reduce masticatory muscle spasm and myalgia. A great advantage of home passive motion exercises by patients is that their own proprioception can be used to achieve the maximum stretch without creating significant pain.

Reduction of inflammation and pain

If the patient attempts to function on inflamed synovial tissues, more inflammation is stimulated. For this reason, it is often quite difficult to reduce temporomandibular joint

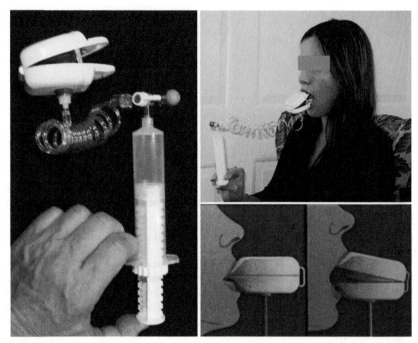

Fig. 10. E-Z Flex II passive jaw motion device uses a gentle air pump mechanism to mobilize the mandible. When the patient depresses the plunger, air from the syringe causes gentle separation of the upper and lower members of the mouthpiece. This device is used in patients with limitation of jaw opening from temporomandibular disorders as well as from other causes. Use of passive motion in patients undergoing radiation therapy to the head and neck for oral and pharyngeal cancer is necessary to prevent radiation-induced trismus. (*Courtesy of* Therapeutic Mobilization Devices, LLC, Great Neck, NY; with permission.)

inflammation as a result of constant use of the TMJ involved in speech, chewing, swallowing, and so on. However, inflammation of synovial tissues must be controlled for the temporomandibular joint to recover normal joint function. The inflammatory process can often be managed with nonsteroidal antiinflammatory medications, such as ibuprofen and naproxen. Unfortunately, it is common for patients to use these medications improperly by discontinuing use of the medication once the pain subsides in conjunction with attempts to resume a normal diet, causing reoccurrence of the symptoms because of persistent joint inflammation. For nonsteroidal antiinflammatory medications to be effective, they must be taken for at least 7 to 14 days, in conjunction with joint unloading, to attempt to reduce synovial inflammation. Some patients benefit from a short course of steroid medications; however, steroids should be used sparingly and generally reserved for acute exacerbations of synovial inflammation that are unresponsive to nonsteroidal antiinflammatory medications. If this course of treatment fails to significantly reduce the symptoms, it is an indication that the synovial inflammation is unlikely to be reversible with standard nonsurgical treatment.

Pain management is a necessary component of patient management. Failure to control pain levels, along with chronic tissue injury, has the potential to lead to central sensitization of ascending nerve pathways that transmit pain, leading to chronic neuropathic pain. This pain leads to symptoms of allodynia, in which nonnoxious stimuli, such as light touch, activate pain pathways leading to the cerebral cortex. An important goal in the management of these patients is to prevent the onset of chronic central neuropathic pain. With the onset of chronic neuropathic pain, local treatment of the diseased joint as well as a reduction in the activity of the central pain pathways is needed. However, successful management of the patient who has developed chronic neuropathic pain is much more difficult, because multiple surgical procedures and repeated trauma to tissues tend to exacerbate central sensitization of the ascending pain pathways.[32–38]

Local anesthetic injections to reduce pain may be helpful in the management of chronic neuropathic pain in conjunction with medications (anticonvulsants, such as gabapentin) that reduce activity of nerve pathways. Narcotic analgesics generally are not recommended in the management of chronic temporomandibular joint pain, because the pain relief is often brief, followed by rebound pain. A short course of narcotic analgesics can be prescribed for the management of postoperative pain. For patients who have complex chronic pain that does not respond to the aforementioned modalities, referral to a pain management specialist is recommended.

Recognize and treat masticatory muscle disorders
Masticatory muscle spasm is common in patients with COHFP, irrespective of the source of the pain, and represents a natural response to immobilize injured tissues. Patients who have severe pain from intra-articular temporomandibular joint pathology will often have significant masticatory muscle spasm and myalgia (muscle pain). Because joint overload from parafunctional masticatory activity is a common factor leading to joint pathology, it is often difficult for the clinician to determine whether the main pathology is intra-articular, with secondary masticatory muscle spasm, or it is masticatory muscle spasm and myalgia, with secondary joint inflammation. Muscle relaxant medications, massage, heat, and passive motion exercises are often helpful in treating chronic masticatory muscle spasm.

Relationship Between TMDs and Headache

Many patients with TMDs complain of headaches. The prevalence of headache in patients with TMD has been reported to be as high as 70% to 85%.[39–41] There is evidence that disorders of the masticatory muscles, related to parafunctional activities such as clenching or nocturnal bruxism, may be related to tension headache.[41–45] Because both headache and TMD symptoms are extremely common, the precise relationship between these 2 conditions is not known. A daily headache that occurs on awakening is often a symptom related to nocturnal bruxism. Patients frequently point to the temporalis muscle region as the primary location of their morning headache. Some patients indicate that stressful periods during the day cause them to clench their teeth and are associated with the symptoms of headache and diffuse jaw pain in the masseter and temporalis regions. If it has been determined that the cause of the headache is masticatory muscle spasm, and other causes of head pain have been ruled out, the treatment is the same as described previously for masticatory muscle disorders. However, it is important for the patient with headache to get a thorough neurologic evaluation to rule out other potential pathologic conditions. Referral to a neurologist and a brain MRI are often a necessary part of the workup.

Principles of Surgical Management of Temporomandibular Joint Disorders

Temporomandibular joint surgery is not a common treatment of routine temporomandibular joint disorders. However, when there is true intra-articular pathology and mandibular dysfunction that does not respond to routine treatment, surgical intervention is likely to be needed. The indications for performing temporomandibular joint surgery in the population of patients with significant temporomandibular joint symptoms and pathologic condition are as follows:

1. The patient has severe pain and/or mandibular dysfunction.
2. The cause of the pain and/or mandibular dysfunction is a diagnosis consistent with significant intra-articular pathology (usually synovitis, osteoarthritis, adhesions).
3. A full course of appropriate nonsurgical therapy has failed to improve the patient's symptoms.

Temporomandibular joint surgery does not necessarily reduce pain (unless if the sensory innervation to the joint is disrupted) but is designed to restore joint structure and function, and patients must understand that the postoperative period requires significant rehabilitation. With proper patient selection, appropriate surgery, and postoperative compliance with passive motion exercises, medications, and reduction of joint loads, most patients will ultimately have significant reduction in pain levels and improvement in mandibular functioning.

The principles of surgical management are as follows:

1. The least invasive procedure with the highest benefit to risk ratio should be performed.
2. Surgical procedures should be designed to remove and/or treat the pathologic tissue that is present.
3. Surgical procedures should assist in the reduction of synovial inflammation. Arthroscopic surgery enables the surgeon to isolate the areas of synovitis and inject a high concentration of antiinflammatory medication under direct vision into the most inflamed synovial tissues.
4. Surgical procedures should result in maximum preservation of the synovium, articular cartilage, and disk.
5. All operative procedures, whether performed under general anesthesia, conscious sedation, or local anesthesia, should be accompanied by the administration of local anesthesia to the surgical site. This administration will prevent barrages of noxious stimuli transmitted by peripheral sensory nerves from reaching the central nervous system.

The surgical options that are available to treat the more common temporomandibular joint disorders include arthrocentesis, arthroscopy, and arthrotomy. For patients who have a joint space, and have a clinical diagnosis of synovitis, osteoarthritis, and/or adhesions, arthrocentesis and arthroscopy are the least invasive surgical options. Arthrocentesis involves the insertion of 2 needles into the superior joint space and irrigating the joint with normal saline or lactated Ringer solution. Arthrocentesis is generally more effective when the onset of symptoms is of a relatively short duration, usually less than 3 months. Arthrocentesis is not effective if there are joint adhesions. Another disadvantage of arthrocentesis is that the actual pathologic condition cannot be visualized. A biopsy specimen cannot be obtained for histopathologic examination. Over recent years, temporomandibular joint arthroscopic surgery is being performed more frequently in an office setting.[46] Arthroscopic surgery has the advantage of permitting direct visualization and treatment of intra-articular pathology and when performed by an experienced surgeon, is minimally invasive. Thus, H.A.I. now rarely performs arthrocentesis because in office, arthroscopic surgery has significant advantages.

Arthroscopic temporomandibular joint surgery has the advantage of being minimally invasive, does not require incisions or sutures, and is associated with a rapid recovery, compared to open joint surgery. The procedure is performed in an ambulatory setting (either in the operating room or in a properly equipped office setting) permitting the patient to recover at home on the same day of the surgery. Once diagnostic arthroscopy has been completed, the areas of pathology can be identified. A second portal of entry enables the surgeon to perform operative procedures under direct vision with the arthroscope being present in one portal and the surgical instruments entering through the second portal. Operative arthroscopic surgery is designed to treat the pathologic condition that is present with maximum preservation of intra-articular tissues (**Fig. 11A–F**). Adhesions are released with miniblades and removed with alligator forceps or motorized shaving instruments. Synovitis is treated by directly isolating the most inflamed tissue and injection of a high concentration of steroid medication in the subsynovial tissues under direct vision. Identifying and treating synovial inflammation is an important part of this procedure. Osteoarthritic fibrillation tissue is removed with forceps and/or motorized shaving instruments. The removal of tissue specimens enables the surgeon to obtain histopathologic confirmation of the correct diagnosis. Occasionally, other uncommon pathologic conditions are diagnosed such as synovial chondromatosis, chondrocalcinosis, and pigmented villonodular synovitis. Anteriorly displaced disks are mobilized to improve translation in the superior joint space. Although there are some arthroscopic surgeons who stabilize the disk in a posterior position through a variety of techniques, H.A.I. opines that this is not necessary or indicated, because there are many asymptomatic individuals with anterior disk position.

Open joint surgery, which formerly was the mainstay of surgical treatment of the patient with intra-articular pathology, still has a place in the armamentarium of the oral and maxillofacial surgeon for the treatment of extensive intra-articular temporomandibular joint pathology. Because less-invasive procedures such as arthroscopy have a proven record of success in treating painful intra-articular pathologies, these modalities should be considered first. However, when the joint space is obliterated by fibrous and/or bony ankylosis, arthrotomy is the surgical treatment of choice. Conditions such as neoplasia (osteochondroma), synovial chondromatosis, and pigmented villonodular synovitis require open joint surgical procedures to remove the pathologic condition and restore joint function. There are numerous methods of reconstructing temporomandibular joints including autogenous reconstruction, distraction osteogenesis, and alloplastic temporomandibular joint reconstruction (**Fig. 12**).

The development of fibrous or bony ankylosis of the temporomandibular joint after arthroplasty is a potential risk of open joint surgery (**Fig. 13**). Because excellent outcomes can be achieved in these patients with a minimally invasive approach involving arthroscopic surgery, the authors believe that arthroplasty with disk repositioning surgery should be avoided.

Surgical outcomes

Studies reporting the outcomes of surgical treatment of temporomandibular joint disorders are usually retrospective cases series. These reports are fairly consistent, with reported success rates ranging from 75% to 90%.[47] Prospective, randomized, double-blind clinical studies are lacking and often impractical because most patients present with severe symptoms and a long history of failed nonsurgical treatments. Those patients who have been referred for a surgical evaluation are focused on treatments designed to relieve their symptoms, and these individuals are unlikely to submit to randomized treatments. Therefore, the published literature forces us to rely on reported case series to evaluate the outcomes of surgical treatment of temporomandibular joint disorders.

Numerous case studies on the outcomes of temporomandibular joint arthroscopy have demonstrated a significant reduction in pain, improved interincisal opening distance, and improved mandibular function without any change in disk position.

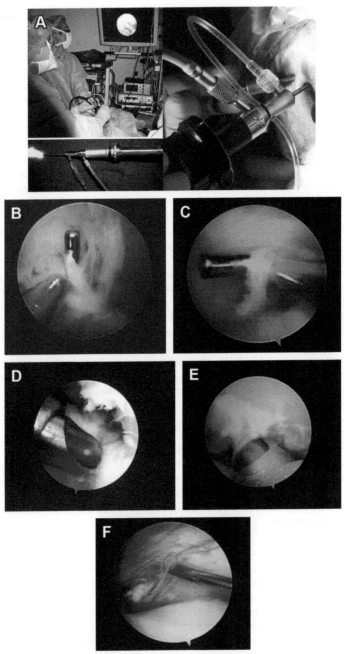

Fig. 11. (*A*) Temporomandibular joint arthroscopy setup. Because of the very small size of this joint, a very delicate arthroscope (usually 1.9 mm diameter or less) is used and special skills are needed by the surgeon to perform this operation successfully. (*B, C*) Operative arthroscopy demonstrating lysis of adhesions. (*D, E*) Operative arthroscopy with removal of pathologic osteoarthritic tissue with a motorized minishaver and a 2.0 full radius blade. (*F*) Direct injection of steroid (betamethasone 6 mg/mL) into areas of synovitis using a #25 gauge spinal needle.

A

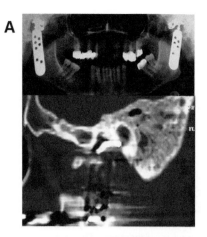

B

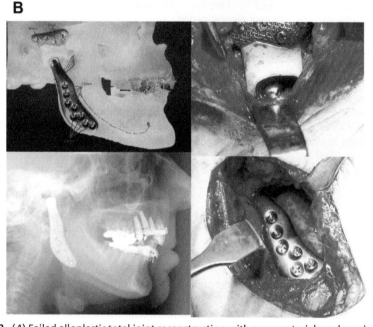

Fig. 12. (A) Failed alloplastic total joint reconstruction with poor materials and surgical technique from 15 years ago. This patient developed a chronic external otitis and mastoiditis because of erosion of the prosthesis into the external auditory canal. This older alloplastic total joint replacement system is no longer on the market. (B) Improved materials and surgical technique have resulted in successful alloplastic total joint replacement. This system (TMJ Concepts, Inc) is custom made on a 3-dimensional plastic model derived from a CT scan before surgical placement. A chrome cobalt condylar head articulates against ultrahigh molecular polyethylene fossa component. The fossa component is stabilized to the temporal bone with a custom-fitted titanium component and titanium screws. The mandibular condylar component is stabilized to the ramus of the mandible with a custom-fitted titanium component and titanium screws.

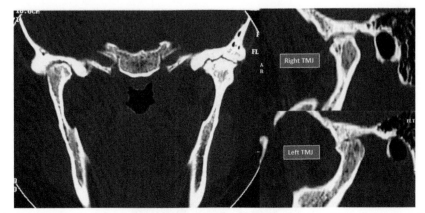

Fig. 13. Fibrous and bony ankylosis after multiple open temporomandibular joint surgeries including arthroplasty, followed by diskectomy. This patient needs chronic pain management and total joint replacement reconstruction.

Although ideal randomized controlled clinical studies evaluating the outcomes of arthroscopy do not exist, case series reports from different investigators have yielded remarkably consistent results. A compilation of 11 studies on the outcomes of arthroscopic surgery have demonstrated a mean success rate of 84%, with a mean reduction in pain levels on the visual analog scale of 4.6 after arthroscopy (mean follow-up 17.1 months) and a mean increase in interincisal opening distance of 10.4 mm.[48–58] These results are consistent with other published results on the outcomes of temporomandibular joint arthroscopy. A recent study compared the results of early versus late arthroscopic temporomandibular joint surgery.[59] Although both the early and late groups have significant reduction in pain and improvement in interincisal opening distance, the earlier group had better outcomes than the late group. This study suggests that prolonged unsuccessful nonsurgical therapy is not conservative and that early intervention with minimally invasive arthroscopic treatment can lead to improved outcomes.

Postoperative rehabilitation
Surgical procedures on the temporomandibular joint that are not followed by an appropriate postoperative rehabilitation regimen are very likely to fail. The surgeon must emphasize to the patient that the postoperative rehabilitation period is crucial in determining the outcome of the surgery. Postoperative rehabilitation designed to restore mandibular range of motion, prevent the formation of adhesions, reduce inflammation, and reduce the etiologic factors such as joint overloading are essential for surgical success.

Conceptually, the first goal after the surgery is to restore a normal mandibular range of motion. However, joint loading (chewing, mandibular parafunction) must be avoided. Although the regimen for each patient is different, based on their postoperative clinical course, the following are the general guidelines that are used. The patient is placed on a nonchew diet for approximately 3 weeks, to prevent loading of intra-articular tissues. This joint unloading is necessary to permit the tissues to recover, because early function and joint overload will precipitate the same factors that caused the initial pathologic condition. If the patient is minimally symptomatic by postoperative week 3, a gradual progression of the diet is permitted, as long as there is no exacerbation of pain or dysfunction. If pain occurs during chewing, the patient is instructed to continue on the nonchew diet for an additional week, until the loads of mastication on the temporomandibular joint are tolerated. If there is no pain during chewing, but if there is soreness in the muscles of mastication after chewing, this is to be expected due to disuse atrophy. Muscle atrophy from a prolonged period of mandibular dysfunction is present postoperatively, and a gradual return to function ultimately builds up the lost muscle strength.

Passive motion exercises are essential in the postoperative period and are necessary to prevent the formation of new adhesions and increase mandibular range of motion. A variety of techniques and devices are available to achieve passive range of motion exercises. H.A.I. prefers the use of E-Z Flex II (H.A.I. is the owner of TMD, LLC, Great Neck, New York, the manufacturer of E-Z Flex II), which uses an air pump mechanism that is gentle and promotes patient compliance (see **Fig. 10**). Other options for passive mandibular motion include other handheld devices, tongue blades, and finger stretching techniques. These exercises are performed thrice daily for 5 to 10 minutes, preceded by moist heat or massage, and followed by ice or massage. Physical therapy may be prescribed, particularly if the patient tends to be noncompliant with the exercises or if the patient's interincisal opening distance is not increasing as expected.

Postoperative pain management usually requires only a few days of narcotic analgesics. Long-term use of narcotics beyond the first postoperative week should be avoided. Nonsteroidal antiinflammatory medications and muscle relaxants (bedtime only) are frequently prescribed. Patients can usually return to their normal activities (work or school) within 4 to 7 days. Once the patient has an adequate range of mandibular motion and reduced pain (usually 4–12 weeks), the passive motion exercises are gradually reduced to twice daily, the consistency of the diet is advanced, and the medications are used as needed. Throughout the postoperative period, avoidance of those factors, such as mandibular parafunction, that contributed to the development of the temporomandibular joint disorder is essential. It is not uncommon for the patient with a high stress lifestyle to do quite well for a period while they are recuperating from the surgery. However, when patients return to their routine daily activities and the same demands and stresses at work or at home are placed on them, mandibular clenching habits return. It is important for the patient to become acutely aware of mandibular parafunction particularly during the day and to develop strategies for recognition and avoidance of habits that cause joint overload.

OTHER DISORDERS AFFECTING THE TEMPOROMANDIBULAR JOINT OF SPECIAL INTEREST TO THE OTOLARYNGOLOGIST
Radiation Fibrosis

Patients with oral and pharyngeal cancers who undergo radiation therapy require special consideration with respect to the importance of maintaining an adequate range of mandibular motion. It is well known that these patients are prone to recurrent cancers or new primary lesions. Thus, maintaining an acceptable interincisal opening distance is necessary to detect recurrent or second primary cancerous lesions at an early stage. Unfortunately, radiation therapy often causes fibrosis of the soft tissues including the muscles of mastication and the temporomandibular joint, resulting in severe restriction in mouth opening. Therefore, it is essential for these patients to perform passive motion exercises on a regular basis before, during, and after radiation therapy (see **Fig. 10**). The goal is to maintain and maximize mandibular range of motion to help offset the effects of radiation fibrosis causing trismus. Once radiation fibrosis and trismus has occurred, it is extremely difficult, if not impossible, to restore mandibular range of motion to an acceptable level. The importance of passive motion mandibular exercises to prevent trismus in patients before radiation therapy is often overlooked. Such overlooking is unfortunate because passive motion therapy is a simple, noninvasive therapy that can prevent or reduce trismus, ultimately improving quality of life and potentially permitting the early detection of oral and pharyngeal cancer.

The Relationship Between Tinnitus and TMDs

The association of tinnitus and other otologic symptoms with TMDs has been controversial, because Costen's article in 1934 reported direct causal relationships between temporomandibular joint disorders and tinnitus/otologia.[1] Objective tinnitus is caused by sounds generated in the body that reach the ear through conduction in body tissue. Subjective tinnitus is much more common, occurs without any physical sound reaching the ear, and is associated with abnormal neural activity generated in the ear, the auditory nerve, or the central nervous system.[60] Subjective tinnitus may occur with hearing loss after exposure to loud noise, after administration of certain drugs, as a symptom of vestibular schwannoma, or as a symptom of Meniere disease. However, most often the cause of tinnitus remains unknown.[60]

Epidemiologic studies have demonstrated tinnitus to be a common symptom in the general population, but with a higher prevalence in patients with TMD symptoms. One study reported the incidence of tinnitus to be 10% to 31% of the general population and up to 85% in the population of patients with TMD symptoms.[61] Another study reported similar findings, with 2 control populations having tinnitus in 13.8% and 32.5%, compared to a 59.6% prevalence of tinnitus in a population of patients with TMD symptoms.[62] The pathophysiological mechanisms between TMD and tinnitus are not well understood, and several attempts have been made to explain the associations.[62–64]

Morphologic and anatomic studies have confirmed a relationship between the middle ear and the temporomandibular joint through the connection between the malleus and the posterior capsule of the joint via the discomalleolar ligament.[65] The structures of the middle ear and TMJ are derived from the first brachial arch (mandibular arch) and thus are anatomically and morphogenically related. The discomalleolar ligament is an intrinsic fibrous ligament that connects the TMJ disk with the malleus of the middle ear. The discomalleolar ligament has fibers that attach to the upper lamina of the bilaminar zone of the articular disk of the temporomandibular joint. These fibers from the discomalleolar ligament attach to the posterosuperior and medial end of the articular disk and enter the middle ear through the most lateral portion of the petrotympanic fissure and the malleolar sulcus, ultimately attaching to the malleus.

The middle ear cavity is connected to the nasopharynx via the eustachian tube. Conditions that impair the opening of the eustachian tube can lead to the sensation of fullness or stuffiness in the ear.[66] Patients can somatically modulate tinnitus with jaw movements, swallowing, and external pressure on the temporomandibular joint.[67–69] The tensor tympani and tensor veli palatini are muscles that are necessary for normal eustachian tube function and are innervated by motor branches of the fifth cranial nerve. The muscles of mastication (masseter, temporalis, as well as medial and lateral pterygoids) are also innervated by the motor division of the fifth cranial nerve. In addition, noxious stimuli that affect the sensory branches of the fifth cranial nerve can affect ear sensations and cause a variety of otologic symptoms. Neural inputs of the trigeminal system are linked to the inner ear via the dorsal cochlear nucleus; thus, the central excitatory effects with the flexing and tightening on the tympanic membrane can bring about sensations of tinnitus and vertigo.[60,67,69] In spite of the close anatomic relationships between the temporomandibular joint, middle ear, eustachian tube, muscles of mastication, muscles of the nasopharynx, and the fifth cranial nerve, the precise mechanisms that produce the symptom of tinnitus remain to be elucidated.

Consistent with Costen's hypothesis are recent reports demonstrating that treatment of TMD symptoms often result in improvement of tinnitus and other otologic symptoms. In a study, 202 patients with TMD with coexisting tinnitus, otalgia, dizziness, and/or vertigo were treated for their TMD symptoms.[70] After satisfactory TMD symptom improvement was obtained, the percentage of subjects reporting significant improvement or resolution of their otologic symptoms was reported as follows: tinnitus 83%, otalgia 94%, dizziness 91%, and vertigo 100%. Other reports have suggested that otologic symptoms and tinnitus may improve with TMD therapy.[64,71–73] Methodological weaknesses of many of these studies have led others to conclude that the lack of prospective, controlled, and randomized studies regarding the effectiveness of TMD treatment as treatment of otalgia and tinnitus in patients with TMD are not well supported.[74] The influence of the placebo effect on otologic symptoms once TMD therapy is instituted cannot be overlooked. In spite of the uncertainty concerning the causal relationship between TMD therapy and otologic symptoms, it is important for the practicing clinician to provide the patient with an appropriate course of management. Therefore, if the patient has otologic symptoms that cannot be explained and if the otolaryngologist suspects the presence of a TMD, it is reasonable for the patient to be referred to a clinician with expertise in the diagnosis and management of TMDs and COHFP. If the consultation confirms the presence of a TMD, treatment of this disorder is certainly appropriate with an ongoing evaluation of the patient's signs and symptoms. If the otologic symptoms resolve, then one may conclude that there was perhaps a relationship between the TMD treatment and the otologic symptoms, although the placebo effect cannot be ruled out. If otologic symptoms persist, it is very important for the diagnosis and management to continue to be reevaluated with further intense workup for the correct diagnosis and course of treatment.

SUMMARY: THE ESSENTIAL ROLE OF THE OTOLARYNGOLOGIST IN DIAGNOSIS AND MANAGEMENT OF TEMPOROMANDIBULAR JOINT AND COHFP DISORDERS: A TEAM APPROACH

The specialist in otolaryngology is a key member of the team of physicians that diagnose and treat COHFP. Otalgia, headache, and facial pain are common symptoms in patients seeking consultation with the otolaryngologist. The challenge for each clinician is to be able to make an accurate diagnosis leading to appropriate timely treatment. Some patients have symptoms, signs, and clinical findings that are specific for local pathology, making diagnosis and treatment relatively clear and straightforward. Patients with COHFP as well as TMDs often have complex histories and clinical findings making it difficult to make an accurate diagnosis. The clinician must constantly reevaluate the patient's response to treatment to help confirm or negate the proposed diagnosis and to adjust treatment regimens accordingly.

When the diagnosis is unclear, referrals to appropriate specialists are a necessary component in the management of the patient with COHFP. Listed below are those specialties that are likely to be included in the management of the patient with chronic orofacial pain:

- Otolaryngology
- Oral and maxillofacial surgery
- Neurology
- Neurosurgery
- Rheumatology

- Psychiatry
- Psychology
- Anesthesiology
- General dentistry
- Endodontics
- Radiology
- Physical therapy
- Alternative medicine

The otolaryngologist should have a relationship with a group of specialists who are available to provide assistance in the diagnosis and management of the patient with COHFP. The clinician must be confident that these specialists are individuals who have the time, expertise, and willingness to take on the challenge of caring for these complex patients.

REFERENCES

1. Costen JB. A syndrome of ear and sinus symptoms dependent upon disturbed function of the temporomandibular joint. Ann Otol Rhinol Laryngol 1934;43(1): 1–15.
2. Kreiner M, Okeson JP, Michelis V, et al. Craniofacial pain as the sole symptom of cardiac ischemia: a prospective multicenter study. J Am Dent Assoc 2007;138(1): 74–9.
3. Scrivani SJ, Keith DA, Kaban LB. Temporomandibular disorders. N Engl J Med 2008;359:2693–705.
4. LeResche L. Epidemiology of temporomandibular disorders: implications for the investigation of etiologic factors. Crit Rev Oral Biol Med 1997;8(3):291–305.
5. Lipton JA, Ship JA, Larach-Robinson D. Estimated prevalence and distribution of reported orofacial pain in the United States. J Am Dent Assoc 1993;124:115–21.
6. Liu F, Steinkeler A. Epidemiology, diagnosis, and treatment of temporomandibular disorders. Dent Clin North Am 2013;57(3):465–79.
7. McCarty WL, Farrar WB. Surgery for internal derangements of the temporomandibular joint. J Prosthet Dent 1979;42(2):191–6.
8. Dolwick MF. Intra-articular disc displacement part I: its questionable role in temporomandibular joint pathology. J Oral Maxillofac Surg 1995;53:1069–72.
9. Moore JB. Coronal and sagittal TMJ meniscus position in asymptomatic subjects by MRI [abstract]. J Oral Maxillofac Surg 1989;47:75.
10. Kircos LT, Ortendahl DA, Mark AS, et al. Magnetic resonance imaging of the TMJ disc in asymptomatic volunteers. J Oral Maxillofac Surg 1987;45:852–4.
11. Trumpy IG, Lyberg T. Surgical treatment of internal derangement of the temporomandibular joint: long-term evaluation of three techniques. J Oral Maxillofac Surg 1995;53:746–7.
12. Quinn JH, Bazan NG. Identification of prostaglandin E2 and leukotriene B4 in the synovial fluid of painful, dysfunctional temporomandibular joints. J Oral Maxillofac Surg 1990;48:968.
13. Shafer DM, Assael L, White LB, et al. Tumor necrosis factor alpha as a biochemical marker of pain and outcome in temporomandibular joints with internal derangements. J Oral Maxillofac Surg 1994;52:786.
14. Kopp S. Neuroendocrine, immune and local responses related to temporomandibular disorders. J Orofac Pain 2001;15:9.
15. Ratcliffe A, Israel HA. Proteoglycan components of articular cartilage in synovial fluids as potential markers of osteoarthritis of the temporomandibular joint. In:

Sessle BJ, Bryant PS, Dionne RA, editors. Temporomandibular disorders and related pain conditions, progress in pain research and management, vol. 4. Seattle (WA): IASP Press; 1995. p. 141–50.

16. Israel H, Diamond B, Saed-Nejad F, et al. Correlation between arthroscopic diagnosis of osteoarthritis and synovitis of the human temporomandibular joint and keratan sulfate levels in the synovial fluid. J Oral Maxillofac Surg 1997;55:210.

17. Kubota E, Imamura H, Kubota T, et al. Interleukin 1 beta and stromelysin (MMP3) activity of synovial fluid as possible markers of osteoarthritis in the temporomandibular joint. J Oral Maxillofac Surg 1997;55:20.

18. Kubota E, Kubota T, Matsumoto J, et al. Synovial fluid cytokines and proteinases as markers of temporomandibular joint disease. J Oral Maxillofac Surg 1998;56:192.

19. Israel H, Diamond B, Saed-Nejad F, et al. Osteoarthritis and synovitis as major pathoses of the temporomandibular joint: comparison of clinical diagnosis and arthroscopic morphology. J Oral Maxillofac Surg 1998;56:1023–8.

20. Stegenga B, DeBont LG, Boering G. Osteoarthrosis as the cause of craniomandibular pain and dysfunction: a unifying concept. J Oral Maxillofac Surg 1989;47:249–56.

21. Stegenga B, DeBont LG, Boering G, et al. Tissue responses to degenerative changes in the temporomandibular joint: a review. J Oral Maxillofac Surg 1991;49:1079–88.

22. Chang H, Israel H. Analysis of inflammatory mediators in TMJ synovial fluid lavage samples in symptomatic patients and asymptomatic controls. J Oral Maxillofac Surg 2005;63:761–5.

23. Shibata T, Murakami KI, Kubota E, et al. Glycosaminoglycan components in temporomandibular joint synovial fluid as markers of joint pathology. J Oral Maxillofac Surg 1998;56:209.

24. Israel H, Saed-Nejad F, Ratcliffe A. Early diagnosis of osteoarthrosis of the temporomandibular joint: correlation between arthroscopic diagnosis and keratan sulfate levels in the synovial fluid. J Oral Maxillofac Surg 1991;49:708–11.

25. Israel H, Langevin CJ, Singer M. The relationship between temporomandibular joint synovitis and adhesions: pathogenic mechanisms and clinical implications for surgical management. J Oral Maxillofac Surg 2006;64:1066–74.

26. Salter RB. The biologic concept of continuous passive motion of synovial joints. The first 18 years of basic research and is clinical application. Clin Orthop 1989;242:12.

27. Akeson WH, Amiel D, Ing D, et al. Effects of immobilization on joints. Clin Orthop 1987;219:28.

28. National Institutes of Health Technology Assessment Conference Statement: management of temporomandibular disorders. J Am Dent Assoc 1996;127:1595–606.

29. Stohler C. Management of the dental occlusion. In: Laskin D, Greene C, Hylander W, editors. Temporomandibular disorders: an evidence-based approach to diagnosis and treatment. Chicago: Quintessence Publishing Company, Inc; 2006. p. 403–11.

30. Kircos LT, Douglas A, Mark AS, et al. Magnetic resonance imaging of the TMJ disc in asymptomatic volunteers. J Oral Maxillofac Surg 1987;45:852.

31. Katzberg RW, Westesson P, Tallents RH, et al. Anatomic disorders of the temporomandibular joint disc in asymptomatic subjects. J Oral Maxillofac Surg 1996;54:147–53.

32. Robinson PP, Boissonade FM, Loescher AR, et al. Peripheral mechanisms for the initiation of pain following trigeminal nerve injury. J Orofac Pain 2004;18(4):287–92.

33. Dubner R, Ren K. Brainstem mechanisms of persistent pain following injury. J Orofac Pain 2004;18(4):299–305.
34. Salter M. Cellular neuroplasticity mechanisms mediating pain persistence. J Orofac Pain 2004;18(4):318–24.
35. Truelove E. Management issues of neuropathic trigeminal pain from a dental perspective. J Orofac Pain 2004;18(4):374–80.
36. Benoliel R, Eliav E, Elishoov H, et al. Diagnosis and treatment of persistent pain after trauma to the head and neck. J Oral Maxillofac Surg 1994;52(11):1138–47.
37. Israel H, Ward JD, Horrell B, et al. Oral and maxillofacial surgery in patients with chronic orofacial pain. J Oral Maxillofac Surg 2003;61:662–7.
38. Milam SB. Failed implants and multiple operations. Oral Surg Oral Med Oral Pathol Oral Radiol Endod 1997;83:156.
39. Magnusson T, Carlsson GE. Comparison between two groups of patients in respect to headache and mandibular dysfunction. Swed Dent J 1978;2:85–7.
40. Andrasik F, Holyroyd KA, Abell T. Prevalence of headache within a college student population: a preliminary analysis. Headache 1979;19:384–7.
41. Jensen R, Olesen J. Oromandibular dysfunction, tension type-headache, cluster headache and miscellaneous headaches. In: Olesen J, Tfelt-Hansen P, Welch KM, editors. The headache. New York: Raven; 1993. p. 479–82.
42. Forssell H, Kangasniemi P. Mandibular dysfunction in patients with muscle contraction headache. Proc Finn Dent Soc 1984;80:211–6.
43. Gelb H, Tarte J. A two year clinical dental evaluation of 200 cases of chronic headache: the cranio-cervical-mandibular syndrome. J Am Dent Assoc 1975;91:1230–6.
44. Heloe B, Heloe LA, Heiberg A. Relationship between sociomedical factors and TMJ symptoms in Norwegians with myofascial pain-dysfunction syndrome. Community Dent Oral Epidemiol 1977;5:207–12.
45. Jensen R, Rasmussen BK, Pedersen B, et al. Muscle tenderness and pressure pain thresholds in headache. A population study. Pain 1993;52:193–9.
46. Israel H, Lee A, Shum J, et al. Temporomandibular Joint Arthroscopy in the operating room versus office: is there a difference in outcomes? [abstract]. J Oral Maxillofac Surg 2010;68(Suppl 9):55–6.
47. Laskin D. Surgical management of internal derangements. In: Laskin D, Greene C, Hylander W, editors. An evidence-based approach to diagnosis and treatment. Chicago: Quintessence Publishing Company, Inc; 2006. p. 469–81.
48. Fridrich KL, Wise JM, Zeitler DL. Prospective comparison of arthroscopy and arthrocentesis for temporomandibular joint disorders. J Oral Maxillofac Surg 1996; 54:816.
49. Sanders B, Buoncristiani R. Diagnostic and surgical arthroscopy of the temporomandibular joint: clinical experience with 136 procedures over a 2-year period. J Craniomandib Disord 1987;1:202.
50. Moses JJ, Poker ID. TMJ arthroscopic surgery: an analysis of 237 patients. J Oral Maxillofac Surg 1989;47:790.
51. Indresano AT. Arthroscopic surgery of the temporomandibular joint: report of 64 patients with long-term follow-up. J Oral Maxillofac Surg 1989;47:439.
52. Israel H, Roser SM. Patient response to temporomandibular joint arthroscopy: preliminary findings in 24 patients. J Oral Maxillofac Surg 1989;47:570.
53. Montgomery MT, Van Sickels J, Harms SE, et al. Arthroscopic TMJ surgery: effects on signs, symptoms and disc position. J Oral Maxillofac Surg 1989;47:1263.
54. McCain JP, Sanders B, Koslin M, et al. Temporomandibular joint arthroscopy: a 6-year multicenter retrospective study of 4,831 joints. J Oral Maxillofac Surg 1992; 50:926.

55. Hoffman DC, Cubillos L. The effect of arthroscopic surgery on mandibular range of motion. Cranio 1994;12(1):11.
56. Murakami K, Hosaka H, Moriya Y, et al. Short-term outcome study for the management of temporomandibular joint closed lock. Oral Surg Oral Med Oral Pathol 1995;80:253.
57. Murakami K, Moriya Y, Goto K, et al. Four-year follow-up study of temporomandibular joint arthroscopic surgery for advanced internal derangements. J Oral Maxillofac Surg 1996;54:285.
58. Chossegros C, Cheynet F, Gola R, et al. Clinical results of therapeutic temporomandibular joint arthroscopy: a prospective study of 34 arthroscopies with prediscal section and retrodiscal coagulation. Br J Oral Maxillofac Surg 1996;34:504.
59. Israel H, Behrman D, Friedman J, et al. Early versus late intervention with arthroscopy for treatment of inflammatory temporomandibular joint disorders. J Oral Maxillofac Surg 2010;68(11):2661–7.
60. Moller AR. Tinnitus: presence and future. Prog Brain Res 2007;166:3–16.
61. Salvetti G, Manfredini D, Barsotti S, et al. Otologic symptoms in temporomandibular disorders patients: is there evidence of an association-relationship. Minerva Stomatol 2006;55(11–12):627–37.
62. Parker WS, Chole RA. Tinnitus, vertigo, and temporomandibular disorders. Am J Orthod Dentofacial Orthop 1995;107(2):153–8.
63. Chole RA, Parker WS. Tinnitus in patients with temporomandibular disorders. Arch Otolaryngol Head Neck Surg 1992;118(8):817–21.
64. Wright EF, Syms CA III, Bifano SL. Tinnitus, dizziness, and non-otologicotalgia improvement through temporomandibular disorder therapy. Mil Med 2000; 165(10):733–6.
65. Rodriguez-Vazquez JF, Merida-Velasco JR, Merida-Velasco JA, et al. Anatomical considerations on the discomalleolar ligament. J Anat 1998;192(4):617–21.
66. Okeson JP. Management of temporomandibular disorders and occlusion. 6th edition. Lexington (KY): Mosby; 2008. p. 164–204.
67. Levine RA, Abel M, Cheng H. CNS somatosensory-auditory interactions elicit or modulate tinnitus. Exp Brain Res 2003;153(4):643–8.
68. Lam DK, Lawrence HP, Tenenbaum HC. Aural symptoms in temporomandibular disorder patients attending a craniofacial pain unit. J Orofac Pain 2001;152(2): 146–57.
69. Shore S, Zhou J, Koehler S. Neural mechanisms underlying somatic tinnitus. Prog Brain Res 2007;166:107–23.
70. Wright EF. Otologic symptom improvement through TMD therapy. Quintessence Int 2007;38(9):564–71.
71. Tullberg M, Ernberg M. Long-term effect on tinnitus by treatment of temporomandibular disorders: a two-year follow-up by questionnaire. Acta Odontol Scand 2006;64(2):89–96.
72. Seedorf H, Leuwer R, Fenske C, et al. The "Costen Syndrome" - which symptoms suggest that the patient may benefit from dental therapy? Laryngorhinootologie 2002;81(4):268–75.
73. deFelicio CM, Melchior Mde O, Ferreira CL, et al. Otologic symptoms of temporomandibular disorders and effect of orofacial myofunctional therapy. Cranio 2008;26(2):118–25.
74. Turp JC. Correlation between myoarthropathies of the masticatory system and ear symptoms (otalgia, tinnitus). HNO 1998;46(4):303–10.

Orofacial Pain: A Primer

Scott S. De Rossi, DMD[a,b,c],*

KEYWORDS

- Orofacial pain • Myofascial pain • Temporomandibular disorder

KEY POINTS

- Orofacial pain refers to pain associated with the soft and hard tissues of the head, face, and neck. It is a common experience in the population that has profound sociologic effects and impact on quality of life.
- New scientific evidence is constantly providing insight into the cause and pathophysiology of orofacial pain including temporomandibular disorders, cranial neuralgias, persistent idiopathic facial pains, headache, and dental pain.
- An evidence-based approach to the management of orofacial pain is imperative for the general clinician.

INTRODUCTION

Orofacial pain refers to pain associated with the soft and hard tissues of the head, face, and neck. The potential origin of orofacial pain includes pulpal and periodontal, vascular, gland, muscle, bones, sinuses, and joint structures. These numerous structures in the head and neck along with their complex innervation account for the wide range of diagnostic possibilities in patients with the complaint of orofacial pain. The diverse potential for pain arising from the vast area of trigeminal innervation accounts for the need for interdisciplinary collaboration in the evaluation and treatment of these complex patients. Orofacial pain is a common experience in the population that has profound sociologic effects and impact on quality of life. It is estimated that one-third of the population of industrialized nations suffers some chronic pain and the oral health care provider will undoubtedly treat patients with orofacial pain. The cost of chronic pain is in the billions of dollars annually in the United States for health

This article originally appeared in Dental Clinics of North America, Volume 57, Issue 3, July 2013.

[a] Department of Oral health and Diagnostic Sciences, College of Dental Medicine, Georgia Regents University, 1120 15th Street, Augusta, GA 30912, USA; [b] Department of Otolaryngology/ Head & Neck Surgery, Medical College of Georgia, Georgia Regents University, 1120 15th Street, Augusta, GA 30912, USA; [c] Department of Dermatology, Medical College of Georgia, Georgia Regents University, 1120 15th Street, Augusta, GA 30912, USA
* Department of Oral health and Diagnostic Sciences, College of Dental Medicine, Georgia Regents University, 1120 15th Street, Augusta, GA 30912, USA.
E-mail address: sderossi@gru.edu

care services, loss of work, decreased productivity, and disability compensation. New scientific evidence is constantly providing insight into the cause and pathophysiology of orofacial pain. An evidence-based approach to the management of orofacial pain is imperative for the general clinician.

PROFESSIONAL RESPONSIBILITY

Pain in the oral and maxillofacial system represents a major medical and social problem in the United States. The US Surgeon General's report on Oral Health in America noted that oral health means more than healthy teeth; it means being free of chronic orofacial pain conditions (http://www.nidcr.nih.gov/DataStatistics/SurgeonGeneral/Report/ExecutiveSummary.htm).

The astute clinician possesses a working knowledge of the basic and clinical science of orofacial pain. To effectively evaluate and treat these patients, the clinician needs to ask questions, analyze answers, further question the patient, and synthesize information. The clinician must perform a proper clinical assessment including a comprehensive head and neck and dental physical examination, neurologic testing, range of motion studies, laboratory evaluation, and perhaps consultations with other health care providers. In addition, the clinician must develop a plan of treatment that is consistent with the standard of care set forth by current scientific literature and evidence. When the scope of care falls beyond the individual expertise of a clinician a team approach should be used and the patient should be referred.

Orofacial pain may be derived from many unique tissues of the head and neck, and subsequently has several unique physiologic characteristics compared with other pain systems, such as back or spinal pain. It is not surprising that accurate diagnosis and effective management of orofacial pain conditions represents a significant challenge for health care providers. Yet, this is an emerging and ever-growing area of dental practice. According to Hargreaves,[1] publications in the field of orofacial pain have demonstrated a steady increase over the last several decades. Robert and colleagues[2,3] published a bibliometric analysis of the scientific literature on pain research that was published in 2008. This paper demonstrated how complex the literature on orofacial pain is, indicating that 975 articles on orofacial pain were published in 275 journals from authors representing 54 countries. One of the biggest barriers for improved patient care and translational research has been the lack of a validated diagnostic criteria and varying terminologies between major groups that study pain.[1] Although efforts have been made to classify patients with temporomandibular disorders with research diagnostic criteria for temporomandibular disorders,[4] headache patients with the International Headache Society criteria, and orofacial pain with the American Academy of Orofacial Pain standards, clinical research suggests that these methods are incomplete for comprehensive diagnosis of patients with orofacial pain.[5,6] It is clear that translational research is necessary to ultimately improve diagnosis and patient care in patients with orofacial pain (**Table 1**).

EPIDEMIOLOGY OF OROFACIAL PAIN

Numerous reports in the scientific literature have attempted to identify the epidemiology of orofacial pain. The 1986 Nuprin Pain Report noted that most Americans experience an average of three or four different kinds of pain annually.[7] Crook and coworkers[8] reported that 16% of the general population suffered pain within a 2-week period. James and colleagues[9] in 1991 reported that greater than 81% of the population reported a significant jaw pain experience over the course of their lifetime. Lipton and coworkers[10] in 1993 noted that 22% of Americans reported orofacial pain within a

Table 1
Classification of pain: scheme for coding chronic pain diagnoses[a]

Axis	Definition
1	Regions (eg, head, face, and mouth)
2	Systems (eg, nervous system)
3	Temporal characteristics of pain (eg, continuous, recurring irregularly, paroxysmal)
4	Patient's statement of intensity: time since onset of pain (eg, mild, medium, severe; $\leq$1 mo; >6 mo)
5	Etiology (eg, genetic, infective, psychological)

[a] International Association for the Study of Pain classification.

6-month period. Although the orofacial pain most commonly experienced by patients and encountered by oral health care providers is toothache, orofacial pain seldom seems to be an isolated complaint.[11] Türp and colleagues[12] noted that more than 81% of patients reporting to an orofacial pain center had pain sources beyond the trigeminal system. Common comorbid conditions include fibromyalgia, chronic fatigue syndrome, headache, panic disorder, gastroesophageal reflux disorder, irritable bowel syndrome, multiple chemical sensitivities, and posttraumatic stress disorder.[13] Often, symptoms for comorbid conditions may differentiate the patient with orofacial pain from patients seeking routine dental care or those with emergent or acute dental pain.[14] It is important that the clinician and the patient work to reveal all pain sources to improve prognosis and ensure appropriate therapy (**Table 2**).[12]

DEFINING PAIN

Orofacial pain is the presenting symptom of a broad spectrum of diseases. Pain is also interdisciplinary. Causes of orofacial pain may include diseases of orofacial structures; psychological abnormalities; referred pain from other sources, such as cervical muscles or intracranial pathology; and often most challenging for the clinician, orofacial pain may occur in the absence of detectable physical, imaging, or laboratory

Table 2
Differential diagnosis of orofacial pain[a]

Intracranial pain disorders	Neoplasm, aneurysm, abscess, hemorrhage, hematoma, edema
Primary headache disorders (neurovascular disorders)	Migraine, migraine variants, cluster headache, paroxysmal hemicrania, cranial arteritis Carotodynia, tension-type headache
Neurogenic pain disorders	Paroxysmal neuralgias (trigeminal, glossopharyngeal, nervus intermedius, superior laryngeal) Continuous pain disorders (deafferentation, neuritis, postherpetic neuralgia, posttraumatic and postsurgical neuralgia) Sympathetically maintained pain
Intraoral pain disorders	Dental pulp, periodontium, mucogingival tissues, tongue
Temporomandibular disorders	Masticatory muscle, temporomandibular joint, associated structures
Associated structures	Ears, eyes, nose, paranasal sinuses, throat, lymph nodes, salivary glands, neck

[a] American Academy of Orofacial Pain classification.

abnormalities.[15] The International Association for the Study of Pain defines pain as an unpleasant sensory and emotional experience associated with actual or potential tissue damage, or described in terms of such damage. Inherent in this definition is that pain is a multidimensional experience encompassing sensory-discriminative, cognitive, motivational, and affective qualities. Suffering goes hand-in-hand with pain and is defined as the negative emotional and psychological state that occurs in response to or anticipation of nociception.[16] It is vital that the clinician remember that pain can be a symptom of the disease to be diagnosed and treated but may also be present in the absence of any physical findings. In essence, physical, psychological, and social factors are mutually influential forces that are able to create an infinite number of pain experiences for the patient.[17] A biologic system that includes anatomic, structural, and molecular substrates of disease interacts with a psychological and social system that includes the effects of motivation and personality on illness and an individual's reaction to it along with a cultural, environmental, and family influence on the expression and experience of pain.[18] Orofacial pain can be acute or chronic. Acute pain begins suddenly and usually does not last long, whereas chronic pain may last for weeks or months. Chronic pain is defined as pain that lasts for more than a month longer than expected based on the illness or injury. It may recur off and on for months and years and may be associated with a chronic disorder, such as cancer, diabetes, or fibromyalgia.[19]

Pain can also be divided into somatic and neuropathic pain. Somatic pain always results from stimulation of nociceptors, because of tissue injury, such as inflammation. Somatic pain ends, however, when underlying tissue injury and inflammation is resolved. The two hallmarks of somatic pain include hyperalgesia and allodynia.[20,21] Hyperalgesia is defined as an increased perception of the painful stimulus after receptor sensitization. Allodynia is the perception of pain in response to a nonnoxious stimuli. Neuropathic pain is considered pain that is initiated or caused by primary lesion or dysfunction in the nervous system.[22–25] Many of the kinds of orofacial pain discussed in this issue fall under this category. Treatment of them requires an understanding of neurophysiology of pain and the identification of sensible treatment goals. Specifically, treatment directed toward rehabilitation and pain control often supersedes treatment directed at a cure. Occasionally, pain may be of a psychogenic origin. Psychogenic pain is often unconscious, involuntary, and may accompany psychiatric disorders or may be an individual's way of dealing with the stresses of their mental illness.[26,27] It is an experience of mental suffering where there is no organic disease or where the organic disease has become overelaborated in its psychological, emotional, and behavioral significance.[27,28]

NEUROPHYSIOLOGY AND ANATOMY OF OROFACIAL PAIN

Nociceptors are responsible for the recognition of proprioception, mechanical stimuli, thermal stimuli, and pain perception.[29] Once stimulated, peripheral nerves direct nociceptive information and convey pain messages to the central nervous system by way of afferent fibers. Speed of transmission depends on the myelination and size of the nerve fibers. The three types of afferents include A, B, and C fibers. A fibers are myelinated and divided into alpha, beta, gamma, and delta. The A-delta fibers carry noxious stimuli that can damage tissues, such as the pain associated with heat. They are rapid conducting small fibers and are responsible for the initial pain of nociception. Fifty percent of C fibers carry afferent noxious stimuli and are polymodal. C fiber stimulation results in initial painless periods followed by diffuse and aching pains. In addition, C fiber nociception interconnects with the limbic system and plays a role in the emotional presentation of pain. In neuropathic pain chronic pain syndromes, the C fiber sensitizes a second high threshold neuron referred to as the wide dynamic range neuron leading to a condition often referred to as spinal windup.[30] This constant and continuous stimulation leads to facilitation of nonnoxious stimuli to a hyperalgesia state leading to relentless pain.[30] Pain can also be modulated by two primary types of drugs that work in the brain: analgesics and anesthetics.[31] The modulation of pain by electrical brain stimulation results from the activation of descending inhibitory fibers that modulate the input and output of various neurons.[30–32] In the central nervous system, much of the information from the nociceptive afferent fibers results from excitatory discharges of multireceptive neurons. The pain information in the central nervous system is controlled by ascending and descending inhibitory systems using endogenous opioids or other endogenous substances, such as serotonin, as inhibitory mediators.[33] In addition, a powerful inhibition of pain-related information occurs at the level of the spinal cord. These inhibitory systems can be activated by various mechanisms including brain stimulation, intracerebral morphine, and peripheral nerve stimulation. Many of the medications used in orofacial pain activate these inhibitory control mechanisms.[34]

To understand and effectively treat orofacial pain, the clinician must have a sound knowledge of the neuroanatomy and physiology of orofacial structures. Most nociceptive impulses are transmitted by the somatic nerves, a significant portion is transmitted by autonomic nerves, and a small portion may be transmitted by motor nerves. There

---

Factors in pain modulation

- Nociceptors
  - Neuroeffector functions
  - Transmission of afferent signals
- Release of neurochemicals when nociceptors respond to noxious stimuli
  - Neuropeptides: substance P and CGRP
  - Excitatory AA: glutamate and aspartate
- Norepinephrine, bradykinin, serotonin, histamine, and prostaglandins
- Endogenous opioids work at receptors in the dorsal horn of the spinal cord and other areas
  - Three receptors: mu (m), kappa, and sigma
    - Most opioids bind to mu receptors
      - Subtype m1: analgesia
      - Subtype m2: respiratory depression, bradycardia, inhibition of gastrointestinal motility
    - Kappa: spinal analgesia without respiratory depression
    - Sigma: produces excitation and dysphoria
- Descending control
  - Responsible for arousal, attention, and emotional stress
  - Altering response to pain
- Modulation of dorsal horn
  - γ-Aminobutryic acid is thought to exert descending control by mediating presynaptic inhibition
  - Responsible for altering response to pain

are unique features of the oral and maxillofacial structures including the temporomandibular joint and masticatory muscles that make an understanding of the anatomy vital in leading to appropriate diagnostic evaluation and management of patients with orofacial pain.[35,36]

The primary sensory innervation of the orofacial structures is the trigeminal system. The trigeminal system oversees the efficacy and tissue integrity of highly integrative orofacial behaviors that are controlled by the cranial nerves and modulated by the autonomic nervous system and greater limbic system.[32] Cranial nerves are extensions of the brain that innervate tissues involved with the trigeminal system directly or indirectly. The largest of the cranial nerves is the trigeminal nerve, which consists of three peripheral branches: (1) the ophthalmic, (2) the maxillary, and (3) the mandibular. Trigeminal nerve is the dominant nerve that relays sensory impulses from the orofacial area to the central nervous system. The regions where these branches collect sensory input conveyed by first-order neurons through the trigeminal ganglia encompass the entire face. The trigeminal nerve principally innervates facial skin, corneas, oral and nasal mucosa, teeth, tongue, masticatory muscles, and meningeal linings (**Fig. 1**). The trigeminal nerve has sensory and motor components. The sensory input converges into the spinal track nucleus of the brainstem.[31–34]

The facial nerve, glossopharyngeal nerve, and vagus nerves, and the upper cervical nerves 2 and 3 also relay sensory information from the face and surrounding area. The facial nerve has a large motor component that supplies the muscles of facial expression, platysma, stapedius, and scalp muscles in addition to a small sensory component that provides taste from the anterior tongue and parotid sensation. The glossopharyngeal nerve provides sensory efferent supply to the mucous membranes of the pharynx, palatine tonsils, and posterior tongue. The tympanic branch supplies sensory information from the middle ear, motor supply the muscles of the pharynx and

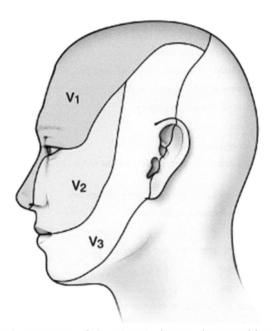

Fig. 1. Braches and innervation of the trigeminal nerve. (*From* Waldman S. Pain review. Philadelphia: Saunders Elsevier; 2009. p. 16; with permission.)

soft palate, and special visceral afferents supply tastebuds of the posterior tongue. The upper for the five cervical nerves provide innervation to the back of the head, lower face, and neck. More importantly, they converge in the brainstem at the trigeminal nucleus (**Table 3**).

A common phenomenon associated with orofacial pain that often confuses the patient and the clinician is heterotopic pain.[37] One of the most important steps the clinician can take in the patient that presents with orofacial pain is determining the site of their pain and whether it coincides with the source of their pain. Primary pain occurs at the source and is often the case in acute injury or infection. This is not a difficult problem to diagnose and treat when other pain sources are absent. Diagnostic dilemmas are encountered and often unnecessary treatment performed when the source of pain is not located in the region of pain perception.[38] This phenomenon is referred to as heterotopic pain. The location where the patient feels the pain, which is easily located by asking the patient to point out the region of the body that is painful, is the site of pain. The source of the pain, however, is the area of the body from which the pain actually originates and may not necessarily be where the patient is experiencing pain. Another diagnostic challenge is referred pain. Referred pain describes pain felt at a location served by one nerve but the source of nociception arrives at the subnucleus caudalis by a different nerve. Convergence by multiple sensory nerves carrying input to the trigeminal spinal nuclei from cutaneous and deep tissues located throughout the head and neck sets the stage for referred pain. This convergence explains how intracranial, neck, shoulder, or throat nociception may actually excite second-order neurons receiving input from facial structures.[39]

Clinicians who evaluate and manage patients with orofacial pain realize a changing role as science clarifies how the central nervous system processes evolve when patients are exposed to chronic stressors. It is vital that practitioners get the entire story, which includes biomedical and psychosocial aspects of their patients' pain experience.[40]

Orofacial pain disorders comprise major and expensive components of health care in the United States. Collectively, they have a high prevalence rate and a large range in pain intensity with commensurate and often significant impact on the quality of life.[41]

Table 3 Cranial and cervical nerves that provide somatic and visceral sensation to the orofacial area	
Nerve	**General Area Served**
V: Trigeminal	Skin of the face, forehead, and scalp as far as the top of the head; conjunctiva and bulb of the eye; oral and nasal mucosa; part of the external aspect of the tympanic membrane; teeth; anterior two-thirds of the tongue; masticatory muscles; temporomandibular joint; meninges of the anterior and middle cranial fossae
VII: Facial	Skin of the hollow of the auricle of the external ear; small area of skin behind the ear
IX: Glossopharyngeal	Mucosa of the pharynx; fauces; palatine tonsils; posterior one-third of the tongue; internal surface of the tympanic membrane; skin of the external ear
X: Vagus	Skin at the back of the ear; posterior wall and floor of external auditory meatus; tympanic membrane; meninges of posterior cranial fossa; pharynx; larynx
Cervical nerve 2	Back of the head extending to the vertex; behind and above the ear; submandibular, anterior neck
Cervical nerve 3	Lateral and posterior neck

Ongoing basic and clinical research focused on acute and chronic orofacial pain conditions is necessary to understand the unique features of this pain system and to develop and evaluate improved ways to treat patients with orofacial pain. Additional research is necessary to establish comprehensive classification schemes for all patients with orofacial pain.[42] It is encouraging to see current research studies incorporating quality-of-life indices, which provide important information on clinical outcomes for patients. The orofacial pain conditions reviewed in this issue represent a highly prevalent spectrum of pain disorders with pain intensities that are observed in many other pain conditions. It is clear, however, that there are unique anatomic, biochemical, and psychological components that provide compelling evidence for specific research and dedicated patient care on orofacial pain.

REFERENCES

1. Hargreaves KM. Orofacial pain. Pain 2011;152:S25–32.
2. Robert C, Wilson CS, Donnadieu S, et al. Bibliometric analysis of the scientific literature on pain research: a 2006 study. Pain 2008;138(2):250–4.
3. Robert C, Wilson CS, Donnadieu S, et al. Evolution of the scientific literature on pain from 1976 to 2007. Pain Med 2010;11(5):670–84.
4. Dworkin SF, LeResche L. Research diagnostic criteria for temporomandibular disorders: review, criteria, examinations and specifications, critique. J Craniomandib Disord 1992;6:301–55.
5. Benoliel R, Birman N, Eliav E, et al. The international classification of headache disorders: accurate diagnosis of orofacial pain? Cephalalgia 2008;28:752–62.
6. Anderson GC, Gonzalez YM, Ohrbach R, et al. The research diagnostic criteria for temporomandibular disorders. VI: future directions. J Orofac Pain 2010;24: 79–88.
7. Sternbach RA. Pain and 'hassles' in the United States: findings of the Nuprin pain report. Pain 1986;27(1):69–80.
8. Crook J, Tunks E, Rideout E, et al. Epidemiologic comparison of persistent pain sufferers in a specialty pain clinic and in the community. Arch Phys Med Rehabil 1986;67(7):451–5.
9. James FR, Large RG, Bushnell JA, et al. Epidemiology of pain in New Zealand. Pain 1991;44(3):279–83.
10. Lipton JA, Ship JA, Larach-Robinson D. Estimated prevalence and distribution of reported orofacial pain in the United States. J Am Dent Assoc 1993;124(10): 115–21.
11. Von Korff M, Dworkin SF, Le Resche L, et al. An epidemiologic comparison of pain complaints. Pain 1988;32(2):173–83.
12. Türp JC, Kowalski CJ, Stohler CS. Temporomandibular disorders–pain outside the head and face is rarely acknowledged in the chief complaint. J Prosthet Dent 1997;78(6):592–5.
13. Clauw DJ. Fibromyalgia: an overview. Am J Med 2009;122:S3–13.
14. Anastassaki A, Magnusson T. Patients referred to a specialist clinic because of suspected temporomandibular disorders: a survey of 3194 patients in respect of diagnoses, treatments, and treatment outcome. Acta Odontol Scand 2004;62: 183–92.
15. Stohler CS. Chronic orofacial pain: is the puzzle unraveling? J Dent Educ 2001; 65(12):1383–92.
16. Hirshberg RM. Pain and suffering: a legal and medical lexicon for the 21st century. Med Law 2012;31(3):339–53.

17. Tenenbaum HC, Mock D, Gordon AS, et al. Sensory and affective components of orofacial pain: is it all in your brain? Crit Rev Oral Biol Med 2001;12(6):455–68.
18. Merrill RL. Central mechanisms of orofacial pain. Dent Clin North Am 2007;51(1): 45–59.
19. Arnold LM, Clauw DJ, Dunegan LJ, et al, FibroCollaborative. A framework for fibromyalgia management for primary care providers. Mayo Clin Proc 2012; 87(5):488–96.
20. Garland EL. Pain processing in the human nervous system: a selective review of nociceptive and biobehavioral pathways. Prim Care 2012;39(3):561–71.
21. Sessle BJ. Peripheral and central mechanisms of orofacial inflammatory pain. Int Rev Neurobiol 2011;97:179–206.
22. Iwata K, Imamura Y, Honda K, et al. Physiological mechanisms of neuropathic pain: the orofacial region. Int Rev Neurobiol 2011;97:227–50.
23. Baron R, Binder A, Wasner G. Neuropathic pain: diagnosis, pathophysiological mechanisms, and treatment. Lancet Neurol 2010;9(8):807–19.
24. Nickel FT, Seifert F, Lanz S, et al. Mechanisms of neuropathic pain. Eur Neuropsychopharmacol 2012;22(2):81–91.
25. Fornasari D. Pain mechanisms in patients with chronic pain. Clin Drug Investig 2012;32(Suppl 1):45–52.
26. Renton T, Durham J, Aggarwal VR. The classification and differential diagnosis of orofacial pain. Expert Rev Neurother 2012;12(5):569–76.
27. Aggarwal VR, Lovell K, Peters S, et al. Psychosocial interventions for the management of chronic orofacial pain. Cochrane Database Syst Rev 2011;(11):CD008456.
28. Williams AC, Eccleston C, Morley S. Psychological therapies for the management of chronic pain (excluding headache) in adults. Cochrane Database Syst Rev 2012;(11):CD007407.
29. Sacerdote P, Levrini L. Peripheral mechanisms of dental pain: the role of substance P. Mediators Inflamm 2012;2012:951920.
30. Staud R, Robinson ME, Price DD. Temporal summation of second pain and its maintenance are useful for characterizing widespread central sensitization of fibromyalgia patients. J Pain 2007;8(11):893–901.
31. Staud R. Abnormal endogenous pain modulation is a shared characteristic of many chronic pain conditions. Expert Rev Neurother 2012;12(5):577–85.
32. Ter Horst GJ, Copray J, Leim R, et al. Projections from the rostral parvocellular reticular formation to pontine and medullary nuclei in the rat: involvement in autonomic regulation and orofacial motor control. Neuroscience 1991;40:735–58.
33. Spetea M. Opioid receptors and their ligands in the musculoskeletal system and relevance for pain control. Curr Pharm Des 2013. [Epub ahead of print].
34. Bialer M. Why are antiepileptic drugs used for nonepileptic conditions? Epilepsia 2012;53(Suppl 7):26–33.
35. Benoliel R, Svensson P, Heir GM, et al. Persistent orofacial muscle pain. Oral Dis 2011;17(Suppl 1):23–41.
36. Bender SD. Temporomandibular disorders, facial pain, and headaches. Headache 2012;52(Suppl 1):22–5.
37. López-López J, Garcia-Vicente L, Jané-Salas E, et al. Orofacial pain of cardiac origin: review literature and clinical cases. Med Oral Patol Oral Cir Bucal 2012; 17(4):e538–44.
38. de C Williams AC, Cella M. Medically unexplained symptoms and pain: misunderstanding and myth. Curr Opin Support Palliat Care 2012;6(2):201–6.
39. Marfurt CF, Rajchert DM. Trigeminal primary afferent projections to "non-trigeminal" areas of the rat central nervous system. J Comp Neurol 1991;303(3):489–511.

40. Giamberardino MA, Affaitati G, Fabrizio A, et al. Myofascial pain syndromes and their evaluation. Best Pract Res Clin Rheumatol 2011;25(2):185–98.
41. Brattberg G, Parker MG, Thorslund M. A longitudinal study of pain: reported pain from middle age to old age. Clin J Pain 1997;13(2):144–9.
42. Mitchell LA, MacDonald RA. Qualitative research on pain. Curr Opin Support Palliat Care 2009;3(2):131–5.

Intraoral Pain Disorders

Joel J. Napeñas, DDS[a,b],*

KEYWORDS

- Caries • Pulpitis • Cracked tooth syndrome • Periapical disease • Alveolar osteitis
- Candidiasis

KEY POINTS

- Dental and pulpal pains are variable in their behavior, can refer to other structures distant from the source, and can mimic other facial pain disorders. Therefore it is essential that all complaints of pain in the mouth and face include ruling out pain of dental origin.
- Periodontal pain is more localizable than pulpal pain, usually by placing pressure apically or laterally on the involved tooth, or through the presence of identifiable clinical abnormality.
- Oral mucosal pain is a superficial somatic pain that is localizable, with the site and source common, and is responsive to local anesthesia in the affected area.
- Pain originating from the bone is due to inflammatory disorders from infection or injury. The severity of pain is related to the degree of confinement of exudate or purulence within the anatomic sites.

INTRODUCTION

Dental and oral diseases are common findings in the general population. Pain associated with dental caries or periodontal disease is the primary reason why most patients seek treatment from dental providers. Many patients who present with a complaint of oral pain have irrefutable clinical decay (**Fig. 1**). However, intraoral pain is not exclusively a result of dental disorders.

This review outlines common somatic intraoral pain disorders, which can originate from disease involving 1 or more broad anatomic areas, the teeth, the surrounding soft tissues (mucogingival, tongue, salivary glands), and bone.

This article originally appeared in Dental Clinics of North America, Volume 57, Issue 3, July 2013.

The author has nothing to disclose.

[a] Division of Oral Medicine and Radiology, Schulich School of Medicine and Dentistry, Dental Sciences Building, Western University, London, ON N6A 5C1, Canada; [b] Department of Oral Medicine, Carolinas Medical Center, PO Box 32861, Charlotte, NC 28232, USA

* Division of Oral Medicine and Radiology, Schulich School of Medicine and Dentistry, Dental Sciences Building, Western University, London, ON N6A 5C1, Canada.

E-mail address: joel.napenas@schulich.uwo.ca

http://dx.doi.org/10.1016/j.ccol.2014.10.010
2352-7986/14/$ – see front matter © 2014 Elsevier Inc. All rights reserved.

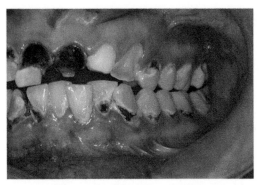

Fig. 1. Rampant caries caused by impaired function of salivary gland.

DENTAL AND PULPAL

When examining pain of dental origin, one must determine if is related to the teeth or pulp directly, or if it is due to irritation of the surrounding periodontal ligament. There is a continuum of pain symptoms that are based on the degree or severity of disease. This continuum ranges from the short, sharp, localizable pain, a physiologic response or warning of noxious stimuli or impending pathologic state, and progresses to the persistent, dull pain that indicates the presence of inflammation, infection, and disease.

Dental and pulpal pain occurs when there is noxious stimulation of the teeth and/or disease affecting the enamel, dentin, or pulpal structures. The disease involves breach of tooth structure attributable to mechanical means (eg, trauma, attrition, abrasion, erosion, iatrogenic) and/or bacteria (ie, caries).

Enamel is avascular, noninnervated, and nonporous, therefore demineralization of or the presence of caries isolated in the enamel is usually painless. Once lesions breach the dentinoenamel junction, pain is experienced through stimuli affecting the dentinal tubules. Myelinated (Aδ) and unmyelinated (C) fibers innervate the pulp. If there is sufficient stimulation (eg, via heat, cold, or pressure), fluid movement in the dentinal tubules activates the low-threshold Aδ fibers, producing the quick, sharp, localized pain. An injured tooth with local inflammation lowers the pain threshold of Aδ fibers. Once there is pulpal involvement and inflammation persists the C fibers are stimulated, producing a more prolonged, dull, and diffuse pain.

A tooth causing pain is initially identified by obtaining a history from the patient, then identifying a tooth with clinical evidence of abnormality (eg, fracture, caries, lost restoration, abrasion). An attempt is then made to increase the pain through noxious stimulation of the tooth in question via mechanical (eg, percussion, biting), thermal (eg, cold and heat), electric (eg, electric pulp testing [EPT]), or chemical means. Radiographs can then be taken of the teeth to for pathologic evaluation.

Caries

Caries occurs through bacterial invasion of the tooth structures, resulting in decay caused by formation of acid metabolites. It may occur on enamel, dentin, and cementum on exposed root surfaces. Patients may complain of thermal sensitivity or sensitivity when exposed to sweet or acidic foods. Pain is sharp, localized, and dissipates immediately after removal of the stimuli. Sensitivity derives from lost enamel and increased exposure of dentin and cementum.

Caries is detected and diagnosed both clinically and radiographically (**Fig. 2**). Management of dental caries varies by the size of the lesion as well as the state of the

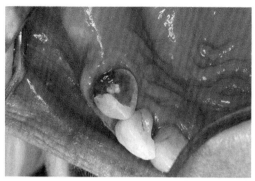

Fig. 2. Carious tooth.

caries. If a lesion is incipient, monitoring and/or topical fluoride placement is adequate. However, if the lesion extends into dentin and is not arrested, removal of the decayed tooth structure and placement of a dental restoration may be required.

Exposed Cementum or Dentin

Exposed cementum or dentin is most commonly caused by incorrect tooth-brushing technique resulting in gingival recession and/or abrasion of enamel (**Fig. 3**). Tooth sensitivity to cold liquids generally results. Pain is also sharp, localized, and dissipates immediately after removal of the cold stimuli. Treatment measures are directed toward limiting dentinal fluid movement by covering the exposed dentin or cementum, which is achieved with oral hygiene instructions to improve tooth-brushing technique, use of desensitizing agents, and sometimes restorations.[1,2]

Pulpal Disease

The most common cause of pulpal pain is dental caries that extends to the pulp; however, other causes include trauma, fracture, exposed dentin or cementum, or premature contact. Acute pulpal pain acts like other visceral type pains, with diffuseness and variability. There may be continuous dull, aching pain with superimposed episodes of pulsing, throbbing, and sharp pain, representing stimulation of the C fibers and the lower threshold of Aδ fibers, respectively. Pulpal pain can be modified by a variety of stimuli including heat, cold, pressure, and head positioning. Teeth that only have pulpal disease are not sensitive to percussion. The specific features of and management strategies for various pulpal disease states are as follows:

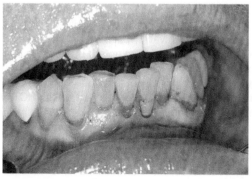

Fig. 3. Exposed cementum on root surfaces.

Normal

Normal pulp has a short response to cold stimuli that subsides almost immediately on removal. There is no evidence of periapical abnormality on radiographs. In the absence of tooth abnormality, no treatment is indicated.

Reversible pulpitis

Reversible pulpitis is characterized by an exaggerated quick, sharp response to cold stimuli, followed by a dull ache that dissipates. There is no complaint of spontaneous pain. Tooth is not tender to percussion, and there is no radiographic evidence of periapical abnormality. Treatment of reversible pulpitis entails removal of the pain-causing stimulus, usually removal of lesion, and restoration of lost tooth structure, as it does not require extirpation of the pulp through root canal therapy (RCT) or extraction of the tooth.

Irreversible pulpitis

Irreversible pulpitis presents as spontaneous, lingering dull ache or constant severe, unrelenting pain; increased pain intensity to noxious stimuli; and positive response to cold and heat stimuli (ie, sharp response followed by dull ache that persists.) Radiographically there may or may not be a thickening in the periodontal ligament (PDL) at the tooth's apex. Treatment requires either RCT or tooth extraction.

Pulpal necrosis

In pulpal necrosis there is no pain and no response to noxious stimuli (cold, heat, or EPT). Radiographs may or may not reveal the presence of a periapical radiolucency. If the infection has extended beyond the apex of the tooth into the surrounding bone (see the section on acute apical periodontitis), a percussion test may be positive. Treatment requires either RCT or extraction.

Cracked Tooth Syndrome

Cracked tooth is defined as incomplete fracture of the dentin that may or may not extend to the pulp.[3] The term cracked tooth syndrome was first introduced by Cameron in 1964, describing when the fractures become symptomatic.[4]

Patient complaints include sharp, momentary pain that is stimulated by biting or releasing, or resulting from exposure to cold food or drinks. The pain in cracked tooth syndrome can be easily localized.[4] Pain sometimes may linger minutes after chewing.[5]

Diagnosis is often difficult because of the lack of clinical and radiographic findings. It is determined through careful history taking and clinical examination. Visual inspection of the tooth should be performed. Tactile inspection with an explorer tip may also be performed. Radiographs should be reviewed with bitewings preferred over periapical films; however, the likelihood of visualizing a cracked tooth on a radiograph is rare (**Fig. 4**). A useful diagnostic aid is transillumination, best performed with use of magnification to better illustrate color changes and clinically significant cracks. Tooth percussion should be performed; however, pain is seldom elicited with percussion in the apical direction. Pain on biting may be noted, but is more commonly noted with release of biting, owing to fluids within dentinal tubules moving toward the pulp.[5]

Treatment of cracked tooth syndrome may include stabilization with an orthodontic band or more permanently with a crown or overlay, or with RCT or extraction of the tooth depending on the extent of the crack.

PERIODONTAL

Periodontal pain (eg, periodontium and alveolar bone) is more localized than pulpal pain, owing to the proprioceptors and mechanoreceptors in the periodontium.[6] Pain

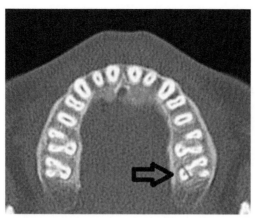

Fig. 4. Fractured palatal root of upper left second molar (*arrow*), as seen on an axial-view computed tomography (CT) image.

caused by chronic periodontal conditions (eg, gingivitis, chronic periodontitis) is generally nonexistent, or may be mild, persistent, or episodic dull pain attributable to inflammation or low-grade infection.

Periodontal pain caused by local factors is localized to affected teeth in which there is inflammation or infection involving the gingiva, periodontium, alveolar bone, or pericoronal tissue. Bacterial infection is usually the causative factor. The bulk of the discussion in this section is focused on these conditions.

Gingival/Periodontal Abscess

Gingival abscesses are relatively uncommon, whereas periodontal abscesses are more common and occur in areas of periodontal disease. Pain complaints can range from low-intensity aches to severe, sharp pain. Pain is made worse by chewing and percussion of adjacent teeth.

Gingival abscesses are confined to the marginal interdental tissue. Both show localized swelling of the gingiva, which may also include alveolar mucosa. Lesions are fluctuant, violacious, and cyanotic or erythematous in appearance, and may or may not be accompanied by drainage via fistula.[7]

Abscesses are caused by the proliferation of periodontal bacterial flora in a diseased periodontal site, although they can also be caused by food or foreign-body impaction or trauma. Abscess microflora contains mostly periodontal pathogens, including *Porphyromonas gingivalis*, *Prevotella intermedia*, *Fusobacterium nucleatum*, *Peptostreptococcus micros* and *Bacterioides forsythus*.[8]

Areas of periodontal disease involve tissue destruction (connective tissue and bone) caused by activation of host inflammatory mediators in response to bacterial microorganisms. The abscess is a focus of purulent exudate in connective tissue, surrounded by infiltration of leukocytes, edematous tissue, and vessels.

Clinical features as described, in conjunction with clinical evidence (eg, deep pockets, horizontal bone loss, gingival edema, and/or erythema) and radiographic evidence of periodontal disease, are sufficient to obtain a diagnosis of a periodontal abscess. Clinical features in the absence of periodontal disease, and a history of trauma, support the diagnosis of a gingival abscess (**Fig. 5**).

Treatment of the abscess entails obtaining purulent drainage, either by incision of the fluctuant area or through the pocket orifice. This action is accompanied by removal

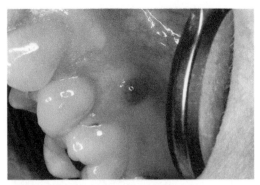

Fig. 5. Gingival abscess on upper left maxillary gingiva.

of the causative agent (eg, foreign body or bacterial foci). Root debridement is performed for periodontal abscesses.

Periapical Disease

Patient complaints include a rapid onset of moderate to severe spontaneous pain that is sharp, throbbing, or aching in nature, pain to percussion of affected teeth, purulence, and/or swelling (**Fig. 6**). Pain is more severe if the abscess is confined to bone; however, if it finds a path into soft tissues and forms a fluctuant pus-filled swelling or a fistula, it can decrease. In more long-standing and chronic cases there may not be any complaints of pain, or only the presence of mild discomfort.

Periapical disease occurs when a bacterial infection of necrotic pulp spreads into the periapical tissues. Virulent bacteria infiltrate the apical PDL, leading to an acute inflammatory reaction.

Diagnostic steps are the same as those outlined for pulpal disease (see earlier discussion). Through clinical examination it must be established that the tooth is nonvital with a necrotic pulp. Periapical diagnoses can be classified as follows.

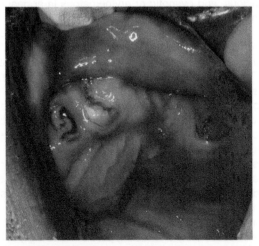

Fig. 6. Abscess on the upper right palate associated with necrotic teeth.

Normal
There is no response to percussion or palpation. Radiographic findings are normal, with intact lamina dura (LD) and uniform PDL space.

Acute (symptomatic) apical periodontitis
This condition is characterized by a complaint of spontaneous pain (moderate to severe). Clinical findings include a nonvital tooth, pain on percussion, and biting of the affected tooth. Radiographs may show widened PDL space and intact LD (**Fig. 7**).

Asymptomatic apical periodontitis
The affected tooth is established as nonvital (eg, no response to cold or EPT) and there is an unremarkable response to percussion or palpation. Radiographic findings include a break in LD, widening PDL space, or the presence of a periapical radiolucency (PARL) (**Fig. 8**).

Acute apical abscess
Acute apical abscess is characterized by a rapid onset of spontaneous pain and swelling of the gingival and alveolar mucosa (unless abscess is confined to bone). Radiographs may or may not show periapical changes.

Chronic apical abscess
This condition is a long-standing focus of infection, usually with little or no discomfort, caused by a path of drainage with a fistula or sinus tract.

Management of periapical disease requires treating the affected tooth via RCT or extraction. If the abscess involves an area of fluctuant swelling, incision and drainage may also be required.

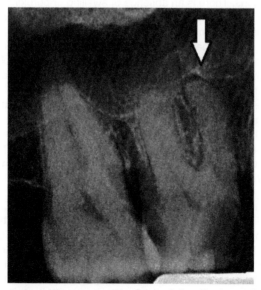

Fig. 7. Widened periodontal ligament at the apex of the distal root (*arrow*) of a carious maxillary first molar. (*Courtesy of* Nader S. Jahshan, DDS, Brantford, Ontario, Canada.)

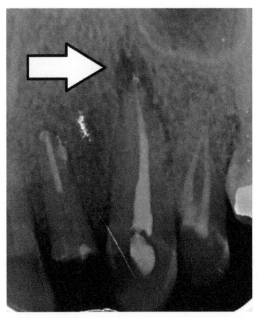

Fig. 8. Periapical radiolucency (*arrow*) on root canal treated upper left canine. (*Courtesy of* Nader S. Jahshan DDS, Brantford, Ontario, Canada.)

Alveolar Osteitis (Dry Socket)

This condition occurs 1 to 5 days after a tooth extraction, and is described by patients as a moderate to severe, deep, continuous, aching, radiating pain that originates in the area of the tooth extraction but may be difficult to localize. It is only partially relieved by analgesic medications. There is an absence of swelling or purulence. Examination of the extraction site reveals exposed bare bone in the tooth socket, which is very sensitive to probing and may emit a foul odor.

Alveolar osteitis occurs when the blood clot in the socket is lost through mechanical means (eg, excessive rinsing or spitting), smoking, or possibly fibrinolytic components in saliva. Thus bare alveolar bone in the socket is exposed to bacteria and food debris, and resultant inflammation and/or infection occurs.

A history of recent tooth extraction, combined with the clinical features, is sufficient to determine a diagnosis.

Treatment entails irrigation and cleansing of the socket to remove bacteria and debris, and application of a topical medicament into the socket to provide analgesia (ie, by cauterizing exposed nerve endings) and antiseptic effects; this is accompanied by more potent oral analgesics for pain.

Periocoronitis

Pericoronitis is inflammation and localized infection of tissue structures surrounding the crown of an impacted tooth, which frequently occurs in the area of fully or partially impacted third molars. Pain is usually continuous, ranges from mild to severe, and can be described as aching, throbbing, and/or sharp, radiating to the ear, throat, and floor of mouth. An erythematous and edematous gingival lesion is seen, and indentation of the opposing tooth is seen frequently. Swelling, purulent discharge, and lymphadenopathy may also be present.

Bacterial growth occurs in the space between the crown of the tooth and the overlying gingival tissue, which may be due to food impaction, trauma (owing to opposing dentition), or inability to clean the site.

Clinical features and the presence of an impacted tooth are sufficient to obtain a diagnosis, which may also be confirmed with radiographs.

Antibiotic therapy is appropriate for proper management. A more conservative approach may involve removal of the operculum overlying the affected tooth; however, hygiene and soft-tissue management in this area is difficult. For prevention, ultimate treatment involves extraction of the affected tooth as well as the tooth in the opposing arch.

ORAL MUCOSAL PAIN

Oral pain related to mucosal disorders is a direct manifestation of changes of the mucosal epithelium. These changes are seen intraorally as vesicle formation, ulcerations, erosions, erythema, pseudomembranes, and/or hyperkeratosis, with hyperalgesia of the affected mucosal tissue.

Pain of mucosal origin is continuous; usually described as raw, stinging, aching, and burning; can be reliably provoked by exposure to stimuli (thermal, mechanical, and chemical); and usually responds to the application of topical or local anesthetic at the site of pain.

Painful oral mucosal disorders may develop as a result of infection (bacterial, viral, or fungal), reactive processes (trauma, allergy, iatrogenic), systemic disorders (autoimmune or metabolic), or dysplasia (cancer). A comprehensive review of mucogingival diseases is beyond the scope of this review; however, select notable and common conditions are briefly discussed.

Oral Candidiasis

Oral candidiasis represents inflammatory conditions caused by infection from the yeast fungi genus *Candida*. The most common cause of oral candidiasis is the species *Candida albicans*. Infection can occur because of change in bacterial flora from antibiotics, lack of saliva, or conditions that impair local or systemic immune function (eg, diabetes, human immunodeficiency virus [HIV]). Acute pseudomembranous candidiasis is the most common form, affecting any intraoral mucosal surface, presenting with superficial, curd-like, white plaques that can be wiped off, overlying an erythematous, eroded, or ulcerated surface (**Fig. 9**). Acute atrophic candidiasis is more painful, with red lesions surrounded by inflamed tissue, with symptoms including oral burning and dysphagia. Chronic atrophic candidiasis appears erythematous and edematous, with a papular surface. Lesions occur on edentulous ridges or palate, frequently under dentures. Chronic hyperplastic candidiasis results in white and/or red hard nodular lesions that cannot be wiped off.

Diagnosis is often made from history and clinical appearance. If a diagnosis is uncertain or the condition arises in immunocompromised patients, a cytologic smear and culture may be performed to identify specific organism.

Oral candidiasis can be addressed with topical medicaments including chlorhexidine rinse, nystatin rinse or ointment, or clotrimazole troches. In refractory cases or in the immunocompromised, systemic medications are used, which include fluconazole, ketoconazole, and itraconazole.

Herpes Simplex Virus

Herpes simplex virus (HSV) infection can cause an acute primary or recurrent oral infection through two different strains, HSV-1 and HSV-2. Primary herpetic

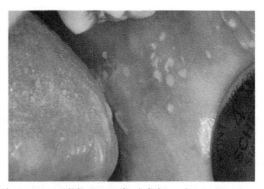

Fig. 9. Pseudomembranous candidiasis on the left buccal mucosa.

gingivostomatitis occurs in those who have not been previously exposed to the virus (eg, children or adolescents). It initially presents with a painful, severe, generalized gingival inflammation, followed by oral vesicles, accompanied by systemic manifestations including fever, malaise, and lymphadenopathy. After initial infection, which in most cases is subclinical, the virus remains latent or dormant within the trigeminal ganglion. Reactivation causes secondary or recurrent herpes stomatitis, which presents as painful vesicle eruptions, typically occurring on keratinized tissue (eg, lips, gingiva, tongue, hard palate) (**Fig. 10**). These eruptions may be preceded by prodromal tingling or burning sensations. Vesicles are quickly ruptured, resulting in a yellow ulceration with erythematous borders. Healing occurs within 1 to 4 days. Treatment of primary herpetic gingivostomatitis is supportive (fluids, nutrition, and analgesia). For recurrent herpes stomatitis, topical pencyclovir and oral valacyclovir (2 g twice a day for 1 day in the early prodromal stages) have been shown to decrease the severity and length of outbreak.[9,10] Other considerations include topical docosanol and oral acyclovir.

Herpes Zoster (Shingles)

Herpes zoster is an oral infection attributable to the varicella zoster virus, which causes chicken pox. Higher-risk individuals include the elderly and immunocompromised. The virus remains latent and dormant in nerve tissue, with the trigeminal

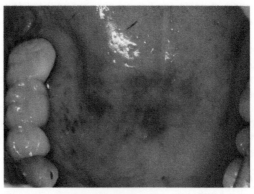

Fig. 10. Herpes simplex virus lesions on the hard palate. Ulcerations remain after bursting of vesicles.

ganglion involved in 10% to 15% of cases, among which 80% involves the ophthalmic division (V1).[11] It is characterized by prodromal symptoms of pain, burning, and tingling, followed by vesicular eruption, rupture, and ulceration in the distribution of the trigeminal nerve within 1 week of onset (**Fig. 11**). Eruptions can be seen both intraorally and extraorally on the skin. Diagnosis is made by history and clinical presentation. Treatment involves systemic antivirals such as acyclovir, valacyclovir, and famciclovir, accompanied by analgesics. Oral corticosteroids are also used to decrease the severity and duration of pain.[12] The most common complication of herpes zoster is post-herpetic neuralgia, a neuropathic condition causing continuous intractable pain that is burning and aching in nature.

Necrotizing Periodontal Disease

Necrotizing periodontal disease encompasses both necrotizing ulcerative gingivitis (NUG) and necrotizing ulcerative periodontitis (NUP). Although the exact etiology is unknown, spirochetes and fusiform bacteria are implicated, and factors include stress, tobacco use, poor oral hygiene, and impaired immunity. The condition presents as a continuously painful, erythematous, and edematous gingiva with punched-out erosion of the interdental papilla, often covered with a gray necrotic pseudomembrane. A fetid odor is common, and systemic symptoms (eg, malaise, low-grade fever) may be present. Diagnosis is obtained through history and clinical symptoms. Treatment consists of mechanical debridement, antibiotic therapy (chlorhexidine rinse, metronidazole, tetracycline, doxycycline), and management of underlying periodontal disease.

Recurrent Aphthous Stomatitis

Recurrent aphthous stomatitis (RAS) is the most common ulcerative condition of the oral cavity.[13] Ulcers most commonly occur in nonkeratinized mucosa (eg, lips, labial and buccal mucosa, ventral tongue, floor of mouth, and soft palate). Pain is continuous and is described as burning and aching, with pain that is disproportionate to the size of the lesions. Lesions can appear solitary or multiple, showing as a yellow ulceration with erythematous border (**Fig. 12**). The exact etiology of RAS is unknown; however, precipitating factors include certain foods, trauma, stress, hormones, nutritional or hematinic deficiencies, and contents of oral hygiene products.[14] Diagnosis is generally elicited by history and clinical presentations, and may include attempts to identify any underlying causes, which may entail history of foods and oral care products as well as blood work. Lesions typically last for 7 to 10 days, followed by complete healing.

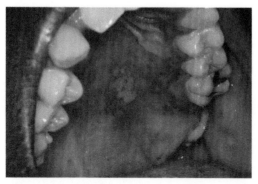

Fig. 11. Herpes zoster lesions on the left hard palate. Lesions are unilateral, following the distribution of the second branch of the trigeminal nerve (V2).

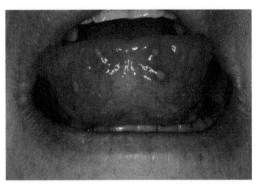

Fig. 12. Recurrent aphthous stomatitis. Multiple ulcerations on the ventral tongue.

Treatment is based on palliation, with topical anesthetics as an option.[15] Other topical agents, primarily aimed at curbing inflammation, include topical tetracyclines and chlorhexidine rinse. Topical steroids are used to possibly decrease the length and severity of symptoms.[16] In refractory, recurrent, and more severe cases, or in the immunocompromised (eg, HIV), systemic immune modulators such as oral corticosteroids, dapsone, pentoxifylline, and thalidomide are used.

Lichen Planus

Lichen planus is a dermatologic disease that often affects the oral mucosa. There are two forms: reticular lichen planus, which is most often asymptomatic, and erosive lichen planus, which is the type more likely to be symptomatic and characterized by burning, or pain when eating or drinking. Reticular lichen planus often shows white lines or striae (often in a reticular or lace-like pattern), or plaques or papules, overlying an area of erythema. Erosive lichen planus is characterized by erythematous areas with ulceration, usually bordered by white striae (**Fig. 13**). Affected areas are the buccal mucosa, tongue, gingiva, palate, and vermillion border. The characteristic reticular pattern is enough of a clinical presentation to obtain a diagnosis; however, biopsy may be required to obtain a diagnosis through histopathologic confirmation. Treatment is indicated only if the patient is symptomatic, and usually consists of

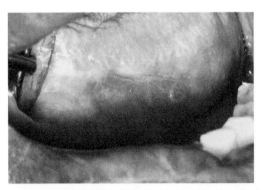

Fig. 13. Erosive lichen planus. Area of erythematous ulceration on the left lateral tongue, surrounded by white plaque and striae.

topical corticosteroids. Other considerations include topical tacrolimus or cyclosporine, or intralesional steroid injections in refractory areas.

Immunobullous Diseases

The immunobullous diseases include pemphigus vulgaris (PV) and mucous membrane pemphigoid (MMP), also known as cicatricial pemphigoid. Autoantibodies cause damage to the epithelium and underlying connective tissue. Patients' chief complaint is continuous oral soreness in affected areas. Clinical presentation of both includes vesicles, erosions, and ulceration in the oral mucosa and skin, with oral manifestations often being the first symptom to appear (**Figs. 14** and **15**). MMP also can affect the eyes, esophagus, and laryngeal and vaginal mucosa. Diagnosis is obtained through biopsy of both lesional and perilesional tissue, with the latter being used for staining for autoantibodies through direct immunofluorescence. In addition, patients' serum is collected to perform an indirect immunofluorescence analysis. MMP can be responsive to potent topical steroid therapy. Treatment of PV or refractory MMP involves systemic corticosteroids and other systemic immune modulators.

Cancer

Orofacial pain may be induced by malignant disease and its therapy. Pain has been reported in at least 50% of patients before, during, and at the end of cancer therapy, some persisting up to 1 year after the completion of therapy.[17]

Squamous cell carcinoma comprises 90% of intraoral malignancies, which in turn comprise 5% of all malignancies in the United States.[18] Pain from intraoral cancers can be due to long-standing ulcerations (**Fig. 16**), secondary infection, stimulation of nerve endings, or infiltration into adjacent peripheral nerve. Pain may be accompanied by paresthesia or hypoesthesia. Other clinical features include loose teeth, occlusal changes, bony expansion, and restricted jaw and/or tongue movement. Such symptoms must be viewed with high suspicion for malignancy when accompanied by pain, requiring further workup (eg, imaging studies, tissue biopsy) to obtain the correct diagnosis.

Oral Mucositis

Oral mucositis (OM) is a painful and debilitating side effect of cancer therapy, including chemotherapy, radiation therapy (to the head and neck), and hematopoietic stem cell transplantation for patients with hematologic malignancies. OM is characterized by erythema, ulceration, and pseudomembrane formation and shedding (**Fig. 17**). More

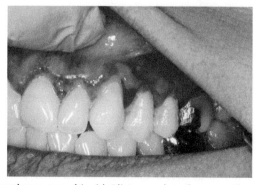

Fig. 14. Mucous membrane pemphigoid. Blisters and erythema on the maxillary gingiva.

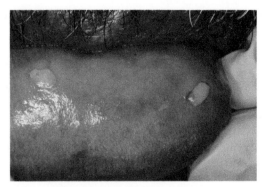

Fig. 15. Pemphigus vulgaris. Blisters on the labial mucosa.

than 40% of patients undergoing cancer chemotherapy contract some form of OM, and more than 60% develop a severe form of oral mucositis from radiation therapy and stem cell transplantation, with up to half of individuals requiring modification or interruption of their cancer treatment and/or parenteral analgesia.[19,20]

Treatment of OM is generally palliative with topical analgesic rinses, oral and parenteral analgesics, and supportive measures (eg, fluids, nutrition).

BONE
Osteomyelitis

Acute osteomyelitis occurs when an inflammatory process (usually infectious) spreads through the medullary spaces of the bone. Signs and symptoms include significant pain and sensitivity in the affected jaw area, swelling, fever, lymphadenopathy, and leukocytosis. This presentation may be accompanied by paresthesia, drainage, or exfoliation of bony sequestra. Chronic osteomyelitis may have swelling, pain, sinus formation, and periods of pain followed by remission. Diagnosis is obtained by combination of clinical symptoms and through imaging studies, which show ill-defined radiolucencies in the affected bone. Treatment entails drainage (in the presence of abscess formation) and antibiotic therapy. For refractory chronic osteomyelitis surgical intervention is required, involving removal of affected bone through curettage and, in more severe cases, resection.

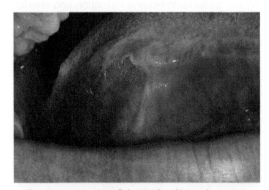

Fig. 16. Squamous cell carcinoma. Painful, nonhealing ulceration on the right lateral tongue that was confirmed as squamous cell carcinoma after biopsy and pathologic diagnosis.

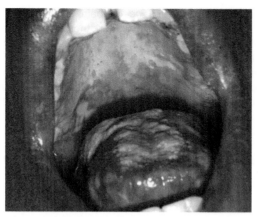

Fig. 17. Oral mucositis in a patient undergoing cancer chemotherapy.

Osteonecrosis

Osteonecrosis occurs because of hypoxia, hypovascularity, and hypocellularity of the bone. Osteoradionecrosis (ORN) and bisphosphonate osteonecrosis (BON) involve the formation of necrotic bone in the oral cavity in response to exposure to radiation therapy and bisphosphonate therapy, respectively. In addition, other, nonbisphosphonate drugs have been implicated in causing osteonecrosis. It is characterized by the presence of nonhealing area of exposed bone of at least 6 months' duration (**Fig. 18**).

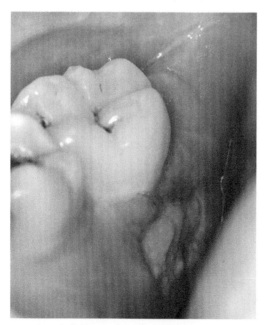

Fig. 18. Osteoradionecrosis. Painful area of exposed bone on the right posterior lingual area in a patient who had undergone radiation therapy to the head and neck.

Clinical manifestations and symptoms include pain, swelling, reduced jaw mobility, bony destruction, and purulent drainage when there is secondary osteomyelitis. Risk factors for ORN include radiation dosages higher than 60 Gy, dental disease, postradiation dental extractions, and previous cancer resection.[21] BON occurs in patients on oral bisphosphonates for osteoporosis; however those having been on intravenous bisphosphonate therapy for cancer involving the bone are at considerably higher risk and incidence.[22] Because of their nonhealing nature, treatment of both ORN and BON is challenging, and there is no established effective treatment regimen. Management strategies include analgesia, long-term topical and systemic antibiotic therapy for secondary infections, pentoxifylline, and hyperbaric oxygen therapy. Surgical considerations include removal of affected bone by curettage or resection and vascularized bone containing pedicle flap, although surgery may exacerbate the condition.

Maxillary Sinusitis

Toothache may be a presenting symptom of maxillary sinusitis, the most common causes of which are upper respiratory tract infection and allergic rhinitis.

Acute sinusitis

Clinical features include: headache; fever; facial pain over affected sinus; clear, mucoid, or purulent thick or thin anterior nasal or posterior pharyngeal discharge; pain over the cheekbone; toothache and tenderness to percussion of multiple maxillary teeth; periorbital pain; and pain during positional changes (increased pain when upright, decreased pain when supine).

Chronic sinusitis

Clinical features include: facial pressure and pain; sensation of obstruction, headache, and sore throat; lightheadedness; and generalized fatigue.

When normal (commensal) sinus flora is augmented, potential for infection is increased. Most common bacteria implicated are *Streptococcus pneumoniae* and *Haemophilus influenzae*. As the maxillary sinus is in close proximity to the maxillary posterior teeth, 10% of maxillary sinusitis cases may result from odontogenic sources, including infection or manipulation of posterior teeth.[23]

Clinical features, along with imaging studies (radiographs, computed tomography [CT], magnetic resonance imaging), aid in obtaining a diagnosis. Radiographically, increased radiopacities are seen in the sinus (**Fig. 19**).

Treatment is targeted at symptoms and includes decongestants, antihistamines, mucolytic agents, α-adrenergic agents, corticosteroids, and analgesics. Antibiotic

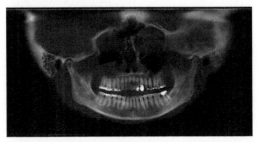

Fig. 19. Panoramic view of a CT image showing radio-opacities in the right maxillary sinus. (*Courtesy of* Richard H. Haug DDS, Charlotte, NC.)

use is indicated in cases of moderate to severe pain, persistence beyond 7 days, and purulent discharge.

SALIVARY GLAND ABNORMALITY
Bacterial Sialadenitis

Bacterial sialadenitis is a bacterial infection of the salivary gland. Clinical features include swollen and painful salivary glands, more often unilateral, with induration and erythema on the overlying skin. It most commonly occurs in patients with reduced salivary flow. Reduced salivary flow decreases mechanical flushing, leading to increased colonization of bacteria in the salivary gland ducts. Predominant bacterial species include *Staphylococcus aureus*, *H influenza*, *Streptococcus viridans*, *S pneumoniae*, *Escherichia coli*, and *Fusobacterium*, *Prevotella*, and *Porphyromonas* species.[24]

Oral Sialoliths

Oral sialoliths (salivary stones) are calcified material that forms within the major salivary glands. Most commonly they occur in the submandibular glands (80%–90%), followed by the parotid (5%–15%) and sublingual glands (2%–5%). Symptoms are based on the degree of obstruction of the duct and the presence of secondary infection. Pain may be accompanied by swelling and ulceration, and may be accompanied by fistulas and purulent drainage when secondary infection occurs. Radiographs (occlusal) and CT scans may show sialoliths; however, they are not always calcified enough to show up on these images (**Fig. 20**). Sialography and sialoendoscopy may also be used.

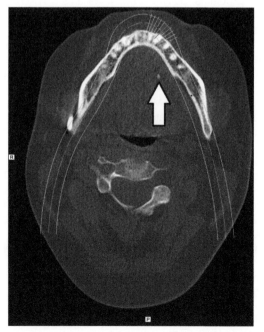

Fig. 20. Sialolith (*arrow*) seen on an axial-view CT image. (*Courtesy of* Richard H. Haug DDS, Charlotte, NC.)

Treatment in the acute phases for bacterial sialadenitis and sialoliths with secondary infection is mainly supportive, with use of analgesics, hydration, antibiotics, and parasympathomimetics to stimulate salivary flow. For sialoliths, surgical removal of the salivary stone may also be indicated.

ACKNOWLEDGMENTS

Special thanks to Dawnyetta Marable, MD, DMD, for her significant contribution in the assembly of this article. Also a special mention to Andrea Herman, Leigha Christenbury Hernandez, and Katherine Tuori for their assistance.

REFERENCES

1. Orchardson R, Gillam DG. The efficacy of potassium salts as agents for treating dentin hypersensitivity. J Orofac Pain 2000;14(1):9–19.
2. Trowbridge HO, Silver DR. A review of current approaches to in-office management of tooth hypersensitivity. Dent Clin North Am 1990;34(3):561–81.
3. Mathew S, Thangavel B, Mathew CA, et al. Diagnosis of cracked tooth syndrome. J Pharm Bioallied Sci 2012;4(Suppl 2):S242–4.
4. Turp JC, Gobetti JP. The cracked tooth syndrome: an elusive diagnosis. J Am Dent Assoc 1996;127:1502–7.
5. Berman LH, Hartwell GR. Diagnosis. In: Cohen S, Hargreaves K, editors. Pathways of the pulp. 9th edition. St Louis (MO): Mosby; 2006. p. 1–39.
6. Van Steenberghe D. The structure and function of periodontal innervation. A review of the literature. J Periodontal Res 1979;14(3):185–203.
7. Abrams H, Jasper SJ. Diagnosis and management of acute periodontal problems. In: Falace DA, editor. Emergency dental care: diagnosis and management of urgent dental problems. Baltimore (MD): Williams & Wilkins; 1995. p. 137–42.
8. Herrera D, Roldan S, Gonzalez I, et al. The periodontal abscess. I. Clinical and microbiological findings. J Clin Periodontol 2000;27(6):387–94.
9. Spruance SL, Rea TL, Thoming C, et al. Penciclovir cream for the treatment of herpes simplex labialis. A randomized, multicenter, double-blind, placebo-controlled trial. Topical Penciclovir Collaborative Study Group. JAMA 1997; 277(17):1374–9.
10. Spruance SL, Jones TM, Blatter MM, et al. High-dose, short-duration, early valacyclovir therapy for episodic treatment of cold sores: results of two randomized, placebo-controlled, multicenter studies. Antimicrob Agents Chemother 2003;47: 1072–80.
11. Ragozzino MW, Melton LJ 3rd, Kurland LT, et al. Population-based study of herpes zoster and its sequelae. Medicine (Baltimore) 1982;61:310–6.
12. Eaglestein WH, Katz R, Brown JA. The effects of early corticosteroid therapy in the skin eruption and pain of herpes zoster. J Am Med Assoc 1970;211:1681–3.
13. Ship JA, Chavez EM, Doerr PA, et al. Recurrent aphthous stomatitis. Quintessence Int 2000;31:95–112.
14. Scully C, Gorsky M, Lozada-Nur F. The diagnosis and management of recurrent aphthous stomatitis: a consensus approach. J Am Dent Assoc 2003;134:200–7.
15. Eisen D, Lynch DP. Selecting topical and systemic agents for recurrent aphthous stomatitis. Cutis 2001;68:201–6.
16. Porter SR, Scully C, Pedersen A. Recurrent aphthous stomatitis. Crit Rev Oral Biol Med 1998;9(3):306–32.
17. Epstein JB, Hong C, Logan RM, et al. A systematic review of orofacial pain in patients receiving cancer therapy. Support Care Cancer 2010;18(8):1023–31.

18. Barasch A, Safford M, Eisenberg E. Oral cancer and oral effects of anticancer therapy. Mt Sinai J Med 1998;65(5–6):370–7.
19. Sonis ST. Oral complications. In: Holland JF, editor. Cancer medicine. 4th edition. Philadelphia: Williams & Wilkins; 1997. p. 3255–64.
20. Schubert MM, Sullivan KMJ, Truelove EL. Head and neck complication of bone marrow transplantation. Develop Oncol 1991;36:401–27.
21. Katsura K, Sasai K, Sato K, et al. Relationship between oral health status and development of osteoradionecrosis of the mandible: a retrospective longitudinal study. Oral Surg Oral Med Oral Pathol Oral Radiol Endod 2008;105:731–8.
22. Migliorati CA, Woo SB, Hewson I, et al. A systemic review of bisphosphonate osteonecrosis (BON) in cancer. Support Care Cancer 2010;18(8):1099–106.
23. Lee KC, Lee SJ. Clinical features and treatments of odontogenic sinusitis. Yonsei Med J 2010;51(6):932–7.
24. Fox PC, Ship JA. Salivary gland diseases. In: Greenburg MS, Glick M, Ship JA, editors. Burket's oral medicine. 11th edition. Hamilton (Canada): BC Decker; 2008. p. 191–222.

Acute and Chronic Low Back Pain

Nathan Patrick, MD, Eric Emanski, MD, Mark A. Knaub, MD*

KEYWORDS

- Acute low back pain • Chronic low back pain • Patient education
- Treatment protocols

KEY POINTS

- Numerous factors put patients at risk for the development of chronic back pain, including age, educational status, psychosocial factors, occupational factors, and obesity.
- Evaluation of patients with back pain includes completing an appropriate history (including red-flag symptoms), performing a comprehensive physical examination, and, in some scenarios, obtaining imaging in the form of plain radiographs and magnetic resonance imaging.
- Treatment of an acute episode of back pain includes relative rest, activity modification, nonsteroidal anti-inflammatories, and physical therapy.
- Patient education is also imperative, as these patients are at risk for further episodes of back pain in the future.
- Chronic back pain (>6 months' duration) develops in a small percentage of patients. Clinicians' ability to diagnose the exact pathologic source of these symptoms is severely limited, making a cure unlikely. Treatment of these patients should be supportive, the goal being to improve pain and function rather than to "cure" the patient's condition.

MAGNITUDE OF THE PROBLEM

Low back pain is an extremely common problem that affects at least 80% of all individuals at some point in their lifetime, and is the fifth most common reason for all physician visits in the United States.[1–3] Approximately 1 in 4 adults in the United States reported having low back pain that lasted at least 24 hours within the previous 3 months, and 7.6% reported at least 1 episode of severe acute low back pain within a 1-year period.[4,5] In addition, low back pain is a leading cause of activity limitation and work absence (second only to upper respiratory conditions) throughout much

This article originally appeared in Medical Clinics of North America, Volume 98, Issue 4, July 2014.

Department of Orthopaedic Surgery, Penn State–Milton S. Hershey Medical Center, 30 Hope Drive, Building A, Hershey, PA 17033, USA

* Corresponding author.

E-mail address: mknaub@hmc.psu.edu

of the world, resulting in a vast economic burden on individuals, families, communities, industry, and governments.[6–9] In 1998, total incremental direct health care costs attributable to low back pain in the United States were estimated at $26.3 billion.[10] Furthermore, indirect costs related to days lost from work are substantial, with nearly 2% of the work force of the United States compensated for back injuries each year.[11]

RISK AND PROGNOSTIC FACTORS

Factors that play a role in the development of back pain include age, educational status, psychosocial factors, job satisfaction, occupational factors, and obesity. Age is one of the most common factors in the development of low back pain, with most studies finding the highest incidence in the third decade of life and overall prevalence increasing until age 60 to 65 years. However, there is recent evidence that prevalence continues to increase with age with more severe forms of back pain.[1,12] Other studies show that back pain in the adolescent population has become increasingly common.[13]

An increased prevalence of low back pain is associated with patients of low educational status.[1] Lower educational levels are a strong predictor of more prolonged episode duration and poorer outcomes.[14] Psychosocial factors such as stress, anxiety, depression, and certain types of pain behavior are associated with greater rates of low back pain. The presence of these conditions also increases the risk that a patient's episode of back pain will last long enough to be considered chronic.[1,15] Likewise, patients who are dissatisfied with their work situation are at risk of having an acute episode of back pain transition to a chronic situation.[16] Occupational factors, specifically the physical demands of work, are also associated with an increased prevalence of low back pain. Matsui and colleagues[17] found the point prevalence of low back pain to be 39% in manual workers, whereas it was found in only 18.3% of those with sedentary occupations. A more recent systematic review found manual handling, bending, twisting, and whole-body vibration to be risk factors for low back pain.[18] Lastly, obesity, or a body mass index of more than 30 kg/m^2, has been connected with an increased incidence of low back pain.[1,19]

PRESENTATION

For most patients, an episode of acute low back pain is a self-limited condition that does not require any active medical treatment.[5] Among those who do seek medical care, their symptoms and disability improve rapidly and most are able to return to work and normal activities within the first month.[20] Up to 1 in 3 of these patients, however, report persistent back pain of at least moderate intensity 1 year after an acute episode, and 1 in 5 reports substantial limitations in activity.[21]

Initial evaluation of patients with back pain should begin with a focused history. Key aspects of this should include: duration of symptoms; description of the pain (location, severity, timing, radiation, and so forth); presence of neurologic symptoms (weakness or alterations in sensation or pain) or changes in bowel and bladder function; evidence of any recent or current infection (fever, chills, sweats, and so forth); previous treatments; and pertinent medical history (cancer, infection, osteoporosis, fractures, endocrine disorders). Key facets of the history are listed in **Box 1**. Some historical facts, referred to by many as red-flag symptoms, may be a harbinger of a dangerous clinical situation (**Box 2**). When present, these symptoms should raise the level of suspicion of the provider that this patient is presenting with more than a simple, benign episode of acute low back pain. In patients presenting with 1 or more of these red flags, there is a 10% chance that they have a serious underlying

---

Box 1
Historical factors that must be considered in the evaluation of a patient with low back pain

Duration

Acute low back pain: less than 4 weeks

Subacute low back pain: 4 weeks to 3 months

Chronic low back pain: more than 3 months

Pain Description

Location (cervical, thoracic, lumbar, sacral)

Severity (pain scale, type of pain, activities affected)

Timing (morning, evening, constant, intermittent)

Aggravating and relieving factors (ambulation/rest, sitting/standing/laying, inclines/declines, back flexion/extension)

Radiation (dermatomal or nondermatomal)

Deficits

Motor weakness

Sensory changes (numbness, tingling, paresthesias, dermatomal or nondermatomal)

Urinary or bowel incontinence, urgency, or frequency

Risk Factors

Age

Educational status

Psychosocial factors

Occupation

Body mass index

Medical History

Cancer

Recent or current infection

Osteoporosis and history of other fractures

Endocrine disorders

Previous spinal surgeries

---

source of their symptoms of low back pain. These patients should have plain radiographs taken of their lumbar spine to rule out serious structural abnormality. In a patient in whom an infectious cause is considered, plain radiographs may be normal early in the disease process. A white blood cell count, erythrocyte sedimentation rate, and C-reactive protein should be obtained. Elevation of these inflammatory parameters should prompt evaluation with magnetic resonance imaging (MRI), with and without contrast, of the lumbar spine.

Patient-completed pain diagrams are useful adjuncts in evaluating patients with acute or chronic low back pain, and are especially useful for those with radicular complaints. Patient outcomes measures such as the Oswestry Disability Index can give insight into how patients' symptoms are affecting their life, and can be useful to track treatment progress.

> **Box 2**
> **Red-flag symptoms**
>
> The presence of any of these historical factors in a patient presenting with low back pain may indicate a serious underlying disorder and should prompt a more rapid and thorough evaluation of the patient.
>
> Age >50 years
>
> Systemic symptoms: fever, chills, night sweats, fatigue, decreased appetite, unintentional weight loss
>
> History of malignancy
>
> Nonmechanical pain (pain that gets worse with rest): night pain
>
> Recent or current bacterial infection, especially skin infection or urinary tract infection
>
> Immunosuppression
>
> History of intravenous drug use
>
> Failure of response to initial treatment/therapy
>
> Prolonged corticosteroid use or diagnosis of osteoporosis
>
> Trauma

PHYSICAL EXAMINATION

Physical examination of the patient with low back pain is a necessity during the office visit. The examination should focus on determining the presence and severity of neurologic involvement. At the conclusion of the visit, the clinician should also attempt to place the patient's back pain into 1 of 3 categories: nonspecific low back pain, back pain associated with radiculopathy or spinal stenosis, or back pain associated with a specific spinal cause.[22,23] Table 1 lists common spinal causes of back pain with associated historical and physical examination findings, in addition to imaging recommendations. Although the physical examination is an essential part of the visit, it rarely provides the clinician with a specific diagnosis for the cause of the patient's symptoms. An examination begins with observation of the patient, typically starting when the clinician enters the examination room and involves noting how the patient acts during the history taking. Visual inspection of the patient's thoracic and lumbar spine, and the posterior pelvis, is accomplished by having the patient in a gown. Assessment for any skin abnormalities or asymmetry around the lumbar spine should be performed. Palpation of the bony elements of the spine and the posterior pelvis in addition to the paraspinal muscles can help localize the patient's complaints. Obvious deformities such as significant scoliosis or a high-grade spondylolisthesis may be discovered with observation and/or palpation in a nonobese patient. Assessment of spinal motion can be difficult in a patient with acute low back pain, but should be attempted. Limitations in specific directions should be noted, as should any worsening of symptoms with specific motions. Unfortunately, the assessment of motion has not proved to be reliable between observers and does not provide the clinician with a specific diagnosis.

A complete neurologic examination is performed, and should include both upper and lower extremity function. Subtle examination findings in the upper extremities, such as hyperreflexia or a positive Hofmann sign, could indicate a more proximal cause (cervical spinal cord compression/dysfunction) of a patient's lower extremity neurologic complaints or bowel/bladder dysfunction. Manual muscle strength testing should be performed of the major muscle groups of the lower extremity to include the myotomes of the lumbar nerve roots (Table 2). Muscle strength should be recorded using a scale of 0 to 5 (**Table 3**). Sensory examination should be performed with reference to the lumbar dermatomes (see **Table 2**). Side-to-side comparison of sensation to light touch and pinprick should be performed in all patients. Assessment of proprioception and vibration sense can be included in select patients in whom central processes or lesions are suspected. Patellar and Achilles deep tendon reflexes are helpful in differentiating central nervous system abnormalities (indicated by hyperactive reflexes) from lumbar nerve root or peripheral nerve problems (hypoactive reflexes expected). The presence of a Babinski sign (upward-moving great toe when the plantar-lateral surface of the foot is scraped) should alert the examiner to the probability of a more central issue. Functional muscle strength should be assessed by asking the patient to stand from a seated position without the assistance of the upper extremities (assessing functional strength of quadriceps). Asking the patient to squat from a standing position can also assess the functional strength of the quadriceps. Having the patient stand on the heels and toes can assess the strength of the ankle dorsiflexor and plantarflexor musculature. A single-leg toe raise can be used to diagnose subtle weakness of the gastrocnemius-soleus complex.

Straight-leg raise (SLR) and cross-SLR tests are not useful in patients with complaints of only low back pain. Nearly all patients with low back pain will have an increase in their symptoms with these maneuvers. These tests are helpful in patients with radiating leg pain in an attempt to differentiate true radiculopathy from other causes of leg pain. For an SLR test to be considered positive, the patient must have a reproduction of the radiating leg pain distal to the knee on the side that is being tested. A positive cross-SLR test occurs when the patient's radicular pain below the knee is reproduced while the contralateral leg is extended at the hip and knee. Positive results for the SLR test have high sensitivity (91%; 95% confidence interval [CI] 82%–94%) but is not specific (26%; 95% CI 16%–38%) for identifying a disc herniation. The cross-SLR test is more specific (88%; 95% CI 86%–90%) but not sensitive (29%; CI 24%–34%).[24] Both SLR and cross-SLR tests are designed to evaluate for compression of the lower (L4-S1) lumbar nerve roots. The femoral stretch test is a similar provocative maneuver that aims to create tension in the upper lumbar roots (L2 and L3) in an attempt to reproduce L2 or L3 radicular symptoms in the anterior thigh.

The physical examination must also evaluate for other potential sources of the patient's pain. Nonmusculoskeletal causes of back pain should be considered, as should nonspinal, musculoskeletal causes. A partial list of nonmusculoskeletal abnormalities that may cause back pain is shown in **Box 3**. The sacroiliac (SI) joints and the hips should be examined to assess whether these structures are contributing to a patient's symptoms. Simple internal and external rotation of the hip in either the supine or seated position places the hip joint through a range of motion that will likely reproduce the patient's pain if it is originating in the hip joint. The SI joint can be loaded or stressed with the Patrick test or the FABER test, whereby the patient's hip is placed into flexion, abduction, and external rotation. This test is typically performed with the patient in the supine position and the lower extremity placed into a "figure-4" position. The Patrick test is positive if it reproduces the patient's back pain on the side that is being examined. A positive test, though not diagnostic of an SI joint problem, should at least alert the examiner to the possibility that the SI joint may be contributing to the patient's symptoms.

Psychosocial issues play an important role in both acute and chronic low back pain. Patients with abnormal psychometric profiles are at greater risk for development of chronic back pain. In addition, they are more likely to be functionally affected (or disabled) by their symptoms of back pain. Screening for depression can be performed in an attempt to identify patients who are at risk. Psychological overlay is often found in

Table 1
Common spinal causes of back pain with associated historical factors, physical examination findings, recommended imaging modalities, and any additional diagnostic testing

Etiology	Key Features	Imaging	Additional Studies
Muscle strain	General ache or muscle spasms in the lower back, may radiate to buttock or posterior thighs; worse with increasing activity or bending	None	None
Disc herniation	Pain originating in the lower back with dermatomal radiation to the lower extremity; relieved by standing and worsened with sitting; may be accompanied by motor/sensory changes	Symptoms present <1 mo: none; Symptoms present >1 mo or severe/progressive: MRI	None
Lumbar spondylosis	Generalized back pain worse immediately after waking up; improvement throughout the day; pain fluctuates with activity and may worsen with extension of the spine	Symptoms present <1 mo: plain radiographs	None
Spinal stenosis with neurogenic claudication	Back pain with radiculopathy that is often worsened with extension/standing and improved with flexion/sitting; may be accompanied by motor/sensory changes	Symptoms present <1 mo: none; Symptoms present >1 mo or severe/progressive: MRI	None
Spondylolisthesis	Back pain that may radiate down one or both legs and is exacerbated by flexion and extension; may be accompanied by motor/sensory changes	Symptoms present <1 mo: none; Symptoms >1 mo or severe/progressive: plain radiographs	None
Spondylolysis: stress reaction or stress fracture of pars interarticularis	One of the most common causes of back pain in children and adolescents	Symptoms present <1 mo: none; Symptoms >1 mo or severe/progressive: plain radiographs	None

(continued on next page)

Table 1
(continued)

Etiology	Key Features	Imaging	Additional Studies
Ankylosing spondylitis	More common in young males; morning stiffness; low back pain that often radiates to the buttock and improves with exercise	Anterior-posterior pelvis radiographs	ESR, CRP, HLA-B27
Infection: epidural abscess ± osteomyelitis	Severe pain with an insidious onset that is unrelenting in nature; night pain; presence of constitutional symptoms; history of recent infection; may have radiculopathy or be accompanied by motor/sensory changes	Plain radiographs and MRI	CBC, ESR, CRP
Malignancy	History of cancer with new onset of low back pain; unexplained weight loss; age >50 y; may have radiculopathy or be accompanied by motor/sensory changes	Plain radiographs and MRI	CBC, ESR, CRP, PTH, TSH, SPEP, UA, UPEP
Cauda equina syndrome	Urinary retention or fecal incontinence; decreased rectal tone; saddle anesthesia; may be accompanied by weakness	MRI	None
Conus medullaris syndrome	Same as cauda equina, but often accompanied by upper motor neuron signs (hyperreflexia, clonus, etc)	MRI	None
Vertebral compression fracture	History of osteoporosis or corticosteroid use; older age	Plain radiographs	1,25-Dihydroxyvitamin D_3
Trauma	Variable examination pending the severity of the injury; may be accompanied by motor/sensory changes	Lumbosacral radiographs, CT, ± MRI	None

Abbreviations: CBC, complete blood count; CRP, C-reactive protein; CT, computed tomography; ESR, erythrocyte sedimentation rate; HLA-B27, human leukocyte antigen B27; MRI, magnetic resonance imaging; PTH, parathyroid hormone; SPEP, serum protein electrophoresis; TSH, thyroid-stimulating hormone; UA, urinalysis; UPEP, urine protein electrophoresis.

Table 2
Lower extremity myotomes, dermatomes, and reflexes by lumbar nerve root

Lumbar Nerve Root	Muscle Group	Sensory Distribution	Deep Tendon Reflex
L2	Hip flexor	Anterior medial thigh	None
L3	Quadriceps	Anterior thigh to knee	Patellar
L4	Anterior tibialis	Medial calf/ankle	Patellar
L5	Extensor hallicus longus	Lateral ankle/dorsum of foot	None
S1	Gastrocnemius/soleus/peroneals	Plantar-lateral foot	Achilles

these patients, which can cloud their physical examination. Assessing for Waddell signs can be useful in determining if there is a nonorganic cause of the patient's symptoms.[25,26] The presence of 1 or more of these findings on examination increases the possibility that the patient has a nonstructural source of the symptoms (**Box 4**). As a word of caution, the presence of Waddell signs does not exclude an organic cause of low back pain; rather, it points to the need for further psychological evaluation of the patient.

IMAGING

Evidenced-based treatment guidelines have long established that most patients presenting with an episode of acute low back pain do not need any imaging. Most of these patients will have improvement in their clinical symptoms within a few days to a week, even in the absence of any active treatment. In addition, imaging (including MRI) is not likely to reveal an exact pathologic diagnosis in the most patients. Overutilization of imaging in the evaluation of acute low back pain leads to increased health care expenditures in a patient population that will likely improve on its own. In addition, imaging in these patients frequently leads to the diagnosis of degenerative disc disease, which allows the patient to adopt the sick role. The thought that one has a "disease" leads the patient to change his or her behavior, and many begin to exhibit fear-avoidance behavior. This term refers to patients' fear that they are going to do something that will injury or worsen their "diseased" back; therefore they decrease their physical activity, which culminates in being detrimental to their recovery. The preferred approach is to reassure patients that they will likely get better without any active medical intervention and that imaging, including MRI, will not reveal an exact pathologic diagnosis in most patients.

Imaging is indicated in patients who present with red-flag symptoms or in those whose symptoms persist despite 4 to 6 weeks of conservative treatment. Standing plain radiographs of the lumbar spine are the initial imaging modality of choice.

Table 3
Grading system for muscle power on manual muscle strength testing

Grade	Description
0	No contraction
1	Muscle flicker/twitch
2	Able to fire muscle with gravity removed
3	Able to fire muscle against force of gravity
4	Able to fire muscle against some resistance
5	Normal strength against resistance

Box 3
Nonmusculoskeletal causes of back pain

Nonmusculoskeletal causes of pain must be considered in patients being evaluated for back pain.

Genitourinary

   Nephrolithiasis

   Pyelonephritis

   Prostatitis

   Endometriosis

   Ovarian cysts

Gastrointestinal

   Esophagitis

   Gastritis and peptic ulcer disease

   Cholelithiasis and cholecystitis

   Pancreatitis

   Diverticulitis

   Other intra-abdominal infections

Cardiovascular

   Abdominal or thoracic aortic aneurysm

   Cardiac ischemia or myocardial infarction

Neurologic

   Intramedullary spinal cord tumors

Though not likely to reveal the exact pathologic cause of a patient's symptoms, these images will rule out troubling disorder such as fracture, tumor, or infection. With these diagnoses largely excluded with plain radiographs, most patients with low back pain do not require further imaging. MRI should be used in patients with neurologic

---

Box 4
Signs of nonorganic abnormality

Waddell's signs, when present, can indicate a psychological component of chronic low back pain.

Tenderness tests: superficial and/or diffuse tenderness and/or nonanatomic tenderness

Simulation tests: based on movements, which produce pain, without actually causing that movement, such as axial loading on the top of the head causing low back pain and pain on simulated lumbar spine rotation

Distraction tests: positive tests are rechecked when the patient's attention is distracted, such as a straight leg raise test with the patient in a seated position

Regional disturbances: regional strength or sensory changes that do not follow accepted neuroanatomy

Overreaction: subjective signs regarding the patient's demeanor and overreaction to testing

From Waddell G, McCulloch J, Kummel E, et al. Nonorganic physical signs in low-back pain. Spine 1980;5:117–25.

complaints or in those for whom the clinician has a high level of suspicion for an occult fracture, tumor, or early infection. MRI is a highly sensitive imaging modality, but lacks specificity when a patient's complaint is axial pain. Degenerative changes are found in many asymptomatic subjects, and these changes increase in frequency with increasing age. Therefore, it is impossible to attribute a patient's back pain to a degenerative disc or an arthritic facet joint, given that they are present in most asymptomatic subjects.

Other imaging modalities that are used in patients with back pain include computed tomography, myelography, and bone scans. The indications for these tests are limited and fall outside the scope of this article. Provocative lumbar discography is a highly debated topic within the community of spine care providers. The senior author believes that discography has poor positive predictive value for successful surgical outcomes when it is used to determine whether a patient is a candidate for surgical intervention for axial low back pain. As a result, discography is not used during the evaluation of patients with chronic low back pain. Other spine surgeons routinely use discography to determine if a patient is a candidate for spinal fusion for "discogenic" low back pain, and many patients agree to have this diagnostic test performed and subsequently undergo spinal fusion in an attempt to improve their axial low back pain. Successful outcomes occur in only 40% to 60% of patients undergoing this type of procedure. Because of these poor results, the senior author does not perform spinal fusion procedures on patients with isolated low back pain and only degenerative changes on imaging.

TREATMENT

An exhaustive discussion of the treatment options available for acute and chronic low back pain is beyond the scope of this article. Most acute episodes of low back pain will resolve within 6 to 8 weeks even in the absence of active treatment. Relative rest, activity modification, nonsteroidal anti-inflammatory drugs (NSAIDs), chiropractic manipulation, and physical therapy are all treatment options in the acute and subacute phase of this clinical syndrome. These treatment modalities probably do not result in a significant change in the natural history of the condition, but do provide the patient with some active treatment modalities while the episode runs its natural course. Initial management of an episode of low back pain should include relative rest, cessation of pain-provoking activities, and a limited course of medications. NSAIDs, acetaminophen, tramadol, muscle relaxants, antidepressants, and opioids are frequently used in the treatment of both acute and chronic back pain. In patients with chronic axial pain, the use of simple analgesics, such as acetaminophen or tramadol, in combination with an antidepressant, appears to have the greatest efficacy.[27] Long-term opioid use for the treatment of chronic low back pain appears to be safe but only modestly effective in this patient group. These patients have only small functional improvements from the use of the medication, and are at risk for the adverse effects of opioid use including central nervous system depression, constipation, development of tolerance, and aberrant behavior. NSAIDs are perhaps the most commonly used single class of medications for back pain symptoms. NSAIDs are as effective as other medication classes but harbor the potential for gastrointestinal side effects. Their safety for long-term use in the setting of hypertension and/or cardiovascular disease has been questioned.

Adjunctive treatment options include physical therapy, a period of immobilization, and local treatment modalities that may include heat, ice, ultrasound, massage, and transcutaneous electrical nerve stimulation. Alternative treatment options may include spinal manipulation, acupuncture, yoga, and other exercise-based therapy programs. These alternative therapies lack conclusive scientific evidence supporting their efficacy in the treatment of acute or chronic back pain. Despite this, there are patients who pursue these options, and many benefit to at least some extent. Physical therapy or exercise-based programs tend to focus on core muscle strengthening and aerobic conditioning. No differences have been found when comparing the effectiveness of supervised with home-based exercise programs.

Spinal injections have a limited role in the treatment of chronic, mechanical low back pain. There is some evidence that intralaminar epidural steroid injections may play a small role in the short-term treatment of this patient population. Some patients may also benefit from facet injections or facet blocks when other conservative treatment modalities have been exhausted.

For those unfortunate few who fail to improve and fall into the category of chronic back pain, modern medicine has failed to provide any effective treatments. Despite many advances in medicine, clinicians' ability to diagnose the exact source of a patient's axial back pain is extremely limited. Therefore, our ability to treat this clinical entity is poor. Many surgeons believe that there are some patients who suffer from chronic back pain who would improve with surgical treatment of their symptoms. The problem lies in our inability to determine which individual patient will benefit from surgery and which will be left with ongoing pain and disability. The goals of treatment for these patients should move away from a "cure" and focus on lessening symptoms and the effects they have on the patient, in addition to improving function.

SUMMARY

Back pain is an extremely common presenting complaint that occurs in upward of 80% of persons. The natural history of acute episodes of back pain is favorable in most patients. Numerous factors put patients at risk for the development of chronic back pain, including age, educational status, psychosocial factors, occupational factors, and obesity. Evaluation of these patients includes completing an appropriate history (including red-flag symptoms), performing a comprehensive physical examination, and, in some scenarios, obtaining imaging in the form of plain radiographs and MRI. Treatment of an acute episode of back pain includes relative rest, activity modification, NSAIDs, and physical therapy. Patient education is also imperative, as these patients are at risk for further episodes of back pain in the future. Chronic back pain (>6 months' duration) develops in a small percentage of patients. Clinicians' ability to diagnose the exact pathologic source of these symptoms is severely limited, making a cure unlikely. Treatment of these patients should be supportive, the goal being to improve pain and function rather than to "cure" the patient's condition.

REFERENCES

1. Hoy D, Brooks P, Blyth F, et al. The epidemiology of low back pain. Best Pract Res Clin Rheumatol 2010;24:769–81.
2. Chou R, Qaseem A, Snow V, et al, Clinical efficacy assessment Subcommittee of the American College of Physicians, American College of Physicians, American Pain Society Low Back Pain Guidelines Panel. Diagnosis and treatment of low back pain: a joint clinical practice guideline from the American College of Physicians and the American Pain Society. Ann Intern Med 2007;147(7):478–91.
3. Hart LG, Deyo RA, Cherkin DC. Physician office visits for low back pain. Frequency, clinical evaluation, and treatment patterns from a U.S. National Survey. Spine 1995;20:11–9.

4. Deyo RA, Mirza SK, Martin BI. Back pain prevalence and visit rates: estimates from U.S. national surveys, 2002. Spine 2006;31:2724–7.
5. Carey TS, Evans AT, Hadler NM, et al. Acute severe low back pain. A population-based study of prevalence and care-seeking. Spine 1996;21:339–44.
6. Lidgren L. The bone and joint decade 2000-2010. Bull World Health Organ 2003; 81(9):629.
7. Steenstra IA, Verbeek JH, Heymans MW, et al. Prognostic factors for duration of sick leave in patients sick listed with acute low back pain: a systematic review of the literature. Occup Environ Med 2005;62(12):851–60.
8. Kent PM, Keating JL. The epidemiology of low back pain in primary care. Chiropr Osteopat 2005;13:13.
9. Thelin A, Holmberg S, Thelin N. Functioning in neck and low back pain from a 12-year perspective: a prospective population-based study. J Rehabil Med 2008;40(7):555–61.
10. Luo X, Pietrobon R, Sun SX, et al. Estimates and patterns of direct health care expenditures among individuals with back pain in the United States. Spine 2004;29: 79–86.
11. Andersson GB. Epidemiological features of chronic low-back pain. Lancet 1999; 354:581–5.
12. Dionne CE, Dunn KM, Croft PR. Does back pain prevalence really decrease with increasing age? A systematic review. Age Ageing 2006;35(3):229–34.
13. Jeffries LJ, Milanese SF, Grimmer-Somers KA. Epidemiology of adolescent spinal pain: a systematic overview of the research literature. Spine 2007;32(23):2630–7.
14. Dionne CE, Von Korff M, Koepsell TD, et al. Formal education and back pain: a review. J Epidemiol Community Health 2001;55(7):455–68.
15. Linton SJ. A review of psychological risk factors in back and neck pain. Spine 2000;25(9):1148–56.
16. van Tulder M, Koes B, Bombardier C. Low back pain. Best practice & research. Clin Rheumatol 2002;16(5):761–75.
17. Matsui H, Maeda A, Tsuji H, et al. Risk indicators of low back pain among workers in Japan: association of familial and physical factors with low back pain. Spine 1997;22(11):1242–8.
18. Hoogendoorn WE, van Poppel MN, Bongers PM, et al. Systematic review of psychosocial factors at work and private life as risk factors for back pain. Spine 2000; 25(16):2114–25.
19. Webb R, Brammah T, Lunt M, et al. Prevalence and predictors of intense, chronic, and disabling neck and back pain in the UK general population. Spine 2003; 28(11):1195–202.
20. Pengel LH, Herbert RD, Maher CG, et al. Acute low back pain: systematic review of its prognosis. BMJ 2003;327:323.
21. Von Korff M, Saunders K. The course of back pain in primary care. Spine 1996; 21:2833–7 [discussion: 2838–9].
22. Deyo RA, Rainville J, Kent DL. What can the history and physical examination tell us about low back pain? JAMA 1992;268:760–5.
23. Bigos S, Bowyer O, Braen G, et al. Acute low back problems in adults. Clinical practice guideline No. 14. AHCPR Publication No. 95–0642. Rockville (MD): Agency for Health Care Policy and Research, Public Health Service, U.S. Department of Health and Human Services; 1994.
24. Devillé WL, van der Windt DA, Dzaferagić A, et al. The test of Lasègue: systematic review of the accuracy in diagnosing herniated discs. Spine 2000; 25:1140–7.

25. Waddell G, McCullock JA, Kummel E, et al. Nonorganic physical signs in low-back pain. Spine 1980;5(2):117–25.
26. Hoppenfeld S. Physical examination of the spine and extremities. Norwalk (CT): Appleton-Century-Crofts; 1976. p. 164–229.
27. Malanga G, Wolff E. Evidence-informed management of chronic low back pain with nonsteroidal anti-inflammatory drugs, muscle relaxants, and simple analgesics. Spine J 2008;8(1):173–84.

Back Pain in Adults

Jonathan A. Becker, MD[a,b,]*, Jessica R. Stumbo, MD[a,b,c]

KEYWORDS

- Back pain • Lumbar spine • Disk herniation • Imaging • Therapeutics
- Pharmacotherapy

KEY POINTS

- Back pain is common with most experiencing full relief of symptoms with minimal intervention within 4 to 6 weeks.
- The initial patient history and examination should focus on identifying any "red flags" that lead the clinician to suspect more severe pathology, such as cancer, infection, fracture, or cauda equina syndrome.
- For most patients, there is no indication for imaging of the lumbar spine and obtaining early studies does not improve outcomes.
- Radiographs are the initial imaging modality of choice, but rarely yield a definitive diagnosis.
- In nearly all complicated cases of back pain, MRI is the most useful imaging modality.
- NSAIDs are commonly used as a first-line therapy for back pain, but carry significant gastrointestinal, renal, and cardiovascular side effects.
- Despite their frequent use for more severe cases of back pain, there is only variable evidence regarding the effectiveness of opioids and systemic corticosteroids.
- Physical therapy is recommended when pain persists for more than 2 to 3 weeks. There is no standard protocol and the evidence supporting specific modalities is limited.
- Epidural steroid injections have been shown to provide a moderate short-term benefit for those with back and leg pain.
- Back surgery is indicated for the minority of patients, but provides the greatest benefit for those with sciatica, pseuoclaudication, or spondylolisthesis.

INTRODUCTION AND EPIDEMIOLOGY

Low back pain is a common problem accounting for a staggering use of the health care system with direct and indirect costs exceeding $100 billion per year in the United

Disclosures: None.
This article originally appeared in Primary Care: Clinics in Office Practice, Volume 40, Issue 2, June 2013.
[a] Primary Care Sports Medicine Fellowship, Jewish Hospital and University of Louisville, Louisville, KY, USA; [b] Department of Family and Geriatric Medicine, University of Louisville, Louisville, KY, USA; [c] Centers for Primary Care, 215 Central Avenue, Suite 205, Louisville, KY 40208, USA
* Corresponding author. Department of Family and Geriatric Medicine, 201 Abraham Flexner Way, Suite 690, Louisville, KY 40202.
E-mail address: jon.becker@louisville.edu

States.[1] To illustrate, low back pain is the second most common reason for a physician visit, it accounts for 2% to 3% of all physician visits, and 25% of all adults in the United States report at least 1 day of pain over a 3-month period.

For most, this is a self-limited condition with 90% experiencing full relief of symptoms with minimal intervention.[2] However, nearly one-third experience pain in excess of 6 months[3] and one-fourth experience a recurrence within 1 year.[1] The prevalence of low back pain has been increasing since 1990 with patients more likely to seek care, require multiple visits, and report chronic pain. Those with chronic pain are more likely to become less physically active and report higher levels of disability.[4]

As in the general population, low back pain is common in athletes. Although overall prevalence is unknown, published rates in competitive athletes range from 1% to 30%.[5] In young and healthy populations, participation in sports seems to be a risk factor for back pain with athletes having a higher incidence compared with those who are sedentary. However, in former elite athletes, there seems to be a lower lifelong incidence.[5,6]

There are specific activities that carry a higher prevalence of low back pain, especially those that involve repetitive hyperextension, such as gymnastics, diving, volleyball, golf, or football (offensive line). Throwing athletes, such as quarterbacks and pitchers, also seem to be at higher risk for back issues. Most of these cases are self-limited and do not cause any alteration in activity. However, low back pain is the most common reason for lost time in a competitive athlete.[5,6]

HISTORY

Regardless of the level of activity of the patient, the history should focus on identifying any "red flags" for a severe pathology. Low back pain is such a common problem that an accurate history may be the only reliable way to determine if the patient's pain is from a benign cause rather than one necessitating rapid diagnosis and treatment. These causes include cancer, cauda equina syndrome, infection, and fracture. A patient's low back pain is not attributable to a spinal abnormality or disease state in 85% of cases so a rigorous work-up is not indicated unless there are clues in the history or physical examination. Even in the presence of a "red flag," only a minority of patients have significant pathology.[3,6–8]

The evaluation of all patients presenting with low back pain starts with a detailed history. At the minimum, it should include the onset, duration, location, and frequency of the pain. Attention should be paid to any clues of a neurologic deficit, radicular pain, spinal stenosis, or an inflammatory condition. Any history of a back injury, use of prior treatments, and their efficacy is also important to review. Perhaps more than in other conditions, a thorough psychosocial history should be taken with emphasis on substance abuse, injury litigation, workmen's compensation, job dissatisfaction, or psychiatric issues.

The history is crucial to finding any underlying "red flags" for more severe processes, such as cancer, vertebral fracture, cauda equina syndrome, or infection. The following should yield concern for neoplasm: any prior history of cancer or metastases; pain unrelieved by rest or when supine; systemic symptoms, such as fever, night sweats, or weight loss; advanced age (>50 years old); and greater than 6 weeks of pain. Those with a history of trauma, osteoporosis (or anything that affects bone health), substance abuse, long-term corticosteroid use, and the elderly are at higher risk for a vertebral fracture. Cauda equina syndrome should be considered if there are bowel or bladder symptoms; sudden onset of pain; or any progressive loss of neurologic function, such as loss of sensation or weakness. Spinal infection may present in the setting of prior lumbar surgery; unrelenting pain not relieved with rest; fever;

immunosuppression; long-term corticosteroid use; intravenous drug use; or recent infection (eg, urinary tract, tuberculosis).

Other clues in the history may prompt further investigation for specific causes. The combination of back and leg pain, symptoms worse with sitting, the presence of numbness or tingling are all typical of radicular pain from a herniated disk or sciatica. Spinal stenosis may present with leg pain that is in excess of back pain, pain exacerbated by standing or walking, or pain relieved by sitting or flexing the spine. Morning stiffness is the hallmark of an inflammatory condition. Patients may also present with constant pain, concomitant gastrointestinal or dermatologic problems, or the presence of other autoimmune diseases.

When treating athletes, it is crucial to obtain specific information regarding their sports or activities. Age, gender, and level of fitness are all useful pieces of information, but any changes in training patterns should also be noted. Review any changes in their training, such as technique, volume, or intensity. Also be sure to note how their symptoms have affected their ability to participate or their performance. The nature of their activity may also play a role in their pain if it involves hyperextension, throwing, twisting, or running. If the athlete has any condition that affects bone health, it places them at a unique risk for stress fractures. These include any aspects of the female athlete triad, deficiencies in calcium and vitamin D intake, any personal or family history of osteoporosis, or prior corticosteroid use.[6]

PHYSICAL EXAMINATION

Before a cause has been determined for low back pain, the physical examination should include at least the following elements:

- Inspection of the lumbar spine
  - Assess for kyphosis, lordosis, or scoliosis
  - Rashes, wounds, signs of trauma or infection
  - Hair patches, sacral dimple, nevi, cafe au lait spots
- Range of motion
  - Lumbar flexion stresses the anterior spine (disk, vertebrae)
  - Lumbar extension stresses the posterior spine (pars, facets)
- Gait evaluation
  - Limping
  - Foot drop
  - Tandem gait
  - Trendelenburg gait
- Palpation of the spine and paraspinal areas
- Straight leg raise testing for those with leg pain[9]
  - Done with the patient supine, examiner passively raises the leg
  - Recreates radicular pain between 10 and 60 degrees
  - When present, a sensitive, but not specific sign
  - Crossed straight leg raising (testing the unaffected leg) carries a higher sensitivity
- Lower extremity neurovascular examination
  - Strength, sensation, and reflex testing (**Table 1**)
  - Focus on L4-S1 nerve roots because this accounts for nearly all disk pathology[3,9]
  - Diminished reflexes may be normal with advanced age
  - Spinal stenosis may have a similar presentation as vascular disease

Significant vertebral tenderness, limited range of motion, fever, or open wounds may be indicative of infection. Fractures also present with limited range of motion

Table 1
Correlation of physical examination findings with corresponding nerve roots

Nerve Root	Reflex	Strength	Sensory
L4 (L3-L4 disk space)	Patella	Ankle dorsiflexion (tibialis anterior); heel walk	Medial side of the lower leg (medial malleolus)
L5 (L4-L5 disk space)	None	Dorsiflexion of the great toe (extensor hallucis longus)	Lateral aspect of the lower leg and dorsum of the foot
S1 (L5-S1 disk space)	Achilles	Plantar flexion and eversion (peroneus longus and brevis); toe walk (gastrocnemius)	Lateral and plantar side of the foot; lateral malleolus

and marked vertebral tenderness. Progressive neurologic deficits, such as marked weakness, sensory deficits, loss of anal sphincter tone, or saddle anesthesia, yield a concern for cauda equina syndrome. Lymphadenopathy or other abnormal physical examination findings related to potential sites of cancer may be present with neoplasm or malignancy.[6,7,9,10]

IMAGING

For most patients with low back pain, imaging is not warranted and does not improve outcomes.[3,7,11] During the first 4 to 6 weeks of symptoms, the American College of Physicians advises that imaging be delayed unless there are signs or symptoms of a serious underlying "red flag" condition. They, along with the American College of Radiology, have developed criteria for early imaging (**Table 2**).

When imaging the lumbar spine, radiographs are generally the initial test of choice. Although they typically do not provide definitive diagnosis, they can be useful to rule out fractures in the setting of "minor" red flags, such as low-velocity trauma or advanced age. Radiographs may also reveal signs of osteoporosis. For most, magnetic resonance imaging (MRI) is the test of choice for complicated low back

Table 2
Indications for early imaging of the lumbar spine

American College of Physicians Practice Guideline: Indications for Early Imaging in Low Back Pain	American College of Radiology Appropriateness Criteria for Imaging
Progressive neurologic findings	Symptoms >6 wk
Constitutional symptoms	Trauma
Age >50 y old	Age >70 y old (or trauma at >50 y old)
Trauma	Weight loss
History of malignancy	Fever (unexplained)
Osteoporosis	Cancer
Risk factors for infection (steroid use, immunosuppression, intravenous drug use)	Long-term steroid use or osteoporosis Intravenous drug use Immunosuppression Progressive neurologic deficit Disabling symptoms Prior surgery

Data from Chou R, Qaseem A, Owens DK, et al. Diagnostic imaging for low back pain: Advice for high-value health care from the American College of Physicians. Ann Intern Med 2011;154:181–9; and American College of Radiology. ACR Appropriateness Criteria. Low back pain. http://www.acr.org/~/media/ACR/Documents/AppCriteria/Diagnostic/LowBackPain.pdf. Accessed July 9, 2012.

conditions. These include pain for greater than 4 to 6 weeks, the presence of any historical "red flags," concern for spinal stenosis, radicular symptoms, or neurologic findings. MRI has the advantage of provide details of the bony anatomy and the soft tissues.[3,10]

Computerized tomography (CT) is useful for patients who cannot undergo MRI, those with surgical hardware, or if there is a need for precise bony anatomy. Myelography, diskography, and bone scan are reserved for when specific conditions are suspected. Bone scan with single photon emission CT (SPECT) imaging provides the sensitivity of a bone scan along with three-dimensional resolution. This makes SPECT a particularly attractive option for the diagnosis of stress fracture. Unlike traditional bone scan, SPECT scans take images from multiple angles and the data can be manipulated to display the anatomy in thin slices much like CT or MRI. Fire scan is an emerging technology that digitally combines CT in tandem to bone scan with SPECT images. It has the unique ability to provide sensitivity of bone scan with bony detail of CT scan. It is purported to have a unique ability to identify areas of bone turnover in great detail, particularly in facet disease.[12]

Athletes carry a higher suspicion of stress fracture than the general population. In light of that, bone scan with SPECT imaging is frequently used early in the evaluation of back in athletes. However, even in those cases where there is high suspicion for bony abnormality, it has been recommended that MRI remain the preferred modality. MRI identifies the subtle changes of bony injury while also providing further detail regarding other structures, such as intervertebral disks. Further modalities could then be used if the diagnosis remains in question.[13]

DIFFERENTIAL DIAGNOSIS

Tables 3–9 illustrate the differential diagnosis.[3,6,10,14–18]

TREATMENT OPTIONS

Most acute episodes of low back pain resolve with conservative therapy within 4 to 6 weeks. However, 5% to 10% of patients develop chronic symptoms (pain lasting greater than 3 months) for which a uniformly effective treatment regimen is lacking. Decisions are complicated by lack of high-quality randomized controlled trials. The goals of treatment should be to educate patients, decrease pain, improve function, and minimize side effects associated with chosen treatment modalities.

Medications

There are a variety of different classes of medications that can be used in the management of low back pain. A main goal of therapy is to use the lowest effective dose for the shortest period of time necessary.

Nonsteroidal anti-inflammatory drugs

Various nonsteroidal anti-inflammatory drugs (NSAIDs) are used in back pain.[3,10,19–26] A recent large Cochrane review[24] supported the use of NSAIDs as first-line management in the treatment of acute and chronic low back pain without sciatica. This review included 65 randomized controlled studies and found statistically significant results in favor of NSAIDs over placebo for improved functional status, number of patients recovered, and decrease in pain intensity from baseline. The 2008 Cochrane review also examined the effectiveness of NSAIDs and found moderate evidence that NSAIDs are equally effective as paracetamol/acetaminophen for pain relief and global improvement.

Table 3
Common causes of low back pain

Diagnosis	Key Historical and Physical Examination Findings	Diagnostic Studies
Lumbar strain	• Acute onset, possibly an injury • Symptoms worse with activity, relieved with rest • Paraspinal spasm or tenderness	• Only to exclude alternative diagnoses
Disk herniation	• Pain often worse with sitting • Symptoms radiate to lower extremities, typically below the knees • Follows dermatomal pattern • Positive straight leg raise	• MRI if symptoms >4 wk • Electromyography and nerve conduction studies if diagnosis in question
Degenerative disk disease	• Pain worse with flexion or sitting • Chronic pain	• Radiographs • MRI
Facet disease	• Pain worse with extension • Worse with standing or walking	• Radiographs • MRI
Spondylolisthesis	• Leg pain may be greater than back pain • Worse with extension, relieved by flexion • Pain worse with activity	• Radiographs • MRI
Spinal stenosis	• Pain relived by sitting or flexion • Lower-extremity paresthesias, possibly bilateral • Neurogenic claudication (pseudoclaudication) • Elderly	• MRI • CT may be useful to delineate bony anatomy • Vascular studies to rule out claudication

A higher rate of side effects with all NSAIDs is noted when compared with acetaminophen/paracetamol. This is true for nonselective NSAIDs and the cyclooxygenase-2 (COX-2) selective drugs. The Cochrane review from 2008 concluded that NSAIDs were associated with an increased risk of side effects compared with paracetamol with a relative risk of 1.76 (95% confidence interval, 1.12–2.76; N = 309).

Nephrotoxicity is a concern with all NSAIDs, especially in the elderly and those with underlying renovascular disease. Gastrointestinal adverse events including dyspepsia, ulcer disease, and bleeding are also known side effects. In select populations including those with a history of NSAID-induced peptic ulcer disease, coadministration of a proton pump inhibitor with an NSAID had similar efficacy when compared with COX-2 therapy in terms of arthritic pain control and had less dyspepsia than the COX-2 treatment group (15% vs 5.7%).[25]

The risk of adverse cardiovascular events varies with the NSAIDs. Rofecoxib, a COX-2, was removed from the market because of increased cardiovascular events. A meta-analysis published in 2006[26] found an increase in vascular events in not only the COX-2 medications but also the nonselective NSAIDs, specifically ibuprofen and diclofenac. A 42% relative increase in vascular events compared with placebo was found with use of COX-2 inhibitors. Traditional NSAIDs had a vascular event rate similar to COX-2 medications. Of note, naproxen seemed to have less of a risk of vascular events in this meta-analysis compared with placebo and ibuprofen and diclofenac. Caution is advised when prescribing all NSAIDs especially to those with underlying cardiovascular disease or risk factors for cardiovascular disease.

Table 4
Causes of low back pain warranting emergent treatment

Diagnosis	Key Historical and Physical Examination Findings	Diagnostic Studies
Neoplastic: • Myeloma • Spinal cord tumor • Metastases	• Systemic symptoms: fever, weight loss, fatigue • Pain when lying down or night pain • History of cancer	• Radiographs • MRI
Cauda equina syndrome	• Saddle anesthesia • Progressive motor or sensory changes • Urinary retention • Bowel or bladder incontinence • Loss of rectal tone	• MRI
Infection • Osteomyelitis • Diskitis • Epidural abscess	• Fever • Loss of range of motion • History of intravenous drug abuse • Severe pain • Recent surgery or infection • Immunosuppression	• MRI • Complete blood count • Blood culture • Sedimentation rate • C-reactive protein
Fracture	• History of trauma • Low bone mineral density/ osteoporosis • Corticosteroid use • Vertebral tenderness • Elderly	• Radiographs • Additional imaging if diagnosis in question

If a patient does not respond to one NSAID it is worthwhile to try another NSAID of a different class before abandoning NSAIDs as a potential treatment option.

Acetaminophen

Acetaminophen is effective for pain relief and is an option for first-line management of low back pain. It is associated with fewer side effects when compared with NSAIDs. The main concern associated with its use is hepatotoxicity especially in patients with underlying liver disease or alcohol use. Asymptomatic elevations in aminotransferase levels can also occur even in healthy patients especially in doses greater than 4 g per day.[3,10,19–24]

Tramadol

Tramadol acts as a weak opioid receptor agonist and inhibits the reuptake of serotonin and norepinephrine. A 2007 Cochrane review found tramadol to be more effective than placebo for pain control in low back pain. Other studies have demonstrated short-term improvements in pain and function but no long-term studies exist. Most common side effects are headache and nausea. Use with caution in patients with a history of narcotic addiction because of its action at the opioid receptor.[3,10,19–23,27]

Opioids

Too few high-quality studies exist with regards to efficacy of opioids in the management of low back pain. Therefore, use is based on clinical judgment. They are typically not considered a first-line management option. In this author's opinion opioids may be considered a treatment option in patients with severe pain that is not effectively

Table 5
Inflammatory causes of low back pain

Diagnosis	Key Historical and Physical Examination Findings	Diagnostic Studies
Ankylosing spondylitis	• Younger population • Predominantly males • Morning stiffness • Pain relieved by activity • Night pain	• Radiographs • Sedimentation rate • C-reactive protein • HLA-B27
Reactive arthritis	• Aseptic arthritis triggered by an extra-articular infection • History of recent gastrointestinal or genitourinary infection • Lower extremities most commonly involved • Classic triad: uveitis, arthritis, urethritis	• Sedimentation rate • C-reactive protein • HLA-B27 (30%–50%) • Imaging to exclude alternative diagnosis
Psoriatic arthritis	• Asymmetric and distal joint involvement • Frequent sacroiliac joint involvement • History of psoriasis with skin and nail changes	• Radiographs
Inflammatory bowel disease	• Systemic manifestation of inflammatory bowel disease • Does not have to correlate with inflammatory bowel disease flare	• Used to exclude alternative explanation for pain
Transverse myelitis	• Develops over 24 h • Typically thoracic spine involvement • Symptoms usually bilateral and occur below level of the lesion • Presents with weakness and sensory deficits or paralysis	• MRI • Cerebrospinal fluid analysis

controlled by NSAIDs, acetaminophen, or other conservative management options. Pain that interferes with sleep may also warrant consideration for opioid use. Side effects include nausea, constipation, sedation, confusion, addiction, and dependence.[10,21,27–29]

Systemic corticosteroids
These are not recommended for treatment of isolated low back pain because of lack of evidence showing efficacy.[10,20] There is variable evidence regarding use in acute low back pain with radicular symptoms, but they may be of benefit.[3,22] Patients should be educated about potential adverse effects when these medications are used including agitation, irritability, insomnia, and poor glycemic control in those with diabetes mellitus.

Topical analgesics
These agents provide the advantage of avoiding systemic toxicities, but have the limitation of providing treatment to a localized area. Side effects include skin irritation or allergic reaction. Topical analgesics can be used alone or in conjunction with other therapies including oral medications.[30–33]

Table 6
Vascular causes of low back pain

Diagnosis	Key Historical and Physical Examination Findings	Diagnostic Studies
Spinal cord vascular malformation	• Men > women • Typically >50 y old • Progressive radicular symptoms • Psuedoclaudication as in spinal stenosis	• MRI with angiography
Spinal cord infarction	• Rapid onset, often in setting of hypotension or aortic pathology • Pain caused by ischemia • Neurologic deficit ranges from weakness to paresis • Correlates with level of impairment (most common is T8) • History of vascular disorder (eg, vasculitis, hypercoagulable state) • History of diabetes mellitus	• MRI (may be normal for up to 24 h)
Epidural hematoma	• Most often a complication of a procedure (epidural injection or surgery) • Rarely spontaneous • Back or radicular symptoms • Progresses to motor and sensory deficits, possible bowel or bladder involvement	• MRI

Capsaicin, a derivative of cayenne peppers, has shown positive but weak evidence in the treatment of neuropathic and musculoskeletal pain.[30,31] Its proposed mechanism of action is depletion of substance P from the sensory afferent nerve fibers. It must be applied multiple times a day for several weeks to get the full benefit. Topical capsaicin is well tolerated by most, but some experience an intolerable burning sensation. A 2006 Cochrane review[31] reported improvement on the visual analog scale at Days 3 and 14 with regards to acute low back pain and treatment with a topical cream containing capsicum. Similar findings were found for chronic low back pain using a capsicum-containing plaster.

Table 7
Metabolic causes of low back pain

Diagnosis	Key Historical and Physical Examination Findings	Diagnostic Studies
Paget disease	• Aching pain that persists into the night • Bony changes and overgrowth lead to pain and spinal stenosis • Cord compression may lead to ischemia	• Radiographs • Alkaline phosphatase • Tests for increased bone turnover • MRI to exclude alternative cause for symptoms
Osteoporosis	• Any comorbidity affecting bone health • History of low bone mineral density • Family history of osteoporosis	• Imaging to rule out fractures • Bone density (DEXA) scan

Table 8
Miscellaneous causes of low back pain

Diagnosis	Key Historical and Physical Examination Findings	Diagnostic Studies
Episacroiliac lipoma ("back mouse")	• Low back pain described as moving to different locations • Rubbery, mobile mass deep subcutaneous tissue	• Done to rule out alternative diagnoses
Zoster	• Vesicular rash • Dermatomal pattern	• Confirmation with polymerase chain reaction testing or culture
Lyme disease (or other tick-borne illness)	• History of tick bite • Travel to endemic area • Characteristic rash ("target lesion")	• EIA Western blot
Statin-induced myopathy	• Use of statin medications	• Elevated creatinine kinase level

Lidocaine 5% patch is another topical option, but there is no documented evidence regarding effectiveness for the treatment of acute or chronic low back pain. The Food and Drug Administration (FDA) has approved it for the treatment of the pain associated with postherpetic neuralgia. It has also shown potential use for myofascial pain[32,33]; however, more studies are needed. Lidocaine patches are generally well tolerated.

Muscle relaxants

These are effective for short-term symptomatic relief of low back pain especially when combined with NSAID therapy. There is mixed evidence to support long-term use in

Table 9
Extraspinal causes of low back pain

Diagnosis	Key Historical and Physical Examination Findings	Diagnostic Studies
Aortic dissection or aneurysm	• Pulsatile abdominal mass • Hypertension (or hypotension if ruptured)	• Radiographs may reveal abnormality, but CT scan diagnostic
Kidney stone	• History of stones • Hematuria • Pain radiates to groin	• Red blood cells in urine • Radiographs or CT scan
Pyelonephritis	• Fever, systemic symptoms • Costovertebral angle tenderness	• White blood cells or casts in urine
Retroperitoneal hematoma or abscess	• Recent trauma • Anticoagulant use • Fever, immune deficiency • Retroperitoneal tenderness	• CT scan or ultrasound
Psoas abscess	• Psoas sign • Fever, immune deficiency	• CT scan or ultrasound
Splenic rupture or infarct	• Trauma • Viral infection (mononucleosis) • Hemoglobinopathy	• CT scan or ultrasound
Sickle cell crisis	• History of sickle cell disease (or trait)	

chronic low back pain. There is a high rate of side effects including dizziness and sedation.[3,21,29,34]

Antidepressants

Conflicting conclusions exist regarding the efficacy of antidepressants in the treatment of chronic low back pain and they should not be considered first-line therapy. A 2003 systemic review of seven randomized controlled trials[35] concluded that tricyclic antidepressants but not selective serotonin reuptake inhibitors provided moderate symptom reduction for patients with chronic low back pain. However, a 2008 Cochrane review[36] stated antidepressants were no more effective than placebo in the treatment of chronic low back pain.

Amitriptyline, a tricyclic antidepressant, is useful in patients with neurogenic pain. Its role in the treatment of back pain is not well defined, but its sedative qualities make it a good option for nighttime use in patients with sleep disturbances.[10,21,35–37]

Depression screening is recommended in patients with chronic low back pain because these two conditions frequently coexist. In 2010, duloxetine was FDA approved for the treatment of chronic musculoskeletal pain including low back pain.[38]

Herbal therapy

Long-term safety data do not exist but short-term studies show herbal preparations, such as devil's claw, white willow bark, and cayenne, may have a role in the treatment of chronic low back pain.[31]

Others

Anticonvulsants including gabapentin are sometimes used for chronic low back pain complicated by radiculopathy and show possible benefits in some trials. At this time, this is not an FDA-approved indication.[39]

Benzodiazepines are commonly used for muscle relaxation in severe cases. This class of drugs can be associated with abuse, addiction, and tolerance. Therefore, they should be used cautiously.[3,10,21,29,40]

Bed Rest

Activity modification is advocated for the treatment of acute low back pain rather than bed rest and immobilization. Bed rest may be recommended for 1 to 2 days if there is severe pain, but patients should be educated that longer periods of bed rest can be associated with a delayed recovery, joint stiffness, and muscle wasting. Provide patient reassurance and education that it is safe to get out of bed and perform activities as tolerated.[3,19,22,41,42]

Physical Therapy

Referral for a course of physical therapy is typically recommended if symptoms persist for more than 2 to 3 weeks. No standard protocol exists. The variety of interventions and modalities used make comparing studies difficult. Individualized regimens that include therapist supervision, stretching, and strengthening tend to be associated with the best outcomes. The McKenzie method, spine stabilization exercises, and home exercise program all display benefits. Traction therapy is "probably not effective" as a single treatment for low back pain according to the 2010 Cochrane review.[3,10,20,22,29,43]

Topical Cold Versus Heat Therapy

Heat therapy seems to be beneficial in reducing pain associated with acute low back pain. Additional pain relief and improved function are achieved when combined with exercise. Minimal evidence exists for the use of cold therapy in acute low back pain.[3,10,29,44,45]

Transcutaneous Electrical Nerve Stimulation

Based on a 2010 review, current evidence does not support the use of transcutaneous electrical nerve stimulation unit in the management of chronic low back pain. As of 2012, Medicare no longer provides coverage for a transcutaneous electrical nerve stimulation unit for this purpose.[10,46,47]

Lumbar Corsets

Evidence for efficacy is unclear regarding use of lumbar corsets in the management of acute and chronic low back pain. Studies show a possible benefit if a lumbar corset is combined with additional spinal support, such as a heat-moldable plastic insert.[3,10,48]

Injection Therapy

The rates of epidural steroid injections and facet injections rose 271% and 231%, respectively, between 1994 and 2001 in the Medicare population.[49]

Epidural steroid injections

Numerous studies have failed to yield a definitive answer regarding the efficacy of epidural steroid injections with published ranges of efficacy between 18% and 90%.[21,22,49–53] The wide range of published efficacy reflects the lack of standardization in injection technique, patient heterogeneity, and the differences in the methodology of the studies analyzing the data. Moderate short-term benefit in patients with chronic low back pain with radiculopathy has been shown.[50] Injections should always be used in conjunction with a multidisciplinary treatment plan.

In a recent study of National Football League players,[52] epidural steroid injections were found to be safe and effective in the treatment of symptomatic acute lumbar disk herniations and allowed a quick return to play. Loss of practice and game time is of high concern in all athletes but especially so in the professional athlete. Therefore, interventions that provide a more rapid return to play are always being sought. In this study, 17 players who had 27 acute disk herniations that were confirmed on MRI from 2003 to 2010 underwent epidural steroid injections. The outcomes were promising because the success rate for returning the athletes to play was 89% with an average loss of 2.8 practices (range, 0–12). Only three players failed conservative treatment and went on to surgery. Risk factors for failed conservative management in this study were disk sequestration noted on MRI and weakness on physical examination. In patients without radicular symptoms no benefit with epidural steroid injections has been shown.

Facet injections and medial branch nerve blocks

Conflicting evidence exists for the efficacy of intra-articular corticosteroid facet injections and medial branch nerve blocks on short- and long-term pain control for facet-related back pain. However, they may be of benefit.[10,22,51,54,55]

Prolotherapy

Prolotherapy is an injection therapy that is thought to aide in the healing of chronic degenerative soft tissue conditions potentially by triggering an acute inflammatory response.[22,56–58] A variety of injected solutions including dextrose, sodium morrhuate, and phenol have been used. No standardized protocol exists.

A Cochrane review[58] published in 2007 found that prolotherapy alone is not effective in the treatment of chronic low back pain. However, when combined with other interventions it may be of benefit. More studies are needed.

Complementary and Alternative Medicine

This broad group of therapies is a popular addition to traditional medical management for acute and chronic low back pain.[19,20,22,59,60] A total of 45% of individuals with back pain see a chiropractor, 24% use massage therapy, and 11% receive acupuncture. Most patients often fail to disclose use of these treatment options to their health care provider.

More high-quality studies are needed to further elucidate the evidence for these treatment options when used alone or in combination with standard medical treatment. Various modalities exist including acupuncture, mobilization/manipulation, and massage that seem to show promise in the treatment of select individuals with acute and chronic low back pain. The safety profile for most complementary and alternative therapies is acceptable.

Stem Cell Therapy

Autologous mesenchymal stem cell therapy for chronic low back pain caused by degenerative disk disease has shown benefit in animal studies and is now being examined as a treatment option in humans.[61] In a pilot study published in 2011, 10 patients with degenerative disk disease with a preserved external annulus fibrosis who had failed conservative therapy (physical and medical options) underwent mesenchymal stem cell and showed statistically significant improvements in lumbar pain levels and level of disability. Although more research is needed, stem cell therapy is another nonsurgical option on the horizon in the treatment of chronic low back pain.

SPECIAL CONSIDERATIONS FOR ATHLETES

Back pain is the most common reason for time away from sports.[5,6,13,20,22,42] Rates vary among sports and data regarding prevalence compared with the general population are inconsistent. Combined with the lack of high-quality randomized studies, it is difficult to make general recommendations. Nonetheless, some inferences can be made:

- Treatment algorithms for athletes should be similar to the general population.
- Relative rest or time off from sports may be appropriate, but there is no role for bed rest in the treatment of low back pain.
- Earlier imaging does not improve outcomes. Radiographs rarely provide definitive diagnosis. Despite a higher rate of stress fracture than the general population, MRI remains the advanced imaging modality of choice for most athletes.
- Injury-specific and postsurgical return to play guidelines lack standardization.
- Despite the variability in protocols and lack of high-quality data, physical therapy or an exercise program that focuses on spine stabilization and core strengthening are programs with encouraging outcomes.

REFERRAL AND SURGICAL INDICATIONS

Back surgery is indicated for only a minority of patients with low back pain.[10,19,21,62–70] However, the rates of low back surgery in the United Sates are increasing. Patients with persistent pain, despite conservative management or progressive neurologic deficits, should be referred for a surgical evaluation especially in cases of herniated disk, spinal stenosis, and spondylolisthesis. The National Institutes of Health–supported Spine Patient Outcomes Research Trial (SPORT) was designed to evaluate the surgical and nonsurgical treatment of intervertebral disk herniations, degenerative spondylolisthesis, and lumbar spinal stenosis. The SPORT studies were randomized, prospective, multicenter trials that included an observational cohort arm.

Intervertebral Disk Herniation

SPORT participants had to meet strict inclusion criteria, which included symptoms for at least 6 weeks, imaging that supported clinical findings, and neurologic signs.[62–65] The surgical procedure was open discectomy.

Nonsurgical and surgical groups showed improvement. In the intent-to-treat analysis all measures favored surgery; however, this difference was not statistically significant regarding the primary outcome measures (self-reported improvements in impairment and health-related quality of life) but was statistically significant for secondary outcome measures (patient satisfaction, self-rated progress, and improvements in sciatica symptoms). When the randomized group and the cohort group are analyzed together, the as-treated analysis shows a statistically significant improvement in all measured outcomes for the surgery group compared with the nonsurgical patients. Improvements after surgery were maintained at greater than 4 years follow-up. Characteristics that increased the treatment effect of surgery were being married, absence of joint problems, and worsening symptoms from baseline.

Degenerative Spondylolisthesis

The surgical procedure was a posterior laminectomy with or without bilateral single level fusion with or without instrumentation.[66] Inclusion criteria included symptoms for at least 12 weeks and imaging confirmation of degenerative spondylolisthesis.

In a combined as-treated analysis of the randomized group and the cohort group, surgery was favored and demonstrated statistically significant improvements in all primary and secondary outcome measures including pain, improvements in disability and function, and patient satisfaction.

Lumbar Spinal Stenosis

The surgical procedure was a posterior decompressive laminectomy.[63,67,68] All patients had symptoms for at least 12 weeks, had neurogenic claudication or radicular leg symptoms, and imaging showing lumbar spinal stenosis at one or more levels.

Similar to the findings with disk herniation and spondylolisthesis, when a combined analysis is done including the randomized and cohort groups, surgery for symptomatic lumbar spinal fusion was favored in all primary and secondary outcome measures including improvements in pain and function and patient satisfaction when compared with nonsurgical treatment. The improvements were also maintained at the 4-year follow-up.

A systemic review[68] published in 2003 also showed surgery was more effective than continued conservative treatments for patients with symptomatic lumbar spinal stenosis who had underwent at least 3 to 6 months of conservative management. The improvements were seen in pain, function, and quality of life, but not walking ability.

Disk Replacement and Spinal Fusion

Disk degeneration is a common part of the aging process and frequently deemed to be the source of nonspecific chronic low back pain. After patients have failed a trial of conservative management, they are referred to surgery to remove the degenerative disk.

Traditional surgical procedures involve removing the disk and doing a fusion of the inferior and superior vertebrae. New techniques involve disk replacement with a plastic or metal artificial implant.

A recent Cochrane review[69] examined seven randomized controlled trials. Six of the trials compared disk replacement with spinal fusion and one compared disk replacement with nonsurgical treatment. The conclusion of the Cochrane review was that based on the short-term studies that are available, disk replacement is at least equivalent but not superior when compared with fusion with respect to pain control, disability levels, and improved quality of life. In patients with nonspecific chronic low back pain who have failed adequate trials of at least 2 years of nonsurgical interventions, surgery can be considered an option.[70]

ACKNOWLEDGMENTS

The authors thank Dr Melvin Law of Premiere Orthopedics in Nashville, Tennessee, for contributing to and expertly reviewing this article.

REFERENCES

1. Deyo RA, Mirza SK, Martin BI. Back pain prevalence and visit rates: estimates from U.S. national surveys, 2002. Spine 2006;31:2724–7.
2. Croft PR, Macfarlane GJ, Papageorgiou AC, et al. Outcome of low back pain in general practice: a prospective study. BMJ 1998;316:1356–9.
3. Casazza BA. Diagnosis and treatment of acute low back pain. Am Fam Physician 2012;85:343–50.
4. Freburger JK, Holmes GM, Agans RP, et al. The rising prevalence of chronic low back pain. Arch Intern Med 2009;169:251–8.
5. Bono CM. Current concepts review: low back pain in athletes. J Bone Joint Surg Am 2004;86:392–6.
6. Daniels JM, Pontius G, El-Amin S, et al. Evaluation of low back pain in athletes. Sports Health 2011;3:336–45.
7. Chou R, Fu R, Carrino JA, et al. Imaging strategies for low back pain: systemic review and meta-analysis. Lancet 2009;373:463–72.
8. Bhangle SD, Sapru S, Panush RS. Back pain made simple: an approach based on principles and evidence. Cleve Clin J Med 2009;76:393–9.
9. Cochrane Collaboration. Physical examination for lumbar radiculopathy due to disc herniation in patients with low back pain. New York: John Wiley & Sons Ltd; 2010.
10. Chou R, Qaseem A, Snow V, et al. Diagnosis and treatment of low back pain: a joint clinical practice guideline from the American College of Physicians and the American Pain Society. Ann Intern Med 2007;147:478–91.
11. Chou R, Qaseem A, Owens DK, et al. Diagnostic imaging for low back pain: advice for high-value health care from the American College of Physicians. Ann Intern Med 2011;154:181–9.
12. Willick SE, Kendall RW, Roberts ST, et al. An emerging imaging technology to assist in the localization of axial spine pain. PM&R 2009;1:89–92.
13. Ganiyusufoglu AK, Onat L, Karatoprak O, et al. Diagnostic accuracy of magnetic resonance imaging versus computed tomography in stress fractures of the lumbar spine. Clin Radiol 2010;65:902–7.
14. Healy PJ, Helliwell PS. Classification of the spondyloarthropathies. Curr Opin Rheumatol 2005;17:395–9.
15. Kaplin AI, Krishnan C, Deshpande DM, et al. Diagnosis and management of acute myelopathies. Neurologist 2005;11:2–18.

16. Cheshire WP, Santos CC, Massey EW, et al. Spinal cord infarction: etiology and outcome. Neurology 1996;47:321–30.
17. Wang VY, Chou D, Chin C. Spine and spinal cord emergencies: vascular and infectious causes. Neuroimaging Clin N Am 2010;20:639–50.
18. Hadjipavlou AG, Gaitanis LN, Katonis PG, et al. Paget's disease of the spine and its management. Eur Spine J 2001;10:370–84.
19. Deyo RA, Weinstein JN. Low back pain. N Engl J Med 2001;344:363–70.
20. Petering RC, Webb C. Treatment options for low back pain in athletes. Sports Health 2011;3:550–5.
21. Last AR, Hulbert K. Chronic low back pain: evaluation and management. Am Fam Physician 2009;79:1067–74.
22. Shen FH, Samartzis D, Andersson GB. Nonsurgical management of acute and chronic low back pain. J Am Acad Orthop Surg 2006;14:477–87.
23. Carragee EJ. Persistent low back pain. N Engl J Med 2005;352:1891–8.
24. Roelofs PD, Deyo RA, Koes BW, et al. Non-steroidal anti-inflammatory drugs for low back pain. Cochrane Database Syst Rev 2008;(1):CD000396. http://dx.doi.org/10.1002/14651858.CD000396.pub3.
25. Lai KC, Chu KM, Hui WM, et al. Celecoxib compared with lansoprazole and naproxen to prevent gastrointestinal ulcer complications. Am J Med 2005;118:1271–8.
26. Kearney PM, Baigent C, Godwin J, et al. Do selective cyclo-oxygenase-2 inhibitors and traditional non-steroidal anti-inflammatory drugs increase the risk of atherothrombosis? Meta-analysis of randomized trials. BMJ 2006;332:1302.
27. Deshpande A, Furlan AD, Mailis-Gagnon A, et al. Opioids for chronic low-back pain. Cochrane Database Syst Rev 2007;(3):CD004959. http://dx.doi.org/10.1002/14651858.CD004959.pub3.
28. Martell BA, O'Connor PG, Kerns RD, et al. Systematic review: opioid treatment for chronic back pain: prevalence, efficacy, and association with addiction. Ann Intern Med 2007;146:116–27.
29. Kinkade S. Evaluation and treatment of acute low back pain. Am Fam Physician 2007;75:1182–8.
30. Mason L, Moore RA, Derry S, et al. Systemic review of topical capsaicin for the treatment of chronic pain. BMJ 2004. http://dx.doi.org/10.1136/bmj.38042.506748.EE.
31. Gagnier JJ, van Tulder MW, Berman BM, et al. Herbal medicine for low back pain. Cochrane Database Syst Rev 2007;(2):CD004504. http://dx.doi.org/10.1002/14651858.CD004504.pub3.
32. Kroenke K, Krebs EE, Bair MJ. Pharmacotherapy of chronic pain: a synthesis of recommendations from systemic reviews. Gen Hosp Psychiatry 2009;31:206–19.
33. Dalpiaz AS, Lordon SP, Lipman AG. Topical lidocaine patch therapy for myofascial pain. J Pain Palliat Care Pharmacother 2004;18:15–34.
34. Van Tulder MW, Touray T, Furlan AD, et al. Muscle relaxants for nonspecific low back pain: a systemic review within the framework of the Cochrane collaboration. Spine 2003;28:1978–92.
35. Staiger TO, Gaster B, Sullivan MD, et al. Systemic review of antidepressants in the treatment of chronic low back pain. Spine 2003;28:2540–5.
36. Urquhart DM, Hoving JL, Assendelft WJ, et al. Antidepressants for non-specific low back pain. Cochrane Database Syst Rev 2008;(1):CD001703. http://dx.doi.org/10.1002/14651858.CD001703.pub3.
37. Machado LA, Kamper SJ, Herbert RD, et al. Analgesic effects of treatments for non-specific low back pain: a meta-analysis of placebo-controlled randomized trials. Rheumatology 2009;48:520–7.

38. Skljarevski V, Desaiah D, Liu-Seifert H, et al. Efficacy and safety of Duloxetine in patients with chronic low back pain. Spine 2010;35:E578–85.
39. Yildirima K, Denizb O, Guresera G, et al. Gabapentin monotherapy in patients with chronic radiculopathy: the efficacy and impact on life quality. J Back Musculoskelet Rehabil 2009;22:17–20.
40. Chou R, Huffman LH. American Pain Society guideline on the evaluation and management of low back pain. Glenview (IL): American Pain Society; 2007.
41. Vroomen P, de Krom M, Wilmink JT, et al. Lack of effectiveness of bed rest for sciatica. N Engl J Med 1999;340:418–23.
42. Malvivaara A, Hakkinen U, Aro T, et al. The treatment of acute low back pain: bed rest, exercises, or ordinary activity? N Engl J Med 1995;332:351–5.
43. Clarke JA, van Tulder MW, Blomberg SE, et al. Traction for low-back pain with or without sciatica. Cochrane Database Syst Rev 2007;(2):CD003010. http://dx. doi.org/10.1002/14651858.CD003010.pub4.
44. French SD, Cameron M, Walker BF, et al. A Cochrane review of superficial heat or cold for low back pain. Spine 2006;31:998–1006.
45. Kettenmann B, Wille C, Lurie-Luke E, et al. Impact of continuous low level heat-wrap therapy in acute low back pain patients: subjective and objective measurements. Clin J Pain 2007;23:663–8.
46. Khadilkar A, Odebiyi DO, Brosseau L, et al. Transcutaneous electrical nerve stimulation (TENS) versus placebo for chronic low-back pain. Cochrane Database Syst Rev 2008;(4):CD003008. http://dx.doi.org/10.1002/14651858. CD003008.pub3.
47. Jacques L, Jensen TS, Rollins J, et al. Decision memo for transcutaneous electrical nerve stimulation for chronic low back pain (CAG-00429N). In: Centers for Medicare and Medicaid Services. 2012. Available at: http://www.cms.gov/medicare-coverage-database/details/nca-decision-memo.aspx?NCAId= 256&ver=1&NcaName=Transcutaneous+Electrical+Nerve+Stimulation+for+Chronic+Low+Back+Pain&bc=ACAAAAAIBAA&. Accessed July 15, 2012.
48. Million R, Nilsen KH, Jayson MI, et al. Evaluation of low back pain and assessment of lumbar corsets with and without back supports. Ann Rheum Dis 1981; 40:449–54.
49. Friedly J, Chan L, Deyo R. Increases in lumbosacral injections in the medicare population 1994 to 2001. Spine 2007;32:1754–60.
50. Benoist M, Boulu P, Hayem G. Epidural steroid injections in the management of low back pain with radiculopathy: an update of their efficacy and safety. Eur Spine J 2012;21:204–13.
51. Staal JB, de Bie R, de Vet HC, et al. Injection therapy for subacute and chronic low-back pain. Cochrane Database Syst Rev 2008;(3):CD001824. http://dx.doi. org/10.1002/14651858.CD001824.pub3.
52. Krych AJ, Richman D, Drakos M, et al. Epidural steroid injection for lumbar disc herniation in NFL athletes. Med Sci Sports Exerc 2012;44:193–8.
53. Cohen SP. Epidural steroid injections for low back pain. BMJ 2011;343:d5310.
54. Boswell MV, Colson JD, Sehgal N, et al. A systemic review of therapeutic facet joint interventions in chronic spinal pain. Pain Physician 2007;10:229–53.
55. Peterson C, Hodler J. Evidence-based radiology (part 1): is there sufficient research to support the use of therapeutic injections for the spine and sacroiliac joints? Skeletal Radiol 2010;39:5–9.
56. Watson JD, Shay BL. Treatment of chronic low back pain: a 1-year or greater follow-up. J Altern Complement Med 2010;16:951–8.

57. Rabago D, Slattengren A, Zgierska A. Prolotherapy in primary care practice. Prim Care Clin Office Pract 2010;37:65–80.
58. Dagenais S, Yelland MJ, Del Mar C, et al. Prolotherapy injections for chronic low-back pain. Cochrane Database Syst Rev 2007;(2):CD004059. http://dx.doi.org/10.1002/14651858.CD004059.pub3.
59. Furlan A, Yazdi F, Tsertsvadze A, et al. Complementary and alternative therapies for back pain II. Evidence Report/Technology Assessment No. 194. Prepared by the University of Ottawa Evidence-based Practice Center under Contract No. 290-2007-10059-I (EPCIII). AHRQ Publication No. 10(11)-E007. Rockville (MD): Agency for Healthcare Research and Quality; 2010.
60. Gay R. Back pain: complementary and alternative medicine module. Am Col Physicians/PIER. 2012. Available at: http://pier.acponline.org/physicians/alternative/camdz417/camdz417.html. Accessed July 15, 2012.
61. Orozco L, Soler R, Morera C, et al. Intervertebral disc repair by autologous mesenchymal bone marrow cells: a pilot study. Transplantation 2011;92:822–8.
62. Pearson A, Lurie J, Tosteson T, et al. Who should have surgery for intervertebral disc herniation? Spine 2012;37:140–9.
63. Asghar FA, Hilibrand AS. The impact of the Spine Patient Outcomes Research Trial (SPORT) on orthopaedic practice. J Am Acad Orthop Surg 2012;20:160–6.
64. Weinstein JN, Lurie JD, Tosteson TD, et al. Surgical versus non-operative treatment for lumbar disc herniations: four-year results for the Spine Patient Outcomes Research Trial (SPORT). Spine 2008;33:2789–800.
65. Tosteson AN, Tosteson TD, Lurie JD. Comparative effectiveness evidence from the spine patient outcomes research trial: surgical versus nonsurgical care for spinal stenosis, degenerative spondylolisthesis, and intervertebral disc herniation. Spine 2011;36:2061–8.
66. Weinstein JN, Lurie JD, Tosteson TD, et al. Surgical compared with nonoperative treatment for lumbar degenerative spondylolisthesis: four-year results in the Spine Patient Outcomes Research Trial (SPORT) randomized and observational cohorts. J Bone Joint Surg Am 2009;91:1295–304.
67. Weinstein JN, Tosteson TD, Lurie JD. Surgical versus non-operative treatment for lumbar spinal stenosis four-year results of the Spine Patient Outcomes Research Trial. Spine 2010;35:1329–38.
68. Kovacs FM, Urrutia G, Alarcon JD. Surgery versus conservative treatment for symptomatic lumbar spinal stenosis: a systemic review of randomized controlled trials. Spine 2011;36:E1335–51.
69. Jacobs W, Van der Gaag NA, Tuschel A, et al. Total disc replacement for chronic back pain in the presence of disc degeneration. Cochrane Database Syst Rev 2012;(9):CD008326. http://dx.doi.org/10.1002/14651858.CD008326.pub2.
70. Airaksinen O, Brox JI, Cedraschi C, et al. Chapter 4. European guidelines for the management of chronic nonspecific low back pain. Eur Spine J 2006;15(Suppl 2):S192–300.

Low Back Pain in the Adolescent Athlete

Arthur Jason De Luigi, DO

KEYWORDS

- Low back pain • Adolescents • Athletes • Spinal injuries

KEY POINTS

- Low back pain is frequently encountered in adolescent athletes.
- The adolescent athlete is at risk for significant structural injuries as well as nonmechanical problems.
- Adolescent athletes who present with low back pain are more likely to have structural injuries and therefore should be investigated fully.
- Any athlete with severe, persisting, or activity-limiting symptoms needs to be evaluated thoroughly.
- It is imperative to complete a comprehensive evaluation of back pain, and a cause such as muscle strain should be a diagnosis of exclusion.

INTRODUCTION

Low back pain is a common problem among adolescent athletes. It is estimated to occur in 10% to 15% of young athletes,[1,2] but the prevalence may be higher in certain sports.[1,3–7] Back pain has been reported as high as 27% in football and between 50% and 86% in gymnastics.[4–6] Although adolescent athletes are undergoing their pubescent changes into adulthood, they cannot be treated like young adults. Therefore, the approach to the treatment of adolescent athletes with low back pain can be difficult and requires thorough understanding of spinal development.

The demographics of adolescents with low back pain varies from that of adulthood, Although there are many conditions that occur in both adolescence and adulthood, there are certain spinal disease/injury processes that are unique to the growing adolescent spine.[8–11] One of the key factors to consider in the adolescent athlete is the ongoing growth and development of the adolescent spine. The growing spine introduces variables into the assessment and management of injuries to the spine that do not exist in the mature and developed spine of the adult population. For example,

This article originally appeared in Physical Medicine and Rehabilitation Clinics of North America, Volume 25, Issue 4, November 2014.

Department of Rehabilitation Medicine, Georgetown University School of Medicine, 3800 Reservoir Road, Washington, DC 20007, USA

E-mail address: Arthur.J.Deluigi@Medstar.net

http://dx.doi.org/10.1016/j.ccol.2014.10.013
2352-7986/14/$ – see front matter

injuries of the pars interarticularis are more common in the adolescent spine, occurring in up to 47% of young athletes,[9] whereas disk-related problems are uncommon in children; only 11% of children have disk-related disease, compared with 48% of adults.[9] Idiopathic pain is also less common in young athletes. Physicians who attribute low back pain in young athletes to simple back strains, without investigations, run the risk of delaying the diagnosis and appropriate treatment of more serious injuries, such as spondylolysis or spondylolisthesis.[8,11] Therefore, it is imperative that the clinician is aware the development of the spine and subsequent variances in injury patterns and frequencies when evaluating the adolescent athlete.

In addition to the structural considerations of the spine, the clinician should also be aware of potential physiologic, psychological, social, and cultural issues that may exist and affect the approach to diagnosis and management of adolescent spine disorders. To treat these athletes appropriately, clinicians need to develop a relationship with the athlete's parents/guardians, coaches, and other potential athletic support staff to facilitate compliance with the activity modifications and treatment necessary to provide optimal rehabilitation to the injured spine. The coordination of care with the athlete's support team facilitates the athlete's recovery, training, and performance.[12]

GROWTH AND DEVELOPMENT OF THE SPINE

There are distinct structural differences of the spine in adolescents from the adult spine, which affect the nature of injury. Compared with the adult spine, the relatively greater hydrophilic nature of the nucleus pulposus of the spine of a child allows for more effective force absorption and central distribution of force transfer to the adjacent vertebrae.[12] However, the composition of the nucleus pulposus begins to change as early as 7 or 8 years old, resulting in a more peripheral force distribution of the disk.[13] There are 3 primary ossification centers of the vertebrae: one in the vertebral body and 2 in the vertebral arch. The 2 ossifications in the center of the vertebral arch typically fuse by 2 to 6 years, and spinal bifida occulta results, caused by failure of fusion of these primary centers.[14,15] Pars interarticularis defects/fractures are more common in the adolescent spine, occurring in up to 47% of young athletes, and are postulated to be caused by incomplete bony maturation present in the neural arch.[9] Biomechanical studies have indicated that the bony strength of the vertebrae, particularly the neural arch, can increase into the fourth or fifth decade of life.[16]

The physes associated with the vertebral end plates facilitate the growth of the vertebral body. Hyaline cartilage adjacent to the nucleus pulposus and physeal cartilage adjacent to the vertebral body comprise the vertebral end plate. A ring apophysis and an end-plate physis comprise the physeal cartilage. The growth of the vertebral body is facilitated by the ring apophysis, which surrounds the periphery of the vertebral body and begins to ossify at 7 or 8 years old,[12] whereas vertical growth of the vertebral body is caused by end-plate physis, which begins to fuse with the vertebral body at about age 14 to 15 years, with final closure occurring around age 21 to 25 years.[12–14]

In addition to understanding the structural aspects of the growing adolescent spine, the clinician needs to be familiar with the variances of pubescent spinal development to assist in the diagnosis and management of spinal injuries. Schmorl nodes occur more frequently in children and adolescents compared with adults. Schmorl nodes are vertebral end-plate herniations of disk material, which are postulated to result from a combination of more central distribution of force via the nucleus pulposus combined with a relatively weak vertebral end plate.[12–15] The adolescent athlete is also at increased risk for apophyseal ring fractures during the ongoing physeal development until ossification.[12]

Another significant variation in injury patterns related to spinal development is disk-related disease in comparing the growing adolescent with mature adults, with the incidence at 11% in children compared with 48% in adults.[9] The proposed pathophysiologic basis for this significant age-related variance is the relative strength of the intervertebral disk compared with that of the adjacent bone in adolescents compared with those in adults.[12-15]

There is a significant variance in individual adolescents in the onset of puberty and the subsequent rate of growth and maturation. The variance between adolescents results in significant differences in size, strength, and skeletal maturity among children of the same chronologic age. Children between 6 and 10 years of age grow about 5 to 8 cm per year and gain about 2 to 3 kg per year.[17] During adolescence, the growth rate increases, leading first to increases in height followed by increases in weight. On average, girls enter adolescent growth spurt and reach their maximal growth velocity about 2 years before boys. Weight gain occurs during the maximal growth in height, with girls gaining about 7 kg in fat-free mass, whereas boys gain about twice this amount.[17]

DEMOGRAPHICS

Although low back pain commonly occurs in the adolescent population, adolescent athletes who participate in specific sports such as football or gymnastics may be at a more substantial risk of pain and structural injury than others at the same chronologic age.[4-6] The overall lifetime prevalence of low back pain by the midteenage years has been found to be 50% or greater in general population studies, with 1-year prevalence rates of 17% to 50%.[12,18-23] In several studies,[12,18-20,22,23] an increase in the prevalence of low back pain with age throughout childhood has been reported, with some of these studies also reporting higher rates of spinal injuries in girls than boys. A definitive connection has yet to be established between physical activity and low back pain, because the previous studies have had a significant variance in their results.[12,20,23-26] In an attempt to provide more objective evidence with the use of an accelerometer to assess activity levels in children and adolescents, Wedderkopp and colleagues[26] did not find any association between physical activity and low back pain. However, several studies[27] have identified an association in adolescents with low back pain between depression and other emotional problems. Another significant risk factor showing a strong correlation was that the development of low back pain during adolescence increased the likelihood for the development of low back pain as an adult in a large-scale twin study.[28]

There is a significant variance in the incidence and the specific spinal pathologic injury in adolescent athletes depending on the specific sport and also the position in a given sport.[12] Contact sports such as football and rugby have a significantly higher incidence of acute injuries from high-energy impacts.[6] In comparison, there is a greater incidence of overuse injuries with sports requiring repetitive flexion, extension, and torsion, such as gymnastics, figure skating, and rowing.[4,5,29] A significantly higher rate of low back pain in a group of female gymnasts and figure skaters and male hockey and soccer players compared with nonathletes has been noted (45% vs 18% over 3 years).[30] However, low back pain spans most sports in the adolescent population and was found to be a significant problem in golfers, rowers, and rugby players.[31-33]

Gymnasts in particular have shown a significantly high incidence of spinal injury (between 50% and 86%) in several studies.[4,5] These findings are limited not only to female gymnasts, because another study of male gymnasts showed that 79% of the male gymnasts had low back pain compared with 38% of their controls.[34] In another study assessing wrestlers, gymnasts, and soccer and tennis players, 65% of these athletes had a history of low back pain, with male gymnasts having the highest frequency, at 85%.[35]

RADIOLOGIC FINDINGS

There have been numerous studies regarding the incidence of radiologic findings in adolescent athletes. The results of these studies have shown that there are high rates of structural abnormalities on imaging studies of adolescent athletes in specific sports. As noted earlier, there was an increased incidence of low back pain symptoms in adolescent athletes who participate in gymnastics, and this trend also continues in the radiologic evaluation of their spines.[12] In a study on the incidence of findings of back pain in male gymnasts, magnetic resonance imaging (MRI) showed statistically significant differences in spinal diseases in gymnasts compared with controls, with findings of thoracolumbar disk degeneration (75% compared with 31%), Schmorl nodes (71% compared with 44%), and injuries to the ring apophysis (17% compared with 0%).[34] These findings were also shown in another study by Goldstein and colleagues,[36] who reported higher rates of various structural abnormalities on MRI studies of elite gymnasts compared with elite swimmers. Another study by Bennett and colleagues[37] performed MRI of the spine of elite female gymnasts, showing apophyseal injuries in almost half and disk degeneration in more than 60%.

Radiographic findings of spinal disease are not limited to adolescent gymnasts. Structural abnormalities on plain radiographs were shown in greater than 60% of the high-school and collegiate football players and in 74% of the rugby players assessed in 2 separate studies by Iwamoto and colleagues.[35,38] Several studies[39–42] have also shown higher rates of spondylolysis in high-level adolescent athletes participating in a variety of sports compared with nonathlete adolescents in the general population. Despite high levels of structural abnormalities on plain films and high rates of reported low back pain for young athletes competing in several sports, longer term follow-up studies[43–45] on many of these athletes did not show any significant increased risk for ongoing low back pain into adulthood compared with the general population.

CONSIDERATIONS IN THE EVALUATION OF LOW BACK PAIN IN THE ADOLESCENT ATHLETE

Injuries to the low back may be caused by an acute traumatic event; however, they are more frequently secondary to overuse injuries caused by chronic repetitive microtrauma.[29] It is imperative to complete a thorough assessment of all adolescent athletes who report symptoms of low back pain to evaluate for the presence of spinal disease. As noted earlier, because of the ongoing growth and development of the adolescent spine, the incidence of specific spinal diseases in adolescent athletes varies from adults. The clinician should also be cognizant of potential nonmechanical causes of low back pain, such as neoplasms, infection, developmental disorders, and systemic inflammatory rheumatisms.[12,28,45–48] One must formulate a strong differential diagnosis and subsequently through the evaluation process develop a rational diagnostic strategy based on a thorough history, review of systems, and physical examination. The clinician should always inquire about any potential red flag symptoms, such as unexplained weight loss, pain at night, pain with recumbency, progressive neurologic deficits, and any loss of bowel or bladder function. In addition, one should inquire about any additional symptoms during a review of symptoms, which may show a systemic process, such as a rheumatic disorder.

RISK FACTORS

As the adolescent athlete undergoes pubescent changes leading to periods of rapid growth, the muscles and ligaments are unable to maintain the pace of the rate of bone growth. This discrepancy places the adolescent athlete at greater risk of injury, as a result of muscle imbalance and a decrease in flexibility.[1,29,49] The skeletally immature spine of adolescent athletes is also vulnerable to injury of the growth cartilage and secondary ossifications centers, because these areas are the weakest link of force transfer and are susceptible to compression, distraction, and torsion injury.[1,7,29]

The vertebral bodies and intervertebral disks comprise the anterior column of the lumbar spine. Epiphyseal growth plates are located at both ends of the vertebral bodies and have overlying cartilaginous growth plates and ring apophyses, which attach to the outer annulus fibrosus. Repetitive flexion may lead to intervertebral disk herniation through the ring apophysis, a secondary ossification center, and injury to the ring apophysis can result in avulsion fractures.[28]

The facet joints, spinous process, and pars interarticularis make up the posterior column of the lumbar spine. Ossification of the posterior column of the spine progresses from anterior to posterior and may be congenitally incomplete in the area of the superior portion of the pars interarticularis of the lower lumbar vertebrae, particularly at the L5 level, predisposing to spondylolytic stress fractures.[1,11] The presence of spina bifida occulta at the lumbosacral junction seems to be an additional risk factor for spondylolysis. Traction from the dorsolumbar fascia and lordotic impingement may affect the growth cartilage of the facet joint and spinous process apophysis of the posterior arch.[1]

Because of the considerable variance in the timing and tempo of growth among children, smaller, less mature athletes may be at higher risk for injury from contact from larger athletes, particularly in contact sports.[11,49]

Several potential risk factors for spinal injury or low back pain in athletes have been identified. These factors include previous low back or lower extremity injuries, incomplete rehabilitation of previous injuries, decreased endurance, lower extremity muscle imbalance, high number of hours of participation per week, and the occurrence of stressful life events. Additional proximate causal factors associated with sports-related injury may include the individual mechanics and skill level associated with sports performance, training patterns, and equipment or facility problems.[47,50]

Training volume and intensity can also cause injuries, particularly when young athletes participate in a sport for longer periods, such as at tournaments and sports camps.[11] However, it is difficult to determine the appropriate amount of training for adolescent athletes, because of the variance in toleration of similar volumes of training. Overuse injuries present more often in athletes experiencing rapid growth,[1,11] suggesting that the volume and intensity of training that an athlete's body can tolerate vary as the athletes grow and mature.[11]

Poor technique, abdominal muscle weakness, hip flexor/hamstring/thoracolumbar fascia tightness, increased femoral anteversion, genu recurvatum, and increased thoracic kyphosis serve as additional risk factors for low back pain. These factors add additional stress to the posterior elements of the spine as a result of increased lumbar lordosis.[1,11]

PREVENTION

Although injuries are a part of sport, there are ways to reduce the risk of injury in young athletes. Recognizing risk factors is a key component to reducing injury.[11] Before the start of a sport season, a preparticipation evaluation may identify certain risk factors, such as previous injuries that have not been fully rehabilitated or muscle weaknesses or inflexibility. These areas can then be addressed before the start of the season. In addition, athletes should start general strength and fitness conditioning several weeks before the start of the season.[49] Increases in the frequency and intensity of training should be gradual, to allow for safe adaptation to the demands of the sport.

During periods of growth, young athletes are prone to loss of flexibility and muscle imbalances, which can predispose them to injury.[11,49] Because of this concern, young athletes should reduce the amount of training and the volume of repetitive motions during growth spurts. Certain sports require maneuvers that place a lot of stress on the posterior spine, such as layback spins in figure skating and walkovers in gymnastics. Athletes may need to limit the number of repetitions of these maneuvers, particularly if pain is associated with these maneuvers. Core strengthening exercises and stretches for tight hamstrings and hip flexors may help reduce the risk of low back pain.[11,49]

Proper technique should be emphasized in all athletes. It is important to correct posture to limit the amount of lordosis of the lumbar spine, which can help prevent injuries to the lumbar spine. In sports requiring lifting, such as pairs skating and dance, proper lifting techniques must be used to prevent back injuries.[11]

In team sports, there can be large discrepancies in the sizes and relative strengths of participants on any given team. Attempts should be made to match athletes in size and strength to prevent injuries from contact with larger, stronger participants.[11,49]

Another important aspect of prevention is recognizing that back pain is not part of the sport. Increasing complaints of pain, particularly if it is interfering with activity, should be taken seriously and addressed early to avoid significant injury.[11]

HISTORY AND PHYSICAL EXAMINATION

A comprehensive history is an essential initial step in the evaluation of adolescent athletes with low back pain. The mode of onset, location, quality, severity, and progression over time of the individual's symptoms provide useful insight into potential causes. Symptoms that remain mild for an extended period before presentation may be suggestive of less significant structural injuries or more indolent underlying processes, whereas more severe, acute, or progressive symptoms may suggest a more substantial structural injury or a rapidly progressive process, such as infection. In addition, the provider should inquire about back pain eliciting any neurologic symptoms and aggravating factors.[12]

The nature of an athlete's specific sport and the position played may also predispose that individual to particular problems as well as the volume of training and level of competition. The timing of injury or pain in relation to the competitive season or training cycle may be relevant for both diagnosis and treatment.[8,11] It is also important to inquire if there have been any recent increases in the training volume or intensity of the athlete. Thorough review of the dietary history, previous injuries, and the menstrual history of female athletes is also of importance.[11]

Primary importance should be placed on the potential of red flag symptoms, such as fever, malaise, unexplained weight loss, pain at night, morning stiffness, bowel or bladder incontinence, and progressive neurologic weakness. Pain at night is often believed to be suggestive of an infectious or neoplastic process.[12,51] Fever, lethargy, weight loss, rashes, headaches, and similar symptoms raise concern for significant systemic processes, including infection and malignancy.[12,48,51] Morning stiffness or additional joint symptoms may suggest a diffuse inflammatory process. A past history or family history of HLA-B27-associated conditions, such as psoriatic arthritis, ankylosing spondylitis, reactive (Reiter) arthritis, or inflammatory bowel disease, may help in determining systemic causes of low back pain.[29]

Isolated axial low back pain without lower extremity symptoms should be viewed differently from a presentation that includes leg pain or neurologic dysfunction, such as numbness, tingling, weakness, or changes in the bowel or bladder. Radicular symptoms such as radiation of pain down the leg and motor or sensory changes suggest the presence of nerve root or cord involvement.[12] Bilateral leg pain suggests bilateral foraminal involvement and should expand the clinician's differential diagnosis. At this point, one should consider and make specific assessment to help differentiate between a significant spondylolisthesis, central canal stenosis, disk herniation in the setting of a congenitally small spinal canal, or a cord process.[12] The presence of lower extremity symptoms does not always mean that they are of spinal origin, and the clinician should also assess for other concomitant nonspinal diseases such as stress fractures, compartment syndrome, or other musculotendinous injuries. The location of the back pain can also significantly affect the differential diagnosis. Thoracic or thoracolumbar pain may be associated with diskogenic processes or Scheuermann kyphosis. Low lumbar pain has many potential causes, including disk disease, central or foraminal stenosis, spondyloarthropathies, and myofascial pain. Pain in the sacral or gluteal region may be more associated with conditions such as sacroiliitis or a sacral stress fracture; however, one still must assess for referred pain from the lumbar facets or nerve root involvement.[12]

After the completion of a thorough history of present illness, the clinician should perform a comprehensive physical examination. The physical examination should be structured to identify significant and specific conditions that were formulated on the differential diagnosis. The result of a thorough history and physical examination should develop a strategic plan of further diagnostic and treatment options.[12]

The physical examination should always be thorough, including inspection of any structural imbalances or asymmetries, lumbar range of motion, lumbosacral and pelvic motion, palpation of the spine, lumbar paraspinals, sacroiliac (SI)/pelvic muscles and joints, and a neurologic examination. It is important to assess lower extremity alignment and function, balance, and spine-specific provocative maneuvers. Gait assessment should be performed to assess for abnormalities such as antalgia, ataxia, or Trendelenberg gait.[12]

The examiner should observe the athlete's spine by having the patient wear a gown open to the back. When observing the athlete from behind it is important in the spine, shoulders, and pelvis to identify that the bony and soft tissue structures on both sides of the midline are symmetric. Visual inspection of the spine should evaluate for the presence of any abnormalities such as hemangiomas, café-au-lait spots, hairy patches, or skin dimples that may indicate spinal disease.[49,52] Inspection should also identify any abnormal curvatures of the spine, such as scoliosis, excessive kyphosis, or lordosis.

Range of motion of the spine should be assessed in flexion, extension, rotation, and lateral flexion (bending). Adolescent athletes should be able to complete forward flexion of the spine and come close to touching their toes without knee flexion. Caution must be used to identify limitation of this motion because of tight hamstrings. Pain with flexion is suggestive of injury to the anterior spinal elements or lumbar muscle strain/spasms. The posterior elements of the spine can be assessed with hyperextension and facet loading (hyperextension with rotation).

Palpation for tenderness of the spine, lumbar paraspinals, and the SI joint is an integral part of the spinal assessment. Myofascial trigger points are taut, palpable bands in the lumbar paraspinal and gluteal muscles, which elicit or trigger the athlete's pain. Tenderness of the SI joint has a positive predictive value for SI disorder.[53]

Special tests include tests for the SI iliac joints, facet joints, and neural tension signs. These tests include FABER (flexion-abduction-external rotation), Gaenslen sign, Gillet test, seated slump test, straight leg raise, Lasègue maneuver, Bragard sign, Lazarević sign, and facet loading.[11,54]

Additional assessment should be completed to assess the hip to rule out hip disease as well as the abdomen to rule out visceral disease. In female athletes, a pelvic examination may be warranted, particularly if menstrual abnormalities are reported by the patient during the history. The neurologic examination should include assessment of motor strength, sensation, and deep tendon reflexes of the lower extremities.

Clearly, other components of a comprehensive physical examination need to be included as medically appropriate, as well. Consideration does need to be given to the potential for significant structural injury, including fracture, and the examination should always be modified appropriately for a given patient to elicit essential information and avoid further harm.

RADIOGRAPHIC EVALUATION OF THE ADOLESCENT SPINE

Spinal imaging should be considered as an additional diagnostic option to assist in establishing a specific diagnosis. There are a variety of different imaging modalities to assist in the diagnostic evaluation, and clinicians need to be familiar with the each of their strengths and limitations. In addition, the clinician should be comfortable with directly assessing the images. Given the relative sensitivities and specificities of the various diagnostic options, the clinician should develop a plan for which imaging modality would provide the most appropriate objective findings based on the formulated differential diagnosis. In addition, the clinician should also consider that the amount of exposure to radiation in the adolescent athlete is of particular concern. Therefore, specific radiographic options should include the risk assessment of radiation exposure versus the potential comparative benefit of the various diagnostic options. The imaging strategies vary based on clinical concerns of the presenting symptoms and findings during the history and physical examination and are discussed in greater detail with each specific spinal condition.[12]

SPECIAL CONSIDERATIONS IN THE ADOLESCENT ATHLETE

Treatment of adolescent athletes involves several specific considerations, as well. The state and demands of physiologic development of the athlete need to be taken into consideration when planning physical training. The psychosocial environment of an injured athlete may also pose challenges for treatment, and the psychological impact of injury can be difficult for athletes and their families. The use of medications may be problematic, as well. There are limited to no data on the effects on children and adolescents of several different medications commonly used to manage pain in adults. Care needs to be taken regarding weight and age in prescribing medications to young athletes, and clinicians need to be aware of any potential conflicts with substance use policies that may apply to an athlete's given sport or level of competition. There are also high rates of use of ergogenic aids and performance-enhancing supplements among adolescent athletes, which introduce the potential for medication interactions, among other problems.[55] The use of these supplements, legal or illegal, may not necessarily be reported to clinicians routinely, and the likelihood of this seems even lower if specific questions regarding their use are not asked.

SPECIFIC SPINAL CONDITIONS AND INJURIES

There are several specific clinical entities that are particularly important to understand in managing young athletes with low back pain. These entities include spondylolysis, spondylolisthesis, posterior element overuse syndrome, diskogenic injuries, vertebral body apophyseal avulsion fracture, Scheuermann kyphosis, SI pain, and other causes of low back pain. These individual conditions are discussed in greater detail in the following sections.[12]

Spondylolysis and Spondylolisthesis

Spondylolysis is a common cause of spinal disease in the adolescent spine and should be considered as a diagnostic possibility in almost every adolescent athlete with significant low back pain. However, it should be high on the differential diagnosis in all athletes who compete in sports involving repetitive extension and rotation, such as gymnastics, figure skating, and rowing.[12] Spondylolysis is definitively the most frequent diagnosis (47%) made in adolescent athletes presenting with low back pain.[9]

Spondylolysis refers to a defect in the pars interarticularis of the vertebral arch, a stress fracture caused by repetitive extension and torsion of the spine, and is most common at L5 and on the left side.[56] Bilateral spondylolysis at the same vertebral level can result in spondylolisthesis. Spondylolisthesis is a separate but related term referring to the anterior displacement of a vertebral body compared with its alignment with the adjacent vertebral body (**Fig. 1**).[12] Spondylolisthesis is graded using the Meyerding scale according to the percentage of slip: grade 1 is a slip of 0% to 25%, grade 2 is 25% to 50%, grade 3 is 50% to 75%, grade 4 is 75% to 100%, and grade 5 is more than 100%.[57]

Spondylolysis and spondylolisthesis are most frequently viewed under the categorization proposed by Wiltse and colleagues.[58] The term isthmic spondylolysis is used to identify those patients who have sustained a lesion in the pars. Isthmic

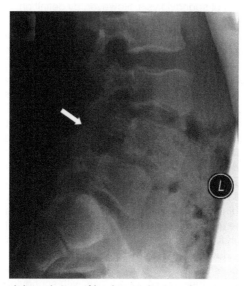

Fig. 1. Plain radiograph lateral view of lumbosacral spine of a young tennis player showing an isthmic spondylolisthesis with bilateral pars defects (*arrow*). (*From* Standaert CJ. Low back pain in the adolescent athlete. Phys Med Rehabil Clin N Am 2008;19(2):292; with permission.)

spondylolysis represents a pars lesion/defect that is believed to be a fatigue fracture of the bone. Most pars lesions identified in many studies occur at L5 (85%–95%).[39,40,42,58,59] In a study of 4243 young athletes with low back pain, Rossi and Dragoni[41] found that about one-half of those with spondylolysis also had concurrent spondylolisthesis. Significant progression of an associated spondylolisthesis is uncommon. There are data[60] to support that there is not any increased risk of progression of spondylolisthesis with sports participation. When there is an increase in the anterior translation of 1 vertebral body on the other, it is usually correlated with an adolescent growth spurt, and typically without any symptoms. Therefore, once spondylolisthesis is identified in the adolescent athlete, the affected individual needs to be monitored radiographically through adolescence to assess for any progression of the spinal disease.[12]

General population studies have shown pars lesions to be a common finding. In a prospective study of plain radiographs in 500 first-grade students, there was an overall prevalence of spondylolysis of 4.4% at age 6 years. All of these lesions identified in this study occurred without any symptoms. These diseases were then followed, and the number increased to 5.2% by age 12 years and 6% by adulthood.[39] Comparatively, another cadaveric study reviewed plain radiographs of 4200 cadaveric spines and found an overall prevalence of 4.2%.[40] However, the incidence of spondylolysis is different in adolescents who compete in athletics; large-scale studies[41,42] of adolescent athletes reported rates of 8% to 14%.

There is definitively a significant variance of the incidence of spondylolysis in athletes who participate in certain sports. Some of the sports with the highest reported frequencies of pars lesions include gymnastics, weight lifting, throwing track and field sports, diving, wrestling, cricket, and crew.[6,41,42,61,62] Sports that involve frequent flexion/extension motions of the lumbar spine, particularly when combined with rotation, may place athletes at more risk for pars fractures.

History and physical examination can be helpful in identifying a clinical pattern suggestive of the diagnosis of spondylolysis. However, by definition, additional spinal imaging is essential establish the diagnosis.

Athletes with spondylolysis typically present with insidious onset of extension-related low back pain.[8,11,12,63,64] The athlete frequently also has an associated reduction in hamstring flexibility. Symptomatic spondylolysis typically presents with axial low back pain without radiation into the legs; however, the athlete may occasionally have radiating pain, numbness, or weakness if the disease affects the nerve roots.[12] The pain typically occurs acutely after a specific traumatic event but may also occur after a relatively mundane event or may progress over time. The typical pain pattern associated with spondylolysis is usually worsened by activity and improved with rest.[12] The athlete may complain of pain with impact, such as running or jumping. It is common for the symptoms to begin to develop toward the end of 1 sports season, subside after the season while the athlete is no longer stressing the area of disease, and then return once the athlete starts training for the next season. The distribution of pain varies depending on whether the lesion is unilateral or bilateral but can lateralize to the side of the unilateral lesion or be more generalized in the low back.[12]

It is uncommon to have associated leg pain, paresthesias, or neurologic loss with isolated spondylosis. However, the presence of these symptoms does not eliminate spondylosis from the differential diagnosis. Rather, these findings should suggest the potential concomitant presence of spondylosis with spondylolisthesis or other diagnoses such as disk herniation in adolescent athletes.[11] There are no pathognomonic findings on physical examination for spondylolysis; however, pain with extension and rotation may suggest disease of the posterior elements such as a pars lesion or facets. A special test to assess for potential spondylolysis is the 1-legged hyperextension maneuver. This maneuver is performed by having the patient stand on 1 leg and leaning backward.[12] The maneuver has been proposed as a means of identifying the presence of a pars lesion, but a recent study of this test[65] concluded that it had low sensitivity and specificity.

Several diagnostic imaging modalities are available for evaluating the pars in an athlete with suspected spondylolysis.[12] However, there is significant controversy regarding the optimal imaging strategy, because of potential risks of radiation exposure in the growing adolescent spine. Given the relatively high prevalence of asymptomatic pars lesions in both the general population of adolescents and adolescent athletes, it is not enough just to visualize a pars lesion. Ideally, there is a clinical picture that is suggestive of disease of the pars, which is supported by the radiographic findings. Optimally, any radiographic pars defect needs to be identified as the source of pain and should be assessed for the potential of the lesion to heal. Therefore, in practical application, the clinician needs to assess the risks of radiation exposure from multiple imaging studies with the benefits of initial diagnosis and subsequent evaluation of pars defect healing.[12]

Historically, plain radiography has been the primary imaging modality used in the identification, diagnosis, and observation of healing of pars lesions based on results of many published studies. The anteroposterior (AP) view may identify anatomic variants or developmental defects such as transitional vertebrae or spina bifida occulta, which is seen frequently in patients with spondylolysis.[66] The lateral view may show spondylolisthesis or a lytic lesion. Typically, a spondylitic lesion seen in plain radiographs appears as a lucency in the area of the pars (see **Fig. 1**).[12] Oblique views may show a stress reaction of the pars interarticularis and is identified as the pathognomonic neck of the Scotty dog lesion.[12] However, the routine use of oblique views is discouraged in adolescent athletes, because of the increased dose of radiation and because only one-third of stress fractures can be identified on plain radiographs.[63,64] Bone scan, single-photon emission computed tomography (SPECT), computed tomography (CT), and MRI have all been shown to be more sensitive than plain radiography in the identification of pars lesions.[67]

Plain radiographs should be followed by nuclear imaging with bone scan or SPECT. Radionuclide imaging, particularly SPECT, can be helpful in the diagnostic evaluation of adolescent athletes with low back pain. Bony lesions in which active bony turnover is occurring are indicated by increased uptake on the bone scan.[8,11,12,63–65] Numerous studies have shown bone scan and SPECT to be more sensitive than plain radiography in the diagnosis of spondylolysis, and it seems to be superior to MRI and CT in this regard, as well.[12,68–75] Multiple studies have also shown that a positive bone scan or SPECT scan correlates with a symptomatic pars lesion.[12,69,76–80] This finding makes SPECT a particularly useful and sensitive screening tool in adolescent athletes with low back pain. However, significant limitation in the use of radionuclide imaging is low specificity, because there are several other abnormalities seen in the posterior elements of adolescents on SPECT or bone scan that do not represent pars lesions.[12,67,71,73,81] Additional imaging, particularly with CT, is generally required to clarify the bony abnormality in a patient with a positive SPECT study (**Figs. 2** and **3A**).[12]

CT can be used to confirm the presence of a pars interarticularis stress fracture and monitor the progress of healing.[8,63] Along with clarifying a bony process identified on nuclear imaging, CT can distinguish between well-corticated fracture margins, termed chronic lesions or nonunions by various investigators, and differing stages of more recent or incomplete fractures.[12,67,75,81–83] The stage of the pars lesion on CT has also been found to be associated with the potential for bony healing.[74,81] In addition,

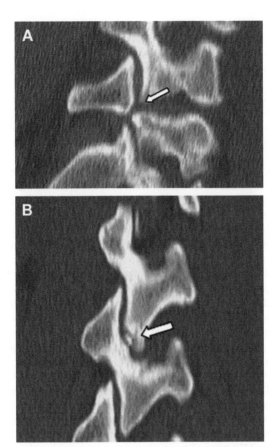

Fig. 2. CT oblique sagittal reformations. (*A*) A chronic pars lesion (*arrow*) with the classic appearance of the neck of the Scotty dog. (*B*) A spondylolytic lesion in the inferior articular process (*arrow*) in a young basketball player confirmed with SPECT. (*From* Standaert CJ. Low back pain in the adolescent athlete. Phys Med Rehabil Clin N Am 2008;19(2):295; with permission.)

in several studies,[12,61,73,75,81,83] several patients have been identified with increased activity in the area of the pars on SPECT but either an incomplete fracture or no fracture noted on CT. This finding seems most consistent with the presence of a stress reaction in the bone without overt fracture and shows the importance of correlating CT findings with nuclear imaging.[12,81] CT involves a higher level of radiation, and is of particular concern in the growing spine of the adolescent athlete. The risk for additional radiation must be weighed with the potential additional clinic benefit provided by CT. Therefore, many reserve CT scans for those not responding to treatment.[11]

Compared with the other imaging modalities, MRI has limitations that hamper its effectiveness as the primary imaging modality for adolescent athletes with low back pain. The main advantages of MRI include the lack of ionizing radiation and the ability to identify disk abnormalities and other types of disease. However, it can be difficult to appreciate cortical detail well at the pars on MRI compared with CT, and it is less sensitive for detecting spondylolysis compared with SPECT bone scan. The important diagnostic findings on MRI in patients with a potential pars lesion are those that are consistent with edema in the area of the pars or pedicle, suggestive of an acute

A   **B**

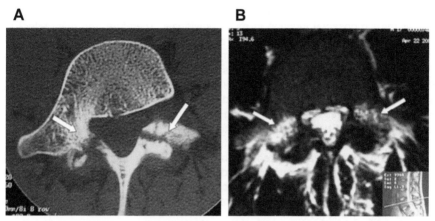

Fig. 3. (*A*) Axial view CT scan showing bilateral pars fractures (*arrows*). (*B*) Axial view CT scan shows unilateral pars fracture *(arrows)* with reactive sclerotic changes on the contralateral side. (*From* Standaert CJ. Low back pain in the adolescent athlete. Phys Med Rehabil Clin N Am 2008;19(2):296; with permission.)

fracture (see **Fig. 3**B).[12] There is a lack of evidence on the clinical implications of these MRI findings. In addition, studies have shown other significant limitations in the ability to identify and appropriately stratify pars lesions based on MRI.[12,65,74] A recent study comparing the relative usefulness of MRI compared with SPECT and CT found that MRI identified only 80% of the pars lesions seen on SPECT.[65] Therefore based on the lack of evidence, and comparative limitations to CT and SPECT, MRI does not seem to be an effective screening tool.[65,74]

Overall, the clinician should develop a definitive diagnostic approach to an adolescent athlete with low back pain who has signs or symptoms suggestive of a spondylolysis. Given the current review of literature, the adolescent athlete should initially be assessed with limited plain films, particularly isolated standing AP and lateral views to identify a spondylolisthesis or gross bony abnormalities, followed by a SPECT study. If the SPECT study is positive, a thin-cut CT (axial sequences 1 mm thick or less) should be obtained through the area of abnormality on SPECT to confirm the diagnosis and to stage the lesion for treatment. If the SPECT study is negative, it is highly unlikely that the athlete has a symptomatic pars defect, and other diagnoses should be considered.[8,11,12,63–75]

In an era of evidence-based medicine, it is interesting to know that there are no controlled trials on the treatment of spondylolysis in adolescent athletes.[12] However, there are several published case series that use a wide variety of treatment approaches. The essential element of care seems to be relative rest.[12] Activity modifications should occur to avoid any activities that cause pain, particularly extension activities. However, the ideal extent of activity restriction involved and the length of time out of sports is unclear.[12] An exercise program should include strengthening of the abdominal muscles, hip flexor and hamstring stretches, and antilordotic exercises.[3,11,49]

Bracing is a particularly controversial issue in the management of spondylolysis.[12] Several investigators[1,8,63,64,66,84,85] advocate the routine use of lumbosacral orthoses of a variety of types in the management of these patients in the early management to limit extension and rotation of the spine. Others[8,86] simply restrict activities without bracing, in conjunction with physical therapy. Biomechanical studies on the effects of lumbosacral bracing show that bracing results in an increase in intervertebral motion at the lumbosacral junction in most individuals. Therefore, the main effect of bracing seems to be a restriction in gross body motion rather than restricting intersegmental mobility.[87,88] The results of outcome studies tend to be similar regarding rates of healing and return to play, regardless of the type or extent of bracing used. Studies[66,82,86,89,90] have shown bony healing with the use of a rigid brace, a soft brace, and no brace. The variance of these findings is what has made the use of specific bracing controversial. It is also surprising that in studies there is little correlation between the extent of bony healing and return to play. Most studies addressing these issues[12,66,83,90–92] show relatively high rates of return to play and lower rates of healing. A recent study[89] that included patients treated with a brace as well as patients treated without a brace did not find any advantage for brace use in terms of achieving bony union. However, another study in young soccer players[93] showed that the best results were obtained with a period of rest from sport for 3 months, regardless of whether bracing was used.

Based on the current evidence, the best initial treatment of all athletes is rest. Ideally, rest should include avoidance of all physical activity and particularly sports beyond that needed for routine daily function.[12] Although there is no evidence showing any specific duration of activity restriction, the consensus is based on the individual clinical response and the appearance of their pars lesion on CT. If CT shows an early or progressive stage lesion, the athlete is advised to rest for 3 months, with subsequent follow-up imaging.[12] However, if the pars lesion has chronic features on CT, the opportunity for bony union is diminished, and rest is advised until the low back pain has subsided.[12,82]

Although anecdotally advocated by some in clinical practice, the routine use of bracing is not uniformly supported by the literature. If bracing is used, bracing continues until the athlete has resumed full activities without pain, and then the brace is gradually weaned until the athlete is participating fully without pain.[12,63,64] As a means of further restricting activity by providing a physical barrier to motion, a rigid brace may be used after 2 or 3 weeks of rest if symptoms are not resolving. After adequate rest for the stage of the lesion and restoration of pain-free range of motion, athletes can be placed in to a comprehensive rehabilitation program.[12]

Generally, rehabilitation for spondylolysis can be started early and progressed depending on symptoms, and generally return to play is about 6 to 8 weeks after the initial injury. The healing time for acute spondylolisthesis requires 2 to 4 months to complete followed by rehabilitation, resulting in return to sport approximately 4 to 6 months after diagnosis.[12] However, the return associated with minimally symptomatic lesions may be sooner during the rehabilitation process.

A patient who has resumed full pain-free activities out of the brace is considered clinically healed. Patients with spondylolisthesis should be followed every 4 to 6 months with standing lateral films until skeletal maturity to assess for progression of slip.[12] Athletes are at low risk for worsening of spondylolisthesis. However, if the slip progresses beyond 50%, or if there are neurologic symptoms or persistent pain, surgical stabilization is indicated.[1,63]

Surgical intervention is rarely required to treat the pain associated with spondylolysis. However, there are potential indications for surgical intervention, including progressive slip, intractable pain, the development of neurologic deficits, and segmental instability associated with pain.[12] Surgical treatment is usually considered the best option for patients with a slip of 50% or greater, and these patients should all undergo surgical evaluation. There are several case series on athletes undergoing surgery with direct pars repair and returning to high-level sports, but considerations about return to play and long-term quality of life need to be factored into decisions on surgical intervention.[12]

As a routine issue, follow-up films are not necessary for patients with a unilateral pars lesion without a spondylolisthesis who do well with conservative treatment. Those with a spondylolisthesis need repeat plain films every 6 to 12 months during the adolescent growth spurts to monitor for possible slip progression. Similarly, this approach can be considered in those with bilateral pars defects, particularly if they are very young at the time of presentation.[12] Repeat imaging with CT can be helpful if it is necessary to determine the extent of healing or progression of the fracture; however, as noted earlier, the risk with additional radiation exposure needs to be assessed. Therefore, if the adolescent is no longer having any more clinical symptoms, the potential risk of increased radiation exposure exceeds the benefit of confirmed radiographic healing. Additional diagnostic evaluation should also be considered in patients who are not responding well to what seems to be appropriate treatment.

Posterior Element Overuse Syndrome

Posterior element overuse syndrome is a constellation of conditions involving muscle-tendon units, ligaments, facet joints, and joint capsules. It is a result from repeated extension and rotation of the spine. It is also called hyperlordotic low back pain, mechanical low back pain, or muscular low back pain.[1,8,9,49,85,94] Posterior element overuse syndrome is the most common cause after spondylolysis of low back pain in adolescents.[65]

Young athletes with posterior element overuse syndrome present with symptoms similar to those of spondylolysis. Pain is associated with extension of the spine and sometimes with rotation. There may be paraspinal muscle tenderness, as well as focal tenderness over the lower lumbar spine, adjacent to the midline. Imaging is typically negative, ruling out spondylolysis.

Management includes ice and nonsteroidal antiinflammatory drugs (NSAIDs) to relieve pain and inflammation. Pain-free activities are permitted, and extension of the spine is avoided. An exercise program emphasizing abdominal strengthening, antilordotic exercises, and hamstring and thoracolumbar stretches should be initiated at home or under the guidance of a physical therapist.[1,8,11,29,85] Although there is insufficient evidence of significant benefit, an antilordotic brace may be helpful in the short-term to provide support and protection.

Disk Disease

Low back pain secondary to disk disease is an uncommon problem in adolescent athletes; however, when it does occur, it can be a significant problem. Acute disk herniations of the nucleus pulposus are uncommon. Adolescents typically present with flexion-based back pain with associated paraspinal muscle spasms, hamstring tightness, and gluteal pain.[1,7,10,11] Compared with the adult population, traditional radicular symptoms are not often initially present.[6,49] In a study comparing adolescents with adults presenting to a sports medicine clinic, Micheli and Wood[9] attributed the low back pain secondary to disk abnormalities in about 50% of the adults compared with only about 10% of the adolescents. Kumar and colleagues[95] reviewed a series of 742 patients undergoing surgery for lumbar disk disease, and adolescents (age <20 years) accounted for only 3.5% of the cases.

Disk disease can result in isolated axial low back pain or radiating pain to the buttocks or lower extremities. The symptoms are generally considered to be worsened by activities involving flexion, rotation, or increases in intra-abdominal pressure.

However, there are no true pathognomonic aspects of the history for diskogenic pain. Similar symptoms can be seen with other types of spine disease, and disk problems can present with other patterns of symptoms. Disk protrusions associated with congenital canal stenosis may represent a distinct problem in athletes with back or leg pain, because there may be an increased risk of neurologic involvement and potentially a less favorable natural history.[7] These athletes may present with a history more consistent with spinal stenosis, including neurogenic claudication. As with all athletes with low back disorders, a comprehensive physical examination including a neurologic evaluation is essential in those with presumed diskogenic abnormalities, to appropriately treat these athletes.

Physical examination of low back pain associated with diskogenic disease shows a decrease in lumbar range of motion, particularly flexion, and positive neural tension signs such as straight leg raise, Lasègue sign, Lazarević sign, Bragard sign, and seated slump test.[54] It is possible to also see decreased reflexes and strength on the affected side of the correlating myotomes. However, the presentation can be variable, with the patient having only axial low back pain until undergoing the provocative examination.[29]

Disk abnormalities on imaging studies are less commonly identified in adolescents than in adults.[12] In a study of 439 13-year-old children from the general population, about one-third were noted to have diskogenic abnormalities on MRI, compared with more than 50% of 40-year-olds in a similar study.[96,97] Athletes who participate in specific sports have been found to have higher rates of degenerative disk changes than the general population.[31,37] Disk herniations in adolescent athletes may also be affected by genetic factors, and the rate of disk herniations occurring in individuals younger than 21 years is 5 times greater in those with a positive family history.[98]

Treatment options for disk injuries in adolescent athletes are similar to those in adults, although there are a few distinct considerations regarding sports participation and age that may be relevant.[12] Overall, almost 90% of patients improve with conservative management.[85,94] Conservative management and nonoperative care are clearly advised as the dominant form of treatment of most adolescent athletes with diskogenic pain.[7,12,47,51,99] Several nonoperative treatment modalities are available, although there is limited study of their effectiveness in the adolescent population. These modalities include physical therapy to address lumbar stability and neuromuscular control, therapeutic modalities, manipulative care, massage, bracing, medications, and interventional spine procedures (eg, epidural injections).[12] In general, it may be best to minimize the use of interventions, medications, and surgery in this population on reviewing the potentials risks versus benefits of some of these treatment options.

Surgical care is generally reserved for those with severe radicular pain who are not responding to optimal conservative management and nonoperative care, having saddle anesthesia or bowel/bladder incontinence as a result of cauda equina involvement, or progressive neurologic loss.[51] Before any consideration of surgical intervention, there should be definitive and clear imaging and other diagnostic findings such as electromyography and nerve conduction studies, which correlate disk and nerve root involvement in the same distribution as the athlete's symptoms. In the care of the adolescent athlete, the clinician and surgeon must take into consideration the balance between the long-term ramifications of surgical intervention on global and spinal health compared with the potential postoperative complications of surgery. Surgical intervention by itself does not guarantee clinical improvement or performance enhancement and should be reserved for clear definitive athletes who have failed conservative management, developed cauda equina symptoms, or have progressive neurologic deficits.[7] As with all other conditions, treatment of disk injuries needs to be directed toward the benefit of the whole individual.

A potential serious complication of disk herniation is cauda equina syndrome, which is caused by the compression of the nerve roots in the lower aspect of the spinal canal.[56] Symptoms of cauda equina syndrome include paralysis of the lower extremities and loss of bowel and bladder function. Cauda equina syndrome is a surgical emergency, and the deficits can remain permanent if not addressed promptly. For this reason, it is imperative to inquire about red flag symptoms in all patients.[11]

Athletes with disk herniation may return to activity once they have attained full pain-free range of motion and full strength and have progressed through sport-specific activities in a controlled setting.[1,49]

Vertebral Body Apophyseal Avulsion Fracture

Activities that involve repetitive flexion and extension of the spine can result in injury to the ring apophysis. Fractures of the cartilaginous ring apophysis may occur, with displacement posteriorly into the spinal canal, along with the intervertebral disk.[11,49] Avulsion fractures occur most often in sports such as gymnastics, wrestling, volleyball, and weight lifting.[11,49] Athletes present with lumbar pain on flexion of the spine. There are usually no associated neurologic symptoms. On examination, both spine flexion and extension are limited. There may be paraspinal muscle spasm. The neurologic examination is usually normal. Lateral radiographs of the lumbar spine may show an ossified fragment in the canal. CT can better identify the fractured apophysis and displaced piece of bone, which may be missed on MRI.[29] Management consists of rest, heat, NSAIDs, and possibly, massage for pain relief. If there are significant neurologic findings resulting from neural compression, the fragment may need to be surgically excised.[11,49,85]

Scheuermann Kyphosis

Another relatively frequent cause of low back pain in adolescents is Scheuermann kyphosis. Scheuermann kyphosis is a developmental condition of uncertain cause affecting the thoracic or thoracolumbar spine and was originally described by Scheuermann in 1921. It is defined by the presence of anterior wedging of at least 5° in 3 consecutive vertebrae, end-plate irregularities, disk space narrowing, and the presence of Schmorl nodes (**Fig. 4**).[12,100,101] The condition has an incidence reported to be 0.4% to 8.3% in the general population and may be more frequent in males than females.[100,101] The mean height in affected individuals tends to be greater than that in the overall population.[101] Although the cause is uncertain, several have been proposed, including mechanical injury, chronic anterior loading, osteoporosis, cartilage abnormalities, and a variety of genetic factors.[51,99,101]

The typical presentation of symptoms in patients with Scheuermann kyphosis is pain, fatigue, deformity, or poor posture. The location of the pain is usually in the area of the deformity and is worsened by activity. It is rare to have any neurologic symptoms or findings with Scheuermann kyphosis. Patients typically present during adolescence, and presentations before age 10 years are uncommon.[51,99–101] The natural history of the disorder is not well understood, but the symptoms often diminish as patients reach skeletal maturity. Adults with a deformity of less than 60° have little chance of having back pain beyond that noted in the general population.[99,101] Physical examination typically shows postural changes, such as lumbar hyperlordosis, and a forward head position caused by increased thoracic kyphosis. The kyphosis in Scheuermann kyphosis is rigid and does not typically correct with extension.[101]

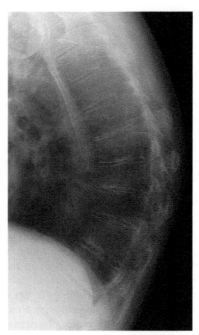

Fig. 4. Plain radiograph, lateral view of the thoracic spine showing the findings associated with Scheuermann kyphosis. Note the multilevel vertebral body wedging, end-plate irregularities, and disk height loss. (*From* Standaert CJ. Low back pain in the adolescent athlete. Phys Med Rehabil Clin N Am 2008;19(2):299; with permission.)

The treatment options for Scheuermann kyphosis depend on the extent of the symptoms and the degree of curvature. Patients with a curve of less than 50° to 60° typically respond well using flexibility and postural exercises in combination with relative rest, antiinflammatories, or bracing. For more substantial curves of 50° to 75° in a skeletally immature patient, bracing should be considered. For those with curves greater than 75°, bracing may no longer be effective and surgical treatment should be considered.[99–101]

Although the kyphosis generally occurs in the thoracic spine, a less common lumbar variant of Scheuermann kyphosis has been described, with end-plate changes, Schmorl nodes, and disk space narrowing as well as vertebral wedging, which occurs less frequently (**Fig. 5**).[12] The lumbar variant is presumed to have a more clearly defined mechanical basis than typical Scheuermann kyphosis and is seen more commonly in athletes participating in sports associated with rapid flexion/extension motions or with heavy lifting.[51,99–101] Although it is often thought of as simply a variant of thoracic Scheuermann kyphosis, some believe that this process may a be a different clinical entity.[101] Pain is typically located at the area of involvement in the thoracolumbar region and exacerbated by activity, particularly lumbar flexion. Examination of the thoracic and lumbar spine typically does not show any marked kyphotic deformity; however, there may be flattening of the lumbar lordosis. The natural history is typically nonprogressive, and treatment involves relative rest, antiinflammatory medication, lumbar stabilization, flexibility, postural training, time, and the use of an orthosis.[99–101]

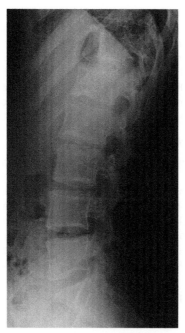

Fig. 5. Plain radiograph lateral view showing the findings associated with the lumbar variant of Scheuermann kyphosis. Again, note the end-plate irregularities, disk height loss, Schmorl nodes, and relative lack of vertebral body wedging. (*From* Standaert CJ. Low back pain in the adolescent athlete. Phys Med Rehabil Clin N Am 2008;19(2):300; with permission.)

SI Joint

The SI joint disperses the forces between the trunk and the lower extremities. This joint can be a source of pain in young athletes, as a result of excessive or reduced motion within the SI joint. Disease of the lumbar spine can alter the mechanics of the lumbar spine, resulting in stress to the SI joints.[11] Inflammation of the SI joint can also result in SI joint pain. SI joint inflammation can occur from infection, such as Reiter syndrome, as well as from seronegative spondyloarthropathies, such as Crohn disease, psoriatic arthritis, and juvenile ankylosing spondylitis. Another cause of SI joint pain is a stress fracture of the sacrum.[11] Athletes with SI joint pain present with extension pain, which is insidious in onset.[8,11]

On examination, pain is localized to the lumbar or buttock region with extension of the spine. They may have poor pelvic stability on Trendelenberg testing. There are several provocative tests that can elicit SI joint pain, including FABER test, Gaenslen, Gillet, and Fortin finger test.[52,53] Palpation elicits tenderness over the affected SI joint.[1,8,11]

Plain radiographs should be considered if symptoms have been present for more than 3 weeks; however, frequently, this imaging is normal. Bone scan may show a stress fracture of the sacrum. MRI can more precisely define the anatomic abnormality. However, the gold standard for diagnosis of SI joint pain is diagnostic intra-articular injection. If infection or a spondyloarthropathy is suspected, blood work, including erythrocyte sedimentation rate, C-reactive protein, rheumatoid factor, antinuclear antibody, and HLA-B27, should be obtained.[11]

Management of SI joint dysfunction includes ice, NSAIDs, activity modification, bracing, physical therapy, osteopathic manipulation, and injections. Ice and NSAIDs help alleviate pain and inflammation. Activities should be restricted to those that do not provoke pain. If a sacral stress fracture is present, protected weight bearing is necessary until pain resolves.[11] Bracing can help stabilize the joint. Physical therapy involves possible manipulation of the SI joint, pelvic stabilization exercises, and hip girdle and abdominal strengthening. SI joint injections, including corticosteroids, prolotherapy, and radiofrequency ablation, are effective in refractory cases.[1,3,8,11]

Other Causes of Low Back Pain

Injury is not the only cause of low back pain in young athletes.[1,11,84,94,102] Infection (diskitis or osteomyelitis), inflammation (seronegative spondyloarthropathies), and tumors (eg, osteoid osteoma, osteoblastoma, bone cysts, Ewing sarcoma, osteogenic sarcoma) can also cause back pain, as well as visceral disease, such as pyelonephritis. A high index of suspicion is necessary to avoid missing these potential reasons for low back pain. Systemic symptoms such as fever, night pain, weight loss, and malaise are red flags for more sinister causes of back pain and should prompt further investigation.[28]

REHABILITATION AND RETURN TO PLAY

Several investigators have described rehabilitation programs for adolescent athletes with low back pain caused by these various lumbar disorders. However, there is insufficient evidence advocating any specific rehabilitation protocols. Nonoperative rehabilitation programs tend to be empirically and anecdotally derived. However, more research into these various programs needs to be performed to determine the most effective means to facilitate recovery and improve function. One of the complexities of developing good evidence-based research on these rehabilitation programs is that both the disease process and the rehabilitation programs are multifactorial. Comprehensive rehabilitation generally addresses several factors affecting the injured athlete and may use additional therapeutic modalities to assist with the recovery and facilitate return to play. Therefore in the clinical setting, it is imperative to establish an early and accurate diagnosis, initiate appropriate acute treatment of injured structures, perform a full assessment of the kinetic chain and athletic technique, and identify environmental or psychosocial barriers to performance.[12] Rehabilitation should progress through a structured, sport-specific program with a focus on specific motions, postures, and activities required in the performance of the athlete's chosen sport. Specific activities, timing, and progression of training in a given athlete depend heavily on the nature of any acute injury and subsequent treatment as well as individual factors related to the athlete that affect performance.[7,12,47,103]

Return to play after injury is allowed when the athlete has been given sufficient time to recover from their acute injury and progressed through a sport-specific rehabilitation program, which also addresses spinal awareness and dynamic postural control. Return to play criteria include full, pain-free range of motion, appropriate aerobic conditioning, normal strength, and a proven ability to perform sports-related skills without pain.[12,104]

When an injured athlete is returning to sport, recommendations must take into account the diagnosis, the sport or activity, the age and skeletal maturity of the child, and the amount of cooperation of the athlete, parents, and coaches in allowing activity modifications during healing.[11,29,49] In general, relative rest is indicated to allow for healing. Activities that cause pain should be avoided until the patient is pain free. Most athletes are able to continue in their sport with modifications of the activity. Once the athlete has attained pain-free range of motion with all activities and has obtained normal strength, they can return to full sport participation.[29]

SUMMARY

Low back pain is frequently encountered in adolescent athletes. The adolescent athlete is at risk for significant structural injuries as well as nonmechanical problems. Adolescent athletes who present with low back pain are more likely to have structural injuries and therefore should be investigated fully. Any athlete with severe, persisting, or activity-limiting symptoms needs to be evaluated thoroughly. It is imperative to complete a comprehensive evaluation of back pain, and a cause such as muscle strain should be a diagnosis of exclusion. Clinicians must have knowledge of the growth and development of the adolescent spine and the subsequent injury patterns and other spinal conditions common in the adolescent athlete. The management and treatment of spinal injuries in adolescent athletes require a coordinated effort between the clinician, patients, parents/guardians, coaches, therapists, and athletic trainers. Treatment should not only help alleviate the current symptoms but also address flexibility and muscle imbalances to prevent future injuries by recognizing and addressing risk factors. Return to sport should be a gradual process once the pain has resolved and the athlete has regained full strength.

REFERENCES

1. d'Hemecourt PA, Gerbino PG II, Micheli LJ. Back injuries in the young athlete. Clin Sports Med 2000;19:663–79.
2. Gerbino PG II, Micheli LJ. Back injuries in the young athlete. Clin Sports Med 1995;14(3):571–90.
3. George SZ, Delitto A. Management of the athlete with low back pain. Clin Sports Med 2002;21:105–20.
4. Hutchison MR. Low back pain in elite rhythmic gymnasts. Med Sci Sports Exerc 1999;31:1686–8.
5. Kolt GS, Kirkby RJ. Epidemiology of injury in elite and subelite female gymnasts: a comparison of retrospective and prospective findings. Br J Sports Med 1999; 33:312–8.
6. Semon RL, Spengler D. Significance of lumbar spondylolysis in college football players. Spine 1981;6:172–4.
7. Watkins RG. Lumbar disc injury in the athlete. Clin Sports Med 2002;21:147–65.
8. Kraft DE. Low back pain in the adolescent athlete. Pediatr Clin North Am 2002; 49:643–53.
9. Micheli LJ, Wood R. Back pain in young athletes. Arch Pediatr Adolesc Med 1995;149:15–8.
10. Trainor TJ, Trainor MA. Etiology of low back pain in athletes. Curr Sports Med Rep 2004;3:41–6.
11. Zetaruk M. Lumbar spine injuries. In: Micheli LJ, Purcell LK, editors. The adolescent athlete. New York: Springer; 2007. p. 109–40.
12. Standaert CJ. Low back pain in the adolescent athlete. Phys Med Rehabil Clin N Am 2008;19(2):287–304.
13. Ferguson RL. Thoracic and lumbar spinal trauma of the immature spine. In: Herkowitz HN, Garfin SR, Eismont FJ, et al, editors. Rothman-Simeone the spine. 5th edition. Philadelphia: Saunders; 2006. p. 603–12.

14. Clark P, Letts M. Trauma to the thoracic and lumbar spine in the adolescent. Can J Surg 2001;44(5):337–45.

15. Commandre FA, Gagnerie G, Zakarian M, et al. The child, the spine and sport. J Sports Med Phys Fitness 1988;28(1):11–9.

16. Cyron BM, Hutton WC. The fatigue strength of the lumbar neural arch in spondylolysis. J Bone Joint Surg Br 1978;60-B:234–8.

17. Malina R. Growth and maturation: applications to children and adolescents in sports. In: Birrer RB, Griesemer BA, Cataletto MB, editors. Pediatric sports medicine for primary care. Philadelphia: Lippincott Williams & Wilkins; 2002. p. 39–58.

18. Burton AK, Clarke RD, McClune TD, et al. The natural history of low back pain in adolescents. Spine 1996;21(20):2323–8.

19. Harreby M, Nygaard B, Jessen T, et al. Risk factors for low back pain in a cohort of 1389 Danish school children: an epidemiologic study. Eur Spine J 1999;8(6):444–50.

20. Kovacs FM, Gestoso M, Gil del Real MT, et al. Risk factors for non-specific low back pain in schoolchildren and their parents: a population based study. Pain 2003;103:239–68.

21. Salminen JJ, Erkintalo M, Laine M, et al. Low back pain in the young. A prospective three-year follow-up study of subjects with and without low back pain. Spine 1995;20(19):2101–7.

22. Taimela S, Kujala UM, Salminen JJ, et al. The prevalence of low back pain among children and adolescents: a nationwide, cohort-based questionnaire survey in Finland. Spine 1997;22(10):1132–6.

23. Troussier B, Davoine P, de Gaudemaris R, et al. Back pain in school children: a study among 1178 pupils. Scand J Rehabil Med 1994;26:143–6.

24. Auvinen J, Tammelin T, Taimela S, et al. Associations of physical activity and inactivity with low back pain in adolescents. Scand J Med Sci Sports 2008;18:188–94.

25. Mogensen AM, Gausel AM, Wedderkopp N, et al. Is active participation in specific sport activities linked with back pain? Scand J Med Sci Sports 2007;17(6):680–6.

26. Wedderkopp N, Leboeuf-Yde C, Andersen LB, et al. Back pain in children. No association with objectively measured level of physical activity. Spine 2003;28(17):2019–24.

27. McBeth J, Jones K. Epidemiology of chronic musculoskeletal pain. Best Pract Res Clin Rheumatol 2007;21(3):403–25.

28. Hestbaek L, Leboeuf-Yde C, Kyvik KO, et al. The course of low back pain from adolescence to adulthood: eight-year follow-up of 9600 twins. Spine 2006;31(4):468–72.

29. Purcell L, Micheli L. Low back pain in young athletes. Sports Health 2009;1(3):212–22.

30. Kujala UM, Taimela S, Erkintalo M, et al. Low back pain in adolescent athletes. Med Sci Sports Exerc 1996;28(2):165–70.

31. Hickey GJ, Fricker PA, McDonald WA. Injuries to elite rowers over a 10-yr period. Med Sci Sports Exerc 1997;29(12):1567–72.

32. Hosea TM, Gatt CJ. Back pain in golf. Clin Sports Med 1996;15(1):37–53.

33. Iwamoto J, Abe H, Tsukimura Y, et al. Relationship between radiographic abnormalities of lumbar spine and incidence of low back pain in high school rugby players: a prospective study. Scand J Med Sci Sports 2005;15:163–8.

34. Sward L, Hellstrom M, Jacobsson B, et al. Disc degeneration and associated abnormalities of the spine in elite gymnasts. A magnetic resonance imaging study. Spine 1991;16(4):437–43.
35. Sward L, Hellstrom M, Jacobsson B, et al. Back pain and radiologic changes in the thoraco-lumbar spine of athletes. Spine 1990;15(2):124–9.
36. Goldstein JD, Berger PE, Windler GE, et al. Spine injuries in gymnasts and swimmers: an epidemiologic investigation. Am J Sports Med 1991;19:463–8.
37. Bennett DL, Nassar L, DeLano MC. Lumbar spine MRI in the elite-level female gymnast with low back pain. Skeletal Radiol 2006;35:503–9.
38. Iwamoto J, Abe H, Tsukimura Y, et al. Relationship between radiographic abnormalities of lumbar spine and incidence of low back pain in high school and college football players. Am J Sports Med 2004;32(3):781–6.
39. Fredrickson BE, Baker D, McHolick WJ, et al. The natural history of spondylolysis and spondylolisthesis. J Bone Joint Surg Am 1984;66:699–707.
40. Roche MA, Rowe GG. The incidence of separate neural arch and coincident bone variations: a survey of 4,200 skeletons. Anat Rec 1951;109:233–52.
41. Rossi F, Dragoni S. The prevalence of spondylolysis and spondylolisthesis in symptomatic elite athletes: radiographic findings. Radiography 2001;7: 37–42.
42. Soler T, Calderon C. The prevalence of spondylolysis in the Spanish elite athlete. Am J Sports Med 2000;28:57–62.
43. Lundin O, Hellstrom M, Nilsson I, et al. Back pain and radiologic changes in the thoraco-lumbar spine of athletes: a long-term follow-up. Scand J Med Sci Sports 2001;11:103–9.
44. Teitz CC, O'Kane JW, Lind BK. Back pain in former intercollegiate rowers; a long-term follow-up study. Am J Sports Med 2003;31(4):590–5.
45. Tsai L, Wredmark T. Spinal posture, sagittal mobility, and subjective rating of back problems in former female elite gymnasts. Spine 1993;18:872–5.
46. Anderson SJ. Assessment and management of the pediatric and adolescent patient with low back pain. Phys Med Rehabil Clin N Am 1991;2(1): 157–85.
47. Bono CM. Low-back pain in athletes. J Bone Joint Surg Am 2004;86:382–96.
48. Hosalkar H, Dormans J. Back pain in children requires extensive workup. Biomechanics 2003;10(6):51–8.
49. Simon LM, Jih W, Buller JC. Back pain and injuries. In: Birrer RB, Griesemer BA, Cataletto MB, editors. Pediatric sports medicine for primary care. Philadelphia: Lippincott Williams & Wilkins; 2002. p. 306–25.
50. Standaert CJ, Herring SA, Cole AJ, et al. The lumbar spine and sports. In: Cole AJ, Herring SA, editors. The low back pain handbook. 2nd edition. Philadelphia: Hanley & Belfus; 2003. p. 385–404.
51. Mason DE. Back pain in children. Pediatr Ann 1999;28(12):727–38.
52. Hoppenfeld S. Physical examination of the lumbar spine. In: Hoppenfeld S, editor. Physical examination of the spine and extremities. Upper Saddle River (NJ): Prentice Hall; 1976. p. 237–63.
53. Fortin JD, Falco FJ. The Fortin finger test: an indicator of sacroiliac pain. Am J Orthop 1997;26(7):477–80.
54. De Luigi AJ, Fitzpatrick KF. Physical examination in radiculopathy. Phys Med Rehabil Clin N Am 2011;22(1):7–40.
55. Dodge TL, Jaccard JJ. The effect of high school sports participation on the use of performance-enhancing substances in young adulthood. J Adolesc Health 2006;39:367–73.

56. Gregory PL, Batt ME, Kerslake RW, et al. Single photon emission computerized tomography and reverse gantry computerized tomography findings in patients with back pain investigated for spondylolysis. Clin J Sport Med 2005;15:79–86.

57. Meyerding HW. Spondylolithesis. Surg Gynecol Obstet 1932;54:371–7.

58. Wiltse LL, Newman PH, Macnab I. Classification of spondylolysis and spondylolisthesis. Clin Orthop Relat Res 1976;117:23–9.

59. Wiltse LL, Widell EH, Jackson DW. Fatigue fracture: the basic lesion in isthmic spondylolisthesis. J Bone Joint Surg Am 1975;57:17–22.

60. Muschik M, Hahnel H, Robinson PN, et al. Competitive sports and the progression of spondylolisthesis. J Pediatr Orthop 1996;16:364–9.

61. Gregory PL, Batt ME, Kerslake RW. Comparing spondylolysis in cricketers and soccer players. Br J Sports Med 2004;38:737–42.

62. McCarroll JR, Miller JM, Ritter MA. Lumbar spondylolysis and spondylolisthesis in college football players: a prospective study. Am J Sports Med 1986;14:404–6.

63. d'Hemecourt P, Zurakowski D, Kriemler S, et al. Spondylolysis: returning the athlete to sports participation with brace treatment. Orthopedics 2002;25:653–7.

64. McTimoney CA, Micheli LJ. Current evaluation and management of spondylolysis and spondylolisthesis. Curr Sports Med Rep 2003;2:41–6.

65. Masci L, Pike J, Malara F, et al. Use of the one-legged hyperextension test and magnetic resonance imaging in the diagnosis of active spondylolysis. Br J Sports Med 2006;40:940–6.

66. Steiner ME, Micheli LJ. Treatment of symptomatic spondylolysis and spondylolisthesis with the modified Boston brace. Spine 1985;10:937–43.

67. Harvey CJ, Richenberg JL, Saifuddin A, et al. Pictorial review: the radiological investigation of lumbar spondylolysis. Clin Radiol 1998;53:723–8.

68. Jackson DW, Wiltse LL, Dingeman RD, et al. Stress reactions involving the pars interarticularis in young athletes. Am J Sports Med 1981;9:304–12.

69. Elliott S, Hutson MA, Wastie ML. Bone scintigraphy in the assessment of spondylolysis in patients attending a sports injury clinic. Clin Radiol 1988;39:269–72.

70. Anderson K, Sarwark JF, Conway JJ, et al. Quantitative assessment with SPECT imaging of stress injuries of the pars interarticularis and response to bracing. J Pediatr Orthop 2000;20:28–33.

71. Bellah RD, Summerville DA, Treves ST, et al. Low back pain in adolescent athletes: detection of stress injury to the pars interarticularis with SPECT. Radiology 1991;180:509–12.

72. Bodner RJ, Heyman S, Drummond DS, et al. The use of single photon emission computed tomography (SPECT) in the diagnosis of low back pain in young patients. Spine 1988;3:1155–60.

73. Congeni J, McCulloch J, Swanson K. Lumbar spondylolysis: a study of natural progression in athletes. Am J Sports Med 1997;25:248–53.

74. Campbell RS, Grainger AJ, Hide IG, et al. Juvenile spondylolysis: a comparative analysis of CT, SPECT, and MRI. Skeletal Radiol 2005;34:63–73.

75. Stretch RA, Botha T, Chandler S, et al. Back injuries in young fast bowlers–a radiologic investigation of the healing of spondylolysis and pedicle sclerosis. S Afr Med J 2003;93:611–6.

76. Lowe J, Schachner E, Hirschberg E, et al. Significance of bone scintigraphy in symptomatic spondylolysis. Spine 1984;9:653–5.

77. Collier BD, Johnson RP, Carrera GF, et al. Painful spondylolysis or spondylolisthesis studied by radiography and single photon emission computed tomography. Radiology 1985;154:207–11.

78. Itoh K, Hashimoto T, Shigenobu K, et al. Bone SPECT of symptomatic lumbar spondylolysis. Nucl Med Commun 1996;17:389–96.
79. Lusins JO, Elting JJ, Cicoria AD, et al. SPECT evaluation of lumbar spondylolysis and spondylolisthesis. Spine 1994;19:608–12.
80. Raby N, Mathews S. Symptomatic spondylolysis: correlation of CT and SPECT with clinical outcome. Clin Radiol 1993;48:97–9.
81. Gregory PL, Batt ME, Kerslake RW, et al. The value of combining single photon emission computerised tomography and computerised tomography in the investigation of spondylolysis. Eur Spine J 2004;13:503–9.
82. Fujii K, Katoh S, Sairyo K, et al. Union of defects in the pars interarticularis of the lumbar spine in children and adolescents: the radiologic outcome after conservative treatment. J Bone Joint Surg Br 2004;86:225–31.
83. Miller SF, Congeni J, Swanson K. Long-term functional and anatomical follow-up of early detected spondylolysis in young athletes. Am J Sports Med 2004;32:928–33.
84. King HA. Back pain in children. Orthop Clin North Am 1999;30:467–74.
85. Brown TD, Micheli LJ. Spinal injuries in children's sports. In: Maffuli N, Chan KM, Macdonald R, et al, editors. Sports medicine for specific ages and abilities. London: Churchill Livingstone; 2001. p. 31–44.
86. Standaert CJ, Herring SA. Spondylolysis: a critical review. Br J Sports Med 2000;34:415–22.
87. Axelsson P, Johnsson R, Stromqvist B. Effect of lumbar orthosis on intervertebral mobility. Spine 1992;17:678–81.
88. Calmels P, Fayolle-Minon I. An update on orthotic devices for the lumbar spine based on a review of the literature. Rev Rhum Engl Ed 1996;63:285–91.
89. Ruiz-Cotorro A, Balius-Matas R, Estruch-Massana AE, et al. Spondylolysis in young tennis players. Br J Sports Med 2006;40:441–6.
90. Blanda J, Bethem D, Moats W, et al. Defects of pars interarticularis in athletes: a protocol for nonoperative treatment. J Spinal Disord 1993;6:406–11.
91. Iwamoto J, Takeda T, Wakano K. Returning athletes with severe low back pain and spondylolysis to original sporting activities with conservative treatment. Scand J Med Sci Sports 2004;14:346–51.
92. Sys J, Michielsen J, Bracke P, et al. Nonoperative treatment of active spondylolysis in elite athletes with normal X-ray findings: literature review and results of conservative treatment. Eur Spine J 2001;10:498–504.
93. Rassi GE, Takemitsu M, Woratanarat P, et al. Lumbar spondylolysis in pediatric and adolescent soccer players. Am J Sports Med 2005;33:1688–93.
94. Sponseller PD. Evaluating the child with back pain. Am Fam Physician 1996;54: 1933–41.
95. Kumar R, Kumar V, Das NK, et al. Adolescent lumbar disc disease: findings and outcome. Childs Nerv Syst 2007;23(11):1295–9.
96. Kjaer P, Leboeuf-Yde C, Sorensen JS, et al. An epidemiologic study of MRI and low back pain in 13-year-old children. Spine 2005;30(7):798–806.
97. Kjaer P, Leboeuf-Yde C, Korsholm L, et al. Magnetic resonance imaging and low back pain in adults: a diagnostic imaging study of 40-year-old men and women. Spine 2005;30(10):1173–80.
98. Ala-Kokko L. Genetic risk factors for lumbar disc disease. Ann Med 2002;34:42–7.
99. Waicus KM, Smith BW. Back injuries in the pediatric athlete. Curr Sports Med Rep 2002;1:52–8.
100. Karol LA. Back pain in children and adolescents. In: Herkowitz HN, Garfin SR, Eismont FJ, et al, editors. Rothman-Simeone the spine. 5th edition. Philadelphia: Saunders; 2006. p. 493–506.

101. Shah SW, Takemitsu M, Westerlund LE, et al. Pediatric kyphosis: Scheuermann's disease and congenital deformity. In: Herkowitz HN, Garfin SR, Eismont FJ, et al, editors. Rothman-Simeone the spine. 5th edition. Philadelphia: Saunders; 2006. p. 565–85.
102. Hollingworth P. Back pain in children. Br J Rheumatol 1996;35:1022–8.
103. Standaert CJ, Herring SA, Pratt TW. Rehabilitation of the athlete with low back pain. Curr Sports Med Rep 2004;3(1):35–40.
104. Herring SA, Kibler WB. A framework for rehabilitation. In: Kibler WB, Herring SA, Press JM, et al, editors. Functional rehabilitation of sports and musculoskeletal injuries. Gaithersburg (MD): Aspen; 1998. p. 1–8.

Evaluation and Treatment of Shoulder Pain

Deborah L. Greenberg, MD

KEYWORDS

- Rotator cuff disease • Subacromial impingement syndrome • Adhesive capsulitis
- Painful arc

KEY POINTS

- Shoulder pain can have a significant impact on function.
- A thorough examination of the shoulder is a necessity.
- Most shoulder pain is due to the structure supporting the shoulder joint.
- Pain relief and exercises are the mainstays of therapy.

INTRODUCTION

Shoulder pain is a common presenting concern in outpatient medical practice. Shoulder problems can significantly affect a patient's ability to work and other activities of daily life such as driving, dressing, brushing hair, and even eating. "The shoulder" consists of a complex array of bones, muscles, tendons, and nerves, making the cause of pain seem difficult to decipher. Shoulder pain can be caused by structures within the shoulder or can arise from problems external to the shoulder. Fortunately, most shoulder pain falls into one of several patterns.

The rotator cuff provides stabilization to the glenohumeral joint, and contributes to mobility and strength of the shoulder. Disease of the rotator cuff is the most common cause of shoulder pain seen in clinical practice. The prevalence of rotator cuff disease increases with age, obesity, diabetes, and chronic diseases that affect the strength of the shoulder such as stroke.[1] An experienced practitioner can often recognize the cause of a patient's shoulder pain with a few questions and a focused examination. Treatment of shoulder pain can be successfully managed by a primary care provider in most cases. Referral to a physical therapist can be important to help improve the patient's mechanics and strength. Early use of imaging studies and specialist referrals are overutilized by primary care providers, and should be limited to specific indications.[2] Consultation with an orthopedic surgeon for fractures and tendon tears will be necessary in some cases.

This article originally appeared in Medical Clinics of North America, Volume 98, Issue 3, May 2014.

The author declares no financial disclosures or conflict of interest.

Division of General Internal Medicine, University of Washington School of Medicine, 4245 Roosevelt Way Northeast, Seattle, WA 98105, USA

E-mail address: debbiegr@u.washington.edu

When evaluating patients with shoulder pain, it is important to understand the anatomy of the region. The major anatomic structures of interest include (**Fig. 1**)[3]:

- Four main bony structures: proximal humerus, clavicle, scapula, and ribs. The acromion, the superior, anterior extension of the scapula, forms the roof of the shoulder.
- Three main joints: glenohumeral, acromioclavicular (AC), sternoclavicular.
- Four rotator cuff muscles/tendons (SITS): supraspinatus (abduction), infraspinatus (external rotation), teres minor (external rotation, adduction), and subscapularis

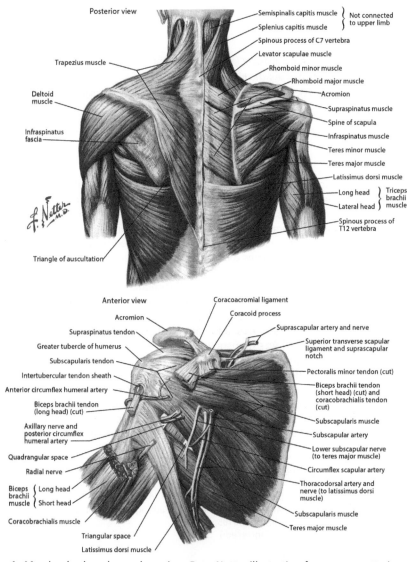

Fig. 1. Muscles: back and scapula region. *From* Netter illustration from www.netterimages. com. © Elsevier Inc. All rights reserved.

(adduction, internal rotation). The supraspinatus and infraspinatus tendons pass through the subacromial space to insert on the greater tubercle of the humerus.
- Bursa: the subacromial bursa provides a cushion as the rotator cuff tendons move below the acromion.
- Surrounding musculature: biceps, deltoid, pectoralis, latissimus dorsi, rhomboids.
- Neurovascular: suprascapular nerve and vessels.

Important Terms

Rotator cuff disease
Rotator cuff disease (RCD) is a term encompassing tendinopathy, partial-thickness tear, or complete tear of one or more of the rotator cuff tendons. RCD also includes subacromial bursitis. In general, the term RCD is used synonymously with subacromial impingement syndrome (SIS).

Subacromial impingement syndrome
SIS is an umbrella term that encompasses rotator cuff tendinopathy and partial tears, as well as subacromial bursitis. The term is meant to convey the proposed etiology of these conditions. Inflammation and pain are caused by compression or impingement of the supraspinatus tendon (most common), infraspinatus tendon, subacromial bursa, biceps tendon, or other structures as they pass through the space between the lateral aspect of the acromion and the humeral head. Functional impingement can occur when there are problems with the mobility and stability of the rotator cuff muscles or the position and movement of the scapula.[4] Risk factors for impingement include repetitive activity above the head, increasing age, and conditions such as stroke and Parkinson disease. These risk factors are related to poor mechanics or decreased strength and stability of the rotator cuff and other supporting muscles. The natural history of SIS is often chronic or with recurrent pain and dysfunction.

Adhesive capsulitis (frozen shoulder)
Chronic pain and reduced active and passive mobility in the glenohumeral joint is associated with a variety of shoulder problems or occur as a primary problem of unknown cause. Adhesive capsulitis typically is seen in patients in their 40s to 60s, but is more common in diabetics in whom it is likely to present at a younger age. Adhesive capsulitis may resolve spontaneously over a period of years, but causes significant pain and functional limitations in the meantime.[5]

SYMPTOMS

Symptoms should be evaluated in the context of the patient as a whole. Age, underlying medical conditions, body habitus and overall strength, and smoking status are all important considerations. A systematic approach to history taking is crucial to avoid missing historical information. The most important factors include:

- Prior condition of shoulder
- Location of current pain:
    Localized or diffuse
    Anterior, lateral, or posterior
- Radiation patterns (clue: radiation past the elbow suggests a neurologic component)
- Timing of pain onset: sudden onset or developed gradually? (clue: came on all at once suggests a tear)[6]
- Associated factors: repetitive stress or recent or prior injury
- Duration: acute (<6 weeks), subacute (6–12 weeks), chronic (>3 months)

- Quality of pain: sharp, dull
- Associated symptoms: weakness, stiffness, crepitus, swelling (clue: fear of recurrence suggests shoulder instability)
- Alleviating and exacerbating factors: pain at night, pain worse with overhead activities (pain at night is a classic symptom for tear but likelihood ratios [LRs] are not significant in systematic review)[7]
- Systemic factors: fever, numbness, weight loss, fatigue, dyspnea, chest pain

Common Symptom Patterns

Subacromial impingement: lateral pain, subacute, worse with movement overhead
Rotator cuff tear: sudden onset, weakness, pain at night
Adhesive capsulitis: distant injury or chronic pain, progressive inability to reach over head, decreased mobility

DIAGNOSTIC TESTS AND IMAGING STUDIES
Physical Examination

The physical examination is used to diagnose the cause of the patient's pain but also to assess functional abilities. Elderly patients in particular may not be able to perform activities of daily living and may require assistance at home. A systematic approach to the examination is essential. The initial physical examination for shoulder pain should focus primarily on the musculoskeletal complex. Additional components of the examination can be performed if there is concern about an extrinsic cause of the patient's shoulder pain.

Observing Both Shoulders for Comparison

Further specific testing can be done based on the results of the initial examination. There are many tests for shoulder mobility and strength. None of the maneuvers has been found to be the ideal test for diagnosis of a particular syndrome or lesion.[8] Abduction maneuvers are recommended, given their better performance in systematic reviews in the diagnosis of specific pathologic conditions of the shoulder.

1. General appearance (**Fig. 2**): Symmetry, bulk, deformities, atrophy above or below the scapular spine. Atrophy in the space below the scapular spine suggests RCD (positive LR 2.0, negative LR 0.61)[7] or injury to the suprascapular nerve.[6]
2. Palpation: Sternoclavicular joint, clavicle, acromioclavicular joint, lateral acromion, biceps tendon in the groove between the greater and lesser tubercle of the humerus. Remember: some patients can be tender at many points but you are trying to recreate the pain that they have been experiencing at home. The anterior joint line can be palpated.
3. General range of motion (ROM)/pain provocation testing: ROM testing identifies limitations in ROM and localizes pain. Start with these basic ROM tests with the patient standing. Test active ROM first and add passive ROM if the patient has pain or limited motion. All maneuvers start from the anatomic position with arms at the side and palms facing forward.

Abduction
Ask the patient to raise the arm from the side (0°) to overhead (**Fig. 3**). Normal ROM is 180°. If the patient has limitation in active ROM, assist with passive ROM. Stand behind the patient and place a hand on the unaffected shoulder. With the other hand support the patient's affected arm just above the elbow. The patient's arm

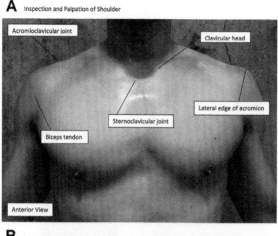

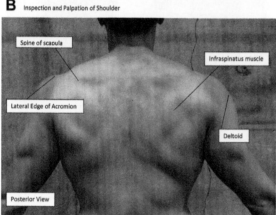

Fig. 2. General appearance of the shoulder. (*A*) Anterior; (*B*) Posterior.

should remain within the horizontal plane. Raise the arm until limited by pain. If pain occurs with active or passive ROM, specify the location (0°–180°).

Pain in the lateral shoulder between 60° and 120° abduction is known as the painful arc, and suggests disease in the rotator cuff or subacromial bursa,[9–11] also known as subacromial impingement. The painful arc is one of the most helpful physical examination findings when considering RCD (positive LR 3.7, negative LR 0.50).[7]

Pain between 120° and 180° suggests a problem with the AC joint.

External rotation
Stand in front of the patient. Ask the patient to hold the arms in front of the body with elbows bent to 90°, palms facing in; ask the patient to hold the elbows against the sides and move the hands outward, parallel to the floor. Normal external rotation is at least 55° and up to 80°. For passive ROM grasp the affected arm proximal to the wrist and externally rotate. Pain or decreased ROM suggests a problem with the teres minor or infraspinatus muscle.

Internal rotation
Stand in front of the patient. Ask the patient to hold the arms in front of the body with elbows bent to 90°, palms facing in; ask the patient to hold the elbows against the

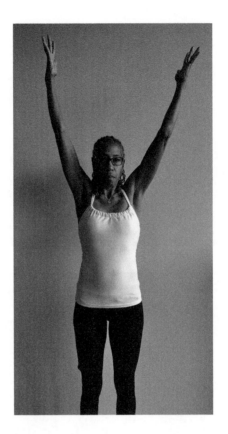

Fig. 3. Abduction.

sides and move the hands inward, parallel to the floor. Normal internal rotation is at least 45°. For passive ROM, grasp the affected arm proximal to the wrist and internally rotate. Pain or decreased ROM suggests a problem with the subscapularis muscle.

Cross-body adduction
Cross-body adduction is also known as the scarf test (**Fig. 4**). The patient reaches the affected arm across the body to the opposite shoulder. Pain in the front of the shoulder suggests AC joint abnormality.

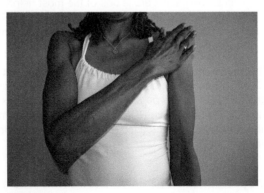

Fig. 4. Cross-body adduction.

- If the basic examination and ROM testing are normal, STOP and consider problems external to the shoulder itself. Pursue more generalized examination: neurovascular examination of the upper extremity, cardiac, pulmonary, abdominal, and neurologic examinations.
- If you are concerned about adhesive capsulitis or glenohumeral arthritis, poorly localized pain, limited range of all active and passive ROM, STOP.
- If you are concerned about AC joint disease, pain over AC joint, pain on abduction, STOP.
- If you are concerned about RCD, further testing for impingement (**Fig. 5**) and strength testing (**Fig. 6**) is required.
- If you are concerned about instability, biceps tendinopathy, or posterior pain, further tests as shown in **Fig. 7** should be considered.

Anteroposterior and Axillary Plain Radiographs of the Shoulder

Radiographs are useful in the setting of trauma, in particular:

- Fall on outstretched arm: fracture of the proximal humerus
- Fall on lateral shoulder: AC joint separation, clavicular or humeral fracture

Radiographs are also useful in evaluating:

- Presence and extent of glenohumeral arthritis, or to differentiate glenohumeral arthritis from adhesive capsulitis in a patient with limited passive ROM
- Presence and extent of AC arthritis
- Shoulder pain in patients with rheumatoid arthritis

Ultrasonography of the Shoulder

Ultrasonography of the shoulder can be used to assess:

- Shoulder dislocation.
- Biceps disorder. Compared with arthroscopy, ultrasonography performs well in the diagnosis of dislocation or subluxation of the long head of the biceps (sensitivity 96%, specificity 100%). Ultrasonography is also reliable for detecting complete tears of the biceps tendon, but may not be adequate for the detection of partial tears (sensitivity 49%, specificity 97%).[12]
- Rotator cuff tears. This modality is operator dependent, but in the hands of a good technician can be as good as magnetic resonance imaging (MRI) for detecting full-thickness tears (sensitivity 92%, specificity 94%) and partial-thickness tears (sensitivity 67%, specificity 94%).[13,14] Summary data for detecting any tear is sensitivity 91% and specificity 85%.[15] Ultrasonography is less expensive than MRI, and is better tolerated and preferred by patients.[16]

Magnetic Resonance Imaging

MRI of the shoulder is indicated for:

- Possible labral tear (trauma, repetitive overhead throwing or playing tennis, catching, or locking)
- Possible rotator cuff tear when quality ultrasonography not available (weakness)

As with ultrasonography, performance characteristics are better for full-thickness tears (sensitivity 84%–96%, specificity 93%–98%) than for partial-thickness tears (sensitivity 35%–44%, specificity 85%–97%).[13] For diagnosing any rotator cuff tear, sensitivity is 98% and sensitivity 79%.[15] MRI allows a better look at the shoulder as a whole, and can be useful if a surgical procedure is planned.

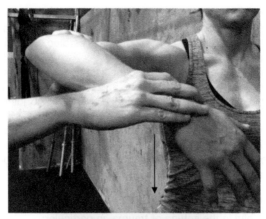

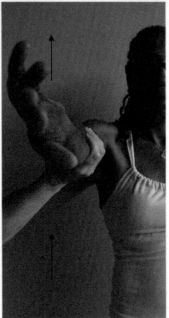

Fig. 5. Additional range of motion/pain provocation tests for suspected impingement. (*A*) Hawkins-Kennedy Impingement Sign:[10] Patient holds arm at 90° flexion with elbow at 90° flexion. Place downward pressure on the forearm and passively internally rotate the arm. (positive LR 1.5, negative LR 0.51).[7] (*B*) Neer's Impingement Sign: The patient internally rotates their hand (thumb toward the ground). Place your hand on the back of the patient's shoulder to stabilize the scapula. Forward flex the patient's straight arm by grasping just below the elbow and lifting. (positive LR 1.3).[7] Full ROM 180°.

Magnetic resonance arthrography (MRA) is better than either ultrasonography or MRI in detecting rotator cuff tears,[17] especially partial-thickness tears. MRA is generally ordered by sports medicine or orthopedic consultants on referral for possible surgical repair in a patient who has not improved with conservative therapy or who has significant strength lost on examination, but in whom a tear was not detected on initial imaging.

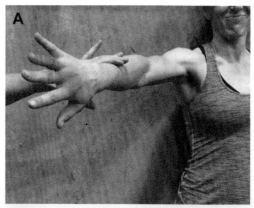

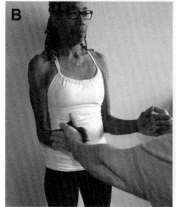 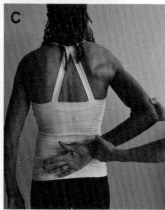

Fig. 6. Strength testing of rotator cuff. (*A*) *Empty Can Test*: Patient starts with a straight arm at 90° abduction. The arm is then brought forward 30° toward center on the horizontal plane and the thumb rotated toward the floor. Apply gentle pressure downward above the elbow while patient attempts to resist this pressure. Pain suggests impingement of the supraspinatus. Weakness suggests a partial- or full-thickness tear.[6] (*B*) *Resisted isometric external rotation*: Patient flexes their arm to 90° and attempts to externally rotate arm against resistance. (positive LR for RCD 2.6, negative LR 0.49).[7] (*C*) *Internal Rotation lag test**: similar to lift-off test. One of the best tests when considering complete tear of subscapularis. Patient places hand on back with elbow at 90°. The examiner lifts the hand off the back. Failure to hold this position is a positive test. (positive LR for full thickness tear 5.6, negative LR 0.04).[7]

Bottom Line

Check radiograph if: trauma or possible arthritis
Check sonogram or MRI if: concern for labral or rotator cuff tear

DIFFERENTIAL DIAGNOSIS

The differential diagnosis is broad and can be aided by the primary location of the pain.

Lateral Shoulder Pain

SIS, rotator cuff tendonitis, subacromial bursitis, full-thickness or partial-thickness tears of the rotator cuff tendons, adhesive capsulitis, multidirectional instability, cervical radiculopathy, proximal humeral fracture, glenohumeral osteoarthritis (**Table 1**).

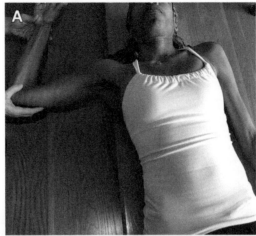

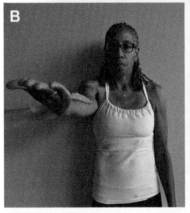
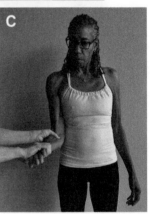

Fig. 7. Further testing if suspecting something other than subacromial impingement syndrome. (*A*) Apprehension Test- patient lies on the table. With their arm positioned off the side of table it is abducted 90° and externally rotated 90° (positive LR 17.2).11 A positive test is patient apprehension in this position. (*B*) Speed's Test: The patient flexes their arm to 90° with palm facing upward. Press downward as the patient resists arm movement. A positive test is pain in area of bicipital groove. (*C*) Yergason's Test: The patient flexes their elbow to 90°. Provide resistance to supination. A positive test is pain in area of bicipital groove.

Anterior Shoulder Pain

RCD, glenohumeral osteoarthritis, AC arthritis, AC separation, biceps tendonitis, adhesive capsulitis, anterior instability, biceps tendon rupture (sudden-onset pain, weakness and swelling), proximal humeral fracture, labral tear (**Table 2**).

Posterior Shoulder Pain

Posterior instability/dislocation, suprascapular nerve entrapment, RCD, labral tear, glenohumeral osteoarthritis, cervical radiculopathy, proximal humeral fracture.

Nonspecific Shoulder Pain

- Polymyalgia rheumatica: older patient, bilateral shoulder pain, full ROM, no weakness, may have hip pain, claudication, fatigue

Table 1
Common causes of lateral shoulder pain

	SIS/RCD	Complete Rotator Cuff Tear	Adhesive Capsulitis
Associated factors	Repetitive movement Stroke Parkinson disease	Long history of shoulder problems Trauma	Diabetes Age
Onset	Subacute to chronic	Acute or chronic with sudden worsening	Subacute to chronic
Other findings	Tenderness below lateral edge of acromion	Pain at night[a] Weakness Catching sensation	Stiffness Significant functional limitations
Range of motion	Full passive ROM	Limited active ROM due to weakness Full passive ROM	Decreased active and passive ROM
Pain with range of motion	[a]Painful arc ± External rotation ± Internal rotation	Often in setting of impingement, thus similar findings possible	Pain with ROM on multiple maneuvers
Weakness	No	Yes Drop-arm test Other tests (see **Fig. 6**)	No
Atrophy	No	Maybe	Maybe

Acute: ≤6 weeks; subacute: 6–12 weeks; chronic: ≥3 months.
Abbreviations: RCD, rotator cuff disease; ROM, range of motion; SIS, subacromial impingement syndrome.
[a] Classic symptom but likelihood ratios not significant in systematic review.[7]

- Cervical radiculopathy: pain below the elbow, numbness or weakness, decreased reflexes
- Glenohumeral osteoarthritis
- Rheumatoid arthritis: stiffness and other joint involvement
- Consider pulmonary, gastrointestinal, and cardiac causes of diaphragm irritation or referred pain

TREATMENT

The goal of treatment is to reduce pain and improve ROM, thus restoring function to the shoulder.

General Measures

- Analgesics: Nonsteroidal anti-inflammatory drugs (NSAIDs) are commonly recommended for the treatment of shoulder pain because of their anti-inflammatory effects. Experience suggests that any commonly used oral analgesics can be used for the treatment of shoulder pain thought to be due to RCD, SIS, AC joint disease, or adhesive capsulitis. There have been no studies comparing oral over-the-counter or prescription acetaminophen with NSAIDs. Thus either can be used, depending on coexistent disease and provider and patient preference.
- Should patients put ice or heat on their shoulder? Ice has traditionally been recommended for painful muscles and joints.[18] There is little evidence to show

Table 2
Differential of anterior shoulder pain

	Biceps Tendonitis	AC Separation	AC Arthritis	Proximal Humeral Fracture	Adhesive Capsulitis	Labral Tear	OA
Associated factors	Age Assoc with SIS	Fall onto lateral shoulder	Repetitive lifting	Age Fall on shoulder or outstretched arm	Chronic progressive pain/stiffness	Repetitive overhead throwing Trauma	Age Prior trauma
Onset	Subacute to chronic	Acute	Chronic	Acute	Subacute to chronic	Acute	Chronic
Specific findings	Tenderness in bicipital groove with internal and external rotation	Unilateral deformity and tenderness of AC joint	Tenderness over AC joint	Bruising	Decreased passive/active ROM	Deep shoulder pain Joint-line tenderness	Stiffness Crepitus Joint-line tenderness
ROM	Normal	Normal except adduction	Normal except adduction	Reluctant to attempt	Decreased passive/active ROM	Normal	Decreased passive/active ROM
Maneuver	Speed Yergason	Cross-arm adduction	Cross-arm adduction	None	Forward flexion reduced	None	None
Initial evaluation	None	Radiograph	Radiograph	Radiograph	None	MRI	Radiograph

Abbreviations: AC, acromioclavicular joint; MRI, magnetic resonance imaging; OA, osteoarthritis; ROM, range of motion; SIS, subacromial impingement syndrome.

whether ice is effective or even counterproductive in the treatment of soft-tissue inflammation. Ice does produce analgesia. Recommend ice for 20 to 30 minutes as often as every 2 hours if it provides relief to the patient. Ice should not be used before vigorous exercise. If ice is not helpful, the patient can try heat.

- Activity and work modification: Patients should limit activities that exacerbate their discomfort, especially overhead movements.

Menu of Additional Therapeutic Options

- Physical therapy: Therapists often use a combination of modalities, which can include manual mobilization, ice, heat, ultrasonography, massage, supervised progressive resistance exercises, electric stimulation, acupuncture, and stretching.
- Exercise therapy: Exercise therapy is generally initiated by a physical therapist. The patient is given instruction on strengthening exercises with movements against gravity and then progressive resistance exercises. The patient then follows a self-management plan at home.
- Manual therapy: Joint and soft-tissue mobilization and manipulation. Manual therapy is thought to break down the adhesions that form between different layers of soft tissue and allow unimpeded movement of the muscle. It can be used alone or in combination with exercises.
- Acupuncture: Needles are placed into specific acupuncture points. Sessions typically last 30 to 60 minutes and are performed 1 to 2 times a week for 4 to 8 weeks. Acupuncture can reduce pain,[19,20] allowing the patient to participate in exercise therapy.
- Subacromial corticosteroid injection: The injection can be guided by ultrasound or by clinical landmarks. There is no difference in safety or efficacy with either approach.[21] The routine use of ultrasound-guided glucocorticoid injection is discouraged, given the excess cost. Patients should not engage in heavy lifting for 2 weeks following an injection.
- Platelet-rich plasma injection: Injection of autologous platelet-rich plasma into the subacromial space. There is no evidence that platelet-rich plasma injections in addition to exercise improve pain or function of the shoulder to a greater extent than exercise alone.[22]
- Immobilization should be avoided unless directed by a surgeon for fracture.
- Botulinum toxin: Intramuscular injection of botulinum toxin A, which may be useful in reducing shoulder pain after stroke and in osteoarthritis of the shoulder.[23]
- Surgical intervention.

Condition-Specific Treatment

SIS/RCD, subacromial bursitis

Bottom Line
1. General measures: ice/heat, oral analgesic, avoid exacerbating activities.
2. Patient should have exercise therapy as part of a home self-management plan or as part of a physical therapist treatment plan.
3. The addition of manual therapy, acupuncture, or a subacromial steroid injection can have added benefit. Consider based on availability, cost, and patient preference.
4. If symptoms fail to improve after 3 months of conservative therapy, referral for surgical intervention can be considered.

The cause of this syndrome is dysfunctional mechanics, primarily of the scapula or rotator cuff muscles, leading to inflammation and pain as tendons and other structure are compressed between the acromion and humeral head. Treatment is designed to reduce pain, allowing sufficient strengthening exercises to correct the mechanical deficiencies.

Exercise therapy is universally recommended for the treatment of SIS and RCD. Exercise can significantly reduce pain and improve function.[24,25] Recommended exercises run the gamut from nonspecific shoulder strengthening to exercises designed to correct the mechanical issues leading to impingement. In one study of patients awaiting surgery for impingement, exercise focusing on eccentric strengthening of the rotator cuff muscles and eccentric/concentric strengthening of the shoulder stabilizers substantially reduced the need to for surgery in comparison with nonspecific shoulder exercises (odds ratio 7.7, 95% confidence interval 3.1–19.4; $P<.001$).[26]

Exercise therapy can be supervised as part of regular visits to a physical therapist, or done independently by the patient at home as part of a self-management plan. Patients willing to participate in self-training typically meet with the therapist initially and then attend 1 to 3 follow-up visits to adjust the exercise plan. Both supervised and independent exercise programs improve symptoms in patients with shoulder pain.[25] Self-management involves fewer visits with the therapist and thus, lower cost. Patients who are willing to adhere to a home program likely have better improvement in pain and function than patients who participate in a more traditional physical therapy program.[27]

Exercise therapy can be combined with manual therapy or acupuncture, or started after a subacromial steroid injection. Manual therapy in addition to exercise may be more effective than exercise alone in reducing pain.[28] Subacromial steroid injection or acupuncture plus home exercise therapy are equally effective at reducing pain and improving function in patients with SIS both short term and after 1 year.[20] Initiation of exercise should be delayed for 2 weeks after a steroid injection.

Surgical decompression, either arthroscopically or as an open procedure, is designed to reduce compression in the subacromial space. Studies have not shown a benefit of surgery over conservative therapy for the reduction of pain or improvement of function in patients with impingement syndrome.[29,30] Given the risks of surgery, this modality should be considered only after conservative therapy has failed.

Rotator cuff tear

Rotator cuff tears can be asymptomatic or can cause significant pain and disability. Patients with a rotator cuff tear who are surgical candidates should be referred to an orthopedic surgeon to discuss the risks and expected benefits of surgical repair. Some patients will recover sufficient pain relief and function without surgery, but the outcome in an individual patient is difficult to predict.[31] Because delayed surgery can cause complications in some patients owing to atrophy and scarring of tissue, patients should be fully informed of their options.

Adhesive capsulitis

Reduction of pain followed by improved ROM is the goal of therapy. Pain reduction can be achieved with a subacromial corticosteroid injection or oral analgesics. Randomized trials have shown that steroid injections and oral NSAIDs, when accompanied by therapeutic exercise, are equally effective in improving pain and function over a period of 6 months.[32] The choice of therapy should be based on patient preference, comorbidities, and availability of treatment options. It is unclear whether manual therapy in addition to other treatments improves outcomes.[28] If the patient is in significant pain, declines injection, and has contraindications to other oral analgesics, oral steroids can reduce pain and improve ROM in the short term, but are unlikely to improve long-term function.[33] Patients should be educated on the time course of recovery. Full recovery can often take as long as 6 to 18 months. Adhesive capsulitis may be self-limited in some patients over a period of months to years.[5] Patients who fail to respond to 3 months of therapy or are unable to participate in therapy because of significant pain can be referred for consideration of imaging-guided capsular distention, manipulation under anesthesia, or other surgical options.

Osteoarthritis of the glenohumeral joint

Initial conservative therapy can include pain relief with analgesics and exercise therapy, although there is limited evidence that these modalities improve function or outcomes. Limited evidence suggests that injectable viscosupplementation can be helpful for some patients.[34] Patients who fail conservative therapy can undergo total arthroplasty of the shoulder joint with hopes of reducing pain and improving function. There are no randomized trials comparing surgical treatment with continued conservative measures in these patients.[35]

Nonspecific shoulder pain/dysfunction

Massage therapy helps improve pain and ROM in short-term studies, especially in patients with posterior shoulder pain and limited internal ROM.[36] There is little evidence that it helps improve function of the shoulder over the long term.[28]

MANAGEMENT
Education

In addition to the specific treatment of shoulder pain, patients should be educated on the cause of their problem and the role of each of the modalities used in treatment. Failure to engage in self-management, particularly rehabilitation exercises, can significantly delay or prevent full return to function.

Prevention

Many shoulder problems are due to repetitive motion with the arms or the lack of strength and mobility. Patients with work-related symptoms should undergo an ergonomic review at work to reduce the risk of persistent problems.[37] All patients should be encouraged to incorporate upper extremity ROM and strengthening to their overall fitness routine.

CASES
Case 1

A 58-year-old man with a history of obesity and diabetes reports pain in his right shoulder over the last several months. He does not remember a specific injury, but is now having difficulty performing his job as a house painter and putting on and taking off his shirt. He has difficulty laying on his right side to sleep. When asked to locate the pain he places his hand over the lateral aspect of his right shoulder. On physical examination he has tenderness below the lateral edge of the acromion. His active ROM is limited to 100° abduction because of the pain, but he has full passive ROM. He has pain with external rotation but no evidence of weakness in his right arm. Hawkins and Neer tests are positive. He has tried ice, a 2-week trial of ibuprofen, and then a 2-week trial of acetaminophen without significant improvement.

Discussion

This patient has a history and examination consistent with SIS. Review his dosing of analgesics to ensure that he tried adequate doses. Further NSAIDs may be contraindicated if he has renal dysfunction. He should be prescribed ice, heat, and then specific exercises with manual therapy, acupuncture, or a subacromial bursa injection.

Case 2

A 63-year-old woman has had pain in her left shoulder for the last 6 months. Pain began while trimming some plum trees in her yard. Initially she had difficulty putting dishes into an overhead cabinet. She has been avoiding all overhead activities for the last 3 months. She finds that her shoulder is stiff and she has difficulty brushing her hair. She is not able to localize her pain to one spot. On examination she has limited active and passive ROM with forward flexion, abduction, internal rotation, and external rotation of her left arm. She does not have weakness.

Discussion

This patient most likely has adhesive capsulitis. If you were concerned about gleno-humeral arthritis, a radiograph would be reasonable to exclude this possibility. Oral analgesics and referral to a physical therapist for exercises is the appropriate initial step.

Case 3

A 74-year-old woman lost her balance while boating. She fell and hit her right shoulder against the seat in the boat. She had immediate pain in her right shoulder, and has been holding her arm against her side in the 3 hours since the accident, as any movement is uncomfortable. Her arm is bruised and she is reluctant to move it. Her pulses and neurologic testing in that arm are intact.

Discussion

No further examination is needed at this point. A radiograph to assess for fracture showed a proximal nondisplaced humeral fracture. After discussion with an orthopedist, she was placed in an arm sling and followed up in the clinic.

FUTURE CONSIDERATIONS AND SUMMARY

Shoulder pain is a common symptom in the adult population. The most common cause of shoulder pain is SIS, reflecting a problem with the rotator cuff or subacromial bursa. Determining the cause of a patient's pain is usually a clinical diagnosis based on careful history taking and physical examination. Limited use of imaging studies will be needed in the setting of trauma, possible glenohumeral arthritis, or when a complete tendon tear is suspected. Therapy is based on pain control and therapeutic exercises in almost all cases. Despite the prevalence of shoulder pain, there is no consensus on the best way to achieve pain control or on the type of exercise most likely to achieve speedy recovery.

REFERENCES

1. Rechardt M, Shiri R, Karppinen J, et al. Lifestyle and metabolic factors in relation to shoulder pain and rotator cuff tendinitis: a population-based study. BMC Musculoskelet Disord 2010;11:165.
2. Buchbinder R, Staples MP, Shanahan EM, et al. General practitioner management of shoulder pain in comparison with rheumatologist expectation of care and best evidence: an Australian National Survey. PLoS One 2013;8:e61243.
3. Thompson JC. Netter's concise orthopaedic anatomy. Chapter 3. Saunders, an imprint of Elsevier Inc; 2002. p. P75–107 Copyright © 2010.

4. Arce G, Bak K, Bain G, et al. Management of disorders of the rotator cuff: pro-ceedings ISAKOS upper extremity community consensus meeting. Arthroscopy 2013;29:1–11.

5. Ewald A. Adhesive capsulitis: a review. Am Fam Physician 2011;83:417–22.

6. Jobe FW, Jobe CM. Painful athletic injuries of the shoulder. Clin Orthop Relat Res 1983;(173):117–24.

7. Hermans J, Luime JJ, Meuffles DE, et al. Does this patient with shoulder pain have rotator cuff disease? The rational clinical examination systematic review. JAMA 2013;310(8):837–47.

8. Hanchard NC, Lenza M, Handoll HH, et al. Physical tests for shoulder impinge-ments and local lesions of bursa, tendon or labrum that may accompany impingement. Cochrane Database Syst Rev 2013;(4):CD007427.

9. Kessel L, Watson M. The painful arc syndrome: clinical classification as a guide to management. J Bone Joint Surg Br 1977;59(2):166–72.

10. Hawkins RJ, Kennedy JC. Impingement syndrome in athletes. Am J Sports Med 1980;3:151–8.

11. Hegedus EJ, Goode AP, Cook CE, et al. Which physical examination tests pro-vide clinicians with the most value when examining of the shoulder? Update of a systematic review with analysis of individual tests. Br J Sports Med 2012;46: 964–78.

12. Armstrong A, Teefey SA, Wu T, et al. The efficacy of ultrasound in the diagnosis of long head of the biceps tendon pathology. J Shoulder Elbow Surg 2006;15:7–11.

13. Gazzola S, Bleakney RR. Current imaging of the rotator cuff. Sports Med Arthrosc 2011;19:300–9.

14. Teefey SA, Rubin DA, Middleton WD, et al. Detection and quantification of rotator cuff tears. Comparison of ultrasonographic, magnetic resonance imaging, and arthroscopic findings in seventy-one consecutive cases. J Bone Joint Surg Am 2004;86:708–16.

15. Lenza M, Buchbinder R, Takwoingi Y, et al. Magnetic resonance imaging, mag-netic resonance arthropathy and ultrasonography for assessing rotator cuff tears in people with shoulder pain for whom surgery is being considered. Cochrane Database Syst Rev 2013;(9):CD009020.

16. Middelton WD, Payne WT, Teefey SA, et al. Sonography and MRI of the shoulder: comparison of patient satisfaction. Am J Roentgenol 2004;183:1449–52.

17. de Jesus JO, Parker L, Frangos AJ, et al. Accuracy of MRI, MR arthropathy, and ultrasound in the diagnosis of rotator cuff tears: a meta-analysis. Am J Roent-genol 2009;192:1701–7.

18. Swenson C, Sward L, Karlsson J. Cryotherapy in sports medicine. Scand J Med Sci Sports 1996;6:193–200.

19. Green S, Buchbinder R, Hetrick S. Acupuncture for shoulder pain. Cochrane Database Syst Rev 2005;(18):CD005319.

20. Johansson K, Bergstrom A, Schröder K, et al. Subacromial corticosteroid injec-tion or acupuncture with home exercises when treating patients with subacromial impingement in primary care—a randomized controlled trial. Fam Pract 2011;4: 355–65.

21. Bloom JE, Rischin A, Johnston RV, et al. Image-guided versus blind glucocorti-coids injection for shoulder pain. Cochrane Database Syst Rev 2012;(9): CD009147.

22. Kesikburun S, Tan AK, Yilmaz B, et al. Platelet-rich plasma injections in the treat-ment of chronic rotator cuff tendinopathy: a randomized controlled trial with one-year follow-up. Am J Sports Med 2013;41(11):2609–16.

23. Singh JA, Fitzgerald PM. Botulinum toxin for shoulder pain. Cochrane Database Syst Rev 2010;(9):CD008271.
24. Hanratty CE, McVeigh JG, Kerr DP, et al. The effectiveness of physiotherapy exercises in subacromial impingement syndrome: a systematic review and meta-analysis. Semin Arthritis Rheum 2012;42:297–316.
25. Littlewood C, Ashton J, Chance-Larsen K, et al. Exercise for rotator cuff tendinopathy: a systematic review. Physiotherapy 2012;98:101–9.
26. Holmgren T, Hallgren H, Öberg E, et al. Effect of specific exercise strategy on need for surgery in patients with subacromial impingement syndrome: randomized controlled study. BMJ 2012;344:e787.
27. Littlewood C, Malliaras P, Mawson S, et al. Self-managed loaded exercises versus usual physiotherapy treatment for rotator cuff tendinopathy: a pilot randomized controlled trial. Physiotherapy 2014;100(1):54–60.
28. Ho CC, Sole G, Munn J. The effectiveness of manual therapy in the management of musculoskeletal disorders of the shoulder: a systematic review. Man Ther 2009;14:463–74.
29. Gebremariam L, Hay EM, Koes BW, et al. Effectiveness of surgical and postsurgical interventions for the subacromial impingement syndrome: a systematic review. Arch Phys Med Rehabil 2011;92:1900–13.
30. Dorrestijn O, Stevens M, Winters JC, et al. Conservative or surgical treatment for subacromial impingement syndrome? A systematic review. J Shoulder Elbow Surg 2009;18:652–60.
31. Pegreffi F, Paladini P, Campi F, et al. Conservative management of rotator cuff tear. Sports Med Arthrosc 2011;19:348–52.
32. Dehghan A, Pishgooei N, Salami MA, et al. Comparison between NSAID and intra-articular corticosteroid injection in frozen shoulder of diabetic patients; a randomized clinical trial. Exp Clin Endocrinol Diabetes 2013;121:75–9.
33. Buchbinder R, Green S, Youd JM, et al. Oral steroids for adhesive capsulitis. Cochrane Database Syst Rev 2006;(4):CD006189.
34. American Academy of Orthopedic Surgeons. The treatment of glenohumeral joint osteoarthritis. Guideline and evidence report [online]. 2009. Available at: http://www.aaos.org/research/guidelines/gloguideline.pdf. Accessed February 25, 2014.
35. Singh JA, Sperling J, Buchbinder R, et al. Surgery for shoulder osteoarthritis. Cochrane Database Syst Rev 2010;(10):CD008089.
36. Yang J, Chen S, Hsieh C, et al. Effects and predictors of shoulder muscle massage for patients with posterior shoulder tightness. BMC Musculoskelet Disord 2012;13:46–53.
37. Hoe VC, Urquhart DM, Kelsall HL, et al. Ergonomic design and training for preventing work-related musculoskeletal disorders of the upper limb and neck in adults. Cochrane Database Syst Rev 2012;(15):CD008570.

Evaluation and Treatment of Musculoskeletal Chest Pain

Amba Ayloo, MD*, Teresa Cvengros, MD, CAQSM, Srimannarayana Marella, MD

KEYWORDS

- Musculoskeletal chest pain • Costochondritis • Stretching exercises
- Pectoralis muscle pain • Fibromyalgia • Myofascial pain • Evaluation • Treatment

KEY POINTS

- Costochondritis is one of the most common causes of musculoskeletal chest pain.
- Stretching exercises have been shown to be effective in relieving the pain in costochondritis.
- Rib fractures, either traumatic or stress fractures, can be a source of chest pain.
- Slipping rib syndrome may occur in children with chronic chest and abdominal pain.
- Muscle strains may cause musculoskeletal chest pain, with intercostal muscle strains being the most common.
- Pectoralis muscle injury needs accurate and early diagnosis for optimal functional recovery in athletes.
- Myofascial pain and fibromyalgia are other causes of musculoskeletal chest pain.
- Herpes zoster should be considered in elderly patients with nonspecific musculoskeletal chest pain.
- It is important to assess all patients with chest pain for non-musculoskeletal causes of pain that could cause increased morbidity or mortality if not identified promptly.

INTRODUCTION

Chest pain is one of the most common reasons for seeking medical attention worldwide. In the United States alone, there are about 7.16 million visits annually to the emergency room with chest pain and most of these patients have noncardiac causes of chest pain.[1] Chest pain accounts for 1% to 3% of office visits to the primary care

This article originally appeared in Primary Care: Clinics in Office Practice, Volume 40, Issue 4, December 2013.
Funding Sources: None.
Conflict of Interest: None.
Family Medicine Residency Program, Department of Family Medicine, Mount Sinai Hospital, California Avenue at 15th Street, Chicago, IL 60608, USA
* Corresponding author.
E-mail address: ambaayloo@gmail.com

provider. Of these visits, 21% to 49% of patients are diagnosed with musculoskeletal chest pain, making it the most common cause of chest pain.[2]

Causes of chest pain include cardiovascular, pulmonary, musculoskeletal, gastro-enterologic, and psychogenic. Pain can also radiate to the chest from the shoulders, cervical and thoracic spine, lower neck, and structures below the diaphragm (**Fig. 1**).[3]

An important mechanism of chest pain may be referred pain from intrathoracic structures, including the heart, lungs, and esophagus.[3] Pain occurs because free nerve endings that transmit pain from visceral thoracic structures, including the heart, synapse on the same spinal cord dorsal horn interneurons that receive afferent input from the skin, muscles, and joints. The convergence of visceral and somatic pain fibers on the same interneurons causes the referred visceral pain that is perceived in somatic areas remote from involved viscera.[2] Thus, it can sometimes be difficult to delineate the precise cause of chest pain as musculoskeletal or visceral in origin.[2]

It is important to rule out visceral causes of chest pain, including cardiac, esopha-geal, or pulmonary causes, such as angina, myocardial infarction, malignancies, or pulmonary embolism, before definitively diagnosing musculoskeletal chest pain.[3,4] For example, anginal pain may occur along with underlying costochondritis or subacromial bursitis, which may influence the distribution of anginal pain.[3] In middle-aged and elderly patients with strong, relevant risk factors for cardiac disease, it is recommended to order an electrocardiogram, echocardiogram, and even stress

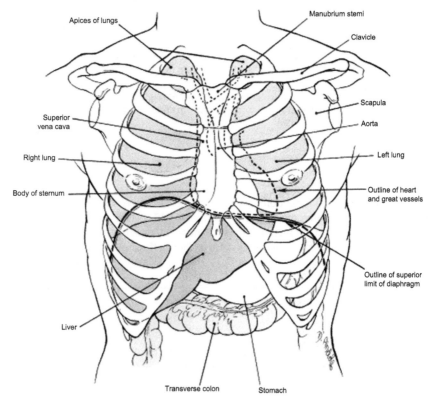

Fig. 1. Diverse origins and causes of chest pain. (*From* Cava JR, Sayger PL. Chest pain in chil-dren and adolescents. Pediatr Clin North Am 2004;51(6):1553–68. Philadelphia: Elsevier; with permission.)

testing as necessary to definitively rule out cardiac causes of chest pain before treating for musculoskeletal chest pain.[3,4]

Musculoskeletal chest pain includes pain related to the anterior chest wall bony and cartilaginous structures, chest wall musculature, and the thoracic spine.[3] In addition, other causes of pain may include skin conditions, neoplasms, and infections of chest wall structures, metabolic causes (vitamin D deficiency),[5] and rheumatologic disorders (**Box 1**).[3,6] The term chest wall syndrome refers to nontraumatic causes of musculoskeletal chest wall pain, which may include diagnoses such as costochondritis, atypical chest pain, and cervicothoracic angina.[7] A good history and physical examination are crucial to accurately diagnosing musculoskeletal chest pain (**Box 2**, **Table 1**).[3]

MUSCULOSKELETAL CHEST PAIN RELATED TO BONY AND CARTILAGINOUS STRUCTURES OF THE CHEST WALL
Costochondritis and Tietze Syndrome

These are conditions characterized by pain and tenderness in costochondral junctions. The comparative characteristics between the 2 conditions are listed in **Table 2**.[3,4]

Box 1
Diverse causes of musculoskeletal chest pain

- **Pain related to bony and cartilaginous structures of the chest wall**

  Costochondritis

  Tietze syndrome

  Rib pain

  - Fractures related to trauma

  - Stress fractures

  Slipping rib syndrome

  Painful xiphoid syndrome

- **Pain related to muscles**

  Muscle strains

  - Pectoralis muscle strains

  - Injuries to internal oblique/external oblique muscles

  - Serratus anterior muscle injury

  Myofascial pain

  Fibromyalgia

  Precordial catch syndrome

  Epidemic myalgia

- **Pain related to thoracic spine**

  Thoracic disc herniation

- **Miscellaneous causes of chest wall pain**

  Skin-related conditions

  - Herpes zoster

  - Neoplasms

  SAPHO syndrome

Table 1
Key points in history taking

Pain[3]	Onset	Usually acute or insidious
	Location	Well localized
	Character	Nonsqueezing, reproducible
	Duration	May become chronic
	Precipitating factor	By posture or movement
	Aggravating factor	
	Relieving factor	
History of acute or repeated excessive activity		
Recent or remote trauma[3]		

Data from Fam AG, Smythe HA. Musculoskeletal chest wall pain. Can Med Assoc J 1985;133:379–89.

Box 2
Key points in physical examination

Thorough systematic examination of anterior and posterior chest wall for

Swelling

Erythema

Heat

Tenderness

Neurologic examination to rule out compressions of nerve roots originating in lower cervical or thoracic segments of spinal cord

Sensory disturbances

Muscular strength

Peripheral reflexes of upper and lower extremities

Data from Fam AG, Smythe HA. Musculoskeletal chest wall pain. Can Med Assoc J 1985;133:379–89.

The possible mechanism of pain is believed to be mechanical derangement, muscular imbalance, or neurogenic inflammation.[8] The pathogenesis of costochondritis is unclear. Because of its frequent association with other primary causes of chest pain, including anginal pain, it is important, especially in patients with relevant risk factors, to rule out any associated cardiac chest pain.[4]

Chest pain involving costochondral joints has also been described in association with vitamin D deficiency.[5] The mechanism involved is believed to be defective bone mineralization caused by lack of vitamin D. This mechanism is shown by findings of rachitic rosary in children with rickets and tenderness of costochondral joints in adult patients

Box 3
Prevalence of costochondritis

Emergency room	30% of chest pain visits were because of costochondritis
Primary care office	20% of chest pain visits were because of musculoskeletal chest pain
	Of these visits, 13% were because of costochondritis

Data from Proulx AM, Zryd TW. Costochondritis: diagnosis and treatment. Am Fam Physician 2009;80(6):617–21.

Table 2
Comparisons between costochondritis and Tietze syndrome

Characteristics	Costochondritis	Tietze Syndrome
Signs of inflammation	Absent	Present
Swelling	Absent	Presence or absence indicate severity of problem
Joints affected	Multiple and unilateral >90% Usually second to fifth costochondral junctions involved (Fig. 2)	Usually single and unilateral Usually second and third costochondral junctions involved[3,9,10]
Prevalence[4]	Relatively common (Box 3)	Uncommon
Age group affected	All age groups, including adolescents and elderly	Common in younger age group
Nature of pain	Aching, sharp, pressure like	Aching, sharp, stabbing initially, later persists as dull aching
Onset of pain	Repetitive physical activity provokes pain, rarely occurs at rest[11]	New vigorous physical activity such as excessive cough or vomiting, chest impact[9]
Aggravation of pain[9]	Movements of upper body, deep breathing, exertional activities	Movements
Association with other conditions	Seronegative arthropathies, angina pain[12]	No known association
Diagnosis	Crowing rooster maneuver[3] and other physical examination findings	Physical examination, exclude rheumatoid arthritis, pyogenic arthritis[2,3]
Imaging studies	Chest radiograph, computed tomography scan, or nuclear bone scan to rule out infections or neoplasms if clinically suspected[4]	Bone scintigraphy and ultrasonography can be used for screening for other conditions[10,11]
Treatment	Reassurance, pain control, NSAIDs, application of local heat and ice compresses, manual therapy with stretching exercises.[8,13] Corticosteroid or sulfasalazine injections in refractory patients[12]	Reassurance, pain control with NSAIDs,[3,9] and application of local heat. Corticosteroid and lidocaine injections to the cartilage, or intercostal nerve block in refractory patients[3,10]

Abbreviation: NSAIDs, nonsteroidal antiinflammatory drugs.

with osteomalacia. Low vitamin D should be suspected in people with poor dietary intake of vitamin D or limited exposure to sunlight. Supplementation of vitamin D was associated with improvement of chest pain and overall quality of life. Further studies are needed to definitively associate vitamin D deficiency and costochondritis.[5]

Evaluation
Physical examination helps in diagnosis. The "crowing rooster" maneuver reproduces the pain of costochondritis (Fig. 3).

Treatment
Conservative treatment is generally recommended (see Table 2). Stretching exercises have been studied recently in the treatment of costochondritis. In a retrospective open

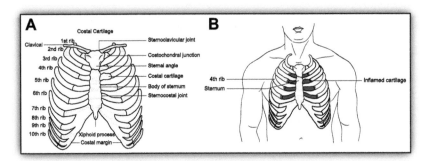

Fig. 2. Rib cage with costal cartilages and inflamed cartilages in costochondritis. (*A*) Labeling of rib cage. (*B*) Inflammation of coastal cartilages.

study of patients with a definitive diagnosis of costochondritis who were taking nonsteroidal antiinflammatory drugs (NSAIDs) in the last 2 to 3 months, there was statistically significant improvement in pain in the study group treated with exercises and NSAIDs, compared with the group on NSAIDs only (**Fig. 4**).[8]

Rib Pain

Rib pain can be caused by swelling, erosions, and trauma causing fractures (**Figs. 5 and 6**).[3,14]

Evaluation

There is usually a history of initial vague chest pain that increases with inspiration, with movements of the chest and upper limb movements.[3,14] Dull, aching pain is more localized around the scapula, neck, and clavicle and may radiate to the sternum in first rib fractures.[15] Physical examination reveals point tenderness at the site of trauma, with or without local swelling on palpation.[14–16]

It is important to suspect and look for trauma to underlying viscera, including lung contusions, injury to liver, spleen, kidney, or any pneumothorax or hemothorax in multiple rib fractures and also in fractures of the first 4 or last 2 ribs, because these are not commonly seen. Child abuse should always be suspected in any child presenting with rib fractures, especially in infants and toddlers, because routine causes of injury and

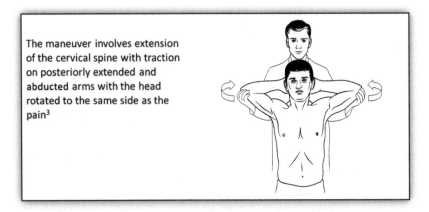

The maneuver involves extension of the cervical spine with traction on posteriorly extended and abducted arms with the head rotated to the same side as the pain[3]

Fig. 3. Crowing rooster maneuver.

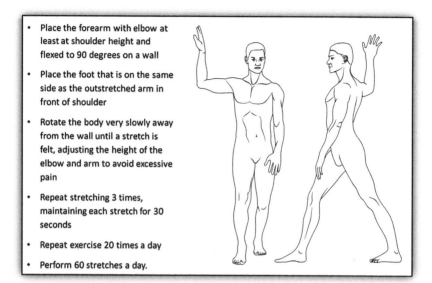

- Place the forearm with elbow at least at shoulder height and flexed to 90 degrees on a wall

- Place the foot that is on the same side as the outstretched arm in front of shoulder

- Rotate the body very slowly away from the wall until a stretch is felt, adjusting the height of the elbow and arm to avoid excessive pain

- Repeat stretching 3 times, maintaining each stretch for 30 seconds

- Repeat exercise 20 times a day

- Perform 60 stretches a day.

Fig. 4. Stretching exercises for costochondritis.

trauma in children do not cause rib fractures (**Fig. 7**). Imaging studies can help in diagnosing or confirming the fracture (**Box 4**).[15–18]

Treatment
Symptomatic treatment with good pain control for at least 3 weeks is generally recommended for non–sports related injuries.[14] Deep breathing is encouraged to prevent lung collapse, atelectasis, and lung infections. Splinting, local nerve blocks, and anesthetic injections are not routinely indicated because of poor efficacy and the associated risk of causing pneumothorax.[14] For athletes with first rib fractures, rest is recommended until

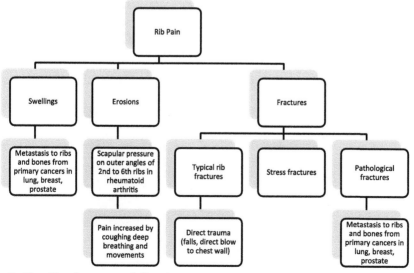

Fig. 5. Algorithm for causes of rib pain.

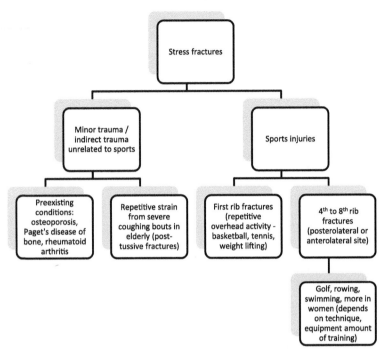

Fig. 6. Algorithm for causes of stress fractures.

symptoms resolve, followed by a gradual return to overhead activity, with correction of technique and biomechanical modification. Full recovery may take up to a year.[16,18] Fractures of the fourth to eighth ribs may need pain control and rest, with gradual return to activity at 4 to 6 weeks, then full activity as tolerated at 8 to 10 weeks.[16]

Slipping Rib Syndrome

This condition occurs when interchondral fibrous attachments between the lower ribs, usually the 9th and 10th ribs, are inadequate, or rupture and loosen, allowing costal cartilage tips to curl up and override the inner aspect of the rib above, impinging on the intercostal nerve.[20,21] It is a recognized cause of chronic pain syndrome in children with recurrent pain in the lower chest and upper abdomen, but is less common compared with adults because of more flexible chests in children.[21] Repetitive trunk

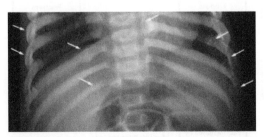

Fig. 7. Rib fractures in a child (*arrows*). (*From* Rubio EI. How do you read these images? Hone your interpretive skills. Rib fractures in a child. 2008. Available at: http://www.pediatricsconsultantlive.com/display/article/1803329/1405067. Accessed March 30, 2013; with permission.)

Box 4
Rib fracture imaging findings

Radiographs show a fracture line in about a half to two-thirds of fractures

In cases with no initial radiographic evidence of fracture, a healing callus may be seen after a few weeks on the radiograph or ultrasonogram

Triple phase bone scan or magnetic resonance imaging (MRI) may be used for early diagnosis.

Data from Refs.[3,15–17,19]

---

motion in athletes involved in sports such as running can cause slippage of a hypermobile rib under the superior rib, causing nerve impingement and pain.[15,16]

There may be a remote history of trauma.[2] Pain is insidious in onset, severe, sharp, and felt in the abdominal wall or anterior costal cartilage. It may be felt as local somatic pain or as visceral pain, which may mimic biliary colic, peptic ulcer disease, and renal colic.[3,16,21]

Evaluation

Diagnosis is clinical. Examination shows increased tenderness and mobility of the anterior end of the costal cartilage, with an occasional painful click over the tip of affected cartilage. This pain can be reproduced by the hooking maneuver (**Fig. 8**).[2,16,20–23]

Treatment

Reassurance, pain control with analgesics, and avoidance of movements and positions that cause the loose costal cartilage to move upwards suddenly and provoke pain are recommended.[2,16,22] Strapping and local infiltration of lidocaine and corticosteroids for intercostal nerve block may be needed, more commonly in children.[16,20–22] Subperichondrial resection of involved costal cartilages is reserved for refractory cases in children (**Box 5**).

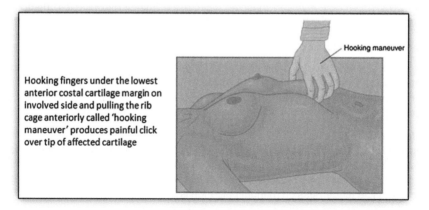

Hooking fingers under the lowest anterior costal cartilage margin on involved side and pulling the rib cage anteriorly called 'hooking maneuver' produces painful click over tip of affected cartilage

Hooking maneuver

Fig. 8. Hooking maneuver for slipping rib syndrome. (*From* Waldman S. Atlas of pain management injection techniques. 3rd edition. Philadelphia: Saunders; 2013. p. 274–6, with permission; and *Data from* Koren W, Shahar A. Xiphodynia masking acute myocardial infarction: a diagnostic cul-de-sac. Am J Emerg Med 1998;16(2):177–8.)

Box 5
Subperichondrial resection

It is important to mark the point of maximum tenderness on the patient while they are awake and supine before going to the operating room

Affected cartilage is excised and perichondrium is preserved

Surgery can be performed as an outpatient procedure

Cryotherapy can help decrease postoperative pain[21]

Data from Fu R, Iqbal CW, Jaroszewski DE, et al. Costal cartilage excision for the treatment of pediatric slipping rib syndrome. J Pediatr Surg 2012;47(10):1825–7.

Painful Xiphoid Syndrome

Painful xiphoid syndrome is characterized by pain and tenderness in the region of the xiphoid cartilage. Pain may be low substernal or epigastric, with radiation to the precordium or abdomen.[3,16]

Evaluation

Painful xiphoid syndrome is a diagnosis of exclusion. Clinical examination by exerting pressure on xiphoid cartilage reduplicates the pain and tenderness. It is important to definitively rule out other serious causes of chest pain, such as myocardial infarction, before reaching this diagnosis.[24]

Treatment

Symptomatic treatment with good pain control is generally recommended. Local injections of corticosteroids or lidocaine are recommended in refractory cases. Surgical excision of xiphoid cartilage is reserved for severe cases.[3]

MUSCULOSKELETAL CHEST PAIN RELATED TO MUSCLES

Muscle strains comprise one of the most common causes of musculoskeletal chest pain. They are usually acute in onset, caused by trauma or overuse.[3] Gradual onset of the muscle pain has also been reported as a result of tension or anxiety in the patient.[2] The commonly involved muscles include the intercostal muscles, pectoralis muscles, internal and external oblique muscles, and serratus anterior muscles.

Intercostal Muscle Strains

Intercostal muscles are the most commonly affected muscles, in almost 50% of patients,[2] followed by the pectoralis muscle group. There may be a history of excessive exertion of untrained muscles with activities like painting a ceiling, chopping wood, or coughing, and in sports with intense upper body activity, such as rowing.[3,16]

Evaluation

Diagnosis is clinical, based on a good history and physical examination. Localized pain or tenderness over the affected muscle groups is seen, which increases with stretching or contracting the involved muscles with activities such as deep inspiration and coughing.[3,16] Muscle tenderness on manual palpation is the most common finding.

Treatment

Reassurance, local application of heat, or use of analgesics for good pain control are recommended, along with avoiding activities that cause recurrence of the pain. Local injections of lidocaine or corticosteroids are reserved for refractory cases.[3,15,16]

Pectoralis Muscle Strains

The pectoralis muscle is one of the most important muscles for various movements of the upper limbs and chest wall (**Fig. 9**).[25] Tears to the pectoralis muscle can be caused by direct blow or indirect trauma.[26–28] The tears can be classified by either cause or location of tear (**Figs. 10** and **11**). Indirect injury occurs when muscle under full tension is subjected to additional stress (eccentric muscle contraction), causing high-grade injuries in athletes in sports such as weight lifting or rugby.[29] Non–sports injury occurs most commonly because of forced abduction with extension or external rotation during a fall or when lifting weights.[25,30]

Evaluation

History and physical examination can help in diagnosis, but imaging is usually advised for correct diagnosis, because clinical assessment can be misled by hematoma or muscle injury.[25] Tears can present as sudden pain in the arm or shoulder accompanied with an audible pop, followed by swelling and ecchymosis. Inspection shows loss of the anterior axillary fold and asymmetry when compared with the other side with palpation of a defect on the side of injury. Loss of arm adduction may be a subtle but important finding in athletes such as weight lifters.[25] Radiographs at initial assessment may show soft tissue swelling with absent pectoralis shadow. Ultrasonography and MRI are modalities of choice and help in making correct decisions about optimal management (**Box 6**).[25]

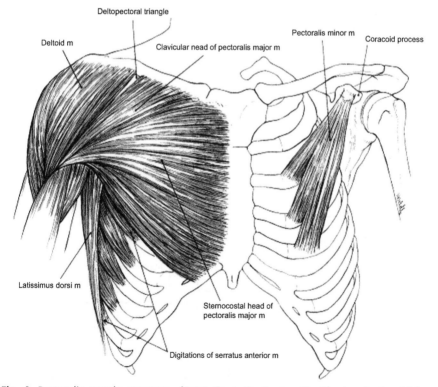

Fig. 9. Pectoralis muscle structure. (*From* Cava JR, Sayger PL. Chest pain in children and adolescents. Pediatr Clin North Am 2004;51(6):1553–68. Philadelphia: Elsevier; with permission.)

Classification of pectoralis muscle injury (tear)

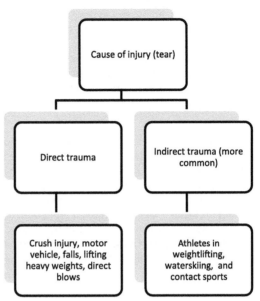

Fig. 10. Algorithm for pectoralis muscle injury based on cause of injury. (*Data from* Hopper MA, Tirman P, Robinson P. Muscle injury of the chest wall and upper extremity. Semin Musculoskelet Radiol 2010;14(2):122–30.)

Treatment

Proper documentation and determination of injury site and mechanism determine the management (**Box 7**).[25,29]

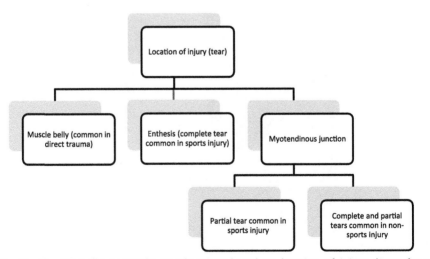

Fig. 11. Algorithm for pectoralis muscle injury based on location of injury. (*Data from* Hopper MA, Tirman P, Robinson P. Muscle injury of the chest wall and upper extremity. Semin Musculoskelet Radiol 2010;14(2):122–30.)

Box 6
Ultrasonography and MRI for diagnosis of pectoralis muscle tears

Ultrasonography is helpful in initial rapid assessment of acute muscle injury and surrounding structures when performed by an experienced clinician[30]

MRI is gold standard for:

Accurate assessment of site and severity of injury and bony structures

Identifying patients who benefit most from surgery

Data from Hopper MA, Tirman P, Robinson P. Muscle injury of the chest wall and upper extremity. Semin Musculoskelet Radiol 2010;14(2):122–30.

Injuries to Internal Oblique/External Oblique Muscles

Injuries at the rib and costal cartilage insertion of internal and external oblique muscles are commonly referred to as side strains (**Fig. 12**).[31] They are uncommon, mostly seen in athletes such as bowlers (cricket), javelin throwers, rowers, swimmers, or ice hockey players. The mechanism of injury is muscle lengthening followed by sudden eccentric contraction.[14,25,31,32] The injury is particularly seen in cricket fast bowlers and is seen in the nonbowling arm.[14]

Evaluation

Physical examination elicits pain and tenderness over the lower 4 costal cartilages, increased by resisted side flexion to the affected side.[31] Diagnosis is clinical, but imaging helps in evaluating the severity of injury and in determining the course of management (**Box 8, Figs. 13** and **14**).[25]

MRI may show hematoma, periosteal stripping, or any stress injury to the underlying rib.[31] It is particularly useful in assessing acute concomitant injury to external oblique muscles. It can help in the follow-up of patients who failed to respond to conservative measures, but can be complicated by respiratory motion artifact.[25,33]

Treatment

Conservative treatment is recommended, with rest, strengthening exercises, and return to activity gradually. A period of 4 to 6 weeks may be needed for complete return

---

Box 7
Treatment of pectoralis muscle tears

Early surgical intervention[25,29,30]:

Complete pectoralis major tendon avulsion at humeral attachment

Helps athletes in early return to sports

Optimum functional recovery

Good cosmetic results

Nonsurgical treatment[29]:

Muscular or musculotendinous tears

Low-grade partial tears

Older, sedentary patients for whom loss of strength may not cause significant impairment or debility

Data from Hopper MA, Tirman P, Robinson P. Muscle injury of the chest wall and upper extremity. Semin Musculoskelet Radiol 2010;14(2):122–30.

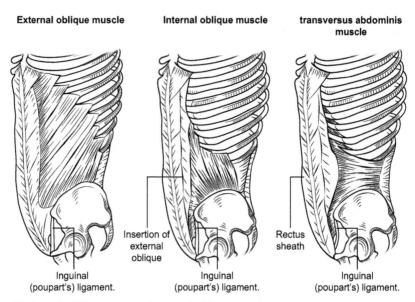

External oblique muscle   **Internal oblique muscle**   **transversus abdominis muscle**

Insertion of external oblique

Rectus sheath

Inguinal (poupart's) ligament.

Inguinal (poupart's) ligament.

Inguinal (poupart's) ligament.

Fig. 12. Insertion of external and internal oblique muscles.

to activity, especially in fast bowlers.[14] Reoccurrence of injury is common, especially in the first 2 years of initial injury.[14]

Serratus Anterior Muscle Injury

Serratus anterior muscle injury is seen in athletes involved in sports such as rowing and weight lifting caused by overuse. Pain is typically located around the medial border of the scapula on the affected side and may radiate to the anterior chest.[15]

Evaluation

Diagnosis is clinical. Physical examination shows reproducible typical pain on resisted scapular protraction.[15]

Treatment

Improvement is seen with rest from activities that increase the pain, but may take several weeks.[15]

Box 8
Ultrasonographic findings in internal oblique muscle injury

Acute injury shows:

Hematoma

Fluid between muscle layers

Loss of normal architecture

Gap in the insertion of the internal oblique into costal cartilages and ribs (see **Fig. 14**)

Not sensitive to assess chronic injury and small muscle tears[32]

Data from Hopper MA, Tirman P, Robinson P. Muscle injury of the chest wall and upper extremity. Semin Musculoskelet Radiol 2010;14(2):122–30; and Obaid H, Nealon A, Connell D. Sonographic appearance of side strain injury. AJR Am J Roentgenol 2008;191(6):W264–7.

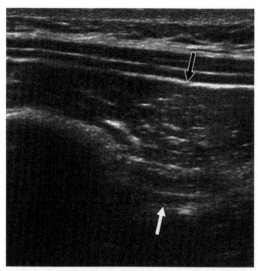

Fig. 13. Ultrasonographic appearance of normal external oblique (*black arrow*) and internal oblique (*white arrow*) muscles. (*From* Obaid H, Nealon A, Connell D. Sonographic appearance of side strain injury. AJR Am J Roentgenol 2008;191(6):265. Available at: http://www.ajronline.org/doi/full/10.2214/AJR.07.3381. Accessed March 12, 2013; with permission.)

Myofascial Pain

As the name implies, myofascial pain is defined as pain originating from muscles or fascia. This type of pain is described as dull and aching, with a stiff feeling. It may be caused by muscle injury or overuse.[34] Myofascial pain may be aggravated by

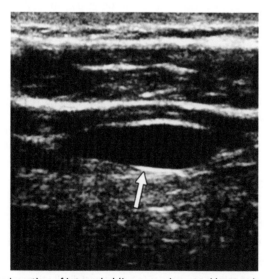

Fig. 14. Gap in the insertion of internal oblique muscle caused by tear (*arrow*). (*From* Obaid H, Nealon A, Connell D. Sonographic appearance of side strain injury. AJR Am J Roentgenol 2008;191(6):265. Available at: http://www.ajronline.org/doi/full/10.2214/AJR.07.3381. Accessed March 12, 2013; with permission.)

muscle use, postural imbalance, cold, anxiety, and psychological stressors.[35] What defines myofascial pain clinically is the identification of a trigger point.[34] A trigger point is "a hyperirritable spot in skeletal muscle that is associated with a hypersensitive palpable nodule in a taut band" of muscle.[36] Additional clinical features of trigger points are listed in **Box 9**.[34,35,37]

Trigger points in the pectoral major and minor muscles, intercostal muscles, anterior serratus muscles, scalenus muscles, and sternalis muscles can be a source of pain referred to the chest wall.[35,38,39] For example, trigger points in the pectoral major or minor muscle may cause ipsilateral chest pain that radiates down the ulnar side of the arm. Sternalis muscle trigger points may cause a deep substernal ache.[35] Myofascial trigger points are common yet often not identified or treated properly, because the initial training of so few medical providers includes adequate education in their identification and treatment.[37]

Evaluation

Carefully examine the chest wall and cervical muscles for active trigger points. The physical examination skills for identifying trigger points are not commonly taught in medical training, and practice is required in order to become competent at this skill. Myofascial pain may not be the sole reason for the pain, but may be a contributing factor in some cases. Therefore, evaluation for other causes of pain is important.[34]

Treatment

It is important to address postural and ergonomic factors and proper stretching and strengthening of muscles when treating myofascial pain. There are several options for local treatment of active trigger points (**Box 10**).[34,37]

Medications that may be helpful include NSAIDs, tricyclic antidepressant drugs, or muscle relaxants, particularly tizanidine (Zanaflex). Consider referral to a provider with experience in treating trigger points and myofascial pain. If myofascial pain is not treated appropriately and underlying predisposing factors are not addressed, it may lead to chronic pain syndromes such as fibromyalgia, through the mechanism of central sensitization.[34]

Fibromyalgia

Fibromyalgia is a distinct complex clinical syndrome that belongs to a group of clinical syndromes characterized by chronic pain, called the central sensitization syndromes.[40–42] The other members of this group include restless leg syndrome, functional gastrointestinal disorders, and chronic fatigue syndrome. Fibromyalgia and other central sensitivity syndromes are characterized by a range of symptoms that include chronic pain, sleep disturbances with decreased rapid eye movement

---

Box 9
Trigger points

Tender ropelike induration in muscle

May produce a twitch response, which is contraction of the muscle, when palpated or needled

May cause restricted range of motion or weakness in the affected muscle

May cause radiation of pain or parasthesias in a myotomal distribution

Firm pressure on a trigger point for at least 5 seconds may elicit referred pain in a myotomal distribution

> **Box 10**
> **Local treatment of trigger points**
>
> Ischemic pressure
>
> Injection of trigger point with anesthetic solution such as lidocaine (wet needling)
>
> Injection of trigger point without anesthetic (dry needling)
>
> Stretching the muscle while spraying with vapocoolant

sleep, other somatic symptoms, and psychological symptoms.[43] The current hypothesis is that these syndromes represent a spectrum of disorders that result in expression of different symptoms over time, as a result of a complex interplay of various psychological, social, and biological factors, called the biopsychosocial model.[44]

According to various studies that evaluated the prevalence of fibromyalgia in patients with musculoskeletal causes of noncardiac chest pain, prevalence ranges between 2.7% and 30%.[9] Both fibromyalgia and noncardiac chest pain seem to share the same pathogenesis of long-standing pain hypersensitivity, which presents as allodynia and hyperalgesia.[40] The other accompanying somatic and visceral complaints are believed to be caused by hypothalamic-pituitary-adrenal axis abnormalities and autonomic dysfunction.[45] Mechanism of central sensitization with somatic or visceral hypersensitivity manifests as noncardiac chest pain in patients with fibromyalgia.[46]

Fibromyalgia is characterized by chronic widespread pain, unexplained somatic symptoms, which include nonrestorative sleep, dysesthesias, cognitive difficulties, dizziness, syncope, dry mouth, and headaches, and psychological symptoms, such as anxiety or depression.[47] Another characteristic feature of fibromyalgia is the presence of specific points of tenderness at 9 symmetric body sites (**Fig. 15**). It is more common in women, in those 50 years or older, and in those with low educational and household income levels.[48]

Evaluation

History and physical examination are important in diagnosing fibromyalgia. The American College of Rheumatology (ACR) established diagnostic and severity criteria in 1990, which were revised in 2000 (**Box 11**).

Treatment

Various pharmacologic and nonpharmacologic treatments have been shown to be beneficial in fibromyalgia (**Box 12**).

A holistic approach that addresses the various symptoms of fibromyalgia including pain, fatigue, sleep, and mood disorders has been shown to be effective and deliver the most effective results in the long-term.[52]

Precordial Catch Syndrome

Precordial catch syndrome is an uncommon condition characterized by episodes of localized, stabbing, or sharp pain catches in the anterior chest, usually in the left parasternal area or near the cardiac apex in healthy young individuals.[3,53] Pain occurs in a bent-over or slouched position and is increased by deep breathing. It is relieved by shallow respirations and by correcting posture. Local tenderness is absent. The cause is believed to be intercostal muscle spasm caused by postural defects.[3]

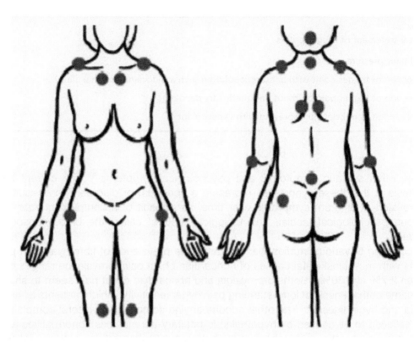

Fig. 15. Tender points in fibromyalgia. (*From* Shipley M. Chronic widespread pain and fibromyalgia syndrome. Medicine 2010;38(4):202–4; with permission.)

Evaluation

Precordial catch syndrome is a diagnosis of exclusion.

Treatment

Reassurance, correcting postural defects, and good pain control are generally recommended.[3,53]

Epidemic Myalgia

Epidemic myalgia is also called devil's grip, caused by acute viral illness with pain in the chest wall and epigastrium.[3] The usual causes are the group B coxsackie viruses, which usually affect intercostal and upper abdominal wall muscles, and rarely the pleura. A prodrome of 1 to 10 days is followed by severe, sharp pain in the lateral chest

---

Box 11
Diagnostic and severity criteria for fibromyalgia

ACR criteria (1990)[49]: presence of chronic widespread pain and tenderness at 11 of 18 body sites

Chronic widespread pain is presence of pain in the upper and lower body, axial skeletal, and left and right sides for at least 3 months, without any history of lesion or trauma to explain the symptoms

ACR revised criteria (2000)[50]: presence of chronic widespread pain and a symptom severity scale (includes fatigue, cognitive disturbances, nonrestorative sleep, and other somatic symptoms)

New criteria offer greater sensitivity for diagnosis of fibromyalgia

---

Box 12
Treatment of fibromyalgia

Pharmacologic treatment: for pain control

- Antidepressants: amitryptiline, cyclobenzaprine, fluoxetine[51]

- Opiates: tramadol

- Central nervous system agents: gabapentin, pregabalin

Nonpharmacologic treatment

- Graded aerobic exercise regimen[52]: helps with pain, avoid overexhaustion

- Sleep evaluation and treatment: helps with nonrestorative sleep and to correct other sleep problems, such as obstructive sleep apnea

- Cognitive behavioral therapy: promotes and reinforces positive behaviors, helps with treatment of pain, fatigue, and other somatic symptoms

Treatment of other coexisting symptoms (psychological, somatic, such as gastrointestinal, etc)

---

wall in adults or the upper abdomen in children. Pain is increased by breathing, coughing, and other thoracic movements and lasts 3 to 7 days, with frequent recurrences.[3]

Evaluation

Diagnosis is usually clinical, with good history and physical examination, with local tenderness of involved muscle groups. Isolation of the virus from the throat or feces or showing increasing titer levels of type-specific neutralizing antibodies can confirm the diagnosis.[3]

Treatment

Symptomatic treatment with good pain control is recommended.[3]

MUSCULOSKELETAL CHEST PAIN RELATED TO THORACIC SPINE

Acute Thoracic Disc Herniation in Athletes

Thoracic disc herniation does not have a typical clinical presentation and most commonly presents as a nonspecific, often acute-onset, midline pain in the thoracic area. It can be unilateral or bilateral. It can be intermittent or constant and may be increased by coughing and straining.[54] Radicular distribution of pain depends on the thoracic spinal segment involved and may be followed by sensory and motor disturbances caused by spinal cord compression. The usual cause is believed to be degeneration, although acute trauma has to be considered in young patients, especially in athletes.[54]

Evaluation

MRI is the imaging of choice and shows thoracic disc herniation.[54]

Treatment

Conservative management is successful in most patients. Selective spinal root or intercostal nerve blockade and epidural steroid injections are used. If there is no improvement in symptoms after 2 to 3 months, or if there is progression of symptoms with new neurologic deficits, operative treatment is recommended, with a success rate of about 80%.[54]

Long-term prognosis is considered to be good, but recurrences of pain and other symptoms are not uncommon. It is important to explain the possibility of recurrent pain to patients, especially young athletes, because it can cause them to prematurely end their sporting careers.[54]

MISCELLANEOUS CAUSES OF MUSCULOSKELETAL CHEST PAIN
Herpes Zoster of the Chest Wall

Herpes zoster is caused by the reactivation of the latent varicella zoster virus, which has been dormant in dorsal root ganglion of the spinal cord since the initial chicken pox infection.[55] About 50% of elderly patients older than 80 years are believed to develop this infection over their lifetime.[55] It presents as a vesicular eruption of the skin, and is dermatomally distributed. The rash is usually unilateral and confined to a single dermatome, but involvement of multiple, bilateral dermatomes is seen. Severe pain is a hallmark of herpes zoster and often precedes, accompanies, and follows resolution of rash (**Box 13**).[56]

Involvement of thoracic dermatomes, especially in elderly patients, can cause diagnostic confusion with cardiac and pulmonary causes of pain, particularly before development of the rash.[62,63] Rash usually involves thoracic dermatomes with grouped vesicles and pustules present on erythematous base. Infection typically resolves completely in 4 weeks. Scarring and depigmentation in the area of the rash may be seen.[6]

Evaluation

Diagnosis during the prodromal phase before appearance of skin lesions is difficult.[6,64] A history of varicella zoster in the past and hyperesthesia and skin tenderness on physical examination that follows a dermatomal distribution are clues to the diagnosis.[6,64] A dermatomally distributed skin rash with grouped vesicles and pustules on an erythematous base is diagnostic (**Fig. 16**). Clinical diagnosis can be confirmed by Tzanck smear (swabs from the base of the vesicles show varicella zoster virus DNA on polymerase chain reaction testing).

Treatment

Pain control and antivirals are mainstays of treatment (**Box 14**).

SAPHO Syndrome

SAPHO syndrome is a chronic disease that is characterized by association of synovitis, acne, pustulosis, hyperostosis, and osteitis.[68] It usually presents with cutaneous manifestations (neutrophilic eruptions, such as palmoplantar pustulosis and hidradenitis suppurativa) and aseptic inflammatory bone lesions with associated findings that include hyperostosis and arthritis of adjacent joints (osteoarthropathy).[69] SAPHO syndrome has a predilection to affect the bony structures of the anterior chest, including

---

Box 13
Characteristics of pain in herpes zoster

Preherpetic neuralgia: prodromal pain that precedes the development of skin eruption (usually by 4 days)[56,57]

- Leads to diagnostic confusion depending on the dermatomes affected

- Fever, malaise, and skin tenderness over affected area may accompany the pain

Postherpetic neuralgia: pain that persists or is recurrent more than 1 month after the onset of initial herpes zoster infection[58]

- More common in elderly women with history of severe prodromal pain and severe skin rash

- Pain is debilitating and resistant to treatment[58,59]

Zoster sine eruption: prodromal pain is not followed by skin eruption

- Leads to diagnostic difficulties[60,61]

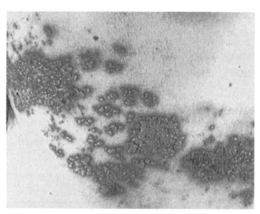

Fig. 16. Dermatomal distribution of herpes zoster skin rash. (*From* Swartz MH. Textbook of physical diagnosis: history of examination. Philadelphia: Saunders; 2009. p. 137–95; with permission.)

the sternum and medial end of clavicle. Anterior chest pain is one of the most common symptoms.[69]

The pathogenesis of SAPHO syndrome is unclear. One of the proposed mechanisms is a possible autoimmune response triggered by a microorganism producing sterile inflammation in the joints and bones.[69–71] *Propionibacterium acnes* is the most commonly cultured microorganism in skin and bone specimens obtained from patients with SAPHO syndrome.[72] Genetic factors and stress are other important factors that are correlated with the syndrome.[69–71]

Evaluation

Although there are no validated criteria, standard diagnostic criteria agreed on by most clinicians and researchers can be used in diagnosis (**Box 15**).[73]

Laboratory findings are nonspecific and include mild leukocytosis, mild anemia, and an increased erythrocyte sedimentation rate. Serum levels of complement C3 and C4 may be increased or normal and serum IgA levels are usually increased.[69]

Treatment

Symptomatic relief with NSAIDs and analgesics are the mainstay of therapy. Corticosteroids, sulfasalazine, and isotretinoin have been used in some cases. Use of tumor necrosis factor inhibitors (such as infliximab and etanercept) and immunomodulators (such as leflunomide and methotrexate) have been proposed in some studies.[69,72,74,75]

Box 14
Treatment of herpes zoster
Start treatment with antiviral agents (acyclovir, valcyclovir) within 72 hours of appearance of skin eruption and continue for 7 days[65]
Postherpetic neuralgia: gabapentin, pregabalin, topical agents (capsaicin cream) and tricyclic antidepressants are commonly recommended[59,66]
Epidural injections of steroid and local anesthetic are used in selective cases[67]

Box 15
Standard diagnostic criteria for SAPHO syndrome

Local bone pain with gradual onset

Multifocal lesions involving long tubular bones and spine

Failure to culture an infectious microorganism

Neutrophilic skin eruptions (palmoplantar pustulosis, nonpalmoplantar pustulosis, psoriasis vulgaris, or severe acne)

Protracted course for several years, with exacerbations and improvement with antiinflammatory drugs

Data from Schuster T, Bielek J, Dietz HG, et al. Chronic recurrent multifocal osteomyelitis (CRMO). Eur J Pediatr Surg 1996;6(1):45–51.

SUMMARY

Musculoskeletal chest pain can be a cause of significant morbidity and anxiety for a patient. Better understanding of the various causes of musculoskeletal chest pain can help prevent unnecessary testing and anxiety for patients and ensure timely treatment.

REFERENCES

1. National Hospital Ambulatory Medical Care Survey: 2009 Emergency Dept Summary Tables–Table 10. 2009. Available at: http://www.cdc.gov/nchs/data/ahcd/nhamcs_emergency/2009_ed_web_tables.pdf. Accessed February 20, 2013.
2. Stochkendahl MJ, Christensen HW. Chest pain in focal musculoskeletal disorders. Med Clin North Am 2010;94(2):259–73.
3. Fam AG, Smythe HA. Musculoskeletal chest wall pain. Can Med Assoc J 1985;133:379–89.
4. Proulx AM, Zryd TW. Costochondritis: diagnosis and treatment. Am Fam Physician 2009;80(6):617–21.
5. Oho RC, Johnson JD. Chest pain and costochondritis associated with vitamin D deficiency: a report of two cases. Case Rep Med 2012;2012:375730.
6. Muir J, Yelland M. Skin and breast disease in the differential diagnosis of chest pain. Med Clin North Am 2010;94(2):319–25.
7. Verdon F, Burnand B, Herzig L, et al. Chest wall syndrome among primary care patients: a cohort study. BMC Fam Pract 2007;8:51.
8. Rovetta G, Sessarego P, Monteforte P. Stretching exercises for costochondritis pain. G Ital Med Lav Ergon 2009;31(2):169–71.
9. Semble EL, Wise CM. Chest pain: a rheumatologist's perspective. South Med J 1988;81(1):64–8.
10. Kamel M, Kotob H. Ultrasonographic assessment of local steroid injection in Tietze's syndrome. Br J Rheumatol 1997;36:547–50.
11. Habib PA, Huang GS, Mendiola JA, et al. Anterior chest pain: musculoskeletal considerations. Emerg Radiol 2004;11:37–45.
12. Freeston J, Karim Z, Lindsay K, et al. Can early diagnosis and management of costochondritis reduce acute chest pain admissions? J Rheumatol 2004;31:2269–71.
13. Rabey MI. Costochondritis: are the symptoms and signs due to neurogenic inflammation. Two cases that responded to manual therapy directed towards posterior spinal structures. Man Ther 2008;13:82–6.

14. Singer K, Fazey P. Thoracic and chest pain. In: Brukner P, Khan K, editors. Clinical sports medicine. 4th edition. Sydney (Australia): McGraw Medical; 2012. p. 449–62.
15. Karlson KA. Thoracic region pain in athletes. Curr Sports Med Rep 2004;3(1): 53–7.
16. Gregory PL, Biswas AC, Batt ME. Musculoskeletal problems of the chest wall in athletes. Sports Med 2002;32(4):235–50.
17. Sik EC, Batt ME, Heslop LM. Atypical chest pain in athletes. Curr Sports Med Rep 2009;8(2):52–8.
18. Coris EE, Higgins HW. First rib stress fractures in throwing athletes. Am J Sports Med 2005;33(9):1400–4.
19. Dragoni S, Giombini A, Di Cesare A, et al. Stress fractures of the ribs in elite competitive rowers: a report of nine cases. Skeletal Radiol 2007;36(10):951–4.
20. Fu R, Iqbal CW, Jaroszewski DE, et al. Costal cartilage excision for the treatment of pediatric slipping rib syndrome. J Pediatr Surg 2012;47(10):1825–7.
21. Mooney DP, Shorter NA. Slipping rib syndrome in childhood. J Pediatr Surg 1997; 32(7):1081–2.
22. Udermann BE, Cavanaugh DG, Gibson MH, et al. Slipping rib syndrome in a collegiate swimmer: a case report. J Athl Train 2005;40(2):120–2.
23. Heinz GJ III, Zavala DC. Slipping rib syndrome: diagnosis using the "hooking manuever". JAMA 1977;237(8):794–5.
24. Koren W, Shahar A. Xiphodynia masking acute myocardial infarction: a diagnostic cul-de-sac. Am J Emerg Med 1998;16(2):177–8.
25. Hopper MA, Tirman P, Robinson P. Muscle injury of the chest wall and upper extremity. Semin Musculoskelet Radiol 2010;14(2):122–30.
26. Kretzler HH Jr, Richardson AB. Rupture of the pectoralis major muscle. Am J Sports Med 1989;17(4):453–8.
27. Wolfe SW, Wickiewicz TL, Cavanaugh JT. Ruptures of the pectoralis major muscle. An anatomic and clinical analysis. Am J Sports Med 1992;20(5): 587–93.
28. Bak K, Cameron EA, Henderson IJ. Rupture of the pectoralis major: a meta-analysis of 112 cases. Knee Surg Sports Traumatol Arthrosc 2000;8(2):113–9.
29. Hanna CM, Glenny AB, Stanley SN, et al. Pectoralis major tears: comparison of surgical and conservative treatment. Br J Sports Med 2001;35(3):202–6.
30. Rehman A, Robinson P. Sonographic evaluation of injuries to pectoralis muscles. AJR Am J Roentgenol 2005;184(4):1205–11.
31. Humphries D, Jamison M. Clinical and magnetic resonance imaging features of cricket bowler's side strain. Br J Sports Med 2004;38(5):E21.
32. Obaid H, Nealon A, Connell D. Sonographic appearance of side strain injury. AJR Am J Roentgenol 2008;191(6):W264–7.
33. Connell DA, Jhamb A, James T. Side strain: a tear of internal oblique musculature. AJR Am J Roentgenol 2003;191(6):1511–7.
34. Bennett R. Myofascial pain syndromes and their evaluation. Best Pract Res Clin Rheumatol 2007;21(3):427–45.
35. Alvarez DJ, Rockwell PG. Trigger points: diagnosis and management. Am Fam Physician 2002;65(4):653–60.
36. Simons DG, Travell JG, Simons LS. Glossary. In: Travell & Simons' myofascial pain and dysfunction: the trigger point manual, vol. 1, 2nd edition. Baltimore (MD): Williams & Wilkins; 1999. p. 1–10.
37. Simons DG. Understanding effective treatments of myofascial trigger points. J Bodyw Mov Ther 2002;6(2):81–8.

38. Moseley GL. Pain: why and how does it hurt?. In: Brukner P, Khan K, editors. Clinical sports medicine. 4th edition. Sydney (Australia): McGraw-Hill; 2012. p. 41–53.
39. Choi YJ, Choi SU, Shin HW, et al. Chest pain caused by trigger points in the scalenus muscle: a case report. Korean J Anesthesiol 2007;53(5):680–2.
40. Nielsen LA, Henriksson KG. Pathophysiological mechanisms in chronic musculoskeletal pain (fibromyalgia): the role of central and peripheral sensitization and pain disinhibition. Best Pract Res Clin Rheumatol 2007;21(3):465–80.
41. Yunus MB. Role of central sensitization in symptoms beyond muscle pain and the evaluation of a patient with widespread pain. Best Pract Res Clin Rheumatol 2007;21:481–97.
42. Almansa C, Wang B, Achem SR. Noncardiac chest pain and fibromyalgia. Med Clin North Am 2010;94(2):275–89.
43. Moldofsky H. The significance of dysfunctions of the sleeping/waking brain to the pathogenesis and treatment of fibromyalgia syndrome. Rheum Dis Clin North Am 2009;35(2):275–83.
44. Ferrari R. The biopsychosocial model: a tool for rheumatologists. Baillieres Best Pract Res Clin Rheumatol 2000;14:787–95.
45. Crofford LJ, Pillemer SR, Kalogeras KT, et al. Hypothalamic-pituitary-adrenal axis perturbations in patients with fibromyalgia. Arthritis Rheum 1994;37:1583–92.
46. Hollerbach S, Bulat R, May A, et al. Abnormal processing of esophageal stimuli in patients with noncardiac chest pain (NCCP). Neurogastroenterol Motil 2001; 12(6):555–65.
47. Clouse R, Carney RM. The psychological profile of non-cardiac chest pain patients. Eur J Gastroenterol Hepatol 1995;7:1160–5.
48. Wolfe F, Ross K, Anderson J, et al. The prevalence and characteristics of fibromyalgia in the general population. Arthritis Rheum 1995;38(1):19–28.
49. Wolfe F, Smythe HA, Yunus MB, et al. The American College of Rheumatology 1990 criteria for the classification of fibromyalgia. Report of the Multicenter Criteria Committee. Arthritis Rheum 1990;33:160–72.
50. Wolfe F, Clauw D, Fitzcharles MA, et al. Clinical diagnostic and severity criteria for fibromyalgia [abstract]. Arthritis Rheum 2009;60(Suppl 10):S210.
51. Hauser W, Bernardy K, Ucelyer N, et al. Treatment of fibromyalgia syndrome with anti-depressants: a meta-analysis. JAMA 2009;301(2):198–209.
52. Goldenberg DL, Burckhardt C, Crofford L. Management of fibromyalgia syndrome. JAMA 2004;292(19):2388–95.
53. Gumbiner CH. Precordial catch syndrome. South Med J 2003;96(1):38–41.
54. Baranto A, Borjesson M, Danielsson B, et al. Acute chest pain in a top soccer player due to thoracic disc herniation. Spine 2009;34(10):E359–62.
55. Johnson RW. Herpes zoster and postherpetic neuralgia: a review of the effects of vaccination. Aging Clin Exp Res 2009;21(3):236–43.
56. Johnson RW. Zoster associated pain: what is known, who is at risk and how can it be managed? Herpes 2007;14(Suppl 2):30–4.
57. Gilden DH, Dueland AN, Cohrs R, et al. Preherpetic neuralgia. Neurology 1991; 41:1215–8.
58. Jung BF, Johnson RW, Griffin DR, et al. Risk factors for postherpetic neuralgia in a patient with herpes zoster. Neurology 2004;62(9):1545–51.
59. Zareba G. Pregabalin: a new agent for the treatment of neuropathic pain. Drugs Today (Barc) 2005;41(8):509–16.
60. Barrett AP, Katelaris CH, Morris JG, et al. Zoster sine herpete of the trigeminal nerve. Oral Surg Oral Med Oral Pathol 1993;75(2):173–5.

61. Schuchmann JA, McAllister RK, Armstrong CS, et al. Zoster sine herpete with thoracic motor paralysis temporally associated with thoracic epidural steroid injection. Am J Phys Med Rehabil 2008;87(10):853–8.
62. Goh CL, Khoo L. A retrospective study of the clinical presentation and outcome of herpes zoster in a tertiary dermatology outpatient referral clinic. Int J Dermatol 1997;36(9):667–72.
63. Franken RA, Franken M. Pseudo-myocardial infarction during an episode of herpes zoster. Arq Bras Cardiol 2000;75(6):523–30.
64. Morgan R, King D. Characteristics of patients with shingles admitted to a district general hospital. Postgrad Med J 1998;74(868):101–3.
65. Dworkin RH, Johnson RW, Breuer J, et al. Recommendations for the management of herpes zoster. Clin Infect Dis 2007;44(Suppl 1):S1–26.
66. Saarto T, Wiffen PJ. Antidepressants for neuropathic pain. Cochrane Database Syst Rev 2005;(4):CD005454. http://dx.doi.org/10.1002/14651858.CD005454. pub2.
67. Van Wijck AJ, Opstelten W, Moons KG, et al. The PINE study of epidural steroids and local anaesthetics to prevent postherpetic neuralgia: a randomized controlled trial. Lancet 2006;367(9506):219–24.
68. Chamot AM, Benhamou CL, Kahn MF, et al. Acne-pustulosis-hyperostosis-osteitis syndrome. Result of a national survey. 85 cases. Rev Rhum Mal Osteoartic 1987; 54:187–96.
69. Zigang Z, Ying L, Yuanyuan L, et al. Synovitis, acne, pustulosis, hyperostosis and osteitis (SAPHO) syndrome with review of the relevant published work. J Dermatol 2011;38(2):155–9.
70. Grossman ME, Rudin D, Scher R. SAPHO syndrome: report of three cases and of the literature. Cutis 1999;64:253–8.
71. Earwaker JW, Cotton A. SAPHO: syndrome or concept? Imaging findings. Skeletal Radiol 2003;32:311.
72. Hurtado-Nedelec M, Chollet-Martin S, Nicaise-Roland P, et al. Characterization of the immune response in the synovitis, acne, pustulosis, hyperostosis, osteitis (SAPHO) syndrome. Rheumatology 2008;47:1160–7.
73. Schuster T, Bielek J, Dietz HG, et al. Chronic recurrent multifocal osteomyelitis (CRMO). Eur J Pediatr Surg 1996;6(1):45–51.
74. Gupta AK, Skinner AR. A review of the use of infliximab to manage cutaneous dermatoses. J Cutan Med Surg 2004;8:77–89.
75. Robert I, Matthias L, Costakis G, et al. Mechanism of action for leflunomide in rheumatoid arthritis. Clin Immunol 1999;3:198–208.

Practical Approach to Hip Pain

Christopher Karrasch, MD, Scott Lynch, MD*

KEYWORDS

- Hip pain • Labral tear • FAI • Osteoarthritis

KEY POINTS

- Detailed history including age, onset of symptoms, location of pain, history of trauma or overuse, duration of symptoms, rheumatologic conditions, and previous therapy is important in narrowing the differential diagnosis.
- Owing to the high sensitivity and specificity of magnetic resonance imaging (MRI) in detecting common injuries, it has become the modality of choice in diagnosing soft tissue abnormality of the hip, but it must be used with prudence because it may reveal pathologic condition that are asymptomatic and could lead to overtreatment.
- Initial treatment centers on analgesia, nonsteroidal antiinflammatory drugs (NSAIDs), cryotherapy, physical therapy, and, if necessary, a brief period of immobilization.
- Intra-articular anesthetic/cortisone injections can be both diagnostic and therapeutic.
- Timely diagnosis is important because time to operative intervention can have a significant effect on surgical outcomes, patient recovery, and satisfaction.

INTRODUCTION

Musculoskeletal ailments are the presenting complaint in nearly 21.5% of visits in the primary care office[1] and 13.8% of emergency room visits.[2] Diagnosis and treatment of hip pain, especially in young patients, is an evolving field. The differential diagnosis is vast for pain about the hip and can be caused by a wide spectrum of pathologic conditions. Recently, there has been a large focus on the labrum and its associated pathologies, which are usually referred to as femoroacetabular impingement (FAI). Like any new diagnosis, there becomes a rush to attribute any and all unexplained pain to the newly discovered pathologic condition. This rush causes a loss of focus on other potential causes of pain, often to the detriment of the patient. Such has

This article originally appeared in Medical Clinics of North America, Volume 98, Issue 4, July 2014.
Department of Orthopaedic Surgery, Penn State Milton S. Hershey Medical Center, Pennsylvania State University College of Medicine, 30 Hope Drive, Hershey, PA 17033, USA
* Corresponding author. Penn State Hershey Medical Center, Bone and Joint Institute, Pennsylvania State University College of Medicine, 30 Hope Drive, PO Box 859, Hershey, PA 17033.
E-mail address: slynch@hmc.psu.edu

been the case with labral tears and FAI. One must resist this temptation and continue to adhere to the fact that a good history and examination are the cornerstones of diagnosis and thus start from the perspective of a large differential diagnosis. A general diagnostic knowledge of the pathologic condition and overall treatment strategies is paramount to avoid long-term disability and progression of disease caused by a delay in appropriate treatment.

HISTORY

A comprehensive history helps narrow the differential diagnosis. A detailed history should include the following aspects: patient age; onset, nature, and location of pain; referred pain; precipitating or provoking causes; mechanical symptoms (ie, snapping, popping, locking, reduced range of motion); ability to bear weight; history of a traumatic event; congenital or childhood hip deformities; recent alterations in activity level; previous musculoskeletal injuries and/or surgeries; underlying rheumatologic conditions; and systemic symptoms.

Differentiating intra-articular from extra-articular causes of pain is important. Many extra-articular pathologies can be mimickers of hip pain but may not be directly associated with the hip joint itself.[3] Categorizing hip pain makes synthesizing a differential diagnosis more systematic, objective, and accurate. Simply asking a patient to point with 1 finger where the pain is can help guide a differential diagnosis. **Box 1** presents various pathologic conditions categorized into intra-articular, extra-articular, and mimickers that can be presenting causes of hip pain at the clinic.

Patients with intra-articular pathology typically complain of pain in the groin and may have mechanical symptoms such as catching, popping, or clicking.[4] Such patients often have difficulty with torsional or twisting activities, prolonged sitting, and rising from a seated position and greater difficulty on inclined surfaces when compared with level ones.[5-7] An acute change in pain and inability to bear weight should raise concern for more serious hip pathology and prompt an urgent referral to an orthopedist or the emergency room.

PHYSICAL EXAMINATION

Examination of the painful hip can be challenging. Although the literature focuses on many provocative maneuvers for specific pathology, the physical examination should begin with the basics of any musculoskeletal evaluation: observation, palpation, range of motion, motor strength, sensation, vascularity, stability, and provocative maneuvers. As with any musculoskeletal examination, the affected limb should be compared with the unaffected limb.

A systematic approach to the physical examination helps limit undiagnosed pathologic condition.[8] A positional approach in which specific examinations are performed with the patient in standing, seated, supine, lateral, and prone positions has been described by Martin.[9] This approach allows good flow through the examination with less patient discomfort and repetitive positional changes.[10] During an examination, many provocative maneuvers can be performed to assess for intra-articular joint pathology. A single test on its own is not diagnostic, but multiple maneuvers in combination with a thorough history increase the accuracy of a clinical diagnosis.[11]

Standing Position

General overall ligamentous laxity should be assessed. The ability to touch thumbs to the forearm and hyperextend the elbow and knee recurvatum are signs of increased laxity, which predisposes affected individuals to hip instability and pain. The patient's

---

Box 1
Common causes of pain around the hip

Intra-articular

Osteoarthritis

Labral tears

Femoroacetabular impingement

Loose bodies

Chondral lesions

Avascular necrosis

Septic arthritis

Fracture

Ligamentum teres tears

Extra-articular

Trochanteric bursitis

Iliotibial band snapping

Iliopsoas tendonitis/snapping

Piriformis syndrome

Stress fracture

Other non-hip-related causes

Sports hernia

Osteitis pubis

Adductor strain

Abdominal/pelvic viscera

Lumbar radiculopathy

Adapted from Tibor LM, Sekiya JK. Differential diagnosis of pain around the hip joint. Arthroscopy 2008;24:1407–21.

---

gait should be evaluated and any abnormalities as well as the patient's overall mechanical alignment (varus/valgus) should be documented. A limp can be caused by pain, limb length discrepancy, or weakness. A Trendelenburg gait is seen when the patient has weak abductor musculature. The patient compensates by laterally leaning his or her thorax over the affected hip to keep the center of gravity over the stance leg. The Trendelenburg test is performed by asking patients to stand on their affected leg. If the abductors are weak, the pelvis droops to the contralateral side.[12] Patients' pelvis should be assessed for obliquity by placing hands on the iliac crests. The iliac crests should be parallel to the floor, and if not, a block should be placed under the foot of the lower crest to evaluate for limb length discrepancy as the cause for the obliquity. The spine should be assessed and any excessive scoliosis, lordosis, kyphosis, or stiffness should be documented. The sacroiliac joints should be palpated for tenderness.

Seated Position

With the patient in sitting position, the neurologic status, including sensory, motor, and reflexes (**Table 1**); skin; and circulation, should be evaluated.

Table 1
Motor and sensory testing for major peripheral nerves of lower extremity

Nerve	Motor	Sensory
Genitofemoral (L1–L2)	None	Proximal anteromedial thigh
Lateral femoral cutaneous (L2–L3)	None	Lateral thigh (meralgia paresthetica)
Obturator (L2–L4)	Thigh/hip adduction	Inferomedial thigh
Superior gluteal (L5)	Thigh abduction	None
Inferior gluteal (L5–S2)	Hip extension	None
Posterior femoral cutaneous (S1–S3)	None	Posterior part of the thigh
Femoral (L2–L4)	Hip flexion/knee extension	Anteromedial thigh, medial leg and foot (saphenous)
Deep peroneal	Ankle and great toe dorsiflexion	Dorsal first web space
Superficial peroneal	Hindfoot eversion	Dorsal lateral foot
Tibial nerve (L4–S3)	Ankle plantarflexion	Plantar surface foot

Supine Position

An abdominal examination including palpation of all 4 quadrants should be performed to screen for acute visceral pathology that can mimic hip pain such as splenic or liver laceration, appendicitis, pelvic inflammatory disease, hernias, and so forth. Palpation should be done laterally over the greater trochanter, the anterior part of the hip, along the inguinal ligament, and pubis for tenderness as well as warmth and any enlarged lymph nodes. Generally, intra-articular hip pathology is not tender to palpation. Muscular strains, tendinitis, and bursitis are tender. Range of motion, both passive and active, should be assessed (**Table 2**).

The Thomas test assesses for hip flexion contractures and is performed by flexing both hips and allowing the affected lower extremity to extend to lay flat on the table.[13] Normal range of motion allows a patient to lay the leg flat on the table with the other hip flexed. Inability to lay the affected leg flat on the table is a positive result of examination and suggests a hip flexion contracture. A straight leg raise against resistance (Stinchfield test) loads the anterolateral joint and produces intra-articular joint pain. The impingement test is performed by flexing, adducting, and internally rotating the hip. Pain can indicate FAI and labral pathology and has been shown to be sensitive in up to 95% of patients with labral tears.[14] However, it is not very specific, because many other disorders also have pain with this maneuver. The flexion, abduction, and external rotation (FABER) test can elicit pain stemming from the sacroiliac and hip joints. Once in the FABER position, extending, adducting, and internally rotating the leg while palpating the anterior part of the hip may elicit a palpable snap that suggests iliopsoas snapping syndrome.[15]

Table 2
Normal hip range of motion

Flexion (tested supine)	120°–135°
Extension (tested prone)	20°–30°
Abduction/adduction (tested supine)	45°–50°/20°–30°
Internal/external rotation (supine with hip at 90°)	30°/50°

Lateral Position

The greater trochanter should be palpated. If tender, the likely diagnosis is trochanteric bursitis or iliotibial (IT) band pathology. The Ober test is performed by flexing and abducting the hip with the knee at 90° and then extending and adducting the hip.[16] If the lower extremity stays in abduction then the IT band is tight. Snapping of the IT tendon, as it passes over the greater trochanter, may be reproduced by extending and externally rotating the hip from a flexed and internally rotated position.[17] The piriformis syndrome is assessed by adducting and internally rotating the hip putting the piriformis muscle on stretch; this can compress the sciatic nerve, reproduce the posterior part of the hip and thigh pain, and sometimes cause tingling or numbness in the sciatic distribution.[18]

Prone Position

Extension as well as internal/external rotation of the hip should be tested. Ely test is performed by passively flexing the knee. Flexing of the hip suggests a tight rectus femoris muscle.[9]

DIAGNOSTIC TEST/IMAGING

Orthogonal radiographs including anterior/posterior (A/P) radiograph of the pelvis and a cross-table lateral view of the proximal femur are the essential initial imaging studies to evaluate the hip. Radiographs are relatively inexpensive, widely available, and can quickly triage hip complaints that may require immediate treatment by an orthopedic surgeon such as a gross fracture or chronic conditions such as osteoarthritis (OA). The A/P radiograph of the pelvis must be critically evaluated to ensure that it is an appropriate examination. On an appropriately performed pelvic A/P radiograph the coccyx should be in line with and 1 to 2 cm above the pubic symphysis to ensure that there is no inletization or rotation. Radiographs can also screen for FAI. Acetabular retroversion makes the hip prone to acetabular overcoverage (pincer deformity) that can cause impingement and pain.[19] This condition can be seen on the A/P pelvic radiograph as the described crossover or posterior wall sign (**Fig. 1**). However, the A/P radiograph must be appropriate because the crossover or posterior wall sign can be overcalled on a pelvic film that is inletized (**Fig. 2**). Obtaining a false profile view may help to delineate acetabular overcoverage further.[20,21] On the cross-table lateral view, the sphericity of the femoral head can be quantified using the described α-angle (**Fig. 3**).[22] An increased α-angle is seen with an aspherical femoral head (cam lesion), which can predispose patients to impingement, labral tears, and early OA.[6,7,23] Plain radiographs can also evaluate for hip deformities such as hip dysplasia (**Fig. 4**) and slipped capital femoral epiphysis as well as other pathologic conditions such as osteitis pubis (**Fig. 5**), which may be causes of pain around the hip.

Ultrasonography is becoming more readily available and can evaluate both intra- and extra-articular ailments. This modality can be used in real time dynamically to evaluate pathologic conditions such as bursitis, snapping hip, hematoma, hip effusions, paralabral cyst formation, as well as nonhip pathology such as hernias, abscess, tumor, and lymphadenopathy.[24] Ultrasonography predictably provides anatomic verification for injections and/or aspirations and improves accuracy of placement for both intra-articular and extra-articular pathologies.[25–28]

Computed tomographic (CT) scans can be helpful in evaluating the anatomic position and orientation of the acetabulum, and to assess for excess femoral anteversion. Three-dimensional reconstructions can be helpful in surgical planning and in further characterizing acetabular retroversion, but, in general, these are not necessary in

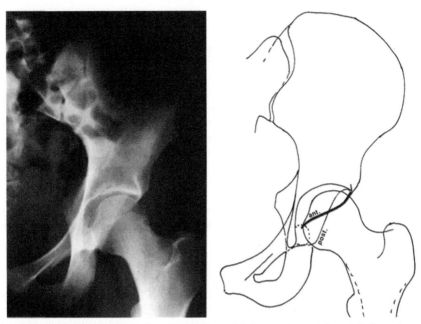

Fig. 1. This is a cropped A/P radiograph of the pelvis in a patient with acetabular retroversion. The crossover or posterior wall sign is outlined.

the primary workup of hip pain. These reconstructions can aid in the diagnosis of occult fractures when a patient is unable to obtain an MRI secondary to a pacemaker, certain cardiac stents, or other pathologic condition that excludes them from the study. MRI has been shown to be superior to CT scans in defining occult and stress fractures about the hip.[29]

MRI of the hip is the most sensitive and specific imaging modality for pathology about the hip. MRI is expensive and should be used with prudence because it can uncover presumed pathologic condition that may be asymptomatic.[30] When prescribing

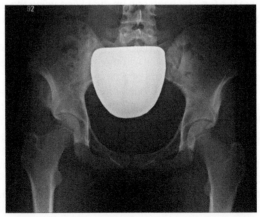

Fig. 2. A/P radiograph of the pelvis that is inletized giving a false sense of a crossover sign, although there is no true acetabular retroversion.

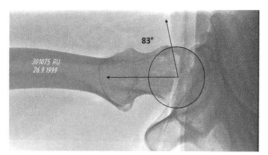

Fig. 3. Cross-table lateral view with a labeled increased α-angle indicating a significant cam lesion and asphericity of the femoral head. Normal α-angle is less than 50° to 55°. MRI of the same hip with concomitant labral tear.

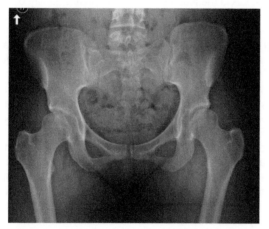

Fig. 4. A/P radiograph of the pelvis demonstrating bilateral hip dysplasia.

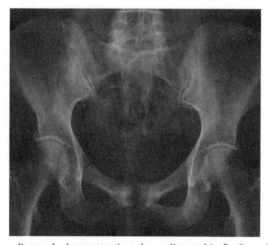

Fig. 5. A/P pelvic radiograph demonstrating the radiographic findings in chronic osteitis pubis with sclerosis and bone remodeling of the pubic symphysis.

an MRI of the hip, it should be ensured that it is an isolated hip MRI and not an MRI of the pelvis because they are vastly different and this mistake can lead to delayed diagnosis as well as increased cost. However, if the clinical diagnosis is more suggestive of adductor strain, osteitis pubis, or sports hernia, an MRI of the pelvis is indicated because an isolated hip MRI may not fully evaluate these pathologic conditions. To rule out intra-articular hip pathology, an MRI with an arthrogram (MRA) can be a powerful tool. When ordering the MRA, patients must be prescribed an intra-articular injection of anesthetic such as bupivacaine and asked to pay particular attention to their pain immediately after the study. Pain relief from the anesthetic has been shown to have a 90% predictability of an intra-articular abnormality.[31]

DIFFERENTIAL DIAGNOSIS/TREATMENT
OA

Of all joint diseases, OA is the leading cause of impaired quality of life, disability, and lost work days in the United States.[32,33] Symptoms are insidious, but may wax and wane in severity, and are felt predominantly in the groin. This condition is the first on the differential for an elderly patient with chronic hip pain. Generally, the pain is exacerbated with activity and improves with rest. Risk factors include female gender, obesity, history of high-demand work (such as farming), high-impact competitive athletics, higher bone density, developmental abnormalities (dysplasia, Legg-Calvé-Perthes disease, slipped capital femoral epiphysis, and FAI), and a family history.[34–40]

The hallmarks on physical examination are decreased passive and active range of motion that is associated with pain. Patients generally lose internal rotation range of motion first. Radiographically, there is joint space narrowing, subchondral sclerosis, and in later disease, bone cysts. Radiographs include weight-bearing A/P pelvic and cross-table lateral views of the proximal femur. These radiographs are to be an adjunct to the history and physical examination while ruling out other conditions. Radiographs should not be relied on independently because radiographic severity does not necessarily correlate with functional disability.[41]

Treatment of OA is based on symptoms, with the goal of pain relief and improved physical function. At present, neither is there any cure for OA nor is there any cartilage regeneration pharmacologics or procedure.[42] Antiinflammatories (NSAIDs) are currently the mainstay of nonoperative management. Patients should be encouraged to stay as active as they can be as well as initiate an exercise program. In a recent meta-analysis of the literature, an approach combining exercises to increase strength, flexibility, and aerobic capacity was significantly more effective in improving limitation in function than a program having no regimented exercise.[43] Intra-articular cortisone injections are effective both therapeutically and diagnostically for those who fail NSAIDs alone. These injections can be administered every 3 to 4 months without a significant increase in cartilage compromise. In the setting of OA once patients have exhausted NSAIDs, physical therapy, and intra-articular cortisone injections, the next step in treatment is a total hip arthroplasty. To obtain the most reliable outcomes, patients should be referred to high-volume surgeons and centers specializing in joint replacement.[44]

Labral Tears

The labrum of the hip is a fibrocartilagenous ring that forms a rim around the articular surface of the acetabulum. Although it has minimal mechanical properties for distributing forces over the articular surface of the acetabulum, it acts as a gasket and creates an important hydraulic seal in the hip joint to provide stability via negative pressure.[45,46] The labrum has neuroreceptors and may have a functional role in proprioception.[47] The blood supply of the labrum is limited to the peripheral ring nearest the acetabulum where healing of repairs can occur.[48] Tears of the labrum can become symptomatic and present with a combination of dull and sharp pain in the groin that is often made worse with activity and prolonged sitting.[14] Activities that cause repetitive loading of the joint, specifically pivoting and hip flexion, increase the risk of labral tears predisposing individuals such as athletes to pathologic condition.[14] Acute subluxations, dislocations, or trauma can cause a tear in the labrum and must be differentiated from labral tears secondary to associated chronic conditions such as dysplasia, FAI, iliopsoas impingement, OA, or acetabular anteversion/retroversion.[49] These secondary tears are thought to be much more common.

On physical examination, maneuvers that assess intra-articular pathology such as log roll, hip range of motion, flexion adduction, and internal rotation reproduce pain in the groin. A/P radiograph of the pelvis and cross-table lateral radiograph are indicated and can help to delineate other pathologies as described above. A hip MRA (**Fig. 6**) is the most sensitive and specific test to diagnose labral tears, approaching 90% and 100%, respectively.[50,51] Patients with a labral tear on MRI who report significant pain relief from the intra-articular anesthetic administered during the test have a significantly increased probability that the labral tear is symptomatic. Hip MRI results must be critically analyzed in conjunction with a clinical history and examination because most labral tears, including those in athletes, are asymptomatic.[30] Nearly all patients older than 70 years have MRI-positive labral pathology that is degenerative in nature and related to degenerative arthritis and age.[52]

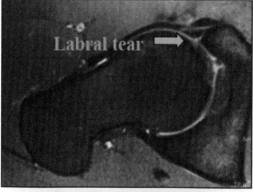

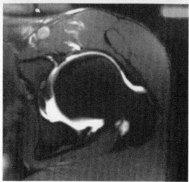

Fig. 6. MRI with intra-articular gadolinium of the hip depicting an anterior labral tear.

Treatment begins with conservative measures including NSAIDs, activity modification, physical therapy, and intra-articular cortisone injections. Once conservative therapy has failed, open versus arthroscopic surgical intervention may be indicated, including labral repair or debridement (**Fig. 7**). Clinical improvement in hip symptoms after surgery has been reported from 68% to 82% in the literature.[5,53,54]

FAI

In normal hip anatomy, the acetabulum and proximal femur articulate without abutment or impingement through a physiologic range of motion. FAI occurs when there is abnormal anatomy of the acetabulum and/or femoral head-neck junction that results in abnormal contact between the two. On the acetabular side, this abnormal contact is a result of acetabular overcoverage of the proximal femur and is termed pincer impingement. This impingement can be caused by a deep acetabulum (coxa profunda), or anterior overcoverage due to acetabular retroversion. A normal femoral head-neck junction is spherical. An aspherical femoral head-neck junction can lead to abutment at the end ranges of hip motion and is termed cam impingement. An aspherical femoral head-neck junction can be caused by various pathologic conditions including slipped capital femoral epiphysis, malunion or malreduced femoral neck fractures, femoral retroversion, and coxa vara. Most frequently, the aspherical portion of the femur is the anterolateral head-neck junction.[55] Although these 2 types of FAI have been described as separate entities, often patients have a combination of both. These nonanatomic relationships leading to impingement can cause pain, decreased range of motion, labral tears, chondral defects of the acetabulum, and eventual OA.[6,7]

Patients are generally young to middle aged and present with pain in the groin provoked by activity. Pain comes on insidiously and often is present for months to years. Prolonged sitting, movements requiring flexion and internal rotation such as getting in and out of cars, and getting up from seated positions often cause pain.[55]

On physical examination, a straight leg raise against resistance loads the anterolateral joint and produces intra-articular joint pain. Pain with the impingement test (flexion, adduction, and internal rotation) can indicate FAI.

Radiographic evaluation to assess for FAI includes an A/P view, a cross-table lateral view with the hip internally rotated 15° (see **Fig. 3**), and in some cases, a false profile

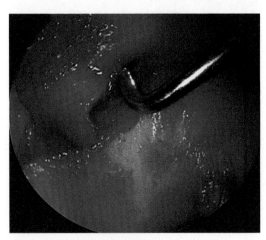

Fig. 7. Arthroscopic hip procedure demonstrating a labral tear.

view (**Fig. 8**).[56] The A/P view evaluates for acetabular overcoverage (pincer), and the cross-table lateral view evaluates for asphericity of the femoral head-neck junction (cam). The α-angle is measured off the lateral view by fitting a best fit circle to the femoral head. Then a point in the circle is centered and an angle is created from the femoral shaft to the leading edge of asphericity that deviates from the best fit circle (see **Fig. 3**). A normal α-angle is less than 50° to 55°, and an angle greater than this is considered a cam lesion. An α-angle greater than 65° is associated with a higher incidence of chondral defects.[57] On the A/P film, a crossover or posterior wall sign can be seen when the acetabulum is retroverted (see **Fig. 1**). Normally the shadows of the posterior and anterior acetabular walls do not cross. A crossover or posterior wall sign indicates anterosuperior acetabular overcoverage.[19] An MRI can further delineate FAI as well as evaluate for concomitant chondral lesions, labral tears, or other intra-articular pathology.

Treatment of FAI includes NSAIDs, activity modification, physical therapy, and, if necessary, intra-articular cortisone injections. When conservative measures fail, surgical intervention may be warranted, which can be done through an open procedure (**Fig. 9**) or an arthroscopic procedure, with both yielding good results. With recent arthroscopic technology and technique advancements, arthroscopic acetabular osteoplasty and femoral head-neck resection has become the treatment of choice in most cases.

Snapping Hip

The painful snapping hip (coxa saltans) can be difficult to diagnose and treat.[58] The condition can be systematically categorized into intra-articular (labral tears, loose bodies, chondral defects, etc), internal (iliopsoas snapping), and external (IT band snapping). Differentiating the location of the condition is predicated on a thorough history, physical examination, and diagnostic imaging.

External snapping is caused by a thickened or tight IT band snapping over the greater trochanter of the proximal femur. More often than not, the snapping is

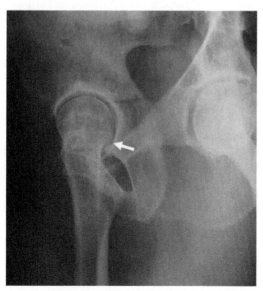

Fig. 8. False profile view of the hip depicting acetabular overcoverage or pincer deformity. Arrow pointing to associated posterior inferior joint space narrowing.

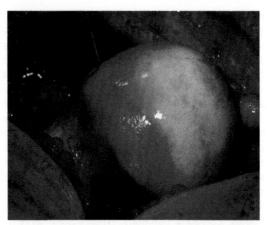

Fig. 9. Open surgical dislocation of the hip demonstrating an aspherical femoral head or cam deformity. The femoral head is more mushroom shaped compared to the normal, which is spherical.

nonpainful. In symptomatic cases, it is often associated with trochanteric bursitis.[59] Most often it is found in middle-aged women or running athletes. The thickened posterior portion of the IT band snaps over the greater trochanter from posterior to anterior when the hip goes from an extended to a flexed position. This snapping can be painful when the bursa is inflamed. Patients often have pain over the greater trochanter that radiates down the lateral thigh and have difficulty sleeping on the affected side. Patients often complain of the feeling that their hip is giving out.

On examination the patient may be able to reproduce the snapping actively, and this may be palpated or observed grossly. The patient has pain with palpation of the greater trochanter if the bursa is inflamed. If the patient is unable to reproduce the snapping, the IT tendon may be palpated as it passes over the greater trochanter during active hip motion. This palpation is done by starting the hip flexed and internally rotated, and then extending and externally rotating the leg.[17] IT band tightness should be assessed with the Ober test by flexing and abducting the hip with the knee at 90° and then extending and adducting the hip.[16] If the lower extremity stays in abduction then the IT band is tight.

Newer advances in ultrasonographic techniques have made it the imaging modality of choice if the clinical examination is unclear. Sometimes IT band snapping can be seen dynamically during an ultrasonography, providing a definitive diagnosis.

The mainstay of treatment is antiinflammatory medications, physical therapy for stretching of the IT band, and if necessary, corticosteroid injections. This treatment resolves symptoms in most cases, but for those who fail conservative treatment referral to an orthopedic surgeon is warranted. Historically, an open surgery has been performed to create tendon relaxing incisions in the IT band over the greater trochanter. It is important that surgery maintains the structural integrity of the abductor mechanism or patients can have abductor weakness that can affect their gait.[60] More recently, endoscopic techniques have been developed with similar good results in eliminating external snapping in most cases.[61]

Internal snapping of the hip is caused by the iliopsoas tendon snapping over the femoral/acetabular capsule or more commonly over the pectineal eminence of the pelvis. The iliopsoas is a powerful hip flexor formed by the confluence of the iliacus and psoas muscles that inserts on the lesser trochanter of the femur. Approximately

10% of the active population has asymptomatic snapping of the iliopsoas tendon. Painful snapping is a sign of either acute iliopsoas tendonitis or more chronic tendinopathy. Such snapping may be caused by repetitive microtrauma, and is seen with a higher incidence in runners, athletes, and elite ballet dancers.[17,62] Patients complain of clicking/popping that can be audible and is felt in the anterior region of the groin. Because the psoas muscle originates from the back, patients often concomitantly complain of low-back pain.[63]

On physical examination, the patient may be able to actively re-create the snapping. Passively the snapping is best evaluated in the supine position by taking the hip from a flexed, abducted, and externally rotated position down to an extended and internally rotated position while palpating over the anterior part of the groin. The snap of the iliopsoas tendon may be grossly palpable, very subtle, or not felt at all with the patient simply feeling an internal snap.

Dynamic ultrasonography is the imaging modality of choice and can be both diagnostic and a means for a therapeutic/diagnostic injection.

Treatment consists of NSAIDs, physical therapy, and if needed, corticosteroid injections. Response to an injection provides improved predictability that surgical intervention will be successful in patients who fail conservative measures.[64] Arthroscopic iliopsoas tendon release has become the surgical treatment of choice secondary to the minimally invasive approach and addresses associated intra-articular pathology.

Pubalgia

A wide spectrum of conditions can lead to pubic pain, including orthopedic (sports hernia, osteitis pubis, adductor strains, etc) as well as nonorthopedic (true hernias, genitourinary pathology, endometriosis, pelvic inflammatory disease, abdominal strains, etc) pathologies. A thorough knowledge of the pelvic anatomy is important in making the diagnosis.

Sports hernia is caused by a tear in the inguinal floor that does not result in a clinically obvious hernia but results in chronic groin pain.[65] Various injury mechanisms have been described, from simultaneous trunk hyperextension and thigh hyperabduction, which causes shearing forces, to muscular imbalances between strong thigh muscles and a concomitantly week abdominal core.[3] Athletes who participate in sports requiring repetitive twisting and torque of the proximal thigh and lower abdominal musculature (hockey, soccer, rugby, etc) are at a higher risk of occurrence.[65] The pain comes on insidiously and often radiates into the adductors, perineum, inguinal ligament, or testicular area and can be provoked by sudden movements such as sprints, quick cuts, sit-ups, or even coughing and sneezing.[3] Periods of rest typically improve symptoms.

On examination there is no appreciable hernia, but tenderness may be elicited around the conjoined tendon, pubic tubercle, external inguinal ring, or posterior inguinal canal. Having the patient perform a Valsalva maneuver may reproduce the pain.

Osteitis pubis is on a continuum with sports hernia and develops when there are increased forces on the symphysis pubis, which can be from repetitive stresses and/or the pull of pelvic musculature. Patients have specific pain located over the pubic symphysis and are generally tender over the symphysis on examination.

Adductor strains/sprains are the most common traumatic causes of groin pain in athletes, with a higher incidence in soccer and ice hockey players.[66] The pain is usually acute, in the groin, and patients can often recall a specific time or incident when the pain started. The acuity may help to differentiate this from a sports hernia and osteitis pubis, which have a more insidious onset. On examination, patients report tenderness to palpation along the adductor complex and have pain with resisted adduction.

Radiographic evaluation in pubalgia can be helpful to rule out fractures or avulsions and can establish a diagnosis of chronic osteitis pubis when the classic bone resorption, irregular contour, and widening of the pubic symphysis is seen (see **Fig. 5**). If there is doubt in diagnosis, an MRI of the pelvis is the most sensitive and specific imaging modality. Patients with athletic pubalgia (sports hernia) often have a secondary cleft sign near the pubic symphysis on MRI (**Fig. 10**).

Treatment of all pubalgia starts with activity modification, NSAIDs, and physical therapy. Treatment of acute adductor strains begins with rest, ice, and compression until the pain is improved. The second step is a regimen focused on range of motion. Once pain-free range of motion is obtained, the patient is advanced to regaining strength, flexibility, and endurance. Osteitis pubis is generally self-limiting, and its treatment should be done following the same protocol as for an adductor strain. True sports hernias may not respond to nonoperative treatment. Surgical intervention for unresolved sports hernias includes repair of the abdominal musculature, inguinal ligament, and its attachments. Historically this has been done either in an open manner or laproscopically using the patient's native tissue. Advances in synthetic materials and technology have produced light-weight mesh that allows both anterior and posterior repairs that allow normalization of the torn anatomy. This technique has been studied and yields excellent results in pain improvement, mobility, and return to previous activities.[67]

Stress Fractures

Stress fractures that can cause hip pain are relatively common in runners and highly competitive athletes. The treatment of stress fractures depends on their location. Most can be treated nonoperatively with activity modification and protected weight bearing. Some specific fractures with a history of poor healing may require surgery. Many patients have a history of a recent increase in activity such as a long run, competition, starting a new season of sport, increase in training, etc. The pain is worse with weight bearing and improves with rest and time.

On examination, the only positive feature may be pain with weight bearing and an altered gait. Patients may have tenderness to palpation over the area, but this may be unreliable.

Radiographs can show evidence of a fracture if it has been chronic with associated sclerosis or bone remodeling in the area of the stress fracture. However, in the early stages of stress fractures, radiographs may have only a 10% sensitivity and are often

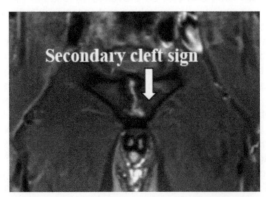

Fig. 10. MRI of the pelvis in the setting of athletic pubalgia with the arrow indicating the secondary cleft sign often seen in the chronic setting.

read as normal.[3,68,69] MRI has been shown to be more reliable than CT scans and is the most sensitive and specific for stress fractures.[29]

Stress fractures of the pubic bones can be treated with activity modification and weight bearing as tolerated. Fractures of the femoral neck are treated with protected weight bearing or surgery depending on their location. If the fracture is on the compression side of the femur during weight bearing (inferior neck), it can be treated with protected weight bearing and has a low incidence of displacement. If the fracture is on the tension side of the femoral neck during weight bearing (superior neck), it has a high incidence of displacement and requires surgical fixation. Displaced femoral neck fractures have a significant incidence of going on to develop avascular necrosis of the femoral head with eventual collapse, arthritis, and probable need for a total hip arthroplasty.

SUMMARY

Hip pain is a common complaint among patients presenting to outpatient clinics. Stratifying patients based on age, acuity, and location (extra-articular vs intra-articular) can help to aid in appropriate imaging and timely referral to an orthopedic surgeon. A thorough history and an organized physical examination combined with radiographs are usually sufficient to diagnose most hip complaints. If the diagnosis remains uncertain, MRI, usually with intra-articular gadolinium, is the imaging modality of choice in diagnosing both intra-articular and extra-articular pathologies.

REFERENCES

1. Månsson J, Nilsson G, Strender LE, et al. Reasons for encounters, investigations, referrals, diagnoses and treatments in general practice in Sweden–a multicentre pilot study using electronic patient records. Eur J Gen Pract 2011;17(2):87–94.
2. McCaig LF, Nawar EW. National Hospital Ambulatory Medical Care Survey: 2004 emergency department summary. Adv Data 2006;(372):1–29.
3. Tibor LM, Sekiya JK. Differential diagnosis of pain around the hip joint. Arthroscopy 2008;24:1407–21.
4. Carreira D, Bush-Joseph CA. Hip arthroscopy. Orthopedics 2006;29:517–23.
5. Byrd JW, Jones KS. Prospective analysis of hip arthroscopy with two year follow up. Arthroscopy 2000;16:578–87.
6. Beck M, Kalhor M, Leunig M, et al. Hip morphology influences the pattern of damage to the acetabular cartilage: femoracetabular impingement as a cause of early osteoarthritis of the hip. J Bone Joint Surg Br 2005;87:1012–8.
7. Ganz R, Parvizi J, Beck M, et al. Femoroacetabular impingement: a cause for osteoarthritis of the hip. Clin Orthop Relat Res 2003;(417):112–20.
8. Shindle M, Voos J, Nho S, et al. Arthroscopic management of labral tears in the hip. J Bone Joint Surg Am 2008;90:2–19.
9. Martin HD. Clinical examination of the hip. Oper Tech Orthop 2005;15:177–81.
10. Braly BA, Beall DP, Martin HD. Clinical examination of the athletic hip. Clin Sports Med 2006;25:199–210.
11. Maslowski E, Sullivan W, Forster-Harwood J, et al. The diagnostic validity of hip provocation maneuvers to detect intra-articular hip pathology. PM R 2010;2: 174–81.
12. Hardcastle P, Nade S. The significance of the Trendelenburg test. J Bone Joint Surg Br 1985;67:741–6.
13. Hoppenfeld S. Physical examination of the spine and extremities. New York: Appleton-Century-Crofts; 1976. p. 143 Physical examination of the hip and pelvis.

14. Burnett RS, Della Rocca GJ, Prather H, et al. Clinical presentation of patients with tears of the acetabular labrum. J Bone Joint Surg Am 2006;88:1448–57.
15. Ilizaliturri V, Villalobos F, Chaidez P, et al. Internal snapping hip syndrome: treatment by endoscopic release of the iliopsoas tendon. Arthroscopy 2005;21: 1375–80.
16. Farr D, Selesnick H, Janecki C, et al. Arthroscopic bursectomy with concomitant iliotibial band release for the treatment of recalcitrant trochanteric bursitis. Arthroscopy 2007;23:905.
17. Winston P, Awan R, Cassidy J, et al. Clinical examination and ultrasound of self-reported snapping hip syndrome in elite ballet dancers. Am J Sports Med 2007; 35:118–26.
18. Windisch G, Braun EM, Anderhuber F. Piriformis muscle: clinical anatomy and consideration of the piriformis syndrome. Surg Radiol Anat 2007;29:37–45.
19. Reynolds D, Lucac J, Klaue K. Retroversion of the acetabulum. A cause of hip pain. J Bone Joint Surg Br 1999;81:281–8.
20. Lequesne M, De Seze S. False profile of the pelvis, a new radiographic incidence for the study of the hip. Its use in dysplasias and different coxopathies. Rev Rhum Mal Osteoartic 1961;28:643–52.
21. Chosa E, Tajima N. Anterior acetabular head index of the hip on false-profile views. New index of anterior acetabular cover. J Bone Joint Surg Br 2003;85: 826–9.
22. Nötzli H, Wyss T, Stöcklin C, et al. The contour of the femoral head-neck-junction as a predictor for the risk of anterior impingement. J Bone Joint Surg Br 2002;84: 556–60.
23. Eijer H, Leunig M, Mahomed M, et al. Crosstable lateral radiograph for screening of anterior femoral head-neck offset in patients with femoro-acetabular impingement. Hip Int 2001;11:37–41.
24. Cho K, Park B, Yeon K. Ultrasound of the adult hip. Semin Ultrasound CT MR 2000;21:214–30.
25. Micu MC, Bogdan GD, Fodor D. Steroid injection for hip osteoarthritis: efficacy under ultrasound guidance. Rheumatology 2010;49:1490–4.
26. Sofka CM, Collins AJ, Adler RS. Use of ultrasonographic guidance in interventional musculoskeletal procedures: a review from a single institution. J Ultrasound Med 2001;20:21–6.
27. Rowbotham E, Grainger A. Ultrasound-guided intervention around the hip joint. AJR Am J Roentgenol 2011;197:122–7.
28. Gilliland CA, Salazar LD, Borchers JR. Ultrasound versus anatomic guidance for intra-articular and periarticular injection: a systematic review. Phys Sportsmed 2011;39:121–31.
29. Chatha H, Ullah S, Cheema Z. Review article: magnetic resonance imaging and computed tomography in the diagnosis of occult proximal femur fractures. J Orthop Surg (Hong Kong) 2011;19:99–103.
30. Silvis M, Mosher T, Smetana B, et al. High prevalence of pelvic and hip magnetic resonance imaging findings in asymptomatic collegiate and professional hockey players. Am J Sports Med 2011;39:715–21.
31. Byrd JW, Jones KS. Diagnostic accuracy of clinical assessment, magnetic resonance imaging, magnetic resonance arthrography, and intra-articular injection in hip arthroscopy patients. Am J Sports Med 2004;32:1668–74.
32. Centers for Disease Control and Prevention (CDC). Prevalence of disabilities and associated health conditions among adults: United States, 1999. MMWR Morb Mortal Wkly Rep 2001;50:120–5.

33. Hootman J, Bolen J, Helmick C, et al. Prevalence of doctor-diagnosed arthritis and arthritis attributable activity limitation-United States, 2003-2005. MMWR Morb Mortal Wkly Rep 2006;55:1089–92.

34. Ganz R, Leunig M, Leunig-Ganz K, et al. The etiology of osteoarthritis of the hip: an integrated mechanical concept. Clin Orthop Relat Res 2008;466:264–72.

35. Gabay O, Hall D, Berenbaum F, et al. Osteoarthritis and obesity. Experimental models. Joint Bone Spine 2008;75:675–9.

36. Spector R, Harris P, Hart D, et al. Risk of osteoarthritis associated with long-term weight-bearing sports: a radiologic survey of the hips and knees in female ex-athletes and population controls. Arthritis Rheum 1996;39:988–95.

37. Cheng Y, Macera C, Davis D, et al. Physical activity and self-reported, physician-diagnosed osteoarthritis: is physical activity a risk factor. J Clin Epidemiol 2000; 53:315–22.

38. Hochber M, Lethbridge-Cejku M, Tobin J. Bone mineral density and osteoarthritis: data from the Baltimore longitudinal study of aging. Osteoarthritis Cartilage 2004; 12:S45–8.

39. Bos S, Slagboom P, Meulenbelt I. New Insights into osteoarthritis: early developmental features of an ageing-related disease. Curr Opin Rheumatol 2008;20: 553–9.

40. Baldes A, Spector T. The contribution of genes to osteoarthritis. Rheum Dis Clin North Am 2008;34:581–603.

41. Hunter D, McDougall J, Keefe F. The symptoms of osteoarthritis and the genesis of pain. Rheum Dis Clin North Am 2008;34:623–43.

42. Steinert A, Nöth U, Tuan R. Concepts in gene therapy for cartilage repair. Injury 2008;39:97–113.

43. Uthman OA, van der Windt DA, Jordan JL, et al. Exercise for lower limb osteoarthritis: systematic review incorporating trial sequential analysis and network meta-analysis. BMJ 2013;347:5555.

44. Katz J, Losina E, Barrett J, et al. Association between hospital and surgeon procedure volume and outcomes of total hip replacement in the United States medicare population. J Bone Joint Surg Am 2001;83:1622–9.

45. Konrath F, Hamel A, Olson S, et al. The role of the acetabular labrum and the transverse acetabular ligament in load transmission in the hip. J Bone Joint Surg Am 1998;80:1781–8.

46. Ferguson S, Bryant J, Ganz R, et al. The acetabular labrum seal: poroelastic finite element model. Clin Biomech 2000;15:463–8.

47. Kim YT, Azuma H. The nerve endings of the acetabular labrum. Clin Orthop Relat Res 1995;(320):176–81.

48. Kelly BT, Shapiro GS, Digiovanni CW, et al. Vascularity of the hip labrum: a cadaveric investigation. Arthroscopy 2005;21:3–11.

49. Robertson WJ, Kadrmas WR, Kelly BT. Arthroscopic management of labral tears in the hip: a systematic review. Clin Orthop Relat Res 2006;455:88–92.

50. Toomayan GA, Holman WR, Major NM, et al. Sensitivity of MR arthrography in the evaluation of acetabular labral tears. AJR Am J Roentgenol 2006;186:449–53.

51. Freedman BA, Potter BK, Dinauer PA, et al. Prognostic value of magnetic resonance arthrography for Czerny stage II and III acetabular labral tears. Arthroscopy 2006;22:742–7.

52. McCarthy J, Noble P, Schuck M, et al. The watershed labral lesion: its relationship to early arthritis of the hip. J Arthroplasty 2001;16:81–7.

53. Farjo LA, Glick JM, Sampson TG. Hip arthroscopy for acetabular labrum tears. Arthroscopy 1999;15:132–7.

54. Santori N, Villar RN. Acetabular labral tears: results of arthroscopic partial limbectomy. Arthroscopy 2000;16:11–5.
55. Larson CM, Stone RM. Arthroscopic Management of Femoroacetabular Impingement. In: Wiesel S. Operative Techniques in Orthopaedic Surgery. Philadelphia: Lippincott Williams & Wilkins; 2011:1(26):213–21.
56. Tannast M, Siebenrock KA. Conventional radiographs to assess femoroacetabular impingement. Instr Course Lect 2009;58:203–12.
57. Beaulé PE, Hynes K, Parker G, et al. Can the alpha angle assessment of cam impingement predict acetabular cartilage delamination? Clin Orthop Relat Res 2012;470:3361–7.
58. Allen WC, Cope R. Coxa saltans: the snapping hip revisited. J Am Acad Orthop Surg 1995;3:303–8.
59. Baker CL, Massie V, Hurt WG, et al. Arthroscopic bursectomy for recalcitrant trochanteric bursitis. Arthroscopy 2007;23:827–32.
60. Byrd JW. Snapping hip. Oper Tech Sports Med 2005;13:46–54.
61. Ilizaliturri VM Jr, Villalobos FE Jr, Chaidez PA, et al. Endoscopic iliotibial band release for external snapping hip syndrome. Arthroscopy 2006;22:505–10.
62. Hölmich P. Long-standing groin pain in sportspeople falls into three primary patterns, a "clinical entity" approach: a prospective study of 207 patients. Br J Sports Med 2007;41:247–52.
63. Little TL, Mansoor J. Low back pain associated with internal snapping hip syndrome in a competitive cyclist. Br J Sports Med 2008;42:308–9.
64. Flanum ME, Keene JS, Blankenbaker DG, et al. Arthroscopic treatment of the painful "internal" snapping hip: results of a new endoscopic technique and imaging protocol. Am J Sports Med 2007;35:770–9.
65. Farber AJ, Wilckens JH. Sports hernia: diagnosis and therapeutic approach. J Am Acad Orthop Surg 2007;15:507–14.
66. Schilders E, Bismil Q, Robinson P, et al. Adductor-related groin pain in competitive athletes. J Bone Joint Surg Am 2007;89:2173–8.
67. Meyers WC, Foley DP, Garrett WE, et al. Management of severe lower abdominal or inguinal pain in high-performance athletes. Am J Sports Med 2000;28:2–8.
68. Mattila VM, Niva M, Kiuru M, et al. Risk factors for bone stress injuries: a follow-up study of 102,515 person years. Med Sci Sports Exerc 2007;39:1061–6.
69. Niva MH, Kiuru MJ, Haataja R, et al. Fatigue injuries of the femur. J Bone Joint Surg Br 2005;87:1385–90.

Anterior Knee Pain in the Athlete

Laurie Anne Hiemstra, MD, PhD, FRCSC[a,b,*], Sarah Kerslake[a,c],
Christopher Irving, MD[a]

KEYWORDS

- Anterior knee pain • Patellofemoral pain • Muscle strength • Quadriceps
- Patellofemoral kinematics

KEY POINTS

- Anterior knee pain has a multifactorial etiology.
- Routine clinical assessment of muscle strength in athletes may not detect deficits, so more challenging functional tests may be required.
- Nonoperative treatment is successful in most cases.
- Strong evidence supports treatment with multimodal physiotherapy.

INTRODUCTION

Anterior knee pain (AKP) is very common, affecting 1 in 4 athletes, 70% of whom are between 16 and 25 years old.[1,2] Considering that the patellofemoral joint is one of the most highly loaded joints in the human body,[3] the prevalence of AKP is not surprising. Athletes with AKP present a significant diagnostic and therapeutic challenge for the sport medicine caregiver. A clear understanding of the etiology of patellofemoral pain in this population is essential in guiding a focused history and physical examination, and achieving appropriate diagnosis and treatment.

The purpose of this clinical review is to provide an assessment framework and a guide for neuromuscular function testing, in addition to an overview of the causes and treatments of AKP in this challenging patient population.

SYMPTOMS

Patients with AKP complain of a variety of symptoms including pain, swelling, weakness, instability, mechanical symptoms, and functional impairment. Pain results from

This article originally appeared in Clinics in Sports Medicine, Volume 33, Issue 3, July 2014.
Disclosures: Dr L.A. Hiemstra is a paid consultant for Conmed Linvatec. Banff Sport Medicine receives unrestricted research support from Conmed Linvatec, Centric Health, Genzyme.
[a] Banff Sport Medicine, PO Box 1300, Banff, Alberta T1L 1B3, Canada; [b] Department of Surgery, University of Calgary, 3330 Hospital Drive NW, Calgary, Alberta T2N 4N1, Canada; [c] Department of Physical Therapy, University of Alberta, 8205 114 Street, Edmonton, Alberta T6G 2G4, Canada
* Corresponding author. Banff Sport Medicine, PO Box 1300, Banff, Alberta T1L 1B3, Canada.
E-mail address: hiemstra@banffsportmed.ca

Clinics Collections 4 (2014) 273–295
http://dx.doi.org/10.1016/j.ccol.2014.10.017
2352-7986/14/$ – see front matter © 2014 Elsevier Inc. All rights reserved.

activities that load the patellofemoral joint, such as climbing up or down stairs, squatting, kneeling, and prolonged flexion of the knee joint.[4]

DIAGNOSTIC IMAGING

Diagnostic imaging including anteroposterior, true lateral, and skyline views should be obtained in all patients with refractory AKP. Computed tomography, magnetic resonance imaging (MRI), or ultrasonography should be considered when the history and physical examination determine that further imaging is required.

Table 1
Example clinical screening and advanced functional screening tests to assess neuromuscular control and strength in athletes presenting with AKP

Basic Strength and Muscle Length	Assessment	Example
Knee extensor strength	Assess in sitting with resistance at ankle and palpation of muscle tone. Can also be assessed as resisted straight leg raise in supine Monitor for lateral deviation of thigh, hip flexion, and/or trunk rotation due to muscle weakness or altered activation patterns[6]	
Hip abductor strength	Assess in side-lying with pelvis stabilized in mid-line and resistance above knee Monitor for hip and/or trunk flexion due to weakness or altered muscle activation patterns[7]	
Hip external rotation strength	Assess in supine with both the hip and knee flexed to 90°. Resist rotation at knee and ankle Monitor for hip flexion and/or poor through-range strength	
Quadriceps muscle flexibility	Assess in prone position with pelvis stabilized while examiner flexes knee. Compare heel with buttock distance Monitor for hip flexion, hip or thigh rotation to attain length[7]	

(continued on next page)

Table 1 (continued)			
Advanced Neuromuscular Lower Limb and Core Control	Assessment	Correct Neuromuscular Control	Poor Neuromuscular Control
Single-leg squat	Tests for core, gluteal, and quadriceps strength and control. Assess depth of squat, dynamic valgus, side flexion of trunk, and pain[8]		
Hop down	Instruct patient to stand on one leg and then hop off step to land 10–15 cm in front of step. Assess quality of movement, and evidence of dynamic valgus, hip drop, or rotation due to poor gluteal and/or core strength, lateral flexion of trunk, etc		
Balance	On BOSU ball or foam block, patient balances for up to 30 s. Compare movement quality, range of motion outside base of support, dynamic valgus, hip drop or rotation, lateral trunk flexion, etc		
Active hip extension	Patient instructed to lift leg 5–10 cm off bed while lying prone. Palpate gluteal and hamstring muscle activation; ideally gluteals should fire first. Assess for excessive motion, use of lumbar lordosis to achieve lift, altered timing of hamstrings and gluteal firing, and hip or trunk flexion		

Patients should be assessed bilaterally to compare limbs and monitor for any aggravation of symptoms.

TREATMENT PRINCIPLES

In all patients who present with AKP, a comprehensive knee, hip, and lower extremity evaluation including assessment of alignment, range of motion (ROM), lower limb and core strength, and functional movement patterns should be completed. Based on these findings, the combination of nonoperative therapy chosen should be selected using best clinical judgment. Nonoperative therapy includes relative rest, controlling inflammation, stimulating the healing response, and correcting biomechanics and neuromuscular control (Table 1).

Relative Rest and Activity Modification

Dye[5,6] challenged the way clinicians view the patellofemoral joint with his theory of the "envelope of function" to describe the pathophysiology of pain in patients with patellofemoral pain without overt abnormality. Dye portrays AKP as the loss of homeostasis of the tissues about the knee, with excessive mechanical overload exceeding the ability of the joint to repair itself in comparison with a homeostatic pain-free environment (**Fig. 1**). In an acute injury, relative rest will allow the tissue to heal and the symptoms will decrease. In more chronic cases, the physiologic responses to overload may cause daily activities to exceed the patient's pain threshold. This scenario represents a substantial therapeutic challenge, and requires significant patient education to rehabilitate the joint with pain-free loading.

The concept of the envelope of function includes 4 zones: disuse, homeostasis, overuse, and structural failure. Dye[5,6] proposed that all joints and musculoskeletal tissues respond to differential loading in one of these 4 zones. The outer limit of the homeostasis zone defines the envelope of function of the joint. The goal of treatment is to maximize the envelope of function as safely and predictably as possible.

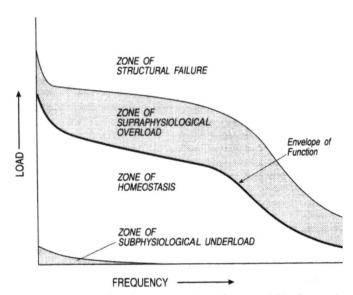

Fig. 1. The 4 different zones of loading across a joint. The area within the envelope of function is the zone of homeostasis. The region of loading greater than that within the envelope of function but insufficient to cause macrostructural damage is the zone of supraphysiologic overload. The region of loading great enough to cause macrostructural damage is the zone of structural failure. The region of decreased loading over time resulting in a loss of tissue homeostasis is the zone of subphysiologic underload. (*From* Dye SF. The pathophysiology of patellofemoral pain: a tissue homeostasis perspective. Clin Orthop Relat Res 2005;436:104; with permission.)

Methods to Control Inflammation

Cryotherapy

Ice packs and cold-therapy units are frequently recommended to athletes to reduce pain and inflammation secondary to AKP. Research has demonstrated the effectiveness of cryotherapy for reducing the internal temperature of the knee joint; however randomized controlled trials (RCTs) specific to AKP are lacking.[7,8] Park and Ty Hopkins[9] used an AKP model to demonstrate that cryotherapy produced a statistically significant reduction in pain. Cold therapy can also decrease the level of prostaglandins in the synovial tissue resulting in decreased inflammation,[10] reduce arthrogenic muscle inhibition caused by swelling,[11] and may facilitate vastus medialis motor neuron activity.[12] Cryotherapy may enable more effective quadriceps strengthening in patients with knee joint abnormality; therefore, despite the current lack of clear research evidence, cryotherapy is recommended as a mainstay of the conservative treatment of AKP.

Anti-inflammatories and analgesics

Medication treatments for AKP commonly include the use of analgesics such as aspirin or acetaminophen, and nonsteroidal anti-inflammatory drugs (NSAIDs). A Cochrane review of pharmacologic treatments for patellofemoral pain found no significant differences in clinical symptoms comparing aspirin with placebo, and limited evidence for the effectiveness of NSAIDs for short-term pain reduction.[13] Another Cochrane review assessing chronic musculoskeletal pain found that topical NSAIDs provided good pain relief, with no difference in efficacy between topical and oral NSAIDs.[14] The use of NSAIDs is controversial because of the absence of a histologic inflammatory response in several AKP abnormalities. There are also concerns that NSAIDs can interfere with the normal healing response of muscles and tendons. Short courses of NSAIDs may be considered when alternative approaches such as exercise, cryotherapy, analgesics, and other modalities have been unsuccessful, or when pain management is essential for participation in rehabilitation.

Methods to Stimulate Healing

Platelet-rich plasma

Platelet-rich plasma (PRP) is blood plasma, rich in platelets and associated bioactive factors, which can be delivered locally to an area that requires augmentation of the healing process.[15]

> "Even though the basic science data supporting the potential beneficial effects of growth factors in augmenting connective tissue healing are promising, the clinical benefits of using PRP to improve functional outcomes has not been universally realized."[15]

PRP injections have been studied for the treatment of tendinopathy and osteoarthritis. Filardo and colleagues[16] reported good medium-term results in the treatment of recalcitrant patellar tendinopathy with multiple PRP injections. The use of PRP has been rated by the American Academy of Orthopaedic Surgeons (AAOS) Clinical Practice Guidelines for the treatment of osteoarthritis of the knee.[17] Based on review of the literature, they were unable to recommend for or against the use of PRP for the treatment of knee osteoarthritis. The AAOS note that the quality of the literature was poor and that clinicians should use their best clinical judgment to make decisions.

Hyaluronic acid

Hyaluronic acid (HA) is a nonsulfated glycosaminoglycan distributed widely throughout connective tissue. Several meta-analyses have shown that HA injections can offer moderate improvement for symptoms of osteoarthritis of the knee. Although side effects have been reported with injections of HA, there is variability in the severity and incidence in the reports.[18–21] The use of HA has been rated by the AAOS Clinical Practice Guidelines for the treatment of knee osteoarthritis.[17] Based on a review of the literature, they were unable to recommend the use of HA for such treatment.

Other therapies

Acupuncture and dry needling have been proposed as effective treatments for AKP. Evidence from 2 RCTs demonstrated a statistically significant reduction in pain following acupuncture, lasting up to 6 months after treatment.[22,23] A few studies have indicated promising results from sclerotherapy and prolotherapy injections, although the lack of high-quality evidence prohibits definitive recommendation for use.[24] Sclerosing agents can be injected into areas of neovascularization, and prolotherapy is proposed to facilitate healing in conditions such as patellar tendinopathy. Systematic reviews and RCTs have demonstrated a lack of supportive evidence for the use of therapeutic ultrasound, iontophoresis, phonophoresis, low-level laser, transcutaneous electrical nerve stimulation, extracorporeal shock-wave therapy, biofeedback, and massage therapies. Recommendation for these treatments in patients with AKP should be based on the likelihood of benefit considering the duration of symptoms and the presenting symptoms.

Improving Lower Extremity Biomechanics

Patellar taping

Patellar taping has been shown to improve pain and function in patients with AKP when used in combination with strengthening exercises.[25–27] However, recent systematic reviews have drawn differing conclusions about the utility of taping for AKP. Warden and colleagues[28] concluded from their meta-analysis that a clinically significant reduction in chronic knee pain occurs with medially directed tape. Bolgla and Boling[29] stated that taping has minimal effect in treating long-term symptoms associated with AKP, but indicated that clinicians may consider patella taping as a short-term treatment to enable patients to perform pain-free exercise. Petersen and colleagues[30] also supported short-term use of a medially directed tape in combination with an exercise program. Callaghan and Selfe[31] determined in their Cochrane review that there was no statistically or clinically significant difference in Visual Analog Scale (VAS) pain scores comparing taping with no taping at the end of the treatment programs. Smith and colleagues[32] indicated that the research is controversial, and that tailoring treatment to the most suitable patients based on presenting characteristics may be the key to treatment success. A clinical trial by Lan and colleagues[33] investigating the response to patellar taping determined that it was an effective treatment for AKP, but was less effective in patients with a higher body mass index, larger lateral patellofemoral angle, and smaller Q-angle. Overall there is minimal evidence that taping significantly alters patellar alignment; however, it may increase the patellofemoral contact area leading to a decrease in pain, and thus enable relatively pain-free completion of exercise programs.[34–37]

Patellofemoral bracing

Similarly to taping, systematic reviews have reached differing conclusions about the outcomes of patellofemoral bracing. A meta-analysis assessing patellar bracing for chronic knee pain concluded there was disputable evidence from 3 low-quality studies regarding the efficacy of patellar bracing.[28] More recently, Swart and colleagues[38] concluded that knee braces offer no additional benefit over exercise therapy for pain and function in patients with AKP. Two reviews have noted the positive results of the Protonics bracing system in AKP, although further trials that examine the bracing system and exercise protocol separately are required.[29,38] Two reviews indicated that there is limited evidence to support the use of braces,[30,32] although Smith and colleagues[32] stated that it may be possible to use braces to reduce AKP onset in populations at risk. Bracing has also been shown in separate studies to decrease pain and improve function in patients with AKP.[39–41] Although the determinants of these positive results are not clear, they may be secondary to redistributed patella stress, enhanced proprioceptive input, and improved neuromuscular control.[29] Lun and colleagues[41] demonstrated that patellar bracing can improve the symptoms of AKP. However, these researchers also found that patellar bracing did not improve the symptoms of AKP more rapidly when added to a lower limb home-strengthening program. A recent quasi-experimental study demonstrated that patellofemoral bracing incorporating an infrapatellar strap significantly reduced pain and improved gait parameters in patients with AKP.[42] To definitively answer this clinical question the heterogeneity of trials, the variety of braces, and the quality of outcome assessment all require attention.

Foot orthotics
There is limited research regarding foot architecture and the use of foot orthotics as a treatment for AKP. It is also important that research has not consistently attributed foot pronation as a risk factor for AKP. Boling and colleagues[43] and Mølgaard and colleagues[44] determined that increased navicular drop was a risk factor for developing AKP; however, other studies have observed decreased foot pronation in association with AKP.[45] A clinical prediction rule, developed to identify patients with AKP most likely to benefit from foot orthoses, determined that individuals most suited to this treatment are older than 25 years, less than 165 cm in height, reporting their worst pain on a VAS at less than 53.3 mm, and with a difference in midfoot width from non–weight bearing to weight bearing of greater than 11 mm.[46] Barton and colleagues[47] demonstrated in an RCT that greater rearfoot eversion is a predictor of the benefit of foot orthotics in patients with AKP. A systematic review by Barton and colleagues[48] concluded that there is limited evidence for the use of prefabricated foot orthoses for short-term improvements in AKP. These investigators also reported that physiotherapy treatment combined with prefabricated foot orthoses is more beneficial than foot orthoses alone. Further well-designed studies focusing on assessment of gait kinematics and lower limb strength before and after interventions are needed to identify the cohort of patients with AKP most likely to benefit from foot orthotics.[29,30]

Stretching
Stretching of the quadriceps, gastrocnemius, and iliotibial band muscles have been investigated for AKP. In theory, tight hamstrings, gastrocnemius, or iliotibial band muscles could increase the patellofemoral joint reaction forces in full knee extension, whereas tight quadriceps could cause the same in full flexion.[49] A recent RCT demonstrated the benefit of quadriceps stretching for reducing pain in AKP, and recommended that this technique be included along with quadriceps strengthening in treatment protocols.[50] Studies investigating lower extremity stretching alone, or in combination with strengthening exercises or other physiotherapy interventions, have demonstrated improved AKP symptoms in up to 60% of patients.[51–55] Proprioceptive neuromuscular facilitation stretching techniques such as contract-relax may be more effective than traditional stretching programs.[56] Flexibility exercises and treatments are recommended as a component of the conservative treatment of AKP.

Strengthening

The effectiveness of exercise for reducing pain and increasing function in patients with AKP is widely supported.[29,30,32,57,58] A meta-analysis of RCTs determined that positive treatment results were evident with exercise interventions including knee extension, squats, stationary cycling, static quadriceps, active straight-leg raise, leg press, and step-up and -down exercises.[58] These investigators recommended a progressive program of daily exercises, including 2 to 4 sets of 10 or more repetitions over an intervention period of 6 weeks or longer. Two recent RCTs assessed the effectiveness of closed kinetic-chain exercises for AKP, and determined that these exercises can reduce pain and improve function.[59,60] Østerås and colleagues[60] also demonstrated that higher-intensity exercise over a 6-week treatment period resulted in statistically significant improvements 1 year after treatment in comparison with a low-intensity program.

A systematic review of conservative management of AKP from 2000 to 2010 concluded that both weight-bearing and non–weight-bearing quadriceps-strengthening exercises are effective for reducing pain in AKP.[29] This finding is consistent with those of the Cochrane review by Heintjes and colleagues[57] from 2003. In the more recent review, Bolgla and Boling[29] noted that although clinicians may prefer weight-bearing exercises to simulate functional activity, the use of non–weight-bearing exercise may be equally beneficial, particularly for patients with marked quadriceps weakness. A recent prospective study investigating weight-training for AKP demonstrated increased knee-muscle strength and patellofemoral joint contact area, potentially reducing mechanical stress in the joint and thereby improving pain and function.[61] One important factor highlighted in recent reviews is that exercises should be pain free.[29,32] The biomechanical stresses at the patellofemoral joint during exercise should be considered by prescribing clinicians, such as patellofemoral joint stress being lower from 90° to 45° of knee flexion during non–weight-bearing exercise, and also lower from 45° to 0° of knee flexion during weight-bearing exercise.[62]

Research protocols that include strengthening of the hip abductors and hip external rotators have reported significant decreases in pain.[29,53,63] A large RCT of military recruits found a 75% reduction in the incidence of AKP when hip exercises were included in training.[55] One study that included hip abductor, external rotator, extensor, and flexor exercises reported comparatively more significant improvements in pain, indicating the need for further study of total hip strengthening in AKP.[64] Bolgla and Boling[29] concluded in their recent systematic review that although hip exercises have been prescribed to obtain strengthening effects (ie, 3 sets of 10–15 repetitions), there is an indication that muscle endurance also needs to be addressed. These investigators stated that clinicians should consider exercise dosage focusing on higher repetitions (ie, 3 sets of 20–30 repetitions), in particular for AKP patients who participate in more demanding activities such as running and jumping.

The treatments available for AKP are numerous but lack evidence for their use, owing to insufficient research quality. The inability to recommend definitive therapeutic treatments for such a common disorder is disappointing, although it must be borne in mind that a lack of quality evidence for specific treatments is not proof that these treatments are ineffective. Each patient will present with unique symptoms and predisposing factors. With improving evidence, it will become increasingly more straightforward to tailor treatments unique to each athlete. Until such times, the authors encourage the use of best clinical judgment and application of available evidence-based medicine.

PATHOLOGY
Patellar Tracking

Abnormal patella tracking has been associated with disorders of the patellofemoral joint, including AKP.[61,65] In some cases deviation from normal tracking may be easily observed, but in other cases the differences may be subtle and therefore not recognized clinically. The patella translates medially in the initial 20° to 30° of knee flexion and then translates laterally[66]; however, there is no consensus regarding the normal amount of patellar tilt or rotation during this excursion.[67] Studies have demonstrated a more lateral patella position during initial flexion in AKP patients, but it is unclear if this deviation is present before the onset of symptoms.[68–70] Patella alta, patellar shape, and altered patellofemoral contact pressures are other potential risk factors for AKP.[69,71,72] Studies of quadriceps muscle function have demonstrated patella maltracking in combination with altered activation of the vastus lateralis (VL) and vastus medialis muscles.[73,74] Increased medial femoral rotation, rather than lateral patella rotation, has recently been demonstrated in AKP patients using weight-bearing MRI.[70] Abnormal patellofemoral alignment and tracking may be risk factors for AKP. However, further studies are needed to identify consistent changes in patellofemoral kinematics and whether these changes are a cause of, or a result of, patellofemoral pain.[65]

Soft-Tissue Pathology

Patellar tendinopathy

Patellar tendinopathy (jumper's knee) affects up to 40% of athletes involved in jumping sports such as volleyball and basketball, and appears to be more prevalent in men than women.[75,76] It can result in significant functional impairment in the athlete and can become chronic in nature, with one prospective study noting that patellar tendinopathy caused more than 50% of athletes to discontinue their sports career.[77] Tendinosis develops in response to chronic overloading of the tendon. Repetitive microtrauma interferes with the normal reparative process of the tendon.[78] Examination often demonstrates tenderness at the attachment of the patellar tendon to the distal pole of the patella. There is commonly palpable thickening of the tendon, and nodules may be palpated throughout the tendon. In less severe cases, functional testing such as squatting or hopping may be required to reproduce the athlete's pain. Ultrasonography may help confirm the diagnosis. There is evidence supporting eccentric strengthening as first-line treatment for patellar tendinopathy,[24,79,80] although systematic reviews have indicated the need for a multimodal approach to rehabilitation.[81,82] Injections have long been used for patellar tendinopathy. Corticosteroid injections may provide short-term benefit, but there is no evidence of long-term benefit and they are generally avoided because of the potential risk of patellar tendon rupture.[83] Studies on the use of PRP in this population demonstrate improvement in symptoms,[16,83] although significant side effects have recently been reported.[84] Studies of sclerotherapy and prolotherapy are currently not of sufficient quality to support definitive recommendation for their use. Surgical options include open, arthroscopic, and percutaneous techniques, and are generally reserved for recalcitrant cases nonresponsive to conservative management. In carefully selected patients surgery can be effective, although failure rates can from 20% to 30%.[85]

Bursitis

There are 11 bursae in the region of the knee joint, the most commonly affected being the prepatellar, infrapatellar, pes anserine, medial lateral collateral ligament, and semimembranosus.[86] In the athletic population common causes include overuse injuries and trauma, but can be associated with rheumatologic conditions, metabolic disorders, infection, and neoplasm. Symptoms and signs of bursitis include activity-dependent pain and focal tenderness over the affected bursa, often with associated swelling, stiffness, warmth, and erythema. Aspiration may be considered to rule out infection or to assess whether fluid analysis is required. Further imaging studies such as radiography, ultrasonography, and MRI may be considered as indicated. Treatment includes relative rest, activity modification, and protective padding over the affected bursa. Treatment to reduce inflammation, including intrabursal corticosteroid injections, may help. Surgery is not commonly required, but should be considered when appropriate nonoperative management has failed.

Pediatric patellar tendon abnormalities
Both attachments of the patellar tendon are subject to overuse or traction disorders in athletes with open growth plates. Osgood-Schlatter disease is a traction apophysitis of the tibial tubercle. The etiology is related to chronic loading of the patellar tendon–tibial tubercle junction, resulting in repeated minor avulsions with subsequent healing and repair attempts.[87] The disease usually occurs during the rapid phase of growth when the tibial tubercle is developing, with a similar prevalence in both genders, and bilateral symptoms are present in up to 30% of cases.[88,89] Sinding-Larsen-Johansson disease is an osteochondrosis of the inferior pole of the patella, and is another cause of AKP in the active adolescent population; it is more common in boys than in girls.[90] Symptoms of these 2 diseases usually include a gradual onset of activity-related pain localized to either the tibial tubercle or distal pole of the patella. Physical examination reveals tenderness and swelling or prominence at the site of injury, and in chronic cases bony irregularities may be palpable. Quadriceps and hamstring tightness are also common findings. Radiographs may be normal, or may show separation, fragmentation, and swelling of soft tissue at the site. Both conditions are usually self-limiting and respond to appropriate nonoperative management, including protective padding, activity modification, and methods to reduce inflammation, although it may take 12 to 24 months for symptoms to resolve.[91] Both long-term sequelae and surgical treatment are uncommon.

Iliotibial band syndrome
Iliotibial band syndrome (ITBS) is a common cause of lateral knee pain in athletes, especially in runners and cyclists, and in other sports such as rowing and swimming.[92–95] The literature surrounding the etiology, pathogenesis, and treatment of ITBS is controversial.[92,93] Current etiologic theories suggest that ITBS is associated with repetitive flexion and extension activities of the knee, in the setting of external and internal risk factors.[96–98] Activity-related pain in athletes is typically localized to the lateral femoral epicondyle (LFE) and/or lateral tibial tubercle.[95,96] Focal tenderness is common over the LFE, and associated swelling and crepitus may be present. Special tests include the Noble compression test to reproduce symptoms, the Ober test to evaluate iliotibial band (ITB) tightness, and the modified Thomas test to evaluate tightness of ITB, iliopsoas, and rectus femoris.[94–96] Treatment in the acute phase includes relative rest and avoidance of repetitive flexion and extension activities, methods to reduce inflammation, and addressing any muscle tightness and weakness.[95,96] A gradual and incremental return to activity is recommended after an athlete has become symptom free, with close monitoring for recurrence of symptoms.[95] Surgical intervention may be considered in cases refractory to conservative management, including arthroscopic debridement and percutaneous or open ITB release.[96]

Infrapatellar fat pad syndrome

Abnormalities related to the infrapatellar fat pad (IFP) can be a common but often over-looked cause of AKP in athletes. The IFP is an intracapsular but extrasynovial structure with rich vascular and nerve supply, and pain arising from IFP disorders can be signif-icant.[99] IFP syndrome may be caused by hemorrhage, inflammation, or impingement of the fat pad, and fibrosis may develop in chronic cases. Symptoms include anterior pain, often localized near the inferior pole of the patella, aggravated by forced exten-sion maneuvers and/or prolonged flexion. Physical examination may include tender-ness and fullness about the patellar tendon, and positive fat-pad impingement signs with forced passive hyperextension of knee and the Hoffa test.[78,100] In chronic cases findings may include catching and snapping, loss of extension, a palpably firm and enlarged fat pad, and decreased ROM of the patella. MRI can demonstrate hemor-rhage, inflammation, and fibrosis within the IFP.[101] Nonoperative treatment including corticosteroid or local anesthetic injections is often successful.[100] Surgical manage-ment includes arthroscopic resection of the IFP, which has been shown to be suc-cessful at relieving symptoms and restoring function.[102,103]

Plica syndrome

Plica syndrome can arise from 4 plicas within the knee: suprapatellar plica, infrapatellar plica, medial plica, and lateral plica. Plicas are present in approximately 20% of the adult population, and are normally asymptomatic.[104,105] Symptom development is most commonly associated with repetitive activity or direct trauma.[106] The medial plica is the most common symptomatic plica in the athlete.[107] When chronic, the plica can become fibrotic and inelastic, resulting in mechanical symptoms and erosive damage to underlying articular cartilage.[108] Typical symptoms may include AKP worsened by repetitive activity or prolonged sitting or standing, locking, catching, snapping, and giv-ing way. Physical examination demonstrates a tender, palpable thickened plica. The mediopatellar plica test has been described as a reliable test for diagnosing medial plica syndrome.[109] Nonoperative treatment has variable reports of success.[51] When indi-cated, arthroscopic resection has enabled successful long-term return to function.[110]

Cartilage Pathology

Chondromalacia patellae is a pathologic diagnosis describing degeneration of the cartilage on the undersurface of the patella.[111] It was originally described by Outer-bridge[112] in 1961 and then modified by the International Cartilage Research Society (ICRS). The ICRS classification is widely used in scientific literature as the reference standard. Chondral lesions of the patella comprise 11% of focal lesions found on arthroscopy.[113] Focal chondral lesions are usually diagnosed on MRI or arthroscopy, and these should initially be treated with activity modification, neuromuscular strengthening and stretching, injections, and other appropriate nonoperative manage-ment. In patients with ongoing pain after nonoperative management, arthroscopy is useful for characterization of the lesion, and may provide some therapeutic effect through debridement. More complex surgical treatment should include careful assessment of the underlying anatomy and biomechanics, such as malalignment and dysplasia. Surgical treatment directed at the lesion includes chondroplasty, microfracture, and chondral resurfacing techniques, such as osteochondral autograft or allograft and autologous chondrocyte implantation. Osteoarthritis of the patella, in contrast to a focal lesion, should be initially treated nonoperatively according to the AAOS Clinical Practice Guidelines.[17] Surgical management is limited, and may include arthroscopy, procedures to offload the patella such as anteromedialization (AMZ) of the tibial tubercle, and patellofemoral arthroplasty.

A subset of patellofemoral osteoarthritis is lateral hyperpressure syndrome, characterized by selective lateral patellofemoral compartment narrowing with patellar tilt. Patients present with pain and tenderness over the lateral patellofemoral joint. Skyline radiographs may show lateral narrowing of the patellofemoral joint space, patellar tilt, and lateral patellar osteophytes. MRI will identify selective lateral patellofemoral chondral damage. Standard nonoperative treatment includes lower extremity strengthening and stretching of lateral knee structures. Injections of HA or PRP may be of benefit in this population. Operative treatment includes correcting or improving biomechanical environment with procedures such as AMZ, lateral release for tilt, osteotomy to correct coronal malalignment, marrow stimulation techniques such as microfracture, and chondral resurfacing options.

Bone Pathology

Osteochondritis dissecans

Osteochondritis dissecans (OCD) is an acquired idiopathic disease of the subchondral bone that leads to death and subsequent collapse of the subchondral bone. The cartilage overlying the bone is unsupported and eventually fails, leading to separation of the cartilage and, eventually, loose body formation. Patients can present with pain at the site of the OCD lesion or with mechanical symptoms from a loose fragment. Diagnosis is generally made with plain radiographs, MRI, or bone scan. Treatment depends on the age of the patient and the stage of the lesion. Skeletally immature patients have excellent healing potential, and up to 66% have been shown to heal with nonoperative management including restricted activity, bracing, and limited weight bearing.[114] Poor prognostic factors include larger lesions, mechanical symptoms, patients approaching skeletal maturity, and MRI findings suggestive of instability.[115] Operative management for stable lesions includes retrograde or antero-grade drilling.[116] For unstable lesions that are reducible, options include fixation with a compression screw or device, or osteochondral plug fixation.[117] A recent systematic review reported a 94.1% healing rate after surgical treatment of OCD lesions.[116] For lesions that require excision there is a variety of cartilage replacement techniques, such as osteochondral autograft or allograft, and autologous chondrocyte replacement.

Stress fractures

Stress fractures, though a less common cause of AKP in the athletic population, are worth mentioning. Approximately half of all lower extremity stress fractures are found in the tibia.[118] Stress fractures have also been described in the proximal fibula,[119] patella,[120] distal femur,[121] and tibial tuberosity.[122,123] Low-risk stress fractures include the posteromedial tibia, femoral diaphysis, and the first to fourth metatarsals.[124] High-risk fractures include the patella, femoral neck, anterior cortex of the tibia, medial malleolus, talus, navicular, fifth metatarsal, and the sesamoids.[125] Stress fractures occur when there is an imbalance between stress or breakdown of bone and the subsequent repair process. Stress fractures of the patella are most often transverse, and occur at the junction of the middle and distal one-third of the patella where the quadriceps tendon transitions into the patellar tendon.[119] Patients can present with a 2- to 3-week history of AKP-type symptoms or with catastrophic failure and a transverse fracture of the patella, with no history of significant trauma.[120] Intrinsic risk factors include menstrual history in women, metabolic conditions, level of fitness and muscle strength, alignment, and bone quality. Extrinsic risk factors include overtraining or a sudden increase in training, diet, and equipment.[126] Physical examination demonstrates tenderness over the site of the stress fracture. Radiographs are the initial imaging modality of choice, but may not show any evidence of stress fracture in the early stages. Radiographic features tend to lag behind clinical symptoms by several weeks. Bone scan and MRI are sufficiently sensitive to show the early changes associated with stress fracture.[127] Treatment includes identifying and modifying any contributing risk factors, and initial rest followed by a gradual, pain-free return to training, starting with nonimpact, followed by low-impact and then regular activities. Operative intervention is aimed at encouraging bone healing with stimulation at the fracture site with or without internal fixation. There is no definitive evidence for the use of other modalities such as bisphosphonates, growth factors, oxygen therapy, bone morphogenic protein, recombinant parathyroid hormone, ultrasound, or magnetic fields in the treatment of stress fractures.[128,129]

Trauma

Direct trauma to the patella occurs in several sports. It may increase intraosseous hyperpressure of the knee and may be an important factor in the etiology of patellofemoral pain.[130] The normal intraosseous pressure in the patella is between 10 and 20 mm Hg,[131,132] but this has been noted to increase to up to 70 mm Hg in conditions where stress is placed on the patella.[133,134] Patellar intraosseous pressure has been measured to be increased in patients with chondromalacia patellae in comparison with controls.[132,134] Raised intraosseous pressure can be the first step in a chain of events that eventually creates structural changes such as degeneration of articular cartilage. Increased intraosseous pressure may be a sign in all patients with patellofemoral pain, or may be an etiologic factor in patients with trauma or direct blow or bone bruise to the patella. However, further research is necessary in this area.

Bipartite patella

Bipartite patella occurs when one of the secondary ossification centers in the patella fails to close. This condition occurs in approximately 2% to 6% of individuals, and is often noted as an incidental finding on imaging. Males are affected more than females, with a ratio of 9:1, and 50% present bilaterally. Type III is the most common (75%), located on the superolateral pole of the patella.[135] Only 2% of bipartite patellae become symptomatic,[136] and often present as AKP after a trauma or direct blow to the patella. The diagnosis is made by plain radiography and palpable tenderness over the synchondrosis. Treatment is initially nonoperative and includes rest, activity modification, and quadriceps stretching. Operative management includes excision of the fragment with repair of the VL to the patella. Results are excellent, and allow a return to activity within 6 weeks.[137]

Patellar Instability

Patients with microinstability of the patella may present primarily with knee pain as the muscles attempt to stabilize the patellofemoral articulation, similar to as occurs in the shoulder where microinstability without gross dislocation can present as pain.[138] Patients can present with no injury history but may display predisposing anatomic factors such as generalized ligamentous laxity, high Q-angle, and valgus alignment.[139] Some patients will describe trauma ranging from mild to severe, but may not demonstrate the typical history of patellofemoral dislocation or ongoing instability. Patients may present with findings typical of patellofemoral instability, or signs of lateral laxity and apprehension may be subtle. Nonoperative treatment should initially include maximizing the neuromuscular function of the lower limb and core. Surgical management includes stabilization of the patella by medial patellofemoral ligament imbrication or reconstruction, in addition to addressing any predisposing anatomic risk factors such as alignment.

Neuromuscular Pathology

Quadriceps muscles

Muscle-strength deficits, diminished neuromuscular control, and altered muscle-firing patterns have been implicated as contributing factors to AKP.[32,140–143] Initially the research focus of AKP was on the quadriceps complex and, specifically, the evidence for a strength or timing imbalance between the VL and vastus medialis oblique (VMO) muscles. Lower peak torque knee extension has been confirmed as a characteristic finding in AKP patients, and has been demonstrated to be a risk factor for developing AKP.[143] One prospective study of chronic AKP patients with 7 years of follow-up determined that restoration of good quadriceps strength and function is essential for recovery.[144] There is also a trend toward a delayed onset of VMO relative to VL in AKP patients, although not all patients demonstrate this VMO-VL dysfunction.[143,145] Pattyn and colleagues[146] recently analyzed the factors that determine AKP outcome from a 7-week program of physical therapy, and determined that patients with a greater quadriceps muscle size, lower eccentric knee strength, and less pain have a better short-term functional outcome.

Hip muscles

Research has also examined hip-muscle weakness as a component of AKP.[147–150] Impaired gluteal muscle function is thought to lead to increased hip joint adduction and internal rotation during activities such as stair climbing, squatting, and sports.[147,148,151] Meira and Brumitt[150] concluded in their systematic review that there is a link between the strength and position of the hip and AKP, and that AKP patients present with a common deficit once symptomatic. A systematic review of hip electromyographic (EMG) studies presented moderate to strong evidence that gluteus medius muscle activity is delayed and of shorter duration during stair ascent and descent in individuals with AKP.[149] This study found some evidence that gluteus medius muscle activity is delayed and of shorter duration during running, and that gluteus maximus muscle activity is increased during stair descent. The investigators recommend that interventions focused on correcting these deficits, such as hip strengthening, biofeedback, or gait retraining, should be included in the treatment and research of AKP.

Muscle flexibility

Reduced lower extremity muscle flexibility has been cited as a characteristic of AKP patients, although study findings have been inconsistent.[141,152,153] Patients with AKP have demonstrated significantly less flexibility of the gastrocnemius, soleus, quadriceps, and/or hamstring muscles when compared with healthy control subjects.[152,154–156] Specific to athletes, a prospective study by Witvrouw and colleagues[155] discovered an association between tight quadriceps and the development of AKP, but not an association with tight hamstring muscles. Reduced iliopsoas and ITB length have also been demonstrated in some studies.[64,157,158]

Functional testing

Because routine clinical assessment of muscle strength in athletes may not detect deficits, more challenging functional tests may be more useful. Functional testing of athletes with AKP has demonstrated decreased performance on vertical jumping,[155] anteromedial lunge, step-down, single-leg press, and balance and reach tests.[153] However, research has not definitively concluded whether this lower functional strength capacity is a risk factor for, or result of, the disorder. A few sport-specific studies have demonstrated other muscle imbalances. An EMG study of trained cyclists showed altered muscle activation patterns in both the quadriceps and hamstring muscle groups in the athletes with AKP.[159] Runners with AKP demonstrate weaker or delayed activation of hip abductor muscles and an associated increase in hip adduction during running.[149,160–162] These results suggest that athletes with AKP are able to demonstrate distinct proximal neuromuscular control strategies.

Summary and recommendations

1. The findings of this clinical review demonstrate the multifactorial nature of AKP in athletes.

2. Most athletes with AKP can be managed nonsurgically.

3. A detailed history and thorough investigation of potential contributing pathology is essential to correctly tailor treatment.

4. Consider patellofemoral instability as a cause of AKP.

5. Perform a thorough lower limb assessment including screening for core strength and functional performance.

6. Ensure that relative rest and activity modification allow the knee to stay within the envelope of function.

7. Rehabilitation should focus on muscle strengthening, flexibility, and neuromuscular control of the core and lower extremity muscles.

8. Use best clinical judgment to select treatments that address the presenting anatomic and neuromuscular characteristics to optimally manage this condition.

9. Carefully progress rehabilitation and/or return to sport while monitoring symptoms.

10. Further high-quality studies are required to determine optimal treatments for AKP, including identification and matching of patient characteristics to effectively tailor care.

REFERENCES

1. DeHaven KE, Lintner DM. Athletic injuries: comparison by age, sport, and gender. Am J Sports Med 1986;14(3):218–24.
2. Devereaux MD, Lachmann SM. Patello-femoral arthralgia in athletes attending a sports injury clinic. Br J Sports Med 1984;18(1):18–21.
3. Dye SF. Functional anatomy and biomechanics of the patellofemoral joint. In: Scott W, editor. The knee. St Louis (MO): Mosby; 1994. p. 381–9.
4. Reilly DT, Martens M. Experimental analysis of the quadriceps muscle force and patello-femoral joint reaction force for various activities. Acta Orthop Scand 1972;43(2):126–37.
5. Dye SF. The knee as a biologic transmission with an envelope of function: a theory. Clin Orthop Relat Res 1996;(325):10–8.
6. Dye SF. The pathophysiology of patellofemoral pain: a tissue homeostasis perspective. Clin Orthop Relat Res 2005;(436):100–10.
7. Sanchez-Inchausti G, Vaquero-Martin J, Vidal-Fernandez C. Effect of arthroscopy and continuous cryotherapy on the intra-articular temperature of the knee. Arthroscopy 2005;21(5):552–6.
8. Warren TA, McCarty EC, Richardson AL, et al. Intra-articular knee temperature changes: ice versus cryotherapy device. Am J Sports Med 2004;32(2):441–5.
9. Park J, Ty Hopkins J. Immediate effects of acupuncture and cryotherapy on quadriceps motoneuron pool excitability: randomised trial using anterior knee infusion model. Acupunct Med 2012;30(3):195–202.

10. Stalman A, Berglund L, Dungnerc E, et al. Temperature-sensitive release of prostaglandin E(2) and diminished energy requirements in synovial tissue with postoperative cryotherapy: a prospective randomized study after knee arthroscopy. J Bone Joint Surg Am 2011;93(21):1961–8.

11. Rice D, McNair PJ, Dalbeth N. Effects of cryotherapy on arthrogenic muscle inhibition using an experimental model of knee swelling. Arthritis Rheum 2009; 61(1):78–83.

12. Hopkins J, Ingersoll CD, Edwards J, et al. Cryotherapy and transcutaneous electric neuromuscular stimulation decrease arthrogenic muscle inhibition of the vastus medialis after knee joint effusion. J Athl Train 2002;37(1):25–31.

13. Heintjes E, Berger MY, Bierma-Zeinstra SM, et al. Pharmacotherapy for patellofemoral pain syndrome. Cochrane Database Syst Rev 2004;(3):CD003470.

14. Derry S, Moore RA, Rabbie R. Topical NSAIDs for chronic musculoskeletal pain in adults. Cochrane Database Syst Rev 2012;(9):CD007400.

15. Arnoczky SP, Shebani-Rad S. The basic science of platelet-rich plasma (PRP): what clinicians need to know. Sports Med Arthrosc 2013;21(4):180–5.

16. Filardo G, Kon E, Di Matteo B, et al. Platelet-rich plasma for the treatment of patellar tendinopathy: clinical and imaging findings at medium-term follow-up. Int Orthop 2013;37(8):1583–9.

17. Brown GA. AAOS clinical practice guideline: treatment of osteoarthritis of the knee: evidence-based guideline, 2nd edition. J Am Acad Orthop Surg 2013; 21(9):577–9.

18. Rutjes AW, Juni P, da Costa BR, et al. Viscosupplementation for osteoarthritis of the knee: a systematic review and meta-analysis. Ann Intern Med 2012;157(3): 180–91.

19. Bannuru RR, Vaysbrot EE, Sullivan MC, et al. Relative efficacy of hyaluronic acid in comparison with NSAIDs for knee osteoarthritis: a systematic review and meta-analysis. Semin Arthritis Rheum 2013. http://dx.doi.org/10.1016/j.semarthrit.2013.10.002.

20. Bellamy N, Campbell J, Robinson V, et al. Viscosupplementation for the treatment of osteoarthritis of the knee. Cochrane Database Syst Rev 2006;(2): CD005321.

21. Miller LE, Block JE. US-approved intra-articular hyaluronic acid injections are safe and effective in patients with knee osteoarthritis: systematic review and meta-analysis of randomized, saline-controlled trials. Clin Med Insights Arthritis Musculoskelet Disord 2013;6:57–63.

22. Jensen R, Gothesen O, Liseth K, et al. Acupuncture treatment of patellofemoral pain syndrome. J Altern Complement Med 1999;5(6):521–7.

23. Naslund J, Naslund UB, Odenbring S, et al. Sensory stimulation (acupuncture) for the treatment of idiopathic anterior knee pain. J Rehabil Med 2002;34(5): 231–8.

24. Gaida JE, Cook J. Treatment options for patellar tendinopathy: critical review. Curr Sports Med Rep 2011;10(5):255–70.

25. Osorio JA, Vairo GL, Rozea GD, et al. The effects of two therapeutic patellofemoral taping techniques on strength, endurance, and pain responses. Phys Ther Sport 2013;14(4):199–206.

26. Paoloni M, Fratocchi G, Mangone M, et al. Long-term efficacy of a short period of taping followed by an exercise program in a cohort of patients with patellofemoral pain syndrome. Clin Rheumatol 2012;31(3):535–9.

27. Crossley K, Cowan SM, Bennell KL, et al. Patellar taping: is clinical success supported by scientific evidence? Man Ther 2000;5(3):142–50.

28. Warden SJ, Hinman RS, Watson MA Jr, et al. Patellar taping and bracing for the treatment of chronic knee pain: a systematic review and meta-analysis. Arthritis Rheum 2008;59(1):73–83.
29. Bolgla LA, Boling MC. An update for the conservative management of patellofemoral pain syndrome: a systematic review of the literature from 2000 to 2010. Int J Sports Phys Ther 2011;6(2):112–25.
30. Petersen W, Ellermann A, Gosele-Koppenburg A, et al. Patellofemoral pain syndrome. Knee Surg Sports Traumatol Arthrosc 2013 [Epub ahead of print]. PMID: 24221245.
31. Callaghan MJ, Selfe J. Patellar taping for patellofemoral pain syndrome in adults. Cochrane Database Syst Rev 2012;(4):CD006717.
32. Smith TO, McNamara I, Donell ST. The contemporary management of anterior knee pain and patellofemoral instability. Knee 2013;20(Suppl 1):S3–15.
33. Lan TY, Lin WP, Jiang CC, et al. Immediate effect and predictors of effectiveness of taping for patellofemoral pain syndrome: a prospective cohort study. Am J Sports Med 2010;38(8):1626–30.
34. Malone T, Davies G, Walsh WM. Muscular control of the patella. Clin Sports Med 2002;21(3):349–62.
35. Christou EA. Patellar taping increases vastus medialis oblique activity in the presence of patellofemoral pain. J Electromyogr Kinesiol 2004;14(4):495–504.
36. Gigante A, Pasquinelli FM, Paladini P, et al. The effects of patellar taping on patellofemoral incongruence. A computed tomography study. Am J Sports Med 2001;29(1):88–92.
37. Derasari A, Brindle TJ, Alter KE, et al. McConnell taping shifts the patella inferiorly in patients with patellofemoral pain: a dynamic magnetic resonance imaging study. Phys Ther 2010;90(3):411–9.
38. Swart NM, van Linschoten R, Bierma-Zeinstra SM, et al. The additional effect of orthotic devices on exercise therapy for patients with patellofemoral pain syndrome: a systematic review. Br J Sports Med 2012;46(8):570–7.
39. Denton J, Willson JD, Ballantyne BT, et al. The addition of the Protonics brace system to a rehabilitation protocol to address patellofemoral joint syndrome. J Orthop Sports Phys Ther 2005;35(4):210–9.
40. Powers CM, Ward SR, Chan LD, et al. The effect of bracing on patella alignment and patellofemoral joint contact area. Med Sci Sports Exerc 2004;36(7):1226–32.
41. Lun VM, Wiley JP, Meeuwisse WH, et al. Effectiveness of patellar bracing for treatment of patellofemoral pain syndrome. Clin J Sport Med 2005;15(4):235–40.
42. Arazpour M, Notarki TT, Salimi A, et al. The effect of patellofemoral bracing on walking in individuals with patellofemoral pain syndrome. Prosthet Orthot Int 2013;37(6):465–70.
43. Boling MC, Padua DA, Marshall SW, et al. A prospective investigation of biomechanical risk factors for patellofemoral pain syndrome: the Joint Undertaking to Monitor and Prevent ACL Injury (JUMP-ACL) cohort. Am J Sports Med 2009; 37(11):2108–16.
44. Mølgaard C, Rathleff MS, Simonsen O. Patellofemoral pain syndrome and its association with hip, ankle, and foot function in 16- to 18-year-old high school students: a single-blind case-control study. J Am Podiatr Med Assoc 2011;101(3):215–22.
45. Thijs Y, Van Tiggelen D, Roosen P, et al. A prospective study on gait-related intrinsic risk factors for patellofemoral pain. Clin J Sport Med 2007;17(6):437–45.

46. Vicenzino B, Collins N, Cleland J, et al. A clinical prediction rule for identifying patients with patellofemoral pain who are likely to benefit from foot orthoses: a preliminary determination. Br J Sports Med 2010;44(12):862–6.
47. Barton CJ, Menz HB, Levinger P, et al. Greater peak rearfoot eversion predicts foot orthoses efficacy in individuals with patellofemoral pain syndrome. Br J Sports Med 2011;45(9):697–701.
48. Barton CJ, Munteanu SE, Menz HB, et al. The efficacy of foot orthoses in the treatment of individuals with patellofemoral pain syndrome: a systematic review. Sports Med 2010;40(5):377–95.
49. Al-Hakim W, Jaiswal PK, Khan W, et al. The non-operative treatment of anterior knee pain. Open Orthop J 2012;6:320–6.
50. Mason M, Keays SL, Newcombe PA. The effect of taping, quadriceps strengthening and stretching prescribed separately or combined on patellofemoral pain. Physiother Res Int 2011;16(2):109–19.
51. Amatuzzi MM, Fazzi A, Varella MH. Pathologic synovial plica of the knee. Results of conservative treatment. Am J Sports Med 1990;18(5):466–9.
52. Crossley K, Bennell K, Green S, et al. A systematic review of physical interventions for patellofemoral pain syndrome. Clin J Sport Med 2001;11(2):103–10.
53. Fukuda TY, Melo WP, Zaffalon BM, et al. Hip posterolateral musculature strengthening in sedentary women with patellofemoral pain syndrome: a randomized controlled clinical trial with 1-year follow-up. J Orthop Sports Phys Ther 2012;42(10):823–30.
54. Rixe JA, Glick JE, Brady J, et al. A review of the management of patellofemoral pain syndrome. Phys Sportsmed 2013;41(3):19–28.
55. Coppack RJ, Etherington J, Wills AK. The effects of exercise for the prevention of overuse anterior knee pain: a randomized controlled trial. Am J Sports Med 2011;39(5):940–8.
56. Moyano FR, Valenza MC, Martin LM, et al. Effectiveness of different exercises and stretching physiotherapy on pain and movement in patellofemoral pain syndrome: a randomized controlled trial. Clin Rehabil 2013;27(5):409–17.
57. Heintjes E, Berger MY, Bierma-Zeinstra SM, et al. Exercise therapy for patellofemoral pain syndrome. Cochrane Database Syst Rev 2003;(4):CD003472.
58. Harvie D, O'Leary T, Kumar S. A systematic review of randomized controlled trials on exercise parameters in the treatment of patellofemoral pain: what works? J Multidiscip Healthc 2011;4:383–92.
59. Ismail MM, Gamaleldein MH, Hassa KA. Closed kinetic chain exercises with or without additional hip strengthening exercises in management of patellofemoral pain syndrome: a randomized controlled trial. Eur J Phys Rehabil Med 2013; 49(5):687–98.
60. Østerås B, Osteras H, Torsensen TA. Long-term effects of medical exercise therapy in patients with patellofemoral pain syndrome: results from a single-blinded randomized controlled trial with 12 months follow-up. Physiotherapy 2013;99(4): 311–6.
61. Chiu JK, Wong YM, Yung PS, et al. The effects of quadriceps strengthening on pain, function, and patellofemoral joint contact area in persons with patellofemoral pain. Am J Phys Med Rehabil 2012;91(2):98–106.
62. Steinkamp LA, Dillingham MF, Markel MD, et al. Biomechanical considerations in patellofemoral joint rehabilitation. Am J Sports Med 1993;21(3):438–44.
63. Earl JE, Hoch AZ. A proximal strengthening program improves pain, function, and biomechanics in women with patellofemoral pain syndrome. Am J Sports Med 2011;39(1):154–63.

64. Tyler TF, Nicholas SJ, Mullaney MJ, et al. The role of hip muscle function in the treatment of patellofemoral pain syndrome. Am J Sports Med 2006;34(4):630–6.
65. Song CY, Lin JJ, Jan MH, et al. The role of patellar alignment and tracking in vivo: the potential mechanism of patellofemoral pain syndrome. Phys Ther Sport 2011;12(3):140–7.
66. Amis AA, Senavongse W, Bull AM. Patellofemoral kinematics during knee flexion-extension: an in vitro study. J Orthop Res 2006;24(12):2201–11.
67. Katchburian MV, Bull AM, Shih YF, et al. Measurement of patellar tracking: assessment and analysis of the literature. Clin Orthop Relat Res 2003;412: 241–59.
68. MacIntyre NJ, Hill NA, Fellows RA, et al. Patellofemoral joint kinematics in individuals with and without patellofemoral pain syndrome. J Bone Joint Surg Am 2006;88(12):2596–605.
69. Salsich GB, Perman WH. Tibiofemoral and patellofemoral mechanics are altered at small knee flexion angles in people with patellofemoral pain. J Sci Med Sport 2013;16(1):13–7.
70. Souza RB, Draper CE, Fredericson M, et al. Femur rotation and patellofemoral joint kinematics: a weight-bearing magnetic resonance imaging analysis. J Orthop Sports Phys Ther 2010;40(5):277–85.
71. Connolly KD, Ronsky JL, Westover LM, et al. Differences in patellofemoral contact mechanics associated with patellofemoral pain syndrome. J Biomech 2009; 42(16):2802–7.
72. Luyckx T, Didden K, Vandenneucker H, et al. Is there a biomechanical explanation for anterior knee pain in patients with patella alta?: influence of patellar height on patellofemoral contact force, contact area and contact pressure. J Bone Joint Surg Br 2009;91(3):344–50.
73. Pal S, Draper CE, Fredericson M, et al. Patellar maltracking correlates with vastus medialis activation delay in patellofemoral pain patients. Am J Sports Med 2011;39(3):590–8.
74. Lin YF, Lin JJ, Jan MH, et al. Role of the vastus medialis obliquus in repositioning the patella: a dynamic computed tomography study. Am J Sports Med 2008; 36(4):741–6.
75. Lian OB, Engebretsen L, Bahr R. Prevalence of jumper's knee among elite athletes from different sports: a cross-sectional study. Am J Sports Med 2005;33(4): 561–7.
76. Zwerver J, Bredeweg SW, van den Akker-Scheek I. Prevalence of jumper's knee among nonelite athletes from different sports: a cross-sectional survey. Am J Sports Med 2011;39(9):1984–8.
77. Kettunen JA, Kvist M, Alanen E, et al. Long-term prognosis for jumper's knee in male athletes. A prospective follow-up study. Am J Sports Med 2002;30(5): 689–92.
78. DeLee J, Drez D, Miller MD. DeLee & Drez's orthopaedic sports medicine: principles and practice. 3rd edition. Philadelphia: Saunders/Elsevier; 2010.
79. Larsson ME, Kall I, Nilsson-Helander K. Treatment of patellar tendinopathy—a systematic review of randomized controlled trials. Knee Surg Sports Traumatol Arthrosc 2012;20(8):1632–46.
80. Jonsson P, Alfredson H. Superior results with eccentric compared to concentric quadriceps training in patients with jumper's knee: a prospective randomised study. Br J Sports Med 2005;39(11):847–50.
81. Malliaras P, Barton CJ, Reeves ND, et al. Achilles and patellar tendinopathy loading programmes: a systematic review comparing clinical outcomes and

identifying potential mechanisms for effectiveness. Sports Med 2013;43(4): 267–86.

82. Woodley BL, Newsham-West RJ, Baxter GD. Chronic tendinopathy: effectiveness of eccentric exercise. Br J Sports Med 2007;41(4):188–98 [discussion: 99].

83. Skjong CC, Meininger AK, Ho SS. Tendinopathy treatment: where is the evidence? Clin Sports Med 2012;31(2):329–50.

84. Bowman KF Jr, Muller B, Middleton K, et al. Progression of patellar tendinitis following treatment with platelet-rich plasma: case reports. Knee Surg Sports Traumatol Arthrosc 2013;21(9):2035–9.

85. Maffulli N, Longo UG, Denaro V. Novel approaches for the management of tendinopathy. J Bone Joint Surg Am 2010;92(15):2604–13.

86. Frontera WR, Silver JK, Rizzo TD. Essentials of physical medicine and rehabilitation: musculoskeletal disorders, pain, and rehabilitation. 2nd edition. Philadelphia: Saunders/Elsevier; 2008.

87. Ogden JA, Southwick WO. Osgood-Schlatter's disease and tibial tuberosity development. Clin Orthop Relat Res 1976;(116):180–9.

88. Kujala UM, Kvist M, Heinonen O. Osgood-Schlatter's disease in adolescent athletes. Retrospective study of incidence and duration. Am J Sports Med 1985; 13(4):236–41.

89. Jarvinen M. Epidemiology of tendon injuries in sports. Clin Sports Med 1992; 11(3):493–504.

90. Medlar RC, Lyne ED. Sinding-Larsen-Johansson disease. Its etiology and natural history. J Bone Joint Surg Am 1978;60(8):1113–6.

91. Krause BL, Williams JP, Catterall A. Natural history of Osgood-Schlatter disease. J Pediatr Orthop 1990;10(1):65–8.

92. Falvey EC, Clark RA, Franklyn-Miller A, et al. Iliotibial band syndrome: an examination of the evidence behind a number of treatment options. Scand J Med Sci Sports 2010;20(4):580–7.

93. van der Worp MP, van der Horst N, de Wijer A, et al. Iliotibial band syndrome in runners: a systematic review. Sports Med 2012;42(11):969–92.

94. Lavine R. Iliotibial band friction syndrome. Curr Rev Musculoskelet Med 2010; 3(1–4):18–22.

95. Baker RL, Souza RB, Fredericson M. Iliotibial band syndrome: soft tissue and biomechanical factors in evaluation and treatment. PM R 2011;3(6):550–61.

96. Strauss EJ, Kim S, Calcei JG, et al. Iliotibial band syndrome: evaluation and management. J Am Acad Orthop Surg 2011;19(12):728–36.

97. Fairclough J, Hayashi K, Toumi H, et al. The functional anatomy of the iliotibial band during flexion and extension of the knee: implications for understanding iliotibial band syndrome. J Anat 2006;208(3):309–16.

98. Ellis R, Hing W, Reid D. Iliotibial band friction syndrome—a systematic review. Man Ther 2007;12(3):200–8.

99. Dye SF, Vaupel GL, Dye CC. Conscious neurosensory mapping of the internal structures of the human knee without intraarticular anesthesia. Am J Sports Med 1998;26(6):773–7.

100. Dragoo JL, Johnson C, McConnell J. Evaluation and treatment of disorders of the infrapatellar fat pad. Sports Med 2012;42(1):51–67.

101. Saddik D, McNally EG, Richardson M. MRI of Hoffa's fat pad. Skeletal Radiol 2004;33(8):433–44.

102. von Engelhardt LV, Tokmakidis E, Lahner M, et al. Hoffa's fat pad impingement treated arthroscopically: related findings on preoperative MRI in a case series of 62 patients. Arch Orthop Trauma Surg 2010;130(8):1041–51.

103. Kumar D, Alvand A, Beacon JP. Impingement of infrapatellar fat pad (Hoffa's disease): results of high-portal arthroscopic resection. Arthroscopy 2007; 23(11):1180–6.e1.
104. Duri ZA, Patel DV, Aichroth PM. The immature athlete. Clin Sports Med 2002; 21(3):461–82, ix.
105. Bellary SS, Lynch G, Housman B, et al. Medial plica syndrome: a review of the literature. Clin Anat 2012;25(4):423–8.
106. Lyu SR. Relationship of medial plica and medial femoral condyle during flexion. Clin Biomech (Bristol, Avon) 2007;22(9):1013–6.
107. Sznajderman T, Smorgick Y, Lindner D, et al. Medial plica syndrome. Isr Med Assoc J 2009;11(1):54–7.
108. Liu DS, Zhuang ZW, Lyu SR. Relationship between medial plica and medial femoral condyle—a three-dimensional dynamic finite element model. Clin Biomech (Bristol, Avon) 2013;28(9–10):1000–5.
109. Kim SJ, Lee DH, Kim TE. The relationship between the MPP test and arthroscopically found medial patellar plica pathology. Arthroscopy 2007;23(12): 1303–8.
110. Weckstrom M, Niva MH, Lamminen A, et al. Arthroscopic resection of medial plica of the knee in young adults. Knee 2010;17(2):103–7.
111. Grelsamer RP, Weinstein CH. Applied biomechanics of the patella. Clin Orthop Relat Res 2001;(389):9–14.
112. Outerbridge RE. The etiology of chondromalacia patellae. J Bone Joint Surg Br 1961;43B:752–7.
113. Hjelle K, Solheim E, Strand T, et al. Articular cartilage defects in 1,000 knee arthroscopies. Arthroscopy 2002;18(7):730–4.
114. Wall EJ, Vourazeris J, Myer GD, et al. The healing potential of stable juvenile osteochondritis dissecans knee lesions. J Bone Joint Surg Am 2008;90(12): 2655–64.
115. Pill SG, Ganley TJ, Milam RA, et al. Role of magnetic resonance imaging and clinical criteria in predicting successful nonoperative treatment of osteochondritis dissecans in children. J Pediatr Orthop 2003;23(1):102–8.
116. Abouassaly M, Peterson D, Salci L, et al. Surgical management of osteochondritis dissecans of the knee in the paediatric population: a systematic review addressing surgical techniques. Knee Surg Sports Traumatol Arthrosc 2013 [Epub ahead of print]. PMID: 23680989.
117. Miniaci A, Tytherleigh-Strong G. Fixation of unstable osteochondritis dissecans lesions of the knee using arthroscopic autogenous osteochondral grafting (mosaicplasty). Arthroscopy 2007;23(8):845–51.
118. Matheson GO, Clement DB, McKenzie DC, et al. Stress fractures in athletes. A study of 320 cases. Am J Sports Med 1987;15(1):46–58.
119. Drabicki RR, Greer WJ, DeMeo PJ. Stress fractures around the knee. Clin Sports Med 2006;25(1):105–15, ix.
120. Mason RW, Moore TE, Walker CW, et al. Patellar fatigue fractures. Skeletal Radiol 1996;25(4):329–32.
121. Milgrom C, Giladi M, Stein M, et al. Stress fractures in military recruits. A prospective study showing an unusually high incidence. J Bone Joint Surg Br 1985;67(5):732–5.
122. Tejwani SG, Motamedi AR. Stress fracture of the tibial tubercle in a collegiate volleyball player. Orthopedics 2004;27(2):219–22.
123. Levi JH, Coleman CR. Fracture of the tibial tubercle. Am J Sports Med 1976; 4(6):254–63.

124. Boden BP, Osbahr DC, Jimenez C. Low-risk stress fractures. Am J Sports Med 2001;29(1):100–11.

125. Boden BP, Osbahr DC. High-risk stress fractures: evaluation and treatment. J Am Acad Orthop Surg 2000;8(6):344–53.

126. Shindle MK, Endo Y, Warren RF, et al. Stress fractures about the tibia, foot, and ankle. J Am Acad Orthop Surg 2012;20(3):167–76.

127. Raasch WG, Hergan DJ. Treatment of stress fractures: the fundamentals. Clin Sports Med 2006;25(1):29–36, vii.

128. Carmont M, Mei-Dan O, Bennell KL. Stress fracture management: current classification and new healing modalities. Oper Tech Sports Med 2009;17(2): 81–9.

129. Young AJ, McAllister DR. Evaluation and treatment of tibial stress fractures. Clin Sports Med 2006;25(1):117–28, x.

130. Medscape General Medicine 1999;(1):1. Available at: http://www.medscape.com/viewarticle/717387.

131. Ficat RP, Philippe J, Hungerford DS. Chondromalacia patellae: a system of classification. Clin Orthop Relat Res 1979;144:55–62.

132. Bjorkstrom S, Goldie IF, Wetterqvist H. Intramedullary pressure of the patella in chondromalacia. Arch Orthop Trauma Surg 1980;97(2):81–5.

133. Arnoldi CC. Patellar pain. Acta Orthop Scand Suppl 1991;244:1–29.

134. Hejgaard N, Diemer H. Bone scan in the patellofemoral pain syndrome. Int Orthop 1987;11(1):29–33.

135. Saupe H. Primäre Krochenmark serelung der kniescheibe. Deutsche Z Chir 1943;258:386–92. http://dx.doi.org/10.1007/BF02793437.

136. Weaver JK. Bipartite patellae as a cause of disability in the athlete. Am J Sports Med 1977;5(4):137–43.

137. Weckstrom M, Parviainen M, Pihlajamaki HK. Excision of painful bipartite patella: good long-term outcome in young adults. Clin Orthop Relat Res 2008; 466(11):2848–55.

138. Ruotolo C, Nottage WM, Flatow EL, et al. Controversial topics in shoulder arthroscopy. Arthroscopy 2002;18(2 Suppl 1):65–75.

139. Hiemstra LA, Kerslake S, Lafave M, et al. Introduction of a classification system for patients with patellofemoral instability (WARPS and STAID). Knee Surg Sports Traumatol Arthrosc 2013 [Epub ahead of print]. PMID: 23536205.

140. Bolgla LA, Malone TR, Umberger BR, et al. Comparison of hip and knee strength and neuromuscular activity in subjects with and without patellofemoral pain syndrome. Int J Sports Phys Ther 2011;6(4):285–96.

141. Fredericson M, Yoon K. Physical examination and patellofemoral pain syndrome. Am J Phys Med Rehabil 2006;85(3):234–43.

142. Halabchi F, Mazaheri R, Seif-Barghi T. Patellofemoral pain syndrome and modifiable intrinsic risk factors; how to assess and address? Asian J Sports Med 2013; 4(2):85–100.

143. Lankhorst NE, Bierma-Zeinstra SM, van Middelkoop M. Factors associated with patellofemoral pain syndrome: a systematic review. Br J Sports Med 2013;47(4): 193–206.

144. Natri A, Kannus P, Jarvinen M. Which factors predict the long-term outcome in chronic patellofemoral pain syndrome? A 7-yr prospective follow-up study. Med Sci Sports Exerc 1998;30(11):1572–7.

145. Chester R, Smith TO, Sweeting D, et al. The relative timing of VMO and VL in the aetiology of anterior knee pain: a systematic review and meta-analysis. BMC Musculoskelet Disord 2008;9:64.

146. Pattyn E, Mahieu N, Selfe J, et al. What predicts functional outcome after treatment for patellofemoral pain? Med Sci Sports Exerc 2012;44(10):1827–33.

147. Prins MR, van der Wurff P. Females with patellofemoral pain syndrome have weak hip muscles: a systematic review. Aust J Physiother 2009;55(1):9–15.

148. Fukuda TY, Rossetto FM, Magalhaes E, et al. Short-term effects of hip abductors and lateral rotators strengthening in females with patellofemoral pain syndrome: a randomized controlled clinical trial. J Orthop Sports Phys Ther 2010;40(11): 736–42.

149. Barton CJ, Lack S, Malliaras P, et al. Gluteal muscle activity and patellofemoral pain syndrome: a systematic review. Br J Sports Med 2013;47(4):207–14.

150. Meira EP, Brumitt J. Influence of the hip on patients with patellofemoral pain syndrome: a systematic review. Sports Health 2011;3(5):455–65.

151. Powers CM. The influence of abnormal hip mechanics on knee injury: a biomechanical perspective. J Orthop Sports Phys Ther 2010;40(2):42–51.

152. Waryasz GR, McDermott AY. Patellofemoral pain syndrome (PFPS): a systematic review of anatomy and potential risk factors. Dyn Med 2008;7:9.

153. Loudon JK, Wiesner D, Goist-Foley HL, et al. Intrarater reliability of functional performance tests for subjects with patellofemoral pain syndrome. J Athl Train 2002;37(3):256–61.

154. Piva SR, Goodnite EA, Childs JD. Strength around the hip and flexibility of soft tissues in individuals with and without patellofemoral pain syndrome. J Orthop Sports Phys Ther 2005;35(12):793–801.

155. Witvrouw E, Lysens R, Bellemans J, et al. Intrinsic risk factors for the development of anterior knee pain in an athletic population. A two-year prospective study. Am J Sports Med 2000;28(4):480–9.

156. White LC, Dolphin P, Dixon J. Hamstring length in patellofemoral pain syndrome. Physiotherapy 2009;95(1):24–8.

157. Hudson Z, Darthuy E. Iliotibial band tightness and patellofemoral pain syndrome: a case-control study. Man Ther 2009;14(2):147–51.

158. Winslow J, Yoder E. Patellofemoral pain in female ballet dancers: correlation with iliotibial band tightness and tibial external rotation. J Orthop Sports Phys Ther 1995;22(1):18–21.

159. Dieter BP, McGowan CP, Stoll SK, et al. Muscle activation patterns and patellofemoral pain in cyclists. Med Sci Sports Exerc 2014;46(4):753–61.

160. Ferber R, Kendall KD, Farr L. Changes in knee biomechanics after a hip-abductor strengthening protocol for runners with patellofemoral pain syndrome. J Athl Train 2011;46(2):142–9.

161. Dierks TA, Manal KT, Hamill J, et al. Proximal and distal influences on hip and knee kinematics in runners with patellofemoral pain during a prolonged run. J Orthop Sports Phys Ther 2008;38(8):448–56.

162. Noehren B, Hamill J, Davis I. Prospective evidence for a hip etiology in patellofemoral pain. Med Sci Sports Exerc 2013;45(6):1120–4.

Plantar Heel Pain

Andrew J. Rosenbaum, MD[a],*, John A. DiPreta, MD[a],
David Misener, BSc(HK), CPO, MBA[b]

KEYWORDS

- Plantar heel pain • Plantar fascia • Plantar fasciitis • Windlass mechanism
- Heel spur • Baxter nerve • First branch lateral plantar nerve
- Extracorporeal shock-wave therapy

KEY POINTS

- Approximately 1 in 10 people are predicted to develop such heel pain during their lifetime.
- Plantar fasciitis is the most common cause of plantar heel pain and is responsible for 80% of the cases.
- Plantar heel pain is usually responsive to conservative interventions, including home stretches, nonsteroidal antiinflammatory drugs, orthoses, night splints, and, at times, corticosteroid injections and extracorporeal shock-wave therapy.
- If conservative measures do not provide pain relief, surgery can be considered.

INTRODUCTION

Plantar heel pain is a very common complaint that can cause significant discomfort and disability. Approximately 1 in 10 people are predicted to develop such heel pain during their lifetime, with more than 2 million individuals undergoing treatment of it annually in the United States.[1,2] Although 1% of all visits to orthopedic surgeons are attributed to heel pain, it is also commonly treated by internists and family practitioners.[3] The annual cost of the evaluation and treatment of plantar heel pain by these providers is estimated at approximately $284 million.[4]

The cause, diagnosis, and effective management of plantar heel pain have challenged practitioners since the early 1800s, when Wood first described plantar fasciitis, citing an infectious origin.[5] In the 1930s, gonorrhea, syphilis, tuberculosis, and streptococcal infections were thought to be responsible.[6] The focus then shifted to plantar fat pad impingement by heel spurs.[7] A plethora of conditions are now acknowledged as causes of plantar heel pain.

This article originally appeared in Medical Clinics of North America, Volume 98, Issue 2, March 2014.

[a] Division of Orthopaedic Surgery, Albany Medical College, 255 Patroon Creek Boulevard, Apartment 1214, Albany, NY 12206, USA; [b] Clinical Prosthetics and Orthotics, 149 South Lake Avenue, Albany, NY 12208, USA
* Corresponding author.
E-mail address: Andrewjrosenbaum@gmail.com

A thorough history and physical examination are crucial to the diagnosis of plantar heel disorders. Although plantar fasciitis is the most common culprit, accounting for 80% of patients with inferior heel pain, the clinician's differential must always include other causes. Mechanical, rheumatologic, and neurologic conditions can all manifest as plantar heel pain. This article reviews the relevant anatomy and biomechanics of the plantar hindfoot, the cause of plantar heel pain, pertinent components of the physical examination, useful diagnostic adjuncts, as well as both conservative and operative treatment modalities.

ANATOMY OF THE PLANTAR FASCIA AND HINDFOOT

The plantar fascia is a broad fibrous aponeurosis that spans the plantar surface of the foot (**Fig. 1**). It originates from the medial and anterior aspects of the calcaneus and helps to divide the intrinsic plantar musculature of the foot into 3 distinct compartments: medial, central, and lateral. Distally, the plantar fascia forms 5 digital bands at the metatarsophalangeal joints. Each digital band then divides to pass on either side of the flexor tendons, inserting into the periosteum at the base of the proximal phalanges.

The plantar fascia has a continuous connection with the Achilles tendon, leading to tightening of the plantar fascia when tensile loads are applied to the tendon. For this reason, Achilles tendon stretching and night splinting have become effective conservative treatments for plantar fasciitis.

The heel's fat pad, first described by Teitze in 1921, is also an integral component of the plantar hindfoot.[8] It is anchored to both the calcaneus and skin, acting as a shock absorber for the hindfoot. It helps to dissipate impact forces caused by heel strike during ambulation, which generates forces up to 110% of one's body weight when walking and 250% of body weight when running.[9] However, after 40 years of age, it begins to degenerate, losing some of its overall thickness and height. With this deterioration, softening and thinning of the fat pad occur, which leads to diminished protection of the heel.[10]

BIOMECHANICS OF THE PLANTAR FASCIA AND HINDFOOT

The foot and its ligaments can be thought of as a truss, with the calcaneus, midtarsal joint, and metatarsals forming the truss's medial longitudinal arch.[11] The plantar fascia acts as a tie-rod, preventing arch collapse via its great tensile strength, particularly during weight bearing. Preservation of the medial longitudinal arch is crucial for ambulation in a systematic and efficient manner. With arch collapse, the appropriate timing of pronation and supination during the gait cycle is altered, leading to inefficient foot function.

The *windlass mechanism* is a term used to describe the role of the plantar fascia in dynamic function during gait; a windlass is the tightening of a rope or cable.[12] As one's toes are dorsiflexed, the plantar fascia tightens, shortening the distance between the calcaneus and metatarsals and elevating the medial longitudinal arch (**Fig. 2**).[13] In the high-arched position, less tension on the truss is required for arch support, as opposed to a low-arched position. In other words, in a high-arched position, there is less tension on the plantar fascia.

CAUSE OF PLANTAR HEEL PAIN

A multitude of mechanical, neurologic, and rheumatologic conditions can manifest as plantar heel pain (**Box 1**). The mechanical causes include derangements of the plantar fascia, calcaneal stress fractures, and heel pad disorders. Although heel spurs are intimately associated with these conditions, they do not directly cause plantar heel

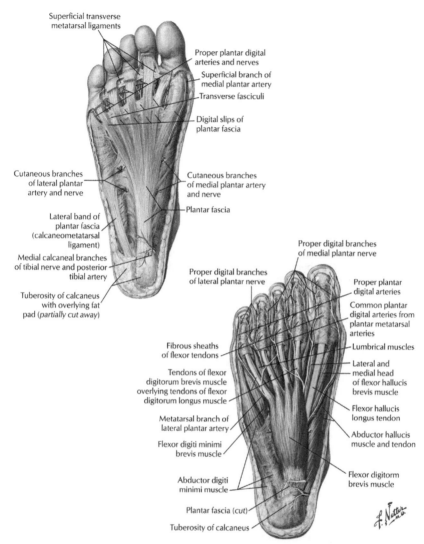

Superficial transverse metatarsal ligaments

Proper plantar digital arteries and nerves

Superficial branch of medial plantar artery

Transverse fasciculi

Digital slips of plantar fascia

Cutaneous branches of lateral plantar artery and nerve

Cutaneous branches of medial plantar artery and nerve

Plantar fascia

Lateral band of plantar fascia (calcaneometatarsal ligament)

Medial calcaneal branches of tibial nerve and posterior tibial artery

Tuberosity of calcaneus with overlying fat pad (*partially cut away*)

Proper digital branches of medial plantar nerve

Proper digital branches of lateral plantar nerve

Proper plantar digital arteries

Common plantar digital arteries from plantar metatarsal arteries

Fibrous sheaths of flexor tendons

Lumbrical muscles

Tendons of flexor digitorum brevis muscle overlying tendons of flexor digitorum longus muscle

Lateral and medial head of flexor hallucis brevis muscle

Metatarsal branch of lateral plantar artery

Flexor hallucis longus tendon

Flexor digiti minimi brevis muscle

Abductor hallucis muscle and tendon

Abductor digiti minimi muscle

Flexor digitorm brevis muscle

Plantar fascia (*cut*)

Tuberosity of calcaneus

Fig. 1. The plantar fascia is a thick band of connective tissue that supports the foot's plantar arch. It originates at the calcaneal tuberosity of the hindfoot, ultimately inserting into the periosteum at the base of the toes' proximal phalanges. (Netter illustration from www.netterimages.com. © Elsevier Inc. All rights reserved.)

pain. Neurologic disorders are typically caused by nerve compression, whereas rheumatoid conditions may present with systemic manifestations. Infection, which was once thought to be the primary cause of heel pain, is not as common as previously thought.

Fascial derangements include rupture and fasciitis. Rupture most often occurs acutely following trauma or athletic competition, whereas plantar fasciitis is a subacute and degenerative process resulting from repetitive and excessive loading of the fascia.

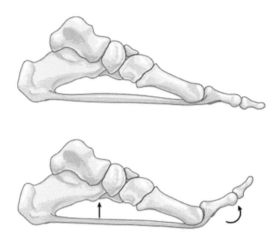

Fig. 2. The windlass mechanism occurs with dorsiflexion of the toes, which leads to tightening of the plantar fascia. (*From* Greisberg J. Foot and ankle anatomy and biomechanics. In: DiGiovanni CW, Greisberg J, editors. Core knowledge in orthopedics: foot and ankle. Philadelphia: Elsevier; 2007; with permission.)

After the metatarsals, the calcaneus is the most common location in the foot for a stress fracture.[14] These injuries most frequently occur in those with osteopenia of the calcaneus and athletes involved in running and jumping sports. Both benign and malignant neoplasms can also cause plantar heel pain. Benign lesions include simple bone cysts, which can weaken bone and cause pathologic fracture. Malignant lesions include primary tumors, of which Ewing sarcoma is the most common, and metastatic disease, including endometrial adenocarcinoma, bronchogenic carcinoma, bladder cancer, and gastric cancer.[15–18]

The deterioration of the fat pad's structural integrity, with advancing age and weight gain, is also thought to contribute to heel pain. Although some think that the progressive thinning of the fat pad is primarily responsible, others have shown an increased thickness to correlate most closely with pain. Further, some think that a reduced elasticity, not fat pad thickness, is the most significant factor.[10,19] Prichasuk[20] found that pad elasticity was reduced in those with pain and that elasticity decreases with increasing age and body weight.

Heel spurs are often associated with heel pain; up to 75% of patients with pain have been shown to have spurs (**Fig. 3**).[21–23] However, spurs are also common in those

---

Box 1
The differential diagnosis of plantar heel pain

- Plantar fasciitis
- Fat pad atrophy
- Partial or complete plantar fascial rupture
- Calcaneal stress fracture
- Plantar nerve impingement
- Hindfoot deformity (cavus or calcaneus)
- Inflammatory enthesopathy

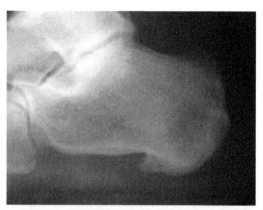

Fig. 3. Lateral radiograph of the hindfoot. A heel spur is evident on the inferior aspect of the calcaneus. (*From* Berkson EM, Greisberg J, Theodore GH. Heel pain. In: DiGiovanni CW, Greisberg J, editors. Core knowledge in orthopedics: foot and ankle. Philadelphia: Elsevier; 2007; with permission.)

without heel pain, suggesting that they are not necessarily the cause of pain.[23] In a randomly chosen sample of 1000 patients, Shmokler and colleagues[21] found a 13.2% incidence of heel spurs but only a 5.2% incidence of heel pain. This finding suggests that both spurs and pain may develop from a common underlying pathologic condition. The work of Kumai and Benjamin[24] supports this notion because their cadaveric study identified degenerative changes within the plantar fascia as the cause of spur formation.

HISTORY AND PHYSICAL EXAMINATION

A comprehensive history is imperative when evaluating patients with plantar heel pain. The patients' general health and past medical history must be reviewed first, identifying any prior treatments for plantar heel pain (ie, medications, injections, therapy, orthoses, surgeries) and the presence of comorbidities. Obesity is an independent risk factor for the development of plantar fasciitis and is present in up to 70% of patients with this disorder.[25,26] It is also important to ask about constitutional symptoms, such as weight loss, fevers, chills, and night sweats, which are findings that suggest a neoplastic or infectious process.

The clinician should inquire into patients' recreational and occupational activities because work-related weight bearing, like obesity, is an independent risk factor for plantar fasciitis.[25] When discussing athletics, the specific sport being played can help differentiate the diagnosis because those who perform running and jumping activities are particularly vulnerable to plantar heel pain. It is also helpful to determine if the pain occurs during heel strike as opposed to push off; if it occurs at the onset of, during, or after activity; and the type of shoe and its insole being used when the pain is present.

A description of the pain and its alleviating and exacerbating factors will assist the clinician in establishing a diagnosis. With the exception of an acute hindfoot fracture or plantar fascia rupture, patients will typically describe the pain as gradual in onset. Of note, those patients with a plantar fascia rupture often have histories of corticosteroid injection.[27,28] Pain that is worse with the first steps in the morning or when standing after prolonged sitting is consistent with plantar fasciitis. These patients may also experience decreased pain with progressive activity, only to have it return later in the day. Constitutional symptoms in the setting of night and/or rest pain suggest either a neoplastic or infectious process. Bilateral plantar heel pain, particularly in conjunction with joint pain and pain at multiple sites of tendon/ligament insertion, suggests that the pain may be related to a rheumatologic process, such as ankylosing spondylitis or Reiter syndrome. With nerve entrapment, patients may describe burning, tingling, or numbness.[29,30]

The physical examination is another critical component of the workup because determination of the location of the pain will facilitate the proper diagnosis. The examination includes a visual assessment of the foot, which may identify swelling, skin breakdown, bruising, or deformity. Palpation of the foot's bony prominences and tendinous insertions near the heel and midfoot must also be done, noting any defects or tenderness; Achilles tendon tightness can contribute to the pain. Observation of ankle and hindfoot range of motion as well as of the foot's posture and arch during weight bearing should also be performed. The physician should also evaluate the patients' spine because an L5-S1 radiculopathy can cause plantar heel pain.

With proximal plantar fasciitis, tenderness over the medial aspect of the calcaneal tuberosity is present. Conversely, distal plantar fasciitis produces pain in the distal aspect of the plantar fascia. Passive dorsiflexion of the toes exacerbates the pain in both the proximal and distal types because this stretches the entire plantar fascia. When a rupture of the plantar fascia occurs, a palpable defect may be evident at the calcaneal tuberosity, along with localized swelling and ecchymosis.[31] Findings suggestive of plantar fibromatosis include pain along the plantar fascia in conjunction with palpable nodules.

A calcaneal stress fracture is diagnosed on physical examination by the squeeze test in which diffuse heel pain is elicited with medial and lateral heel compression. Swelling and warmth may also be present. Neoplastic processes must be considered in the setting of persistent heel pain that is refractory to conservative treatment.

Tarsal tunnel syndrome is a compression neuropathy involving the posterior tibial nerve as it traverses the tunnel. Percussion of the nerve within the tarsal tunnel, as well as simultaneous dorsiflexion and eversion, may reproduce symptoms, which include pain and numbness that radiate to the plantar heel. The findings seen with plantar fasciitis are often similar. However, unlike tarsal tunnel syndrome, patients with plantar fasciitis will have pain with passive toe dorsiflexion. Patients may also present with entrapment of the first branch of the lateral plantar nerve (Baxter nerve, FBLPN). Because of its close proximity to the medial calcaneal tubercle, it is usually present with plantar fasciitis and difficult to distinguish.

Pain that is attributed to the fat pad is centered more proximally than the plantar fascia's origin. It is often associated with erythema and inflammation at the plantar heel. On palpation, it is often softened and flattened.

DIAGNOSTIC ADJUNCTS

The history and physical examination will often reliably diagnose the cause of plantar heel pain. However, when the diagnosis remains unclear, imaging modalities and laboratory studies can be obtained. Plain radiographs provide information about the foot's bony structures and alignment. Weight-bearing anteroposterior and lateral views are standard, with axial and 45° medial oblique views included at times. Heel spurs are commonly seen on the lateral radiographs of patients with plantar heel pain (see **Fig. 3**). A calcaneal lucency, referred to as the *saddle sign* often accompanies the spur, visible just proximal to it on the radiograph.[19] Although soft tissues are poorly visualized on plain radiographs, tumors, osteomyelitis, stress fractures, and fat pad atrophy are sometimes visible.

When a calcaneal stress fracture is suspected, a triple-phase bone scan will have increased uptake. With plantar fasciitis, this too will occur.[32,33] However, the increased uptake in this setting will be localized to the inferomedial aspect of the heel, enabling this test to distinguish the two processes.

Magnetic resonance imaging (MRI) has become a frequently used adjunct in the evaluation of plantar heel pain because it provides great detail of soft tissue structures through its multiplanar capability. Fascial thickening and increased signal intensity within the plantar fascia are typical MRI findings seen with plantar fasciitis. Admittedly, these findings are nonspecific, making MRI most useful for excluding other causes of heel pain. It has been shown that plantar fibromatosis, tumors, infection, and nerve entrapment are all reliably diagnosed with MRI.[34,35]

Ultrasound can identify fascial thickenings and soft tissue edema in the plantar heel and is becoming a commonly used diagnostic tool. In the setting of plantar fasciitis, ultrasound will reveal thickened, hypoechoic fascia. Although the quality of images obtained is operator dependent, some studies suggest that it is superior to MRI, with fat pad edema and degeneration being detected earlier via this modality. Ultrasound is also inexpensive and fast, further distinguishing it from MRI.[36]

When bilateral or recalcitrant heel pain is present, clinicians should order a complete blood count, erythrocyte sedimentation rate, rheumatoid factor, antinuclear antibodies, uric acid, and human leukocyte antigen-B27 studies. These tests may help identify a rheumatologic or autoimmune disorder, such as a seronegative spondyloarthropathy, Behçet syndrome, or inflammatory bowel arthritis.

Nerve conduction velocity and electromyography testing can objectively delineate the severity of a compression neuropathy around the foot and ankle as well as diagnose a spinal radiculopathy or peripheral neuropathy. However, these studies are of more benefit in the diagnosis of tarsal tunnel syndrome than plantar nerve entrapment because the FBLPN is difficult to examine with these tests.[37]

TREATMENT OF PLANTAR HEEL PAIN
Conservative Modalities

Mechanical, rheumatologic, and neurologic sources of plantar heel pain require, and are usually responsive to, a trial of conservative measures. Interventions include home stretching programs and physical therapy, nonsteroidal antiinflammatory drugs (NSAIDs), injections, heel pads, orthoses, night splints, and extracorporeal shockwave therapy (ESWT). In a work by Wolgin and colleagues,[38] 82 of 100 patients' plantar heel pain improved with conservative therapy, and an additional 15 patients were able to work and perform activities despite having mild symptoms. Callison[39] found that 73% of patients treated with nonoperative modalities had significant improvement within 6 months of treatment, whereas only 20% failed to improve.[39] A study by Davies and colleagues[40] also supports nonoperative interventions because they showed that less than 50% of patients who had a surgical procedure for heel pain were completely satisfied with the results.

A home stretching program is the first-line treatment of plantar heel pain. Both plantar fascia–specific and Achilles tendon–based protocols are available. Plantar fascia–specific stretching attempts to recreate the windlass mechanism, whereas Achilles tendon programs attempt to optimize the length of the gastrocnemius-soleus complex. DiGiovanni and colleagues[41] compared these protocols and showed that heel pain was resolved or improved at 8 weeks in 52% of patients treated with a plantar fascia–specific program versus 22% of those performing Achilles tendon exercises. However, at the 2-year follow-up, no difference was evident between the two groups.[41]

NSAIDs are an appropriate treatment of plantar heel pain but are typically prescribed in conjunction with another intervention, such as stretching. The true effectiveness of NSAIDs is, thus, unclear because they are infrequently the sole treatment modality. Although up to 76% of patients report successful outcomes with their use, no study to date has examined their efficacy alone.[38]

Corticosteroid injections are a commonly used treatment of plantar fasciitis, with one study identifying 170 of 233 orthopedic surgeons polled as using steroid injections for heel pain.[42] However, there is limited evidence to suggest that this intervention is effective at providing sustained pain relief. Crawford and colleagues[43] found improved symptoms at 1 month but not at 6 months as compared with a control group. Complications of steroid injection include rupture of the plantar fascia and fat pad atrophy.[27] One's injection technique can reduce the incidence of these complications; the needle should be placed superior to the fascia, from the medial side. This placement spreads the solution across the fascial layer, avoiding the fat pad and plantar nerves.

The injection of botulinum toxin A (BTX-A) is also being used to treat plantar foot pain. Its analgesic and antiinflammatory properties make it an intriguing intervention. In a placebo-controlled, double-blinded study, Babcock and colleagues[44] associated BTX-A injections with significant improvements in pain relief and foot function at both 3 and 8 weeks following treatment. Elizondo-Rodriguez and colleagues[45] have also found BTX-A to be an effective treatment of plantar fasciitis. In their prospective, randomized, double-blinded, and controlled clinical trial, the effectiveness of BTX-A injected into the gastrocnemius-soleus complex was compared with steroid injection into the medial plantar fascia. Over the 6 months that the patients were followed after receiving one of the two aforementioned injections, the group who received the BTX-A was found to have faster and more sustained symptom relief.[45]

Heel pads, foot orthoses, and shoe modifications are adjunctive modalities often used in the treatment of plantar heel pain. From a biomechanical perspective, foot orthoses are designed to place the foot and lower extremity in a more advantageous position by minimizing the existing stresses to the static and dynamic soft tissues of the foot and lower limb; orthoses off-load the plantar fascia, recreate the shape of the heel pad, and decrease excessive pronation.[46–48]

Commonly used orthoses include prefabricated silicone or rubber heel cups and arch supports, felt pads, custom arch supports, the University of California Biomechanics Laboratory orthosis (UCBL), and the supramalleolar ankle foot orthosis (SMO). The UCBL shoe insert is a maximum control foot orthotic that was named after the location in which it was developed, the University of California Berkeley Laboratory in 1967 (**Fig. 4**). It has since been defined as a deep-seated foot orthosis. The UCBL differs from other foot orthoses in that it fully encompasses the heel, which in turn holds the heel, or hindfoot, in a neutral, vertical position. While correcting and holding the heel in a neutral position, the UCBL also controls the inside arch of the foot and the outside border of the forefoot. These 3 corrective forces keep the foot held in a neutral position.

The SMO, as with other orthoses, gets its name for the part of the body for which it encompasses (**Fig. 5**). This orthosis supports the leg just above the medial and lateral malleoli. The SMO is designed to maintain a vertical or neutral heel while also supporting the 3 arches of the foot, which can help improve standing balance and walking. This design also allows for more control of the ankle and foot. It is more supportive than a UCBL but less supportive than a standard ankle foot orthosis (AFO).

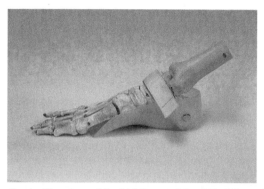

Fig. 4. The UCBL orthosis. (*Courtesy of* David Misener, BSc, CPO, MBA, Albany, NY.)

Shoes are integral to the success of an orthosis because they help to stabilize the orthosis within the shoe and around the foot. A proper shoe provides stability and shock absorption. How a shoe is built also makes a difference in its fit and function. Neutral-arched feet should be placed in shoes with firm midsoles, straight to semi-curved lasts, and moderate hindfoot stability. Low-arched or flat feet should be placed in shoes with a straight last and with motion control to help stabilize the feet. High-arched feet require cushioning and moderate hindfoot stability to compensate for the lack of natural shock absorption.

Ample evidence exists based on subjective pain relief, symptom resolution, and patient satisfaction for the success of orthosis.[49] In a randomized study by Pfeffer and colleagues,[2] 236 patients were randomized into 5 treatment groups: 1 control and 4 with different shoe inserts. Those treated with prefabricated inserts had the largest improvement in heel pain.[2] Roos and colleagues[50] also found foot orthoses to be effective in both the short- and long-term treatment of plantar fasciitis. In this prospective randomized trial, those who used orthoses experienced a 62% decrease in pain at 1 year as compared with patients treated with night splints. Admittedly, other studies have questioned the effectiveness of foot orthoses, identifying only small benefits.[51] Despite this, heel pads and orthoses are powerful tools in the clinician's armamentarium for the treatment of plantar heel pain.

Night splints are designed to prevent shortening of the plantar fascia during long periods of rest, with the goal of alleviating morning start-up pain. The night splint AFO

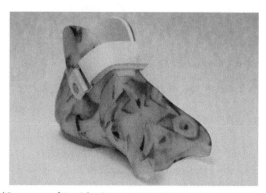

Fig. 5. The SMO. (*Courtesy of* David Misener, BSc, CPO, MBA.)

should be placed in 5° of dorsiflexion. Wapner and Sharkey[52] reported that 11 of their 14 patients improved when splinted in this position. Conversely, Probe and colleagues[53] found no significant benefit in adding night splinting to a standard NSAID and stretching protocol. Casting has also been used to unload the heel and immobilize the plantar fascia, hoping to reduce the repetitive microtrauma associated with plantar fasciitis.

ESWT is indicated for patients who have had at least 6 months of plantar fasciitis heel pain recalcitrant to at least 3 nonsurgical interventions (**Fig. 6**). The powerful shock waves break up scar tissue, stimulate angiogenesis, promote new bone formation, disrupt calcific deposits, and increase cytokine diffusion. Good or excellent results in the setting of chronic heel pain have been reported in 57% to 80% of patients.[54,55] ESWT is often performed under conscious sedation with regional anesthesia. It is well tolerated by patients. The contraindications include patients with hemophilia, coagulopathies, malignancy, and skeletal immaturity.

OPERATIVE TREATMENT

Surgery is indicated in the treatment of plantar heel pain that has failed a minimum of 6 months of conservative modalities (**Box 2**). An open partial release of the plantar fascia is the standard intervention. Although both open and endoscopic techniques have been described, there is no consensus as to the best choice; no studies have been conducted that directly compare these two techniques. Because entrapment neuropathy of the FBLPN presents similarly to plantar fasciitis, decompression of this nerve is frequently performed concurrently. Watson and colleagues[56] reported that 93% of their patients had satisfactory outcomes with partial medial plantar fasciectomy and nerve decompression. When nerve decompression is to be performed, an open approach is advocated because the risk of nerve injury may be higher with endoscopic procedures.[57]

Resection of heel spurs is also performed at times, most commonly in conjunction with the aforementioned procedures. However, Manoli and colleagues[58] reported calcaneal fractures secondary to extensive resection, an unwelcome complication of this procedure. Additionally, the notion that the subcalcaneal spur is the cause of plantar pain has lost popularity in recent years; therefore, this supplementary procedure is being performed less frequently. Fallat and colleagues[59] retrospectively compared percutaneous plantar fasciotomy with open fasciotomy and heel spur resection, determining that the percutaneous procedure

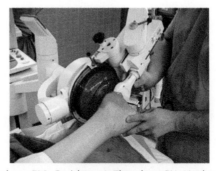

Fig. 6. ESWT. (*From* Berkson EM, Greisberg J, Theodore GH. Heel pain. In: DiGiovanni CW, Greisberg J, editors. Core knowledge in orthopedics: foot and ankle. Philadelphia: Elsevier; 2007; with permission.)

Box 2
Algorithm for the treatment of plantar fasciitis

If history and physical examination consistent with plantar fasciitis, begin

- Home stretching program multiple times daily (either plantar fascia specific or Achilles tendon stretching)

- Wear shoes with good support and a premade or custom-made orthotic

- Trial of NSAIDs

If no improvement

- Reexamine patient and consider alternative diagnoses

- If still consistent with plantar fasciitis, add alternative treatment, such as night splints and corticosteroid injection

If symptoms persist more than 6 months

- Consider shock-wave therapy

- Consider surgery

---

was as effective at relieving the plantar fasciitis pain and that those patients had a faster return to full activity.

Gastrocnemius recession is another procedure that may be indicated for the treatment of plantar fasciitis recalcitrant to conservative interventions. Because limited ankle dorsiflexion, specifically isolated gastrocnemius contracture, is frequently associated with plantar fasciitis, the release of the gastrocnemius can be an effective treatment.[60] Abbassian and colleagues[61] found proximal medial gastrocnemius release to provide complete or significant pain relief in 81% of their patients treated with this. Additionally, none of their patients reported worsening of their symptoms.

SUMMARY

Plantar heel pain is a frequently encountered phenomenon that transcends multiple medical specialties, including orthopedic surgery and primary care. Plantar fasciitis is the most common cause. However, other mechanical, rheumatologic, neurologic, and infectious causes exist; a comprehensive history and physical examination is pivotal to making the correct diagnosis. When the cause remains unclear after the evaluation, diagnostic adjuncts are available and include triple-phase bone scan, MRI, ultrasound, and laboratory studies. Regardless of diagnosis, nonoperative interventions are the mainstay of treatment and include but are not limited to stretching, NSAIDs, orthoses, and steroid injections. Operative intervention is only indicated after 6 months of failed conservative modalities.

REFERENCES

1. Crawford F, Atkins D, Edwards J. Interventions for treating plantar heel pain. Cochrane Database Syst Rev 2000;(3):CD000416.
2. Pfeffer G, Bacchetti P, Deland J. Comparison of custom and prefabricated orthoses in the initial treatment of proximal plantar fasciitis. Foot Ankle Int 1999; 20(4):214–21.
3. Riddle DL, Schappert SM. Volume of ambulatory care visits and patterns of care for patients diagnosed with plantar fasciitis: a national study of medical doctors. Foot Ankle Int 2004;25(5):303–10.

4. Tong KB, Furia J. Economic burden of plantar fasciitis treatment in the United States. Am J Orthop 2010;39(5):227–31.
5. Leach RE, Seavey MS, Salter DK. Results of surgery in athletes with plantar fasciitis. Foot Ankle 1986;7(3):156–61.
6. Chang CC, Miltner LJ. Periostitis of the os calcis. J Bone Joint Surg 1934;16: 355–64.
7. DuVries HL. Heel spur (calcaneal spur). Arch Surg 1957;74:536–42.
8. Pfeffer GB. Plantar heel pain. In: Myerson MS, editor. Foot and ankle disorders. Philadelphia: WB Saunders; 2000. p. 834–50.
9. Perry J. Anatomy and biomechanics of the hindfoot. Clin Orthop Relat Res 1983;(177):9–15.
10. Jahss MH, Kummer F, Michelson JD. Investigations into the fat pads of the sole of the foot: heel pressure studies. Foot Ankle 1992;13:227–32.
11. Hicks JH. The mechanics of the foot. II. The plantar aponeurosis and the arch. J Anat 1954;88(1):25–30.
12. Viel E, Esnault M. The effect of increased tension in the plantar fascia: a biomechanical analysis. Physiother Pract 1989;5:69–73.
13. Kwong PK, Kay D, Voner PT, et al. Plantar fasciitis: mechanics and pathomechanics of treatment. Clin Sports Med 1988;7:119–26.
14. Narvaez JA, Narvaez J, Ortega R, et al. Painful heel: MR imaging findings. Radiographics 2000;20:333–52.
15. Berlin SJ, Mirkin GS, Tubridy SP. Tumors of the heel. Clin Podiatr Med Surg 1990; 7:307–21.
16. Cooper JK, Wong FL, Swenerton KD. Endometrial adenocarcinoma presenting as an isolated calcaneal metastasis. A rare entity with good prognosis. Cancer 1994; 73:2779–81.
17. Bergqvist D, Mattsson J. Solitary calcaneal metastasis as the first sign of gastric cancer. A case report. Ups J Med Sci 1978;83:115–8.
18. Kaufmann J, Schulze E, Hein G. Monarthritis of the ankle as manifestation of a calcaneal metastasis of bronchogenic carcinoma. Scand J Rheumatol 2001;30: 363–5.
19. Amis J, Jennings L, Graham D, et al. Painful heel syndrome: radiographic and treatment assessment. Foot Ankle 1988;9:91–9.
20. Prichasuk S. The heel pad in plantar heel pain. J Bone Joint Surg Br 1994;76: 140–2.
21. Shmokler RL, Bravo AA, Lynch FR, et al. A new use of instrumentation in fluoroscopy controlled heel spur surgery. J Am Podiatr Med Assoc 1988;78:194–7.
22. Snook GA, Chrisman OD. The management of subcalcaneal pain. Clin Orthop Relat Res 1972;82:163–8.
23. Williams PL, Smibert JG, Cox R, et al. Imaging study of the painful heel syndrome. Foot Ankle 1987;7:345–9.
24. Kumai T, Benjamin M. Heel spur formation and the subcalcaneal enthesis of the plantar fascia. J Rheumatol 2002;29:1957–64.
25. Riddle DL, Pullsic M, Pidcoe P, et al. Risk factors for plantar fasciitis: a matched case-control study. J Bone Joint Surg Am 2003;85:872–7.
26. Tahririan MA, Motififard M, Tahmasebi MN, et al. Plantar fasciitis. J Res Med Sci 2012;17:799–804.
27. Acevedo JI, Beskin JL. Complications of plantar fascia rupture associated with corticosteroid injection. Foot Ankle Int 1998;19(2):91–7.
28. Sellman JR. Plantar fascia rupture associated with corticosteroid injection. Foot Ankle Int 1994;15(7):376–81.

29. Schepsis AA, Jones H, Haas AL. Achilles tendon disorders in athletes. Am J Sports Med 2002;30:287–305.
30. Kinoshita M, Okuda R, Morikawa J, et al. The dorsiflexion-eversion test for diagnosis of tarsal tunnel syndrome. J Bone Joint Surg Am 2001;83-A: 1835–9.
31. Ahstrom JP Jr. Spontaneous rupture of the plantar fascia. Am J Sports Med 1988; 16:306–7.
32. Graham CE. Painful heel syndrome: rationale of diagnosis and treatment. Foot Ankle 1983;3(5):261–7.
33. Sewell JR, Black CM, Chapman AH, et al. Quantitative scintigraphy in diagnosis and management of plantar fasciitis (calcaneal periostitis): concise communication. J Nucl Med 1980;21(7):633–6.
34. Theodorou DJ, Theodorou SJ, Resnick D. MR imaging of abnormalities of the plantar fascia. Semin Musculoskelet Radiol 2002;6(2):105–18.
35. Farooki S, Theodorou DJ, Sokoloff RM, et al. MRI of the medial and lateral plantar nerves. J Comput Assist Tomogr 2001;25(3):412–6.
36. Kamel M, Eid H, Mansour R. Ultrasound detection of heel enthesitis: a comparison with magnetic resonance imaging. J Rheumatol 2003;30(4):774–8.
37. Baxter DE, Pfeffer GB. Treatment of chronic heel pain by surgical release of the first branch of the lateral plantar nerve. Clin Orthop Relat Res 1992;(279): 229–36.
38. Wolgin M, Cook C, Graham C, et al. Conservative treatment of plantar heel pain: long-term follow-up. Foot Ankle Int 1994;15(3):97–102.
39. Callison WI. Heel pain in private practice [abstract]. Presented at the Orthopaedic Foot Club. Dallas (TX), April 4, 1989.
40. Davies MS, Weiss GA, Saxby TS. Plantar fasciitis: how successful is surgical intervention? Foot Ankle Int 1999;20(12):803–7.
41. DiGiovanni BF, Nawoczenski DA, Malay DP, et al. Plantar fascia–specific stretching exercise improves outcomes in patients with chronic plantar fasciitis: a prospective clinical trial with two-year follow-up. J Bone Joint Surg Am 2006;88: 1775–81.
42. Fadale PD, Wiggins ME. Corticosteroid injections: their use and abuse. J Am Acad Orthop Surg 1994;2(3):133–40.
43. Crawford F, Atkins D, Young P, et al. Steroid injections for heel pain: evidence of short-term effectiveness. A randomized controlled trial. Rheumatology 1999;38: 974–7.
44. Babcock MS, Foster L, Pasquina P, et al. Treatment of pain attributed to plantar fasciitis with botulinum toxin A: a short-term, randomized, placebo-controlled, double-blind study. Am J Phys Med Rehabil 2005;84:649–54.
45. Elizondo-Rodriguez J, Araujo-Lopez Y, Moreno-Gonzalez JA. A comparison of botulinum toxin A and intralesional steroids for the treatment of plantar fasciitis: a randomized, double-blinded study. Foot Ankle Int 2013;34:8–14.
46. Heiderscheit B, Hamill J, Tiberio D. A biomechanical perspective: do foot orthoses work? Br J Sports Med 2001;35(1):4–5.
47. Kogler GF, Veer FB, Solomonidis SE, et al. The influence of medial and lateral placement of orthotic wedges on loading of the plantar aponeurosis. J Bone Joint Surg Am 1999;81(10):1403–13.
48. Nester CJ, van der Linden ML, Bowker P. Effect of foot orthoses on the kinematics and kinetics of normal walking gait. Gait Posture 2003;17(2):180–7.
49. Gross ML, Davlin LB, Evanski PM. Effectiveness of orthotic shoe inserts in the long-distance runner. Am J Sports Med 1991;19(4):409–12.

50. Roos E, Engstrom M, Soderberg B. Foot orthoses for the treatment of plantar fasciitis. Foot Ankle Int 2006;27:606–11.
51. Landorf KB, Keenan AM, Herbet RD. Effectiveness of foot orthoses to treat plantar fasciitis: a randomized trial. Arch Intern Med 2006;166:1305–10.
52. Wapner KL, Sharkey PF. The use of night splints for treatment of recalcitrant plantar fasciitis. Foot Ankle 1991;12:135–7.
53. Probe RA, Baca M, Adams R, et al. Night splint treatment for plantar fasciitis: a prospective randomized study. Clin Orthop Relat Res 1999;(368):190–5.
54. Helbig K, Herbert C, Schostok T, et al. Correlations between the duration of pain and the success of shock wave therapy. Clin Orthop Relat Res 2001;(387): 68–71.
55. Rompe JD, Schoellner C, Nafe B. Evaluation of low-energy extracorporeal shock wave application for treatment of chronic plantar fasciitis. J Bone Joint Surg Am 2002;84:335–41.
56. Watson TS, Anderson RB, Davis WH, et al. Distal tarsal tunnel release with partial plantar fasciotomy for chronic heel pain: an outcome analysis. Foot Ankle Int 2002;23(6):530–7.
57. Neufeld SK, Cerrato R. Plantar fasciitis: evaluation and treatment. J Am Acad Orthop Surg 2008;16:338–46.
58. Manoli A 2nd, Harper MC, Fitzgibbons TC, et al. Calcaneal fracture after cortical bone removal. Foot Ankle 1992;13(9):523–5.
59. Fallat LM, Cox JT, Chahal R, et al. A retrospective comparison of percutaneous plantar fasciotomy and open plantar fasciotomy with heel spur resection. J Foot Ankle Surg 2013;52:288–90.
60. Patel A, DiGiovanni B. Association between plantar fasciitis and isolated contracture of the gastrocnemius. Foot Ankle Int 2011;32:5–8.
61. Abbassian A, Kohls-Gatzoulis J, Solan MC. Proximal medial gastrocnemius release in the treatment of recalcitrant plantar fasciitis. Foot Ankle Int 2012;33: 14–9.

Nerve Blocks for Chronic Pain

Salim M. Hayek, MD, PhD[a],*, Atit Shah, MD[b]

KEYWORDS

- Nerve block • Chronic pain • Diagnosis • Therapy

KEY POINTS

- Nerve blocks can be performed for a variety of conditions, providing diagnostic and therapeutic modalities.
- Whenever considering nerve blocks, risks and benefits must be considered before intervention.

INTRODUCTION

Nerve blocks are often performed as therapeutic or palliative interventions for pain relief. However, they are often performed for diagnostic or prognostic purposes. When considering nerve blocks for chronic pain, clinicians must always consider the indications, risks, benefits, and proper technique, in order to provide maximal benefit for the patients. Nerve blocks encompass a wide variety of interventional procedures. The most common nerve blocks for chronic pain and that may be applicable to the neurosurgical patient population are reviewed in this article. This article is an introduction and brief synopsis of the different available blocks that can be offered to a patient.

DIAGNOSTIC VERSUS THERAPEUTIC NERVE BLOCKS

In general, nerve blocks may be divided into diagnostic and therapeutic interventions. Pain is a subjective unpleasant sensation, the exact pathophysiology of which is uncertain or multifactorial in most clinical situations. In human beings, chronic pain

This article originally appeared in Neurosurgery Clinics of North America, Volume 25, Issue 4, October 2014.

Disclosures: All authors report and declare no support from any organization for the submitted work; no financial relationships with any organizations that might have an interest in the submitted work in the previous 3 years; no other relationships or activities that could have influenced the submitted work.

[a] Division of Pain Medicine, Department of Anesthesiology, University Hospitals of Cleveland, Case Western Reserve University, 11100 Euclid Avenue, Cleveland, OH 44106, USA; [b] Department of Anesthesiology, Case Western University, 450 East Waterside Drive Unit 1511, Chicago, IL 60601, USA
* Corresponding author.
E-mail address: salim.hayek@uhhospitals.org

is a complex process that is compounded by psychosocial, financial, and sometimes legal matters.[1] When the cause of pain is unclear despite appropriate history taking, physical examination, and imaging or electrodiagnostic studies, diagnostic or prognostic nerve blocks may be in order. For instance, pain originating in the zygapophyseal joints or the sacroiliac joint cannot reliably be diagnosed by clinical examination or imaging studies and diagnostic local anesthetic blocks are frequently called on to confirm the diagnosis.[2,3] However, there are significant limitations to nerve blocks in making the leap from pain relief to establishing that pain is mediated by the targeted nerve, because performance of a nerve block takes into consideration many assumptions:

1. The nerve being blocked is responsible for generation, conduction, or maintenance of the painful stimulus
2. The operator performing the procedure is skilled in the performance of the block
3. The needle is placed in the exact and correct anatomic location
4. The patient does not have anatomic variations or aberrant physiologic or pharmacologic responses to the medication used
5. The volume of the medication injected is appropriate for the nerve/space
6. The medication injected will remain in place and anesthetize only the targeted nerve and no other nerves or structures or act systemically
7. The patient is able to understand and interpret the response to the block appropriately

Nonetheless, when properly performed in the appropriate clinical setting, nerve blocks can provide valuable adjunct information that, when taken together with the patient's complete clinical picture, may help in decision making about the cause of pain.

The most commonly performed diagnostic nerve blocks include:

1. Selective nerve blocks. These may be indicated in the presence of radicular symptoms and questionable or multiple levels of abnormalities on imaging studies. Assessing selective nerve root blocks is challenging given that no loss of cutaneous sensation occurs following surgical division of a single nerve root.[1] Multiple studies attest to the high positive predictive value of selective nerve root blocks and their accuracy is superior to that of imaging and electrodiagnostic testing.[4–7] Nonetheless, accuracy of these blocks awaits authentication in controlled blinded trials.
2. Joint injections. Controlled diagnostic blocks have been used successfully to identify the sacroiliac joint and other joints as a source of pain and represent the most reliable way of diagnosing painful joint syndromes. Sacroiliac joint pain accounts for between 15% and 20% of patients presenting with axial low back pain. Even though their validity has yet to be proved, small-volume local anesthetic blocks are still the most used method for diagnosing sacroiliac joint pain.[8]
3. Medial branch blocks. Medial branches of posterior rami supply zygapophyseal (facet) joints at the same level and the level below. Hence, blocking a single facet joint requires blockade of 2 medial branches. Diagnostic medial nerve branch blocks are the gold standard to establish facet-mediated pain. Lumbar zygapophyseal pain accounts for up to 15% of patients with axial low back pain.[9]
4. Differential nerve blocks. These blocks are often performed in the setting of abdominal or pelvic pain of unknown cause. An anatomic (nerve-by-nerve block) or pharmacologic approach may be used. The pharmacologic approach is preferred and involves epidural blockade of all innervation to the target area (typically T4 level) and evaluation of the pain response as the epidural block resolves. It

is most useful to differentiate organic peripheral pain that would be amenable to further interventions from central pain.[10]

False-positive responses occur with blocks even with the use of imaging. For instance, a placebo response rate of 38% (false-positives) has been shown for uncontrolled lumbar facet joint blocks and a low positive predictive value of 31%.[11] To curtail the rate of false-positive responses, repeat blocks or comparative local anesthetic blocks have been performed, resulting in refinement of diagnostic accuracy.[12,13]

Diagnostic blocks typically provide a patient with relief limited to the duration of action of the local anesthetic used, although longer-lasting responses are occasionally noted.

THERAPEUTIC NERVE BLOCKS

Therapeutic interventions allow longer-term pain relief. The many common therapeutic nerve interventions include epidural steroid injections, radiofrequency ablations, and sympathetic nerve neurolysis.

Epidural Steroid Injection

Introduction
Epidural steroid injections have been used for chronic spinal pain relief for decades. Depositing steroids in the epidural space helps reduce inflammation around nerve roots contributing to pain. Epidural steroids can be delivered by several approaches, including the interlaminar, transforaminal, and caudal approaches.[14,15]

Epidural steroid injection can be performed as a more conservative approach than surgery, when surgery is not indicated or as a palliative bridge to surgery. Epidural injections can benefit a patient when the pain is secondary to disc herniation, discogenic pain, or spinal stenosis.[15] Benefits involve predominantly short-term pain relief, although occasionally long-term pain relief occurs. A series of 3 injections can be done in a 6-month span; however, this standard relates to limiting steroid toxicity. The main concern with repeated epidural steroid injections centers on the amount of total steroid injected and the possibility of causing adrenal suppression and affecting bone reabsorption.[14–16]

Indications
Indications for epidural steroid injection include radiculopathy secondary to disc herniation, isolated spondylotic spurring of the foramina, or neurogenic claudication associated with spinal stenosis.[15]

Efficacy
Moderate to strong evidence exists for interlaminar and transforaminal epidural steroid injections, at least in the short-term relief of radicular pain.[15]

Multiple studies of transforaminal epidural steroid injections in patients with herniated discs, radiculopathy, and stenosis reported significant benefit in pain scores, walking tolerance, and standing.[17,18]

In 2010, the American Society of Anesthesiologist Task Force on Chronic Pain Management published a practice guideline that stated, "Epidural Steroid injections with or without local anesthetics may be used as part of a multimodal treatment regimen to provide pain relief in selected patients with radicular pain or radiculopathy. Shared decision making regarding epidural steroid injections should include a specific discussion of potential complications, particularly with regard to the transforaminal approach."[19]

Procedure
There are multiple approaches to delivering steroid into the epidural space. The interlaminar epidural steroid injection uses a midline approach and delivers medications centrally with some spread to surrounding nerve roots. It is useful in central canal stenosis and in patients with diffuse disorder. The transforaminal approach is a directed injection, either right or left sided, and delivers medication that surrounds the affected nerve root with spread into the anterior epidural space. The caudal approach uses the opening at the sacral hiatus to deliver medication to the lower lumbar spine area. These procedures are done under fluoroscopic guidance and confirmation is obtained with contrast dye before injection of steroid (**Fig. 1**).[15,16]

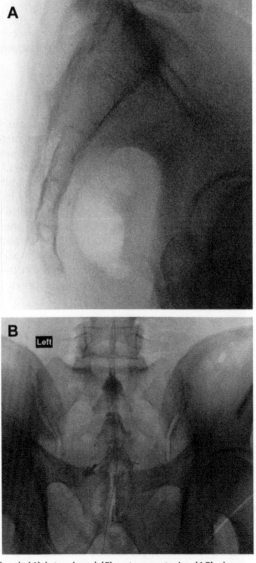

Fig. 1. Caudal epidural; (*A*) lateral and (*B*) anteroposterior (AP) views.

Complications

When considering an epidural steroid injection, the risks versus benefits must be assessed. Potential risks of the procedure include, but are not limited to, dural puncture, postdural headache, bleeding, infection, nerve damage, epidural hematoma, epidural abscess, and paralysis. Transforaminal injections of particulate steroids carry a small but significant risk of embolization of large steroid particles into radicular arteries and from there into arterial spinal cord artery or vertebral arteries. Catastrophic events have occurred, in particular with cervical transforaminal injection of particulate steroids. Nonparticulate steroids are now advocated in transforaminal epidural steroid injections in the cervical region. Even though the risks are low, all patients must be well informed and consented before the procedure.[14–16]

Facet Joint Nerve Blocks

Introduction

Zygapophyseal or facet joints are a source of pain for many patients.[20] A common cause of this joint pain is degeneration and arthritis of the spine and joint.[14,15]

Pain that is caused by facet joints typically presents with axial pain that increases with movement. Pain is worse with bending, extending, and rotational movements. Radiation of pain toward the extremity is an uncommon presentation but pain is often referred to the buttocks or shoulders.[15]

Patients typically have insidious onset of pain over time; however, a subgroup of patients has sudden onset of facet pain that occurs after some sort of trauma or deceleration (whiplash) injury.[16]

Though facet arthropathy is a common finding on imaging, correlation must be made with history and physical examination. When suspicion of facet-related pain is high, a diagnostic medial branch block must be performed to confirm the diagnosis. A unilateral or bilateral approach can be performed, depending on the patient's character of pain.[9] The facet joint is provided with sensory innervation by the medial branch of the posterior primary ramus.[14,16]

Medial branch blocks provide diagnostic value, indicating whether the joint is the pain generator for a patient. Patients are asked to perform movements that normally cause them pain after the procedure and their pain is reassessed. Significant pain relief, 50% or greater, is considered a positive response and a patient can return for a radiofrequency ablation at a later date. Radiofrequency ablation provides a much longer duration of pain relief, averaging about 6 to 9 months in duration.[14,15]

Procedure

A diagnostic medial branch block is conducted with local anesthetic only. Using fluoroscopic guidance, the needles are positioned along the posterior spine at a consistent location where the medial branch is known to travel.[21]

In the cervical region, the needles are advanced toward the middle of the articular pillars. After correct location has been verified, 0.25 mL of local anesthetic is injected. In the thoracic and lumbar regions, after correct location has been verified, 0.5 mL of local anesthetic is injected.[15]

Radiofrequency ablation is performed in a similar manner to medial branch blocks; however, sensory and motor testing is typically performed before the ablation (**Fig. 2**).[15]

Efficacy

Good evidence exists in support of radiofrequency lesioning of the medial branch nerves given that properly performed diagnostic tests have provided significant temporary relief.

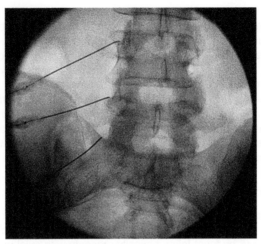

Fig. 2. Medial branch probe positioning; AP view.

Numerous placebo-controlled trials have examined lumbar facet pain and shown that radiofrequency ablation yielded positive results in lumbar pain in selected patients.[22,23]

Complications
Complications include pain at the injection site, injury to spinal nerves, uncomfortable dysesthesia, and sensory loss. Use of fluoroscopic guidance, proper testing before ablation, and performance of the procedure in an awake or minimally sedated patient results in near elimination of major risks.[14,16]

Sympathetic Blocks

Introduction
These are multiple neural pathways that are involved in the perception and maintenance of pain. Following neuronal injury, the sympathetic nervous system is involved in pain perception and maintenance of chronic pain.[14,16]

The sympathetic chain extends from the first thoracic level to the second or third lumbar level. Its target area covers the cervical to the sacral region, providing sympathetic stimulation throughout the body.[14,16] Targeting different sympathetic ganglia allows blockade of sympathetic fibers in various regions throughout the body that may be contributing to or maintaining a patient's chronic pain.[14,16]

Efficacy
Limited evidence exists in support of the use of sympathetic blocks in pain relief of extremity pain.[24–27] There is stronger evidence for efficacy in neurolytic celiac plexus blocks in patients with pancreatic cancer pain.[28–30] There are multiple studies investigating the use of neurolysis in patients with cancer. One study comparing celiac plexus neurolysis versus sham showed significant pain relief at follow-up at 6 weeks.[29] A meta-analysis of 21 retrospective studies in patients undergoing celiac plexus neurolysis reported that 89% of patients received excellent pain relief in the follow-up visit at 2 weeks and 90% of patients received pain relief at the 3-month visit. When investigating superior hypogastric plexus blocks, it has been reported that 70% of patients with pelvic pain associated with cancer received significant pain relief in terms of visual analog scores.[31]

Stellate Ganglion Block

Introduction

The cervical sympathetic trunk contains 3 ganglia: the superior, middle, and inferior cervical ganglia. In 80% of people the lowest cervical ganglia is fused with the upper thoracic ganglion to form the cervicothoracic ganglion, also known as the stellate ganglion.[32] The cervicothoracic ganglion is on or just lateral to the longus colli muscle between the base of the seventh cervical transverse process and the neck of the first rib. The cervicothoracic ganglion receives preganglionic fibers from the lateral gray column of the spinal cord. The preganglionic fibers for the head and neck emerge from the upper 5 thoracic spinal nerves, ascending in the sympathetic trunk to synapse in the cervical ganglia. The preganglionic fibers supplying the upper extremity originate from the upper thoracic segments between T2 and T6 and in turn synapse in the cervicothoracic ganglion.

Procedure

The block is generally conducted at the sixth or seventh cervical vertebra using ultrasonography or fluoroscopic guidance. Ultrasonography allows a physician to visualize the soft tissue, artery, vein, and neural bundle. Fluoroscopy allows better visualization of bony structures.[15]

Regardless of the technique, after appropriate positioning of the needle is confirmed, approximately 2 to 5 mL of 0.25% bupivacaine or ropivacaine are injected. Injection is done slowly, in increments, being aware of any signs of local anesthetic toxicity. Signs of appropriate spread include increased temperature in the affected upper extremity, venodilatation in the ipsilateral arm, nasal congestion, anhidrosis, and Horner syndrome.[14,15] For a successful sympathetic block, a temperature increase in the hand to at least 34°C is recommended to achieve meaningful interruption of the postganglionic sympathetic supply.[33] The many indications for the blockade of the stellate ganglion include, but are not limited to, complex regional pain syndrome of the upper extremity, vascular insufficiency of the upper extremity, hyperhydrosis, acute pain of herpes zoster, postherpetic neuralgia, congenital prolonged QT syndrome (left cervicothoracic ganglion blockade), migraines, tension and cluster headaches, cerebral angiospasm, and cerebral thrombosis **(Fig. 3)**.

Complications

Because of the close proximity of many critical and important structures in the neck, numerous complications are possible. Minor complications include recurrent laryngeal nerve paralysis or phrenic nerve paralysis from local anesthetic spread, and self-resolving somatic block. Pneumothorax may occur, especially on the right side (higher lung apex). Major complications result from intraspinal spread (subdural or epidural injection) typically resulting in ventilatory inadequacy; or from intravascular injection, usually the vertebral artery, with loss of consciousness, convulsions, ventilatory inadequacy, and hypotension. Use of image guidance may curtail many of these complications.

Celiac Plexus

Introduction

The celiac plexus is another sympathetic plexus that is generally found at the level of T12 and L1, just lateral to the aorta. The celiac plexus is formed by a combination of the greater, lesser, and least splanchnic nerves with parasympathetic contribution from the vagus nerve. This important plexus is responsible for conducting afferent

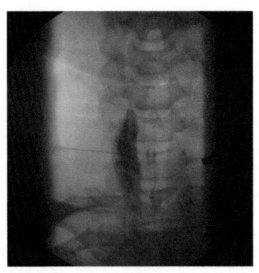

Fig. 3. Stellate ganglion needle positioning; AP view.

visceral pain signals typically covering the abdomen with distal bowel and pelvic structures excluded.[14,16]

Celiac plexus blocks can provide diagnostic value to a physician by identifying pain that is conducted by sympathetic fibers. If a patient receives short-lived significant benefit, the patient may be a candidate for neurolytic celiac plexus block, which has long-lasting benefit in 70% to 90% of patients with visceral pain from upper intra-abdominal malignancies.[14,16]

Neurolytic block is generally performed using alcohol or phenol. Ethyl alcohol is less viscous than phenol and allows easier injection through small-diameter needles. Ethyl alcohol has a high concentration that can be appreciated by patients as pain on injection, and therefore injection of local anesthetic precedes ethanol injection. After injection, alcohol can also cause an inflammatory reaction that can persist and cause pain for a short time after the procedure.[14,16]

Phenol is typically prepared by combining carbolic acid, oxybenzene, hydroxybenzene, phenyl hydroxide, phenylic acid, and phenic acid. Phenol, unlike alcohol, is very viscous and difficult to inject. On injection, patients generally experience little pain.[25]

Procedure

The procedure is conducted under fluoroscopic guidance with the patient in the prone position. Once the needle is in the correct location, confirmation with contrast is obtained. Spread to the anterolateral surface of the aorta is desired.[15]

Diagnostic celiac plexus block is performed before neurolysis. When performing diagnosis, a total volume of 20 to 30 mL of 0.25% bupivacaine is injected. An identical volume is injected when performing neurolysis with frequent aspiration (**Fig. 4**).[15]

Complications

The most common side effects known after celiac plexus block include orthostatic hypotension and diarrhea. Complications include local anesthetic toxicity, kidney injury, pneumothorax, and aortic injury. With neurolysis, complications are similar and also include increased blood alcohol concentration, cardiovascular collapse,

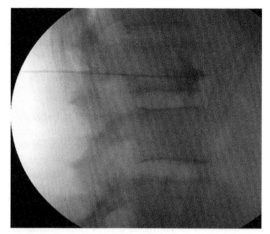

Fig. 4. Celiac plexus needle positioning; lateral view.

and paraplegia.[1–3] Paraplegia may occur secondary to damage or occlusion of the artery of Adamkiewicz and occurs at a rate of 1 in 683 blocks, predominantly with ethanol.[34] However, there has been 1 case report of paraplegia following a neurolytic celiac plexus block with phenol.[35]

Lumbar Sympathetic Block

Introduction
The lumbar sympathetic plexus is involved in pain that is sympathetically maintained in the lower extremities. The lumbar sympathetic chain lies at the level of the second to fourth lumbar vertebral bodies. The most common indication for a lumbar sympathetic block include complex regional pain syndrome of the lower extremity with sympathetically maintained pain. Patients may benefit most when sympathetic plexus block is combined with a treatment plan involving physical therapy; however, evidence is scarce, with only 1 study in children showing short-term relief.[14,16,27]

Procedure
Similar to celiac plexus block, the patient starts in the prone position and the procedure is conducted under fluoroscopic guidance. The needle is typically placed over the inferior portion of the second or third lumbar vertebrae. Once the needle is verified in correct position, 15 to 20 mL of 0.25% bupivacaine or ropivacaine are injected incrementally. Proper spread yields a lower extremity sympathetic block that results in venodilatation and a temperature increase to within $3°C$ of the patient's core temperature.[15,36]

When a patient perceives only short-term benefit from local anesthetic injections, neurolysis can be performed. For neurolysis, phenol or alcohol can be used. Needles are positioned at the level of L2, L3, and L4, which represent the most common location of the lumbar sympathetic chain. After proper positioning has been confirmed, 2 to 3 mL of phenol or alcohol are injected at each site.[15]

Radiofrequency ablation is another option to short-lived pain control with local anesthetic injection. With this approach, radiofrequency probes are inserted over the anterolateral surfaces of the second, third, and fourth lumbar vertebrae.[15,37]

Complications

Complications include local anesthetic toxicity, kidney injury, intrathecal injection, and partial neurolysis of adjacent nerves, including predominantly the genitofemoral nerve.[14–16]

Superior Hypogastric Block

Introduction

The superior hypogastric plexus is responsible for sympathetically maintained pain in the pelvic region, which includes the uterus, vagina, rectum, prostate, and bladder. The plexus is located at the level of the fourth and fifth lumbar vertebrae and first sacral vertebrae.[14,16] Limited evidence exists in support of its use in visceral pelvic pain.

Procedure

Superior hypogastric blocks are performed in a similar manner to lumbar sympathetic blocks with needle placement at the level of the fifth lumbar vertebrae. After correct needle location is confirmed, 8 to 10 mL of 0.25% bupivacaine local anesthetic are injected. The procedure is repeated bilaterally and, for those patients who do not receive significant duration of pain relief, neurolysis can be performed.[15]

Complications

Complications include nerve injury, local anesthetic toxicity, puncture of surrounding organs, bleeding, and partial neurolysis of adjacent nerves.[14–16]

Intercostal Nerve Block

Introduction

Underneath each thoracic rib (T1–T12) runs an intercostal nerve that provides sensory input from the thoracic and abdominal dermatomal regions. These nerves are branches of the anterior primary rami that lie underneath the respective rib in the subcostal groove. The intercostal artery and nerve run alongside the nerve. The location of these 3 structures from superior to inferior typically includes vein, artery, and nerve. Along the course of the intercostal nerve there are multiple branches, such as the posterior, lateral cutaneous, and anterior branches.[14,16]

These nerves can be blocked with local anesthetic or frozen and deactivated with cryoablation. Indications include surgical thoracic pain, rib pain from fracture, neuropathic pain from herpes zoster, and cancer pain attributable to rib metastases.[14,16]

Procedure

Intercostal nerve blocks can be performed using either ultrasonography or fluoroscopic guidance. The block can be performed anywhere along the course of the nerve; however, it is recommended to block the nerves proximal to the branching of the posterior cutaneous nerve to obtain posterior coverage.[15]

Using fluoroscopy, the patient is placed in the prone position. A needle is advanced to the subcostal groove. Careful attention must be paid to the lung anatomy in order to avoid the risk of pneumothorax. Contrast is injected to verify correct placement and 2 to 4 mL of local anesthetic can be injected for diagnostic purposes. The procedure can be repeated at multiple levels; however, be aware of local anesthetic toxicity because both artery and vein are in close proximity.[14,15]

After a positive diagnostic intercostal block, cryoablation can be performed. Cryoablation uses an active probe tip that is cooled to −20°C. Cryoablation damages the vasa nervorum, causing edema and nerve injury. Patients can obtain weeks to months of pain relief, depending on the speed of nerve regeneration. Cryoablation minimizes the risk of neuroma formation and deafferentation pain (**Fig. 5**).[14,15]

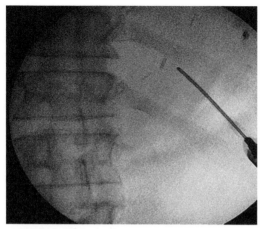

Fig. 5. Intercostal nerve cryoablation needle positioning; AP view.

Efficacy

Studies of intercostal nerve block for pain relief have been reported with positive results. One retrospective study of pain control in patients with cancer reported that 80% of patients received optimal pain control, whereas 56% of patients reported a reduction in their analgesic use. Thirty-two percent of the patients did not have recurrence of pain until the end of their lives.[38]

Complications

Complications include local anesthetic toxicity, infection, pneumothorax, nerve damage, hematoma, and spinal anesthesia.[14–16]

Occipital Nerve Block

Introduction

As the greater occipital nerve or lesser occipital nerve becomes irritated, the patient may experience headaches. Occipital nerve headaches present with paroxysmal pain that can be stabbing in nature. The pain occurs along the distribution of the greater and lesser occipital nerves.[14,16]

Possible causes for occipital nerve headaches include trauma to the nerves, spondylosis, cervical disc disease, myofascial pain, and tumors in the occipital scalp.[14,16]

When approaching a patient with head pain for the first time, a systematic and complete history and physical should be completed. At first, conservative modalities can be attempted, which include massages, physical therapy, heat, ice, nonsteroidal antiinflammatory drugs, muscle relaxants, anticonvulsants, and antidepressants. Patients with significant pain without relief from conservative approaches can be offered occipital nerve blockade if the cause is thought to arise from the occipital nerve.[14,16]

Procedure

The greater occipital nerve arises from the dorsal ramus of the second cervical nerve and passes between the inferior capitis oblique and semispinalis capitis muscles.[14]

The occipital nerve block is performed with the patient in the sitting position. The occipital artery runs lateral to the occipital nerve and is found approximately at one-third the distance between the occipital protuberance and the mastoid process along the nuchal ridge. Palpation of the artery is performed and a needle is inserted just medial to the artery and advanced until bony contact is made along the nuchal ridge. After negative aspiration, approximately 3 to 5 mL of local anesthetic are injected. The lesser occipital nerve can be blocked as well; however, the insertion point is more lateral.[14]

Efficacy

An uncontrolled study of 180 patients with cervicogenic headaches reported that 94% of patients experienced complete relief of their headaches lasting from 10 to 77 days.[39]

Complications

Complications include bleeding, infection, nerve damage, and allergy.[14]

SUMMARY

Nerve blocks can be performed for a variety of conditions, providing diagnostic and therapeutic modalities. Whenever considering nerve blocks, risks and benefits must be considered before intervention. This article discusses a variety of nerve blocks that can be offered to patients when appropriate.

REFERENCES

1. Hogan QH, Abram SE. Neural blockade for diagnosis and prognosis. A review. Anesthesiology 1997;86:216–41.
2. Schwarzer AC, Aprill CN, Derby R, et al. Clinical features of patients with pain stemming from the lumbar zygapophysial joints. Is the lumbar facet syndrome a clinical entity? Spine 1994;19:1132–7.
3. Maigne JY, Aivaliklis A, Pfefer F. Results of sacroiliac joint double block and value of sacroiliac pain provocation tests in 54 patients with low back pain. Spine 1996; 21:1889–92.
4. Schutz H, Lougheed WM, Wortzman G, et al. Intervertebral nerve-root in the investigation of chronic lumbar disc disease. Can J Surg 1973;16:217–21.
5. Dooley JF, McBroom RJ, Taguchi T, et al. Nerve root infiltration in the diagnosis of radicular pain. Spine 1988;13:79–83.
6. Stanley D, McLaren MI, Euinton HA, et al. A prospective study of nerve root infiltration in the diagnosis of sciatica. A comparison with radiculography, computed tomography, and operative findings. Spine 1990;15:540–3.
7. Haueisen DC, Smith BS, Myers SR, et al. The diagnostic accuracy of spinal nerve injection studies. Their role in the evaluation of recurrent sciatica. Clin Orthop Relat Res 1985;(198):179–83.
8. Cohen SP. Sacroiliac joint pain: a comprehensive review of anatomy, diagnosis, and treatment. Anesth Analg 2005;101(5):1440–53.
9. Cohen SP, Srinivasa RN. Pathogenesis, diagnosis, and treatment of lumbar zygapophysial (facet) joint pain. Anesthesiology 2007;106(3):591–614.
10. Garcia J, Veizi E, Hayek S. Differential diagnostic nerve blocks. In: Deer T, editor. Interventional and neuromodulatory techniques for pain management. Philadelphia: Elsevier/Saunders; 2012.
11. Schwarzer AC, Aprill CN, Derby R, et al. The false-positive rate of uncontrolled diagnostic blocks of the lumbar zygapophysial joints. Pain 1994;58:195–200.
12. Barnsley L, Lord S, Bogduk N. Comparative local anaesthetic blocks in the diagnosis of cervical zygapophysial joint pain. Pain 1993;55:99–106.

13. Barnsley L, Lord S, Wallis B, et al. False-positive rates of cervical zygapophysial joint blocks. Clin J Pain 1993;9:124–30.
14. Benzon HT. Essentials of pain medicine. Philadelphia: Elsevier/Saunders; 2011.
15. Rathmell JP. Atlas of image-guided intervention in regional anesthesia and pain medicine. Philadelphia: Wolters Kluwer/Lippincott Williams & Wilkins Health; 2012.
16. Benzon HT, Raj PP. Raj's practical management of pain. Philadelphia: Mosby-Elsevier; 2008.
17. Ghahreman A, Ferch R, Bogduk N. The efficacy of transforaminal injection of steroids for the treatment of lumbar radicular pain. Pain Med 2010;11(8):1149–68.
18. Riew KD, Yin Y, Gilula L, et al. The effect of nerve-root injections on the need for operative treatment of lumbar radicular pain. A prospective, randomized, controlled, double-blind study. J Bone Joint Surg Am 2000;82-A(11):1589–93.
19. Rosenquist RW, Benzon HT, Connis RT. Practice guidelines for chronic pain management: an updated report by the American Society of Anesthesiologists Task Force on chronic pain management and the American Society of Regional Anesthesia and Pain Medicine. Anesthesiology 2010;112:810–33.
20. Kuslich SD. The tissue origin of low back pain and sciatica: a report of pain response to tissue stimulation during operations on the lumbar spine using local anesthesia. Orthop Clin North Am 1991;22(2):181–7.
21. Lau P, Mercer S, Govind J, et al. The surgical anatomy of lumbar medial branch neurotomy. Pain Med 2004;5(3):289–98.
22. Stovner LJ, Kolstad F, Helde G. Radiofrequency denervation of facet joints C2–C6 in cervicogenic headache. a randomized, double-blind, sham-controlled study. Cephalalgia 2004;24:821–30.
23. Van WR, Geurts JW, Wynne HJ. Radiofrequency denervation of lumbar facet joints in the treatment of chronic low back pain. a randomized, double-blind, sham lesion-controlled trial. Clin J Pain 2005;21:335–44.
24. Day M. Sympathetic blocks: the evidence. Pain Pract 2008;8:98–109.
25. Forouzanfar T, Van Kleef M, Weber WE. Radiofrequency lesions of the stellate ganglion in chronic pain syndromes: retrospective analysis of clinical efficacy in 86 patients. Clin J Pain 2000;16:164–8.
26. Price DD, Long S, Wilsey B. Analysis of peak magnitude and duration of analgesia produced by local anesthetic injected into sympathetic ganglia of complex regional pain syndrome patients. Clin J Pain 1998;14:216–8.
27. Meier PM, Zurakowski D, Berde CB, et al. Lumbar sympathetic blockade in children with complex regional pain syndromes: a double blind placebo-controlled crossover trial. Anesthesiology 2009;111(2):372–80.
28. Lillemoe KD, Cameron JL, Kaufman HS, et al. Chemical splanchnicectomy in patients with unresectable pancreatic cancer. A prospective randomized trial. Ann Surg 1993;217(5):447–55.
29. Wong GY, Schroeder DR, Carns PE. Effect of neurolytic celiac plexus block on pain relief, quality of life, and survival in patients with unresectable pancreatic cancer: a randomized controlled trial. JAMA 2004;291:1092–9.
30. Eisenberg E, Carr DB, Chalmers TC. Neurolytic celiac plexus block for treatment of cancer pain: a meta-analysis. Anesth Analg 1995;80:290–5.
31. Plancarte R, Amescua C, Patt RB, et al. Superior hypogastric plexus block for pelvic cancer pain. Anesthesiology 1990;73:236–9.
32. Marples IL, Atkinson RE. Stellate ganglion block. Pain Rev 2001;8:3–11.
33. Malmqvist EL, Bengtsson M, Sorensen J. Efficacy of stellate ganglion block: a clinical study with bupivacaine. Reg Anesth 1992;17:340–7.

34. Davies DD. Incidence of major complications of neurolytic coeliac plexus block. J R Soc Med 1993;86(5):264–6.
35. Galizia EJ, Lahiri SK. Paraplegia following coeliac plexus block with phenol. Case report. Br J Anaesth 1974;46(7):539–40.
36. Tran KM, Frank SM, Raja SN, et al. Lumbar sympathetic block for sympathetically maintained pain: changes in cutaneous temperatures and pain perception. Anesth Analg 2000;90(6):1396–401.
37. Rocco A. Anatomy of the lumbar sympathetic chain for radiofrequency lesioning. Reg Anesth Pain Med 1995;17(1):28.
38. Wong FC, Lee TW, Yuen KK, et al. Intercostal nerve blockade for cancer pain: effectiveness and selection of patients. Hong Kong Med J 2007;13(4):266–70.
39. Anthony M. Cervicogenic headache. Prevalence and response to local steroid therapy. Clin Exp Rheumatol 2000;18(19):59–64.

Spinal Cord Injury Pain

Michael Saulino, MD, PhD[a,b],*

KEYWORDS

- Spinal cord injury • Musculoskeletal pain • Neuropathic pain • Spasticity

KEY POINTS

- Spinal cord injury (SCI)-associated pain has a specific classification approach that assists in guiding treatment strategies.
- SCI-related pain seems to be prevalent, but there is considerable variability in the epidemiology of this condition.
- Evaluation of SCI-associated pain relies heavily on history and is supplemented by a neuromusculoskeletal examination and judicious use of laboratory and radiologic testing.
- Relatively few treatments for SCI-associated pain have been extensively studied.

INTRODUCTION

Although traumatic SCI results in a number of serious impairments including paralysis, sensory loss, and neurogenic bowel/bladder function, perhaps no SCI-associated condition is more vexing to the treating physiatrist than chronic pain. Some of these SCI-related impairments can be accommodated with compensatory strategies, whereas chronic pain, especially neuropathic pain associated with injury to the spinal cord, remains quite recalcitrant. In addition to the expected challenges in treating any chronic pain condition, treatment of SCI-related pain has the difficulty of disruption of normal neural pathways that subserve pain transmission and attenuation. This article attempts to describe the classification, epidemiology, evaluation methods, and treatment strategies for this serious pain syndrome.

CLASSIFICATION

Before 2000, there was no consistent approach to the classification of SCI-related chronic pain. This variability was described by Hicken and colleagues[1] during a review in 2002 in which 29 distinct schemes were described with potentially confusing and inconsistent terminology. By 2008, 3 classifications systems emerged as the leading systems based on their utility, comprehensiveness, validity, and reliability. These

This article originally appeared in Physical Medicine and Rehabilitation Clinics of North America, Volume 25, Issue 2, May 2014.

[a] MossRehab, 60 Township Line Road, Elkins Park, PA 19027, USA; [b] Department of Rehabilitation Medicine, Jefferson Medical College, Thomas Jefferson University, Philadelphia, PA, USA
* MossRehab, 60 Township Line Road, Elkins Park, PA 19027.
E-mail address: saulinom@einstein.edu

schemes included the Cardenas classification,[2] the taxonomy of the International Association for the Study of Pain,[3] and the Bryce-Ragnarsson classification.[4] Through the leadership of Bryce, a unified system was created and published in 2011. The International Spinal Cord Injury Pain Classification (ISCIP) has been adopted by many leading SCI and pain professional associations throughout the world.[5] This classification is visually depicted in **Fig. 1**.

Given the probable ubiquity of the ISCIP classification, some commentary on this approach is warranted. The first tier of this system is divided into nociceptive, neuropathic, other, and unknown categories. The distinction between the nociceptive and neuropathic categories is certainly approximate because the treatment approaches to these syndromes are often vastly different. As discussed later in this article, nociceptive pain can often be addressed by classic physiatric techniques (in the case of musculoskeletal pain) or other medical interventions (in visceral and other nociceptive pain). This fact is in contradistinction to neuropathic pain in which many treatment approaches are either pharmacologic or interventional. The ISCIP classification also demonstrates the continued difficulties of even expert clinicians and scientists to categorize every single pain condition associated with the SCI population, as

Tier 1: pain type	Tier 2: pain subtype	Tier 3: primary pain source and/or pathology (write or type in)
☐ Nociceptive pain	☐ Musculoskeletal pain	☐ _____ e.g., glenohumeral arthritis, lateral epicondylitis, comminuted femur fracture, quadratus lumborum muscle spasm
	☐ Visceral pain	☐ _____ e.g., myocardial infarction, abdominal pain due to bowel impaction, cholecystitis
	☐ Other nociceptive pain	☐ _____ e.g., autonomic dysreflexia headache, migraine headache, surgical skin incision
☐ Neuropathic pain	☐ At-level SCI pain	☐ _____ e.g., spinal cord compression, nerve root compression, cauda equina compression
	☐ Below-level SCI pain	☐ _____ e.g., spinal cord ischemia, spinal cord compression
	☐ Other neuropathic pain	☐ _____ e.g., carpal tunnel syndrome, trigeminal neuralgia, diabetic polyneuropathy
☐ Other pain		☐ _____ e.g., fibromyalgia, complex regional pain syndrome type I, interstitial cystitis, irritable bowel syndrome
☐ Unknown pain		☐ _____

Fig. 1. The International Spinal Cord Injury Pain Classification (ISCIP). (*From* Bryce TN, Biering-Sorensen F, Finnerup NB, et al. International spinal cord injury pain classification: part I. Background and description. March 6–7, 2009. Spinal Cord 2012;50(6):415; with permission.)

demonstrated by the other and unknown categorizations. The reliability of the ISCIP classification has undergone initial testing using a clinical vignette approach by clinicians experienced with SCI who received minimal training in use of the system. The correctness levels varied from 65% to 85% based on the degree of correlation strictness for the various responses.[6] This result confirms the difficulty in assessment and classification of SCI-associated pain.

The relationship of spasticity to pain is complex. Spasticity can limit the range of motion about a joint and result in musculoskeletal pain. Reduction of spasticity may reduce the pain associated with biomechanical pain. However, as noted above, SCI can also produce neuropathic pain. Modulation of spasticity may not be effective in reducing neuropathic pain.[7] It is also relevant to note that some interventions to treat spasticity may also modulate the pain transmission pathways. In addition, the sensory loss in many patients with SCI, especially those with American Spinal Injury Association impairment scale A neurologic levels, may eliminate or substantially reduce the pain responses associated with noxious events. Increased spasticity may be the only harbinger of these events.[8]

EPIDEMIOLOGY

Given the classification ambiguity of chronic SCI-related pain described above, attempts at epidemiology can be problematic. Other potential confounders include oversampling because patients may have more than one pain syndrome, adequate pain description, criteria used for chronicity and severity, traumatic versus nontraumatic differentiation, and appropriate inclusion/exclusion criteria. Dijkers and colleagues[9] executed a review consisting of 42 articles that described the epidemiology of this clinical problem. A wide variance was noted in the literature, with prevalence of SCI-associated pain in the literature varying from 26% to 96% without an apparent clustering around any group of percentages. The quality of the individual study did not seem to significantly influence the reported prevalence rate. More detailed analysis failed to demonstrate appreciable difference in SCI-associated pain prevalence related to gender, injury completeness, or paraplegia versus tetraplegia. Some individual studies have reported trends for these demographic items, but when viewed from the perspective of the entirety of the medical literature, these trends disappear. Pain conditions among individuals with SCI are generally stable over time. Emergence or dramatic change in a chronic pain condition is worthy of new evaluative approach.

EVALUATION

The approach to SCI pain should commence in a manner similar to all chronic pain conditions—history, physical examination, and judicious use of diagnostic testing. Information should be obtained regarding the patient's initial SCI including date, mechanism of injury, associated injuries such as long bone and visceral trauma, description of vertebral column stabilization procedures, and comorbidities of the acute hospitalization and rehabilitation phase of injury. Descriptors should be attained regarding pain history, including time of onset from initial injury, time course, pain location, intensity and quantity, alleviating and aggravating factors, past evaluations, treatments (including effectiveness), and pharmacologic assessment. Inquiry into the presence or change in upper motor neuron signs, such as clonus or spasticity, is reasonable. Functional, occupational, and recreational history should be acquired for 2 reasons. First, these activities may contribute to the development of pain (eg, development of shoulder pain in a wheelchair athlete). Second, the degree of pain interference with these activities will allow the clinician to judge the functional impact of the patient's pain condition. Some degree of psychological assessment is warranted with exploration into possible depression, anxiety, personality disorders, concomitant brain injury, substance use, and cognitive impairment. In selected cases, a more formal psychological assessment, including psychometric testing, by either a psychologist or a psychiatrist may be appropriate. Last, the patient should be queried as to what diagnostic tests have been undertaken previously.

Although not an absolute "red flag," emergence of below-level pain after years or even decades from the initial SCI should be viewed as a concerning sign. For above-level pain syndromes, the typical elements of history should be queried as for the non-SCI patient with added elements that are pertinent to the patient with SCI. A reasonable example of this approach is a patient with SCI who presents with a suspected carpal tunnel syndrome. The patient should be asked questions about sensory symptoms and their distribution with the added elements of wheelchair, crutch, or cane use because use of these devices could be a contributing factor to a suspected median neuropathy. Particular attention should be paid to treatment failures. Some patients may have been exposed to a particular agent but were not given sufficient time or dose that would reasonably be expected to result in a therapeutic response. Other patients may have discontinued use of a medication because of intolerable adverse effects. If these 2 scenarios are present, insufficient response might be overcome with either a rechallenge of prior medications or use of adjuvant therapies to manage side effects.

Pain assessment should have a component of patient self-report. These measures supplement information obtained during the clinical interview and provide a means of evaluating success or failure of treatment strategies. The most commonly used measure of pain, for all types of pain, is the numerical rating scale (NRS). An NRS includes a range of numbers, generally starting from 0 (eg, 0–10 or 0–100), which is anchored to descriptors, for example, no pain at the lowest extreme of the range and worst pain imaginable at the highest extreme. Several studies have established the NRS as a reliable measure of pain intensity.[10] Another typical measure of pain intensity is a visual analog scale, which consists of a line (horizontal or vertical) anchored at either extremes with no pain on one end and another extreme (eg, worst pain imaginable) on the other end. Respondents are instructed to draw a small line that intersects with the scale at the point that represents their pain intensity. The measured distance (eg, in millimeters) from the no pain anchor to the recorded mark represents the subject's pain intensity. Typically, a clinically meaningful change in pain intensity is approximately a 33% decrement in visual analog score (VAS).[11]

Beyond pain intensity, it is reasonable to attempt assessment of pain according to daily activities. Of note, the Initiative on Methods, Measurement, and Pain Assessment in Clinical Trials (IMMPACT) group recommended that measures of pain severity, physical functioning, and emotional functioning be included in all clinical trials of chronic pain interventions.[12] The impact of pain on physical functioning may be obtained through a number by pain interference scales such as the Graded Chronic Pain Disability scale, the Brief Pain Inventory, and the Multidimensional Pain Inventory. These scales have demonstrated reasonable reliability and validity in SCI populations.[13]

Many patients with chronic pain disorders and SCI have comorbid psychological disorders including depression, anxiety, anger, psychosis, eating disorders, substance dependence, cognitive impairment, and personality disorders. The physician should inquire about the existence and severity of these behavioral problems. Cotreatment with mental health professionals is often warranted for more in-depth neuropsychological assessments. Examples of standardized psychological assessments used in these populations include the Beck Depression Inventory and the Patient Health Questionnaire. The latter has demonstrated validity in the SCI population.[14]

The physical examination of the individual with SCI-associated pain should start with the International Standards for Neurologic Classification of Spinal Cord Injury neurologic evaluation.[15] This examination is supplemented by further neurologic testing including reflex testing, assessment of other sensory abnormalities (allodynia, hyperalgesia, and hyperpathia), and evaluation of muscle overactivity (spasms, spasticity, and clonus). Focal examination of a particular pain area would then proceed as a neuromusculoskeletal approach used for pain complaints in all populations. Items to be included are inspection, palpation, active and passive range of motion, and provocative maneuvers. Observation of wheelchair propulsion, posture, and gait may be appropriate in selected patients. Appropriate comfort and fit of assistive devices (cane, walker, and crutch) and orthotic devices should be undertaken if these equipment seem to contribute to the pain syndrome. A survey of mood, behavior, personality, and cognition is certainly reasonable.

Regarding diagnostic testing, above-level syndromes can be evaluated in a manner parallel to the non-SCI patient. Conditions associated with at-level and below-level lesions are more challenging. Imaging of the site of initial spinal region should be considered in these circumstances. Potential examples of pain generators that might be detected include segmental instability or compression about the site of injury, spinal nerve impingement, orthopedic hardware loosening, fluid collections, and syringomyelia. Discussion with the interpreting radiologist is recommended to assist with the choice of imaging modalities. Potential discussion points could include interference of hardware, the need for radiographic contrast (intravenous gadolinium for magnetic resonance imaging [MRI], subarachnoid ionic contrast for computed tomographic [CT] myelogram, etc), and the differentiation of acute from chronic changes. Given the possible unreliability of abdominal/pelvic examinations in an insensate patient, imaging may also be warranted if visceral pain is suspected. In addition to the traditional MRI and CT modalities, specialized techniques may be warranted for potential pain generator relative to neurogenic bowel and bladder (ie, colonoscopy, cystoscopy, urodynamics testing, etc). Triple-phase bone scanning could be appropriate for evaluation of unsuspected fractures or complex regional pain syndrome.[16]

Judicious use of laboratory testing follows a parallel pathway for above-level syndromes and a surveillance approach for at-level and below-level syndromes. Care must be taken with regard to interpretation so as not to "over read" the importance of particular abnormality. An example of this pitfall would be to attribute asymptomatic urinary bacterial colonization as the sole cause of visceral pain. Potential laboratory tests in this population might include a complete blood cell count, erythrocyte sedimentation rate/C-reactive protein levels (to trend an inflammatory process such as abscess), and hormonal assessment (including pregnancy testing). Subtherapeutic vitamin B_{12}[17] and Vitamin D levels[18] have been implicated in neuronal dysfunction in SCI and represent potentially reversible abnormalities.

MANAGEMENT
Nonpharmacologic

A generalized exercise program in the form of global strength training, cardiovascular training, or recreational physical activities has the potential to be beneficial for several SCI-related conditions (eg, spasticity, muscle atrophy, bone health), but its effect on global pain in this population has not been greatly satisfactory. Animal studies have suggested that antinociceptive behaviors can be reduced with weeks of exercise training.[19,20] Extrapolation from these experiments to the human condition has not been straightforward. Some human trials suggest that a long-term exercise program can attenuate global pain complaints,[21] but these effects may not persist if regular exercise is discontinued.[22] More targeted exercise programs for specific pain complaints have a much higher likelihood of success. The best example of this approach is seen with shoulder pain in paraplegic individuals.[23–25]

In addition to generalized and specified exercise programs, referral to physical or occupational therapy may be appropriate for the patient with SCI with musculoskeletal pain in an effort to address biomechanical abnormalities that can be associated with mobility aids. Modification of orthotics, canes, walkers, crutches, and wheelchairs has the potential to influence detrimental ergonomics. Perhaps the best example of this intervention is adjustment of rear wheel of a manual wheelchair in an effort to modify the forces about the shoulder that can occur as a result of wheelchair propulsion.[26]

Acupuncture is popular for both the general and SCI populations. In 1997, a report from the National Institutes of Health supported the use of acupuncture for certain conditions, including pain.[27] Survey assessments have reported that between 15% and 35% of individuals with SCI have tried acupuncture for pain relief with a variable degree of effectiveness. One retrospective review reported that two-thirds of patients treated with acupuncture for below-level neuropathic pain found it effective.[28] Support for acupuncture from prospective studies is limited. Nayak and colleagues[29] reported that approximately half of the patients who received 15 sessions of this modality experienced a clinically meaningful reduction in pain. This study suggested that acupuncture may be more effective in individuals with incomplete injuries or musculoskeletal pain when compared with complete injuries or neuropathic pain. Dyson and colleagues[30] reported that both acupuncture and sham acupuncture groups had reductions in pain ratings when exposed in a double-blind manner.

Pharmacologic

At present, there is only one medication that currently has US Food and Drug Administration (FDA) indication for SCI-associated pain. Pregabalin is a structural derivative of the inhibitory neurotransmitter γ-aminobutyric acid. Pregabalin is an alpha-2-delta ligand that has analgesic, anticonvulsant, anxiolytic, and sleep-modulating activities. Pregabalin binds potently to the alpha-2-delta subunit of voltage-gated calcium channels. It is hypothesized that this binding reduces the influx of calcium into hyperexcited neuron, which in turn results in a reduction in the release of several neurotransmitters, including glutamate, noradrenaline, serotonin, dopamine, and substance P.[31] Siddall and colleagues[32] randomized 137 patients with SCI to either placebo (67 patients) or flexible dosing of pregabalin (70 patients). Roughly half of the patients had complete injuries. The dosing ranged from 150 to 600 mg/d in 2 divided doses. The mean baseline pain score was 6.54 in the pregabalin group and 6.73 in the placebo group. The mean endpoint pain score was lower in the active treatment group (4.62) compared with that in the placebo group (6.27; $P<.001$), with efficacy observed as early as week 1 and maintained for the duration of the study (12 weeks). The average pregabalin dose after the 3-week stabilization phase was 460 mg/d. During this trial, pregabalin was associated with improvements in disturbed sleep and anxiety. The most common adverse events were mild or moderate, typically transient, somnolence and dizziness. Edema was reported in 20% of the pregabalin patients, which resulted in 3 discontinuance episodes, compared to 6% in the placebo group, which resulted in 2 discontinuance episodes. Cardenas and colleagues[33] executed a similar study with 230 patients with 108 patients receiving active drug and 112 patients receiving placebo. This study had a longer duration (16 weeks). Approximately half of the patients had complete injuries. Pregabalin-treated patients experienced a nearly 2-point improvement on a 10-point NRS scale in the intensity of SCI-related pain during the previous 24 hours compared to baseline levels. Similarly, the patients experienced an improvement in disturbed sleep and sleep interference. The average daily dose of pregabalin was 410 mg/d during the dose maintenance period and 357 mg/d over the full treatment period. The most frequent treatment-related adverse effects included somnolence, dizziness, edema, dry mouth, fatigue, and blurred vision. Most adverse effects were mild to moderate in severity and transient in nature. Treatment-emergent peripheral edema was reported in 13.4% of pregabalin-treated patients in this study, resulting in 1 discontinuation. The incidence of edema in this study, as well as the previous study, was comparable with the reported incidence of other neuropathic pain conditions including diabetic peripheral neuropathy and postherpetic neuralgia. Thus, patients with SCI do not seem more susceptible to developing peripheral edema in response to pregabalin than patients with other neuropathic pain conditions.

Before pregabalin release and also at present, gabapentin remains commonly used. Similar to pregabalin, gabapentin is active at voltage-gated calcium channels. This agent has been considered effective in SCI-associated neuropathic pain in several smaller studies. Levendoglu and colleagues[34] reported that gabapentin was more effective than placebo in a crossover study involving 20 patients with paraplegia with neuropathic pain that had been present for more than 6 months. Tai and colleagues[35] conducted a prospective, randomized, double-blind, crossover study on 7 patients who had for more than 30 days postinjury SCI-related pain. This study found a significant reduction in "unpleasant feelings" with gabapentin compared to placebo. Reduction in pain intensity and burning pain trended toward significance, whereas no differences were observed for other pain descriptors. To and colleagues[36] performed a retrospective chart review of 44 patients with SCI-related neuropathic pain examining the effectiveness of gabapentin. About 76% of these subjects reported a reduction in pain intensity. The mean pretreatment VAS was 8.86, which decreased to 4.13 after 6 months of treatment. Last, Putzke and colleagues[37] examined the use of gabapentin in this population with a longitudinal observational study on 27 patients. This group observed a relatively high discontinuance rate (6/27 or 22%). Of the remaining 21 patients, 14 (67%) reported a greater than 2-point reduction in VAS at 6 months. It is reasonable to conclude that gabapentin can be effective in neuropathic pain in SCI-associated neuropathic pain. A recent study of intrathecal gabapentin failed to demonstrate any benefit in an unselected chronic pain population despite promising results from animal data, particularly with neuropathic pain.[38] Although pregabalin has US FDA approval for SCI-related pain, there is no head-to-head trial comparing the effectiveness of gabapentin with that of pregabalin. The affordability of gabapentin may make it the more desirable choice. Many insurers require a trial of gabapentin before approving pregabalin.

The use of antidepressants for below-level neuropathic pain SCI pain has a long-standing tradition. The substantial benefit of tricyclic antidepressants (TCAs) in neuropathic pain has led to this use.[39] Perhaps the most commonly used agent is amitriptyline. There are conflicting results in the medical literature with some studies demonstrating efficacy[40] and other studies demonstrating descriptive minimal efficacy[41] in SCI-associated pain. One comparison trial described a therapeutic benefit of amitriptyline over gabapentin.[40] The so-called second-generation TCAs (ie, secondary amines such as nortriptyline, desipramine, and protriptyline) are preferred because analgesic efficacy is equivalent and tolerability is better compared to those of first-generation TCAs (ie, tertiary amines such as amitriptyline, clomipramine, and doxepin). All TCAs are considered to have a ceiling effect. Thus, once a therapeutic effect is achieved, further dosing increases should be avoided in order to minimize adverse effects.[42]

The most recent additions to antidepressant use for chronic pain are the dual serotonin and norepinephrine reuptake inhibitors. Medications in this class include duloxetine, milnacipran, and desvenlafaxine. Pain modulation seems to be independent of their antidepressant properties. Duloxetine, the first medication approved for use in the United States within this class, has FDA indication for chronic musculoskeletal pain, fibromyalgia, and diabetic neuropathy. A small trial of duloxetine for central neuropathic pain caused by either stroke or SCI failed to show a reduction in pain intensity but did demonstrate changes in other aspects of these chronic pain syndromes, including allodynia.[43] There are no reports of using either milnacipran or venlafaxine for chronic SCI-associated pain. Several serotonin-norepinephrine reuptake inhibitors are in various stages of clinical development for a wide variety of indications.[44]

Opioid medications have been suggested as reasonable options for chronic nociceptive and perhaps neuropathic pain. Perhaps, no other decision in medicine causes more anxiety than prescribing opiates for patients with chronic, noncancer pain. Concerns over diversion, misuse, dependence, addiction, monitoring, and cost can make the analysis of using chronic opiate therapy troublesome for even experienced clinicians.[45] In the patient with SCI, concerns over the potential exacerbation of neurogenic bowel because of opioid-related constipation makes this decision even more challenging. There are several new strategies for the management of opioid-related constipation including peripheral opioid receptor antagonists and prokinetic agents.[46] A review of the use of opioids in neuropathic pain suggested clinical efficacy of this medication class for long-term use. It is relevant to note that this review has a large preponderance of peripheral-based neuropathic pain (diabetic neuropathy or postherpetic neuropathy), but some subjects with SCI were included.[47] There are several developments within the opioid class medications that may be of specific interest to physiatrists treating SCI-related pain. Tapentadol is a centrally acting analgesic with dual mechanisms of action—agonist activity at the mu opioid receptor and inhibition of norepinephrine reuptake. A potential therapeutic advantage of this agent is its utility in neuropathic pain. This benefit has been observed with both low–back pain with a neuropathic pain component as well as diabetic peripheral neuropathy.[48,49] There are no specific reports on the use of this agent in SCI. In addition, this medication may also have therapeutic advantages over other opiates including a lower incidence of withdrawal symptoms as well as decreased frequency of gastrointestinal side effects. However, because of the activity that this agent has with monoamine metabolism, there is a potential to exacerbate or precipitate serotonin syndrome.[50] Another dual-acting product is tramadol, which is a combination of a serotonin and noradrenaline reuptake inhibitor and a mu opioid agonist. This medication is noteworthy because its mechanism of action is distinct from those of other opioids. Tramadol has been shown to demonstrate benefit in osteoarthritis, fibromyalgia, and neuropathic pain; however, there is insufficient evidence to definitely define tramadol as more effective compared with other opioids.[51] A small, randomized controlled trial in SCI-related neuropathic pain demonstrated a positive response to this medication.[52]

The relationship between pain and spasticity is complex. Reduction of spasticity may reduce the pain associated with biomechanical pain. Modulation of spasticity may not be effective in reducing neuropathic pain.[7] There are several oral medications that can accomplish spasticity reduction including baclofen, tizanidine, diazepam, and dantrolene. Of particular interest, tizanidine has a dual mechanism of action: an

α_2-adrenergic agonism at the spinal level and an influence on descending noradrenergic pathways. It is this latter mechanism that may be of particular interest in the management of SCI-related pain.[53] Similarly, botulinum toxins have the potential to reduce muscle overactivity in a focally directed manner. Abobotulinum toxin A has formal FDA indication for adult, upper extremity spasticity after stroke and brain injury, although there are ongoing clinical trials for the other preparations and indications. Over and above their antispasticity activities, botulinum toxins have the capacity to be antinociceptive.[54] However, there are no formal studies examining the effects of botulinum toxin on SCI-related pain independent of their spasticity reduction properties.

Medicinal marijuana and synthetic cannabinoids represent intriguing pharmacologic choices for the management of SCI-associated pain. Cannabis contains 60 or more cannabinoids, the most abundant of which are delta-9-tetrahydrocannabinol (THC) and cannabidiol (CBD). Rintala and colleagues[55] executed a small study with dronabinol on SCI-related neuropathic pain. This agent is a pure isomer of THC. This investigation failed to demonstrate a significant difference in pain intensity compared with an active control. Sativex is a cannabis extract that contains THC + CBD in a fixed ratio, delivered as an oromucosal spray. Sativex has indication for multiple-sclerosis-related spasticity in several countries but not in the United States.[56] A recent study of neuropathic pain associated with multiple sclerosis failed to demonstrate significant differences during the double-blind phase of this trial.[57] There are no specific reports on the use of this agent in SCI-associated pain. There is an ongoing clinical trial examining the use of vaporized cannabis in SCI pain. There are no formal studies examining the use of medicinal marijuana in this patient population despite Cardenas and Jensen[58] reporting that up to 37% of patients with SCI have used marijuana for pain reduction purposes.

Nicotine has been reported to exacerbate SCI-related pain with abstinence resulting in relief. One recent study examined the effect of nicotine in a randomized, placebo-controlled crossover design on the subtypes of SCI-related pain (neuropathic, musculoskeletal, and mixed pain) among smokers and nonsmokers. This study involved 42 subjects of whom two-thirds had paraplegia. Nonsmokers with SCI showed a reduction in mixed forms of pain after nicotine exposure, whereas smokers with SCI reported increase in pain for both mixed and neuropathic pain. This study suggests differential effects on SCI-related pain for smokers and nonsmokers. This observation potentially offers some insight into the mechanisms of SCI-associated pain as well as supports the suggestion of smoking cessation in some patients with SCI.[59]

Interventional

Spinal cord stimulation is defined as posterior epidural stimulation of the dorsal columns. The proposed mechanisms of action of this therapy involve the gate theory of pain, enhancement of parasympathetic activity, inhibition of sympathetic activity, upregulation of descending inhibitory pathways, and downregulation of ascending pain pathways. There have been many case reports documenting both success and failure of this technology for this pain syndrome. Shaw[60] has presented a meeting abstract in which 12 patients with SCI received dorsal column stimulation for treatment of pain. The patients with complete injuries had variable success; however, none of them experienced paresthesias at stimulation above their injury. In the incompletely injured patients, paresthesias were experienced at varying levels of stimulation intensity. The patients with incomplete SCI had a higher degree of pain relief than those with complete SCI; however, 1 patient with complete SCI, who had been injured for less than 2 years, had complete relief of pain.[60] Lagauche and colleagues[61] executed a review of this modality in SCI-related pain and failed to find a consistently positive therapeutic effect.

Intrathecal drug delivery provides direct administration of therapeutic agents to the subarachnoid space where they have enhanced access to receptor sites. Intrathecal baclofen is a well-established technique for reduction of spasticity associated with SCI.[62,63] To the extent that spasticity is related to musculoskeletal pain, this technique has the capacity to attenuate pain in this population. However, the use of intrathecal baclofen as a pure pain-modulating agent is limited.[64] The utility of more traditional intrathecal analgesic agents has not been overwhelmingly successful. Combination therapy with baclofen and clonidine,[65] morphine and clonidine,[66] baclofen and morphine,[67] baclofen and ziconotide,[68] as well as hydromorphone and ziconotide[69] have resulted in varying degrees of success. Intrathecal gabapentin failed to demonstrate a therapeutic effect in a generalized pain population.[38]

A particularly interesting, albeit experimental, neuromodulation approach to SCI-associated pain is oscillating field stimulation. A human trial of a low-voltage, alternating polarity device was undertaken to assess the possibility of this therapy, causing substantive neurologic recovery as suspected from animal studies. Pain was assessed during this trial to insure that this device did not cause pain. Somewhat surprisingly, use of this device was associated with a rather dramatic reduction in pain. After the 15-week treatment phase, VAS scores improved from a mean of 8 to a mean of 2 six months after treatment had been discontinued. No neuropathic pain was reported in any patient. The status of this device is uncertain until a larger, multi-center trial is undertaken.[70]

SUMMARY

SCI pain is clearly a challenging pain syndrome. Each element of this review (classification, epidemiology, evaluation, and management) has demonstrated limitations. Further investigation by clinicians and researchers in both the SCI and pain communities is warranted in an effort to further delineate the nature of this problem and create more effective treatment strategies. Physiatrists are uniquely positioned to participate in this process and should engage in this endeavor whenever possible.

REFERENCES

1. Hicken BL, Putzke JD, Richards JS. Classification of pain following spinal cord injury: literature review and future directions. In: Burchiel K, Yezierski RP, editors. Spinal cord injury pain: assessment, mechanisms, management. Seattle (WA): International Association for the Study of Pain Press; 2002. p. 25–38.
2. Cardenas DD, Turner JA, Warms CA, et al. Classification of chronic pain associated with spinal cord injuries. Arch Phys Med Rehabil 2002;83(12):1708–14.
3. Siddall P, Yezierski RP, Loeser JD. Pain following spinal cord injury: clinical features, prevalence and taxonomy. International Association for the Study of Pain 2000;3:3–7.
4. Bryce TN, Dijkers MP, Ragnarsson KT, et al. Reliability of the Bryce/Ragnarsson spinal cord injury pain taxonomy. J Spinal Cord Med 2006;29(2):118–32.
5. Bryce TN, Biering-Sorensen F, Finnerup NB, et al. International spinal cord injury pain classification: part I. Background and description. March 6–7, 2009. Spinal Cord 2012;50(6):413–7.
6. Bryce TN, Biering-Sorensen F, Finnerup NB, et al. International spinal cord injury pain (ISCIP) classification: part 2. Initial validation using vignettes. Spinal Cord 2012;50(6):404–12.

7. Ward AB, Kadies M. The management of pain in spasticity. Disabil Rehabil 2002; 24(8):443–53.
8. Phadke CP, Balasubramanian CK, Ismail F, et al. Revisiting physiologic and psychologic triggers that increase spasticity. Am J Phys Med Rehabil 2013;92(4): 357–69.
9. Dijkers M, Bryce T, Zanca J. Prevalence of chronic pain after traumatic spinal cord injury: a systematic review. J Rehabil R D 2009;46(1):13–29.
10. Jensen MP, Turner JA, Romano JM, et al. Comparative reliability and validity of chronic pain intensity measures. Pain 1999;83(2):157–62.
11. Hanley MA, Jensen MP, Ehde DM, et al. Clinically significant change in pain intensity ratings in persons with spinal cord injury or amputation. Clin J Pain 2006;22(1):25–31.
12. Dworkin RH, Turk DC, Peirce-Sandner S, et al. Research design considerations for confirmatory chronic pain clinical trials: IMMPACT recommendations. Pain 2010;149(2):177–93.
13. Bryce TN, Budh CN, Cardenas DD, et al. Pain after spinal cord injury: an evidence-based review for clinical practice and research. Report of the national institute on disability and rehabilitation research spinal cord injury measures meeting. J Spinal Cord Med 2007;30(5):421–40.
14. Bombardier CH, Richards JS, Krause JS, et al. Symptoms of major depression in people with spinal cord injury: implications for screening. Arch Phys Med Rehabil 2004;85(11):1749–56.
15. Kirshblum SC, Waring W, Biering-Sorensen F, et al. Reference for the 2011 revision of the international standards for neurological classification of spinal cord injury. J Spinal Cord Med 2011;34(6):547–54.
16. Le Chapelain L, Perrouin-Verbe B, Fattal C, SOFMER French Society for Physical Medicine and Rehabilitation. Chronic neuropathic pain in spinal cord injury patients: what relevant additional clinical exams should be performed? Ann Phys Rehabil Med 2009;52(2):103–10.
17. Petchkrua W, Little JW, Burns SP, et al. Vitamin B12 deficiency in spinal cord injury: a retrospective study. J Spinal Cord Med 2003;26(2):116–21.
18. Hummel K, Craven BC, Giangregorio L. Serum 25(OH)D, PTH and correlates of suboptimal 25(OH)D levels in persons with chronic spinal cord injury. Spinal Cord 2012;50(11):812–6.
19. Hutchinson KJ, Gomez-Pinilla F, Crowe MJ, et al. Three exercise paradigms differentially improve sensory recovery after spinal cord contusion in rats. Brain 2004;127(Pt 6):1403–14.
20. Kuphal KE, Fibuch EE, Taylor BK. Extended swimming exercise reduces inflammatory and peripheral neuropathic pain in rodents. J Pain 2007;8(12): 989–97.
21. Hicks AL, Martin KA, Ditor DS, et al. Long-term exercise training in persons with spinal cord injury: effects on strength, arm ergometry performance and psychological well-being. Spinal Cord 2003;41(1):34–43.
22. Ditor DS, Latimer AE, Ginis KA, et al. Maintenance of exercise participation in individuals with spinal cord injury: effects on quality of life, stress and pain. Spinal Cord 2003;41(8):446–50.
23. Curtis KA, Tyner TM, Zachary L, et al. Effect of a standard exercise protocol on shoulder pain in long-term wheelchair users. Spinal Cord 1999;37(6): 421–9.
24. Nawoczenski DA, Ritter-Soronen JM, Wilson CM, et al. Clinical trial of exercise for shoulder pain in chronic spinal injury. Phys Ther 2006;86(12):1604–18.

25. Mulroy SJ, Thompson L, Kemp B, et al. Strengthening and optimal movements for painful shoulders (STOMPS) in chronic spinal cord injury: a randomized controlled trial. Phys Ther 2011;91(3):305–24.
26. Katalinic OM, Harvey LA, Herbert RD. Effectiveness of stretch for the treatment and prevention of contractures in people with neurological conditions: a systematic review. Phys Ther 2011;91(1):11–24.
27. NIH consensus conference. Acupuncture. JAMA 1998;280(17):1518–24.
28. Rapson LM, Wells N, Pepper J, et al. Acupuncture as a promising treatment for below-level central neuropathic pain: a retrospective study. J Spinal Cord Med 2003;26(1):21–6.
29. Nayak S, Shiflett SC, Schoenberger NE, et al. Is acupuncture effective in treating chronic pain after spinal cord injury? Arch Phys Med Rehabil 2001;82(11): 1578–86.
30. Dyson-Hudson TA, Kadar P, LaFountaine M, et al. Acupuncture for chronic shoulder pain in persons with spinal cord injury: a small-scale clinical trial. Arch Phys Med Rehabil 2007;88(10):1276–83.
31. Gajraj NM. Pregabalin: its pharmacology and use in pain management. Anesth Analg 2007;105(6):1805–15.
32. Siddall PJ, Cousins MJ, Otte A, et al. Pregabalin in central neuropathic pain associated with spinal cord injury: a placebo-controlled trial. Neurology 2006;67(10): 1792–800.
33. Cardenas DD, Nieshoff EC, Suda K, et al. A randomized trial of pregabalin in patients with neuropathic pain due to spinal cord injury. Neurology 2013;80(6): 533–9.
34. Levendoglu F, Ogun CO, Ozerbil O, et al. Gabapentin is a first line drug for the treatment of neuropathic pain in spinal cord injury. Spine (Phila Pa 1976) 2004; 29(7):743–51.
35. Tai Q, Kirshblum S, Chen B, et al. Gabapentin in the treatment of neuropathic pain after spinal cord injury: a prospective, randomized, double-blind, crossover trial. J Spinal Cord Med 2002;25(2):100–5.
36. To TP, Lim TC, Hill ST, et al. Gabapentin for neuropathic pain following spinal cord injury. Spinal Cord 2002;40(6):282–5.
37. Putzke JD, Richards JS, Kezar L, et al. Long-term use of gabapentin for treatment of pain after traumatic spinal cord injury. Clin J Pain 2002;18(2): 116–21.
38. Rauck R, Coffey RJ, Schultz DM, et al. Intrathecal gabapentin to treat chronic intractable noncancer pain. Anesthesiology 2013;119(3):675–86.
39. Sindrup SH, Jensen TS. Efficacy of pharmacological treatments of neuropathic pain: an update and effect related to mechanism of drug action. Pain 1999; 83(3):389–400.
40. Rintala DH, Holmes SA, Courtade D, et al. Comparison of the effectiveness of amitriptyline and gabapentin on chronic neuropathic pain in persons with spinal cord injury. Arch Phys Med Rehabil 2007;88(12):1547–60.
41. Cardenas DD, Warms CA, Turner JA, et al. Efficacy of amitriptyline for relief of pain in spinal cord injury: results of a randomized controlled trial. Pain 2002; 96(3):365–73.
42. Mico JA, Ardid D, Berrocoso E, et al. Antidepressants and pain. Trends Pharmacol Sci 2006;27(7):348–54.
43. Vranken JH, Hollmann MW, van der Vegt MH, et al. Duloxetine in patients with central neuropathic pain caused by spinal cord injury or stroke: a randomized, double-blind, placebo-controlled trial. Pain 2011;152(2):267–73.

44. Stahl SM, Grady MM, Moret C, et al. SNRIs: their pharmacology, clinical efficacy, and tolerability in comparison with other classes of antidepressants. CNS Spectr 2005;10(9):732–47.

45. Hallinan R, Osborn M, Cohen M, et al. Increasing the benefits and reducing the harms of prescription opioid analgesics. Drug Alcohol Rev 2011;30(3):315–23.

46. Walters JB, Montagnini M. Current concepts in the management of opioid-induced constipation. J Opioid Manag 2010;6(6):435–44.

47. Eisenberg E, McNicol E, Carr DB. Opioids for neuropathic pain. Cochrane Database Syst Rev 2006;(3):CD006146.

48. Steigerwald I, Muller M, Davies A, et al. Effectiveness and safety of tapentadol prolonged release for severe, chronic low back pain with or without a neuropathic pain component: results of an open-label, phase 3b study. Curr Med Res Opin 2012;28(6):911–36.

49. Schwartz S, Etropolski M, Shapiro DY, et al. Safety and efficacy of tapentadol ER in patients with painful diabetic peripheral neuropathy: results of a randomized-withdrawal, placebo-controlled trial. Curr Med Res Opin 2011;27(1):151–62.

50. Riemsma R, Forbes C, Harker J, et al. Systematic review of tapentadol in chronic severe pain. Curr Med Res Opin 2011;27(10):1907–30.

51. Leppert W. Tramadol as an analgesic for mild to moderate cancer pain. Pharmacol Rep 2009;61(6):978–92.

52. Norrbrink C, Lundeberg T. Tramadol in neuropathic pain after spinal cord injury: a randomized, double-blind, placebo-controlled trial. Clin J Pain 2009;25(3):177–84.

53. Kamen L, Henney HR 3rd, Runyan JD. A practical overview of tizanidine use for spasticity secondary to multiple sclerosis, stroke, and spinal cord injury. Curr Med Res Opin 2008;24(2):425–39.

54. Wheeler A, Smith HS. Botulinum toxins: mechanisms of action, antinociception and clinical applications. Toxicology 2013;306:124–46.

55. Rintala DH, Fiess RN, Tan G, et al. Effect of dronabinol on central neuropathic pain after spinal cord injury: a pilot study. Am J Phys Med Rehabil 2010; 89(10):840–8.

56. Notcutt W, Langford R, Davies P, et al. A placebo-controlled, parallel-group, randomized withdrawal study of subjects with symptoms of spasticity due to multiple sclerosis who are receiving long-term Sativex(R) (nabiximols). Mult Scler 2012; 18(2):219–28.

57. Langford RM, Mares J, Novotna A, et al. A double-blind, randomized, placebo-controlled, parallel-group study of THC/CBD oromucosal spray in combination with the existing treatment regimen, in the relief of central neuropathic pain in patients with multiple sclerosis. J Neurol 2013;260(4):984–97.

58. Cardenas DD, Jensen MP. Treatments for chronic pain in persons with spinal cord injury: a survey study. J Spinal Cord Med 2006;29(2):109–17.

59. Richardson EJ, Richards JS, Stewart CC, et al. Effects of nicotine on spinal cord injury pain: a randomized, double-blind, placebo controlled crossover trial. Top Spinal Cord Inj Rehabil 2012;18(2):101–5.

60. Shaw E. Clinical outcomes of Spinal cord stimulation (SCS) in patients with chronic spinal cord injury. Neuromoduation 2011;14(5):444–84 [Abstract].

61. Lagauche D, Facione J, Albert T, et al. The chronic neuropathic pain of spinal cord injury: which efficiency of neuropathic stimulation? Ann Phys Rehabil Med 2009;52(2):180–7.

62. Coffey JR, Cahill D, Steers W, et al. Intrathecal baclofen for intractable spasticity of spinal origin: results of a long-term multicenter study. J Neurosurg 1993;78(2): 226–32.

63. Ordia JI, Fischer E, Adamski E, et al. Continuous intrathecal baclofen infusion by a programmable pump in 131 consecutive patients with severe spasticity of spinal origin. Neuromodulation 2002;5(1):16–24.

64. Saulino M. The use of intrathecal baclofen in pain management. Pain Manag 2013;2(6):603–8.

65. Middleton JW, Siddall PJ, Walker S, et al. Intrathecal clonidine and baclofen in the management of spasticity and neuropathic pain following spinal cord injury: a case study. Arch Phys Med Rehabil 1996;77(8):824–6.

66. Siddall PJ, Molloy AR, Walker S, et al. The efficacy of intrathecal morphine and clonidine in the treatment of pain after spinal cord injury. Anesth Analg 2000; 91(6):1493–8.

67. Saulino M. Simultaneous treatment of intractable pain and spasticity: observations of combined intrathecal baclofen-morphine therapy over a 10-year clinical experience. Eur J Phys Rehabil Med 2011;48(1):39–45.

68. Saulino M, Burton AW, Danyo DA, et al. Intrathecal ziconotide and baclofen provide pain relief in seven patients with neuropathic pain and spasticity: case reports. Eur J Phys Rehabil Med 2009;45(1):61–7.

69. Saulino M. Successful reduction of neuropathic pain associated with spinal cord injury via of a combination of intrathecal hydromorphone and ziconotide: a case report. Spinal Cord 2007;45(11):749–52.

70. Walters BC. Oscillating field stimulation in the treatment of spinal cord injury. PM R 2010;2(12 Suppl 2):S286–91.

Management of Chronic Pain Following Nerve Injuries/CRPS Type II

Ian Carroll, MD, MS[a], Catherine M. Curtin, MD[b,c],*

KEYWORDS

• Chronic pain • Complex regional pain syndrome • Neuropathic pain • Nerve injuries

KEY POINTS

• Perioperative interventions can reduce incidence of postoperative chronic pain: prevention is much more desirable than treating complex regional pain syndrome (CRPS)/neuropathic pain.
• There is a critical time window in treating the patient with CRPS/neuropathic pain: early intervention is better.
• Surgeons need to be comfortable beginning treatment of CRPS/neuropathic pain.

Every incision and every fracture injures some sensory nerve. Most of the time, these nerves recover from this insult without long-term consequences; however, for some people, pain continues long after the wounds have healed. This chronic pain then affects quality of life, limits the patient's ability to participate in therapy, and adversely affects functional outcomes. Chronic postoperative pain is a particularly frustrating problem for the surgeon because it is hard to anticipate, ruins a technically perfect procedure, and the surgeon may be unsure of the next steps of treatment. There is much information on chronic pain and its treatment, but this literature is often published outside of surgery and diffusion of this information across disciplines is slow. This article synthesizes some of this literature and provides a systematic presentation of the evidence on pain associated with peripheral nerve injury.

Chronic pain and complex regional pain syndrome (CRPS) are large topics and we have divided this article into sections. When available, we have presented pooled data for each subsection, including consensus statements and systematic reviews. When

This article originally appeared in Hand Clinics, Volume 29, Issue 3, August 2013.
[a] Department of Anesthesia, Stanford University, 450 Broadway, Redwood City, CA 94603, USA;
[b] Department of Surgery, Palo Alto VA, 3801 Miranda Avenue, Palo Alto VA, Palo Alto, CA 94304, USA; [c] Division of Plastic Surgery, Stanford University, Suite 400, 770 Welch RD Palo Alto, CA 94304, USA
* Corresponding author. Division of Plastic Surgery, Stanford University, Suite 400, 770 Welch RD Palo Alto, CA 94304.
E-mail address: curtincatherine@yahoo.com

Clinics Collections 4 (2014) 339–349
http://dx.doi.org/10.1016/j.ccol.2014.10.021

pooled data are not available, we present information from randomized controlled trials (RCTs). Given the diversity and the breadth of the topic, we hope that this overview provides an information foundation and the reviews presented will direct the reader to more detailed information.

DEFINITIONS

The first step when discussing pain is to understand terminology.

Neuropathic Pain

This article focuses on pain associated with nerve injuries: neuropathic pain. The International Association for the Study of Pain (IASP) Neuropathic Pain Special Interest Group has defined neuropathic pain arising as a direct consequence of a lesion or disease affecting the somatosensory system.[1,2] It has typical characteristics that help separate it from other types of pain, such as joint pain from osteoarthritis. A recent Delphi survey of experts defined neuropathic pain as having a clinical history of nerve injury and the pain should demonstrate typical characteristics: (1) prickling, tingling, pins and needles; (2) pain with light touch; (3) electric shocks or shooting pain; (4) hot or burning pain; and (5) Brush allodynia.[3] For the researcher, there are several validated measures to differentiate neuropathic pain.[4] For more detailed information on how to assess neuropathic pain, we refer you to a recent guideline, which provides detailed information on recommended measures.[5]

Chronic Pain

Acute pain after injury is a normal and healthy response. It serves the purpose of limiting activity and protecting the injured areas to allow the tissue to heal. Yet at some point, pain transitions to a pathologic process, no longer serving the protective role, and the pain becomes chronic or intractable. Much effort has been devoted to define when pain has transitioned to this chronic state. Smith and colleagues'[3] consensus study felt neuropathic pain was intractable when the pain persisted despite trials of at least 4 drugs of known effectiveness in neuropathic pain. The most frequently cited definition for chronic pain was produced by the IASP, which states that chronic pain is pain that has persisted beyond the normal tissue healing time and often 3 months is set as the convenient cutoff.[1]

CRPS

The definition of complex regional pain has undergone a long evolution as our understanding of the process has evolved. During the Civil War era, it was known as causalgia. In 1946, this type of pain was referred to as Reflex Sympathetic Dystrophy,[6] and during the 1990s, the nomenclature was changed to the current term: CRPS. There has been much debate on the criteria to make this diagnosis. Both the IASP and a consensus statement called the Budapest criteria present fairly similar lists of what a patient should display to have a diagnosis of CRPS.[7,8] The IASP defines CRPS as a syndrome characterized by a continuing (spontaneous and/or evoked) regional pain that is seemingly disproportionate in time or degree to the usual course of pain after trauma or other lesion. The pain is regional (not in a specific nerve territory or dermatome) and usually has a distal predominance of abnormal sensory, motor, sudomotor, vasomotor edema, and/or trophic findings.[7] This article focuses on the CRPS type II associated with nerve injury; however, it is not hard to imagine that CRPS type I may be mediated by similar pathways by injury to smaller unnamed nerves in the bone and soft tissue.

This diagnosis of CRPS is based on history and physical examination: there is no specific diagnostic test for CRPS. Given that CRPS is a clinical diagnosis, there has been a much research on what clinical signs are most specific to this diagnosis. The IASP guidelines state that the patient must have pain disproportionate to the injury and there is no other diagnosis that explains the pain. **Box 1** presents the most recent clinical criteria for diagnosis of CRPS.[8]

EPIDEMIOLOGY

Severe complex regional pain syndrome is a rare occurrence, but chronic pain after injury to sensory nerves is more frequent. CRPS may be the severe end stage of a spectrum of pain processes after nerve injury. Epidemiologic studies of complex regional pain syndrome are often flawed because of the infrequency of the diagnosis. The largest study was from the Netherlands using a general population database.[9] The investigators looked at 217,000 patients and found the overall incidence of CRPS was 26 per 100,000 person years. Women were affected at least 3 times more often than men and the upper extremity was affected more frequently than the lower limb.

Chronic pain after nerve injury is far more common than CRPS. There are no large studies assessing the incidence of pain after major nerve injury. Case series in brachial plexus injuries have found that nearly all patients experience pain after injury. A recent case series of patients with nerve injuries found a high prevalence of pain (66%), with many having severe pain.[10] Yet even smaller injuries, such as the trauma associated with carpal tunnel syndrome, have a 20% rate of pain at 3 months.[11] Although the pain after carpal tunnel release is not a direct nerve injury, the pain is often burning and the scar is sensitive to light touch: features consistent with a neuropathic process. Many of these may be because of injury to branches of the palmar

---

Box 1
Clinical criteria for complex regional pain syndrome

Must report at least one symptom in 3 of the 4 following categories

1. Sensory: Reports of hyperalgesia and/or allodynia

2. Vasomotor: Reports of temperature asymmetry and/or skin color changes and/or skin color asymmetry

3. Sudomotor/Edema: Reports of edema and/or sweating changes and/or sweating asymmetry

4. Motor/Trophic: Reports of decreased range of motion and/or motor dysfunction (weakness, tremor, dystonia) and/or trophic changes (hair, nail, skin)

Must display at least 1 sign[a] at time of evaluation in at least 2 of the following categories

1. Sensory: Evidence of hyperalgesia (to pinprick) and/or allodynia (to light touch and/or deep somatic pressure and/or joint movement)

2. Vasomotor: Evidence of temperature asymmetry and/or skin color changes and/or asymmetry

3. Sudomotor/Edema: Evidence of edema and/or sweating changes and/or sweating asymmetry

4. Motor/Trophic: Evidence of decreased range of motion and/or motor dysfunction (weakness, tremor, dystonia) and/or trophic changes (hair, nail, skin)

[a] A sign is counted only if it is observed at time of diagnosis.

Data from Harden RN, Oaklander AL, Burton AW, et al. Complex regional pain syndrome: practical diagnostic and treatment guidelines. Pain Med 2013 Feb;14(2):180–229.

cutaneous branch of the median nerve. Thus, for the hand surgeon, understanding methods to prevent and treat chronic pain associated with a nerve injury is important to improve outcomes.

PREVENTION

The hand surgeon should understand preventive measures that can influence the postoperative pain course and identify the patients/procedures that would be at higher risk for postoperative pain so perioperative measures can be instituted. So who is at risk? There has been extensive work to stratify characteristics associated with the development of chronic pain. First is the type of injury. Major nerve trauma bombards the spinal cord and central nervous system with nociceptive stimuli and, not unexpectedly, these patients are at high risk of pain. Then there are also specific injuries, such as distal radius fracture, which have a high rate of development of CRPS.[12] Patient factors also are associated with risk of chronic pain. CRPS is more frequently seen in women.[9] Psychological factors before injury have long been thought to increase the risk chronic pain. The theory is that a patient with an increased basal rate of catecholamines will be more easily sensitized to pain, but the data are lacking and, at this time, the link between psychological traits and CRPS risk is still speculative. One of the most important predictors of high postoperative pain is high preoperative pain level: these patients already have a nociceptive system that is primed. Thus, if the surgeon is caring for a patient with several risk factors, it is helpful to consider perioperative interventions.

The next section reviews perioperative interventions that have data from RCTs that support their role in reducing postoperative chronic pain.

Preemptive use of local anesthetics can reduce the number of patients who have chronic postoperative pain. A study on patients who had breast surgery found that the group that received regional anesthetic block had significantly decreased pain at 1 month, 6 months, and 12 months after surgery when compared with the control group.[13] Another trial found decreased pain months after surgery in the group that had a preoperative block before thoracotomy.[14] There are several other studies indicating that anesthetizing the nerve with local analgesia before incision affects long-term chronic pain.[15]

Vitamin C has also been found to reduce the transition to CRPS after distal radius fractures. Vitamin C is a free radical scavenger, which reduces vascular permeability after trauma. It has also may decrease tumor necrosis factor alpha and interleukin-6, which are important inflammatory cytokines. Zollinger and colleagues[16] evaluated vitamin C in the treatment of distal radius fractures in an RCT of 123 patients. They determined 500 mg of vitamin C for 50 days provided a statistical benefit, with decreased pain in these patients. They next looked at dosing study and found that the odds ratio of developing CRPS after distal radius fracture was 0.22 among those who received vitamin C. Statistically significant benefit was seen at 500 mg per day and 1500 mg per day.[17] Another quasiexperimental study on foot and ankle patients found that after institution of a perioperative vitamin C regimen, the rate for CRPS decreased from 9.6% to 1.7%.[18] These 3 studies support the use of vitamin C at 500 mg per day as part of the perioperative regimen.

There are several other medications that show promise for reducing the transition to chronic pain, including gabapentin and ketamine. There are good data for improvement with these medications in acute pain after surgery, but because of wide heterogeneity in the literature, there is still a lack of evidence on their impact on chronic pain. There is a new meta-analysis of gabapentin and pregabalin, supporting their use for chronic pain.[19] At this time, we would advise the surgeon that these medications may reduce chronic pain and the surgeon should consider using these medications despite weaker levels of evidence. Our algorithm for the perioperative management of pain, based on the available literature, is provided in **Tables 1** and **2.**

TREATMENT

Despite the most meticulous care, the surgeon will still be faced with the patient who has lingering chronic pain well after the soft tissue has healed. If the physician feels the patient meets the criteria for CRPS treatment, referral to a pain specialist should be initiated immediately. However, the reality of practice is such that there is often a delay before a pain specialist sees the patient and thus the hand surgeon should start treatment. In addition, the surgeon may have patients with neuropathic pain who do not fully meet the criteria for CRPS but require additional treatment for their pain. The animal studies are clear that there is a window of opportunity with pain; thus, if a patient is having pain disproportionate to expectations, therapy should be initiated promptly in attempt to break the process.[19] The next paragraph reviews evidence-based treatments for chronic neuropathic pain/CRPS.

The surgeon should always begin with a thorough physical examination to rule out treatable causes of the pain, such as carpal tunnel syndrome. There have been several case series that have shown patients who present with CRPS may have a nerve entrapment that responded to surgical release.[20,21] Practitioners should have a low threshold for obtaining additional electrodiagnostic testing if there is a suspicion of nerve entrapments.

Therapy

The first arm of treatment is therapy and other nonpharmacological modalities, which are keystones in neuropathic pain management. The goal is to provide sensory reorganization and desensitization, and extinguish the pathologic pain pathways. There are a few randomized trials demonstrating benefits for therapy when compared with controls.[22–24] Two meta-analyses looking at physical therapy modalities for the treatment of CRPS have been performed. Although these studies were hindered by the heterogeneity of the literature, they did find evidence that graded motor imagery and mirror therapy reduced pain.[25,26] Acupuncture has been studied as an adjunct treatment for chronic pain. At this point, evidence is lacking for the treatment of CRPS but a

Table 1 Authors' perioperative treatment algorithm	
All Patients	1. Preoperative local anesthetic administration (at site of incision or using a block)
Moderate concern for chronic postoperative pain	1. Preoperative local anesthetics 2. Vitamin C 500 mg daily for 50 d
High concern for chronic postoperative pain (patient with high preoperative pain, nerve manipulation, high anxiety)	1. Preoperative local anesthetics 2. Gabapentin 900 mg 2 h before surgery 3. Gabapentin 300–600 mg 3 times a day for 14–30 d (if tolerated by patient) 4. Vitamin C 500 mg daily for 50 d 5. If a general anesthetic: we ask the anesthesiologist about possibility of intraoperative ketamine administration

Table 2
Authors' treatment algorithm for patient presenting with CRPS/neuropathic pain

New acute CRPS	1. Urgent referral to pain specialist 2. Solumedrol dose pack if acute presentation 3. Gabapentin 300–1200 mg 3 times a day (as tolerated by patient)[a] 4. Vitamin C 500 mg/d 5. Search for occult nerve injury: comprehensive nerve conduction studies and evaluate for sensory nerve injuries easily missed on nerve conduction studies: (1) radial sensory branch injury, (2) palmar cutaneous branch of the median, (3) cutaneous neuromas in scar.
Diffuse neuropathic pain	1. Gabapentin 300–1200 mg 3 times a day (as tolerated by patient)[a] 2. Desipramine 25 mg and increase each week by 25 mg until taking 100–150 mg/d. Goal is serum plasma level 100–300 ng/mL. Desipramine can have cardiac toxicity at higher doses, thus it is not for patients with heart disease or family history of sudden death, and not for patients taking other antidepressants. 3. If not candidate for tricyclic antidepressants because of heart disease, consider duloxetine. Start 20 mg/d and increase to 60–120 mg/d. 4. Start therapy including myofascial releases
Diffuse neuropathic pain (not tolerating or no effect of gabapentin)	1. Desipramine 25 mg and increase each week by 25 mg until taking 100–150 mg/d. Goal is serum plasma level 100–300 ng/mL. Desipramine can have cardiac toxicity at higher doses, thus it is not for patients with heart disease or family history of sudden death, and not for patients taking other antidepressants. 2. If not candidate for tricyclic antidepressants because of heart disease, consider duloxetine. Start 20 mg/d and increase to 60–120 mg/d.
Tender scar to light touch	1. Inject intradermally with bupivacaine, if relief = scar problem 2. Therapy for scar management and desensitization 3. Trial of topicals, such as capsaicin 4. Potential Botox injection[b] 5. Consider scar revision if conservative treatment fails 6. Some scar neuromas are not particularly tender but pain relief occurs with intradermal injection.

[a] Dosing of gabapentin is challenging; there is the balance of getting an efficacious does without having side effects, such as drowsiness, which make the medication intolerable. We titrate up slowly starting 300 mg per day and increasing every other day to a goal of 600 mg 3 times a day. Patients are counseled to stop increasing the dose when side effects become too bothersome (ie, stop at dose they can live with). Some patients just do not tolerate higher doses of gabapentin, we have found that for these patients starting very low (100 mg per day) and slowly titrating up can allow patients to get benefit from this medication.

[b] Botox in painful scars is an off-label use of this medication with only preliminary data at this time.

large study in Germany found that acupuncture reduced pain for a variety of conditions.[27] There are many other modalities that have been described for the treatment of CRPS, but at this time, strong evidence does not exist (eg, myofascial releases, stress loading).

Medications

Pharmacologic treatments are a second arm in management of CRPS and neuropathic pain. During the acute phase of CRPS, corticosteroids have been used as burst therapy, which has been supported in some randomized trials.[28,29] Most other medications that have been studied were in those with a chronic presentation of CRPS/neuropathic pain. A mainstay in treatment for chronic pain is gabapentin, which was originally produced as an antiseizure medication and has become a useful pain management tool.[30] It binds to the alpha-2 delta subunit of presynaptic P/Q-type voltage-gated calcium channels, modulating the traffic and function of these channels. This may directly modulate release of excitatory neurotransmitters from activated nociceptors. Alternatively, some data suggest that gabapentin's antinociceptive mechanism may arise through activation of noradrenergic pain-inhibiting pathways in the spinal cord and brain.[31] Although there are limited data on gabapentin for CRPS, there is a wealth of literature on the treatment of chronic neuropathic pain. A recent Cochrane review looked at gabapentin for those with chronic neuropathic pain and found that gabapentin gave a high level of relief to about a third of the patients with mostly tolerable adverse effects[32]; however one RCT of gabapentin in patients with CRPS I found only mild effect.[33] Gabapentin is a fairly safe medication but has frequent side effects that can be intolerable to the patient. The common side effects are fatigue, dizziness, weight gain, and restlessness. More severe side effects are rare but include changes in mood and suicidal thoughts. We have found that slow initiation of dosing and allowing the patient to hold at the dose where side effects become bothersome has increased patient acceptance of this drug. Pregabalin shares the same mechanism of action and side effects as gabapentin; however, it is absorbed more efficiently by the small intestines when given at higher doses. Switching from gabapentin to pregabalin may therefore be useful in patients who describe partial analgesia at 1200 mg of gabapentin 3 times a day without the occurrence of dose-limiting side effects.

Bisphophonates have some of the best evidence showing benefit in the treatment of CRPS. They were proposed as a treatment for CRPS because they inhibit bone resorption, which is a common finding in patients with CRPS. Several studies have shown benefit from bisphosphonates for CRPS.[34–36] Indeed, a recent review of clinical trials to treat CRPS found that bisphosphonates were the only medications with clear benefits for patients with CRPS.[37] There has been concern that long-term use of bisphosphonates may result in pathologic fractures, but this complication is rare, and for the treatment of CRPS, many patients need only a few months of treatment. Bisphosphonates should be avoided in patients with poor dentition because of the risk of osteonecrosis of the jaw, and patients should be warned to report any jaw, face, tooth, or head discomfort during treatment.

Tricyclic antidepressants (TCAs; amitriptyline, desipramine, and imipramine) are also routinely used in the treatment of neuropathic pain. These medications augment the pain inhibitory pathways and can have other beneficial side effects, such as amitriptyline helping with sleep and desipramine helping with mood. The 2007 Cochrane review confirmed that TCAs were beneficial and these are tolerated well by most patients.[38] Amitriptyline is safe at low doses and can be started while waiting for the patient to be seen by a pain specialist. No one tricyclic is more effective than another, but they all seem to be more effective the higher the dose that the patient is able to tolerate. In this regard, desipramine is particularly helpful because it has the least affinity for the muscarinic cholinergic and histamine receptors that mediate side effects. Patients are therefore often able to tolerate a titration to 100 to 150 mg per day where TCAs are more effective. A typical regimen starts at 25 mg per day and increases by 25 mg each week. However, with high doses there are cardiac side effects. So for the hand surgeon, starting out with 25 mg daily while waiting for a pain specialist is a safe and effective starting strategy.

Topical medications have also been used for chronic pain treatment, including EMLA cream, capsaicin ointment, and lidocaine patches. Capsaicin has good evidence of efficacy in treatment of neuropathic pain. Its mechanism of action was once thought related to substance P but is now thought to arise via the TRPV1 receptor. Overactivation of nociceptors by capsaicin may cause some of these fibers to actually die back from the skin surface. A 1997 meta-analysis of 5 trials determined that capsaicin had a positive effect compared with placebo and a more recent Cochrane review confirmed that capsaicin provided pain relief.[39,40]

Interventions

The third arm of treatment is the more invasive interventions, such as sympathetic blocks and nerve stimulators. Sympathetic blocks have long been used in the treatment of CRPS but the evidence of its effectiveness is lacking. One study found that only 50% of sympathetic block performed actually blocked the sympathetic chain.[41] Nerve stimulators also are used in the treatment of chronic pain. Spinal cord stimulators are the common stimulators used for chronic pain with one RCT demonstrating initial efficacy compared with physical therapy alone, but those gains diminished over time to nonsignificance at 5 years.[42]

Botox is an evolving tool in the treatment of pain. It blocks the acetylcholine release and this seems to reduce pain. It is being used intradermally to reduce pain with some early success and may be useful for cutaneous neuromas.[43]

Finally, it is important to consider peripheral nerve compression in patients with symptoms of CRPS. Placzek and colleagues[44] reported on 8 patients who developed CRPS following upper extremity surgery with clinical concerns for median or combined median and ulnar nerve compression, which were confirmed with electrodiagnostic studies. They were treated with nerve decompression, which resulted in statistically significant decrease in pain and increase in Disabilities of the Arm, Shoulder, and Hand (DASH) scores, with immediate relief of most other symptoms and improvement on motion and grip strength.

SURGICAL PATIENTS WITH CRPS

Management of a patient who has CRPS or chronic pain and may require additional surgical procedure can be challenging, as those with a history of CRPS are at risk for a recurrence/reactivation of their pain with additional trauma and thus this group is approached with caution. The first group of potential surgical candidates would be those patients with CRPS who also have a nerve injury, which is the pain generator. These patients include those with compression neuropathies or painful scar neuromas. Although there is no good evidence, most believe that surgery in this population is appropriate. For these patients, we first attempt conservative treatments (physical therapy, medication, rest, splinting, desensitization). If these fail, then we proceed with surgery. At surgery, we give our entire perioperative regimen, and if possible use an indwelling regional anesthetic catheter for the first few postoperative days. If possible, we limit immobilization and begin therapy shortly after surgery with the idea that it may be important to have the nerve gliding in the operative bed before scarring can tether or compress it. The second group is patients who might need surgery, but have had CRPS in the past. In general, this group should be approached with caution and unless the surgery has a high likelihood of improving quality of life, we would advise patients against surgical intervention.

Every practicing hand surgeon will see patients with chronic neuropathic pain and complex regional pain syndrome. There is much literature on these processes but most is in the anesthesia journals and not always readily accessible to the hand surgeon. We feel that the take-home messages are prevention for those at risk and that initiation of early treatment is something that hand surgeons should be comfortable performing.

REFERENCES

1. IASP Subcommittee on Taxonomy. Classification of chronic pain. Descriptions of chronic pain syndromes and definitions of pain terms. Pain Suppl 1986;3: S1–226.
2. Treede RD, Jensen TS, Campbell JN, et al. Redefinition of neuropathic pain and a grading system for clinical use: consensus statement on clinical and research diagnostic criteria. Neurology 2008;70:1630–5.
3. Smith BH, Torrance N, Ferguson JA, et al. Towards a definition of refractory neuro-pathic pain for epidemiological research. An international Delphi survey of ex-perts. BMC Neurol 2012;12:29.
4. Bennett MI. The LANSS Pain Scale: the Leeds assessment of neuropathic symp-toms and signs. Pain 2001;92:147–57.
5. Haanpää M, Attal N, Backonja M, et al. NeuPSIG guidelines on neuropathic pain assessment. Pain 2011;152(1):14–27.
6. Evans J. Reflex sympathetic dystrophy. Surg Clin North Am 1946;26:780–90.
7. Available at: http://www.iasp-pain.org/Content/NavigationMenu/Publications/ FreeBooks/Classification_of_Chronic_Pain/default.htm. Accessed February 5, 2013.
8. Harden RN, Oaklander AL, Burton AW, et al. Complex regional pain syndrome: practical diagnostic and treatment guidelines. Pain Med 2013;14(2):180–229. http://dx.doi.org/10.1111/pme.12033.
9. de Mos M, de Bruijn AG, Huygen FJ, et al. The incidence of complex regional pain syndrome: a population-based study. Pain 2007;129(1–2):12–20.
10. Ciaramitaro P, Mondelli M, Logullo F, et al. Italian Network for Traumatic Neurop-athies. Traumatic peripheral nerve injuries: epidemiological findings, neuropathic pain and quality of life in 158 patients. J Peripher Nerv Syst 2010;15(2):120–7. http://dx.doi.org/10.1111/j.1529-8027.2010.00260.x.
11. Boya H, Ozcan O, Oztekin HH. Long-term complications of open carpal tunnel release. Muscle Nerve 2008;38(5):1443–6.
12. Puchalski P, Zyluk A. Complex regional pain syndrome type 1 after fractures of the distal radius: a prospective study of the role of psychological factors. J Hand Surg Br 2005;30:574–80.
13. Kairaluoma PM, Bachmann MS, Rosenberg PH, et al. Preincisional paravertebral block reduces the prevalence of chronic pain after breast surgery. Anesth Analg 2006;103(3):703–8.
14. Obata H, Saito S, Fujita N, et al. Epidural block with mepivacaine before surgery reduces long-term post-thoracotomy pain. Can J Anaesth 1999;46(12): 1127–32.
15. Lavand'homme PM, Eisenach JC. Perioperative administration of the alpha2-adrenoceptor agonist clonidine at the site of nerve injury reduces the develop-ment of mechanical hypersensitivity and modulates local cytokine expression. Pain 2003;105(1–2):247–54.

16. Zollinger PE, Tuinebreijer WE, Kreis RW, et al. Effect of vitamin C on frequency of reflex sympathetic dystrophy in wrist fractures: a randomized trial. Lancet 1999; 354(9195):2025–8.

17. Zollinger PE, Tuinebreijer WE, Breederveld RS, et al. Can vitamin C prevent complex regional pain syndrome in patients with wrist fractures? A randomized, controlled, multicenter dose-response study. J Bone Joint Surg Am 2007;89(7): 1424–31.

18. Besse JL, Gadeyne S, Galand-Desmé S, et al. Effect of vitamin C on prevention of complex regional pain syndrome type I in foot and ankle surgery. Foot Ankle Surg 2009;15(4):179–82.

19. Xie W, Strong JA, Meij JT, et al. Neuropathic pain: early spontaneous afferent activity is the trigger. Pain 2005;116(3):243–56.

20. Koh SM, Moate F, Grinsell D. Co-existing carpal tunnel syndrome in complex regional pain syndrome after hand trauma. J Hand Surg Eur Vol 2010;35(3): 228–31.

21. Grundberg AB, Reagan DS. Compression syndromes in reflex sympathetic dystrophy. J Hand Surg Am 1991;16(4):731–6.

22. Oerlemans HM, Oostendorp RA, de Boo T, et al. Traumatic peripheral nerve injuries: epidemiological findings, neuropathic pain and quality of life in 158 patients. J Peripher Nerv Syst 2010;15(2):120–7. http://dx.doi.org/10.1111/j.1529-8027.2010.00260.x.

23. Oerlemans HM, Oostendorp RA, de Boo T, et al. Adjuvant physical therapy versus occupational therapy in patients with reflex sympathetic dystrophy/complex regional pain syndrome type I. Arch Phys Med Rehabil 2000;81(1):49–56.

24. Oerlemans HM, Oostendorp RA, de Boo T, et al. Pain and reduced mobility in complex regional pain syndrome I: outcome of a prospective randomized controlled clinical trial of adjuvant physical therapy versus occupational therapy. Pain 1999;83(1):77–83.

25. Daly AE, Bialocerkowski AE. Does evidence support physiotherapy management of adult Complex Regional Pain Syndrome Type One? A systematic review. Eur J Pain 2009;13(4):339–53. http://dx.doi.org/10.1016/j.ejpain.2008.05.003.

26. Bowering KJ, O'Connell NE, Tabor A, et al. The effects of graded motor imagery and its components on chronic pain: a systematic review and meta-analysis. J Pain 2013;14(1):3–13. http://dx.doi.org/10.1016/j.jpain.2012.09.007.

27. Witt CM, Schützler L, Lüdtke R, et al. Patient characteristics and variation in treatment outcomes: which patients benefit most from acupuncture for chronic pain? Clin J Pain 2011;27(6):550–5. http://dx.doi.org/10.1097/AJP.0b013e31820dfbf5.

28. Christensen K, Jensen EM, Noer I. The reflex dystrophy syndrome response to treatment with systemic corticosteroids. Acta Chir Scand 1982;148(8):653–5.

29. Braus DF, Krauss JK, Strobel J. The shoulder-hand syndrome after stroke: a prospective clinical trial. Ann Neurol 1994;36(5):728–33.

30. Clarke H, Bonin RP, Orser BA, et al. The prevention of chronic postsurgical pain using gabapentin and pregabalin: a combined systematic review and meta-analysis. Anesth Analg 2012;115(2):428–42.

31. Maneuf YP, Luo ZD, Lee K. alpha2delta and the mechanism of action of gabapentin in the treatment of pain. Semin Cell Dev Biol 2006;17(5):565–70.

32. Moore RA, Wiffen PJ, Derry S, et al. Gabapentin for chronic neuropathic pain and fibromyalgia in adults. Cochrane Database Syst Rev 2011;(3):CD007938.

33. van de Vusse AC, Stomp-van den Berg SG, Kessels AH, et al. Randomised controlled trial of gabapentin in Complex Regional Pain Syndrome type 1 [ISRCTN84121379]. BMC Neurol 2004;4:13.

34. Varenna M, Adami S, Rossini M, et al. Treatment of complex regional pain syndrome type I with neridronate: a randomized, double-blind, placebo-controlled study. Rheumatology 2013;52(3):534–42.

35. Varenna M, Zucchi F, Ghiringhelli D, et al. Intravenous clodronate in the treatment of reflex sympathetic dystrophy syndrome. A randomized, double blind, placebo controlled study. J Rheumatol 2000;27:1477–83.

36. Fulfaro F, Casuccio A, Ticozzi C, et al. The role of bisphosphonates in the treatment of painful metastatic bone disease: a review of phase III trials. Pain 1998; 78:157–69.

37. Tran de QH, Duong S, Finlayson RJ. Treatment of complex regional pain syndrome: a review of the evidence. Can J Anaesth 2010;57(2):149–66.

38. Saarto T, Wiffen PJ. Antidepressants for neuropathic pain. Cochrane Database Syst Rev 2007;(4):CD005454.

39. Kingsley WS. A critical review of controlled clinical trials for peripheral neuropathic pain and complex regional pain syndromes. Pain 1997;73(2):123–39.

40. Derry S, Lloyd R, Moore RA, et al. Topical capsaicin for chronic neuropathic pain in adults. Cochrane Database Syst Rev 2009;(4):CD007393.

41. Malmquist EL, Bengtsson M, Sorensen J. Efficacy of stellate ganglion block: a clinical study with bupivacaine. Reg Anesth 1992;17:340–7.

42. Kemler MA, de Vet HC, Barendse GA, et al. Effect of spinal cord stimulation for chronic complex regional pain syndrome Type I: five-year final follow-up of patients in a randomized controlled trial. J Neurosurg 2008;108(2):292–8. http://dx.doi.org/10.3171/JNS/2008/108/2/0292.

43. Ranoux D, Attal N, Morain F, et al. Botulinum toxin type A induces direct analgesic effects in chronic neuropathic pain. Ann Neurol 2008;64(3):274–83. http://dx.doi.org/10.1002/ana.21427.

44. Placzek JD, Boyer MI, Gelberman RH, et al. Nerve decompression for complex regional pain syndrome type II following upper extremity surgery. J Hand Surg Am 2005;30(1):69–74.

Chronic Pelvic Pain

Sharon L. Stein, MD

KEYWORDS

- Chronic pelvic pain • Myofascial pain • Pelvic pain syndrome • Levator syndrome
- Proctalgia fugax

KEY POINTS

- Chronic pelvic pain (CPP) is a difficult problem to treat that affects approximately 15% of women and unknown percentage of men.
- CPP may be difficult to diagnose and treat because causes, evaluation, and treatments may traverse multiple specialties.
- The most common causes for CPP include endometriosis, adhesions, musculoskeletal pain, and neurologic dysfunction.
- Patients with CPP are more likely to have other somatic pain syndromes, constipation, irritable bowel syndrome, or a history of sexual or physical abuse.
- Treatments of CPP are cause-specific. For patients who lack a clear cause, NSAIDs, tricyclic antidepressants, biofeedback, and neuroablative techniques are used.

INTRODUCTION

The evaluation and successful treatment of pelvic pain is a complex problem. Chronic pelvic pain (CPP) may encompass gastroenterologic, urologic, gynecologic, oncologic, musculoskeletal, and psychosocial systems.[1] Subspecialists often lack interdisciplinary training and understanding of the diverse causes needed to evaluate and treat patients. This deficit makes comprehensive evaluation, diagnosis, and treatment difficult, and may frustrate patients who are sent from one specialist to another for further evaluation and diagnosis.

This article attempts to create a multidisciplinary overview for evaluation, testing and treatment options. It reviews the most common causes of CPP and discusses management options. Finally, some obstacles to treatment are reviewed and ways to improve efficiency of evaluation and treatment are suggested.

DEFINITION OF CPP

Pelvic pain is divided into acute and chronic pain. Acute pain is typically caused by a precise cause, such as anal fissure or thrombosed external hemorrhoid. Acute pain

This article originally appeared in Gastroenterology Clinics of North America, Volume 42, Issue 4, December 2013.
Division of Colorectal Surgery, Department of Surgery, University Hospitals Case Medical Center, 11100 Euclid Avenue Lakeside 5047, Cleveland, OH 44106, USA
E-mail address: Sharon.stein@uhhospitals.org

tends to diminish and it resolves with treatment and healing; it is not discussed in this article. In contrast, CPP is described as pain lasting a minimum of 6 months in duration, which may be sudden or gradual in onset and affects "the visceral or somatic system and structures supplied by the nervous system from the 10th thoracic spinal level and below."[2] Because of the broad definition of pelvic pain, the evaluation of pelvic pain extends across many subspecialties and organ systems.

EPIDEMIOLOGY OF CPP

CPP is a ubiquitous disease; in the United States it is estimated that 9 million women between ages 18 and 50 or 15% of the female population suffer from CPP.[3] A study from the United Kingdom demonstrated a CPP rate of 24%, with 33% of women reporting 5 years or greater duration.[4] A study in New Zealand found a prevalence of 25.4%.[5] A 1994 Gallup poll estimated the direct cost of CPP at $881.5 million dollars annually, with 15% of women with CPP noting lost work revenue and 45% reporting decreased work productivity.[3]

Ideally, a specific cause can be elucidated; however, in many cases, a distinct diagnosis is never discovered. Population studies demonstrate between 50% and 61% of all women with pelvic pain lack a clear diagnosis.[3,5] Even patients who undergo diagnostic laparoscopy still lack a diagnosis in 30% to 40% of cases.[6]

An epidemiologic study found that women with CPP are more likely to have a history of spontaneous abortion, military service, nongynecologic surgery, and nonpelvic somatic complaints than controls.[7] Additional studies have demonstrated a correlation with history of multiple sexual partners and psychosexual trauma or abuse.[7–9] CPP subjects are four times as likely to have a history of pelvic inflammatory disease.[10] Subjects with CPP also have a higher incidence of constipation, irritable bowel syndrome (IBS), depression, and anxiety than control groups.

Although CPP is better described and is more prevalent in women, it is not exclusive to the female gender. Chronic prostatitis/chronic pelvic pain (CP/CPP) is a well-described cause of pelvic pain in men. Musculoskeletal disorders may also be present with pelvic pain. As the diagnosis of CPP is better understood and known, it is likely that more men will present with similar complaints.

RELEVANT HISTORY FOR PATIENTS WITH CPP

History is a vital element in evaluation of CPP. Given the complexity of elements involved, a thorough history must include history of gastroenterologic, gynecologic, urologic, musculoskeletal, and pain symptoms. A full review of systems, including infectious diseases, endocrine disorders, and psychiatric disorders, is necessary. The International Pelvic Pain Society provides an extensive history intake form.[11]

A discussion of the character, intensity, radiation, and chronicity of pain should be obtained. Duration of pain, and exacerbating and alleviating factors, should be determined. Daily variation may give clues to the cause. Pelvic congestion syndrome typically increases in intensity as the day progresses, whereas proctalgia fugax tends to awaken the patient at night.

Determining the relationship of pain to each organ system is important. From a gynecologic perspective, correlation with sexual activity is also important. Pain associated with superficial stimulation is more consistent with vaginitis or vulvodynia; whereas deep dyspareunia is consistent with endometriosis or pelvic inflammatory disease. Abnormal vaginal bleeding may be symptomatic of uterine leiomyomas, adenomyosis, or malignancy, and should be evaluated with pelvic ultrasound.

A history of high-risk sexual behavior, multiple partners, and/or genital discharge can suggest pelvic inflammatory disease.

A history of pain or pressure with urination, difficulty emptying, or frequency suggests urologic causes. History of gastrointestinal disorders, including constipation and IBS, can be helpful. Manual evacuation and vaginal digitation are consistent with obstructed defecation. A history of recent trauma or pregnancy may help illuminate a musculoskeletal cause and surgical interventions 3 to 6 months ago may suggest adhesive disease.[12] Copies of colonoscopies, operative reports, or pathologic specimens are crucial. Previous perineal operations, mesh placement, and radiation may suggest iatrogenic causes.

Visceral and somatic pain may be sensed differently. Because visceral innervation of the pelvic structures share common neural pathways, distinguishing the cause of visceral pain may be difficult.[10] Visceral pain is associated with dull, crampy, or poorly localized pain, and may be associated with autonomic phenomena such as nausea, vomiting, and sweating.[13] Somatic pain, in contrast, originates from muscles, bones, and joints, and typically presents according to specific dermatomes. Somatic pain is associated with sharp or dull pain. Neuropathic pain may produce burning, paresthesia, or lancing pain. A history of pain syndromes, or drug or alcohol, abuse may also factor into evaluation and treatment. Janicki[14] has described a centralized sensitization of the pain receptors in patients with CPP and has suggested that understanding this may also be necessary for success.

An evaluation should also determine level of functional disability. The patient's ability to work, engage in daily activities, and emotional and sexual relationships is relevant. A full psychological evaluation should be considered for patients with history of sexual, physical abuse, depression, or anxiety. This does not alleviate the need for physical diagnosis; however, recognition and treatment may be important elements in symptom improvement.

PHYSICAL EXAMINATION

The physical examination encompasses multiple specialty examinations and may be time consuming for the practitioner and difficult for the patient with CPP. The entire examination and evaluation may require several visits to complete. All practitioners should have a chaperone during invasive examinations and at least one member of the medical team should be female.

Before commencing a formal examination, the practitioners should evaluate patient gait, movement, and sitting pose. Patients with pelvic girdle pain or spinal pain may have difficulty ambulating and sit off to one side; the practitioner should question the patient on this.

Specific areas of concern include the abdomen and abdominal wall. Patients should be examined for scars and previous surgeries or complications from surgeries should be reviewed. The abdomen should be palpated for tenderness, masses, or lesions. Distension and bloating may suggest history of constipation or bowel obstruction. The area of greatest abdominal pain should be localized. Performing a Valsalva maneuver or asking the patient to raise her head and legs separates the visceral organs from abdominal wall and may identify pressure points. Flexion of the head reduces abdominal pain and points to a visceral origin; conversely, increasing pain suggests abdominal wall or musculoskeletal origin.

The pelvic examination should commence with visual inspection noting areas of discoloration, dermatologic disorders, or sequelae of infection. A Q-tip examination using light touch is used to evaluate the sensory and neurologic systems of the perineum. Signs of incontinence at baseline or with straining should be noted. Pelvic organ prolapse quantification (Pop-Q) examination should be performed. Rectal prolapse can be noted during propulsive activity as well. Preferably, patients should be examined in both a reclining and standing position for greater sensitivity.

Anteriorly, the urethra and bladder trigone should be evaluated. A mass by the urethra suggests ureteral diverticulum, whereas tenderness and dysuria suggests urethritis, urethral syndrome, or interstitial cystitis (IC). A urinalysis can evaluate for infectious causes of urologic origin. Hematuria is associated with endometriosis. If urinary tract cause is suggested, a cystoscopy with evaluation for Hunner ulcers and a potassium chloride (KCl) sensitivity test to evaluate for IC are warranted. Urodynamics are indicated if urinary dysfunction exists.

In the vaginal compartment, an evaluation for vaginal discharge, Pap smear, and bimanual examination should be performed. Vaginal discharge and cervical motion tenderness are concerning for sexually transmitted diseases and can be further evaluated with cultures or histology. Tenderness may suggest vulvodynia or vaginitis.

A rectal examination should include digital examination and anoscopy to evaluate for lesions. For patients with bleeding, inflammation, or lesions noted on anoscopy, a colonoscopy may be warranted. Fissures, hemorrhoids, fistulas, or abscesses can cause chronic anal pain. Pain on rectal examination without fluctuance can be a sign of an intersphincteric abscess, which may have no external signs.

The musculoskeletal examination should evaluate the abdominal wall and pelvic floor muscles. During vaginal examination, the levator plate should be palpated on both sides of the vagina. A finger is curved over the levators during relaxation and contraction to evaluate for tenderness. The piriformis muscle is palpated through the vagina, cephalad to the ischial spine in a posterior lateral direction. The piriformis is lateral to the bulbospongiosus and transverse perineum that run parallel to the vagina. The internal and external sphincter muscles are evaluated transanally at rest and with contraction. Note should be made of weakness or deficiency. During normal contraction, a slight upward pull should be felt from the coccygeus, puborectalis, and pubovaginalis muscles. During propulsion, descent of the pelvic wall and motility of the rectum should be noted.

The coccyx should be evaluated for coccygodynia. Pain with palpation or mobility is a sign of coccygodynia; a normal coccyx should rotate 25° to 30° without discomfort. External rotation of the leg against resistance may exacerbate the pain. Flexion of the hip and knee against resistance may demonstrate psoas pain. Additional musculoskeletal evaluation includes evaluation of pelvic ring instability, which is particularly common after delivery. Straight leg raise, resisted hip abduction, adduction tests, and posterior provocative pain test may be helpful in evaluating the stability of the pelvic ring.

If the examination fails to elicit a clear cause for their pain, an MRI may be helpful. In a study of subjects with CPP and no specific clinical findings, MRI was able to elucidate a cause in 39% of cases.[15] For the remainder, 36% of subjects were ultimately diagnosed with levator ani syndrome and 25% with unspecified anorectal pain. Other testing includes pelvic ultrasound, cystoscopy, and colonoscopy. In the past, laparoscopy was performed for diagnostic purposes but is no longer indicated.[16]

COMMON CAUSES FOR CPP

The three most common documented findings on laparoscopy for CPP are endometriosis (33%), adhesions (24%), and absence of pathologic condition on laparoscopy (35%).[17] However, hundreds of different causes may cause pelvic pain (**Fig. 1**).

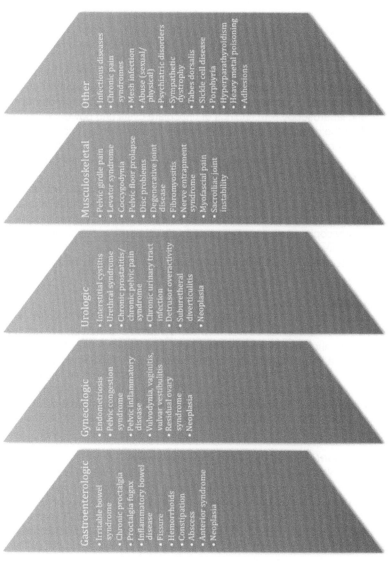

Fig. 1. Some of the causes of CPP.

Because normal pelvic function requires coordinated activity of the muscular, connective, visceral, and neural tissues of the pelvis, dysfunction in any area can create a complex situation that may ultimately manifest itself as pelvic pain.

Gynecologic

Endometriosis
Endometriosis is one of the leading causes of CPP in women. Endometriosis is defined as the presence of endometrial tissue outside of the uterine cavity. Areas of involvement may include proximal or distant sites and may affect gastroenterologic and gynecologic function secondary to local or metastatic invasion.

Typically, patients are nulliparous, in their 20s and 30s, with symptoms correlated with menstrual cycle, including dysmenorrhea and pain. Deep dyspareunia and involuntary infertility are also common. Patients are often diagnosed by symptoms alone, but diagnostic laparoscopy with findings of chocolate cysts and powder puff staining help to confirm the diagnosis. Up to 40% of patients may have no finding at laparoscopy.[16] Severity of pain is not generally correlated with gross or pathologic findings during surgical extirpation.[18] Noninvasive diagnosis is being evaluated using ultrasound and pelvic MRI.[19–23]

Treatment of endometriosis is often hormonal, including oral contraceptives or induced menopause, which may lead to the atrophy of implants and relief of symptoms. Acupuncture has been used with success in some cases.[24,25] Presacral neurectomy or laparoscopic uterine nerve ablation (LUNA) may decrease symptoms; however, these are not endorsed by a recent Cochrane review.[26] Surgical excision, abdominal hysterectomy, and salpingo-oophorectomy may be recommended in refractory cases.

Pelvic congestion
Pelvic congestion is most frequently seen in women between 20 and 30 years old, and is analogous to a scrotal varicocele in men. Symptoms generally worsen before menstruation and increase in severity during the day. Patients may also complain of deep dyspareunia or postcoital pain. Dilated vessels can be seen on imaging such as duplex venography, MRI, or during laparoscopy. Pathologic findings including fibrosis of tunica intima and media are noted with hypertrophy and proliferation of capillary endothelium.[27] Both ovarian suppression and embolic treatment seem to control symptoms, with embolic treatment success varying from 24% to 100% in studies.[28]

Vulvodynia, vaginitis, and vulvar vestibulitis syndromes
Vulvodynia, vaginitis, and vulvar vestibulitis syndromes, as well as clitoral pain, are forms of pain localized to the anterior compartment. It is hypothesized they are caused by stretching of the perivaginal and perivulvar muscles, hormonal changes, or contact irritation. Symptoms are typically intermittent in nature and may be experienced as itching, burning, stinging, rawness, or dyspareunia. Onset may occur after first sexual experience or tampon use, but may also occur after trauma such as delivery or vigorous sexual activity. Laboratory testing is generally performed to rule out infectious and dermatologic causes. A cotton swab or Q-tip test can localize areas of sensitivity. Management generally consists of biofeedback to desensitize the affected region, including application of manual therapy or electrotherapy. Topical agents such as lidocaine or lubricant may be helpful and, in some patients, botulinum toxin type A (Botox) injections are efficacious. Up to 50% of patients may respond to pain medications, such as tricyclic agents, or gabapentin.[29,30] Behavioral therapy

and interventional pain techniques may be helpful in patients who fail to respond to initial treatments.

Urologic

Chronic prostatitis/chronic pelvic pain (CP/CPP)

Although CPP is generally recognized as an entity affecting women, men can also have CPP. In addition to a multitude of musculoskeletal ailments, men can develop CP/CPP. This syndrome was recognized by the National Institute of Health in 1995. It is characterized by CPP and voiding symptoms in the absence of urinary tract infection, anatomic abnormality, or urologic malignancy.[31] Inflammatory and noninflammatory types, depending on the presence or absence of leukocytes in expressed prostatic secretions, have been described. A 2013 review of articles on CP/CPP suggested treatment options and advocated a multimodal therapeutic approach that may include use of alpha-blockers in patients with significant voiding symptoms, and physical therapy or antibiotics for newly diagnosed antimicrobial-naive patients.[32]

Interstitial cystitis (IC)

Symptoms of IC include bladder pain, urinary frequency, urgency, or nocturia. Pain is often present in the suprapubic area but it may occur in the lower back or buttock. Fifty-one percent of women complain of dyspareunia. Concomitant fibromyalgia, vulvodynia, anxiety, and depression are common.[33]

Urinalysis is generally performed to rule out urinary tract infection. On cystoscopy, Hunner ulcers may be seen in the bladder mucosa and a KCl sensitivity test is used to obtain a definitive diagnosis. The KCl sensitivity test evaluates the bladder for increased epithelial permeability that is believed to contribute to IC.[34] This test is positive in up to 75% of patients, although false positives may occur.[35]

First-line treatment of IC is generally nonsteroidal antiinflammatory medication (NSAID), although neither NSAIDs nor opioids have been noted to be effective. Pentosan polysulfate sodium (PPS) is the only treatment of IC approved by the Food and Drug Administration (FDA).[17] PPS is hypothesized to mimic the normal glycosaminoglycan layer that protects the bladder urothelium that is dysfunctional in IC. Treatment is effective in 28% to 32% of patients but may require up to 6 months of treatments.[36,37] Use of PPS in conjunction with tricyclic antidepressants may have better results.[17] Both dimethyl sulfoxide and heparin have been administered as intravesicular injection with limited success, and Botox in combination with hydrodistention has been used with some efficacy.[38,39] Sacral nerve stimulation has been used for patients who failed other therapies.[40]

Urethral syndrome

Urethral syndrome is associated with incomplete emptying and burning during urination, particularly after intercourse. The urethra may be tender on examination. It is believed that urethral syndrome is caused by noninfectious, stenotic, or fibrous changes in the urethra. Urethral syndrome is associated with grand multiparity, delivery without episiotomy, and general pelvic relaxation.[41] Treatment generally consists of diathermy and coagulation.[42]

Gastroenterologic

Irritable bowel syndrome (IBS)

IBS is defined as the chronic presence of abdominal pain or discomfort 3 days or more per month that correlates with stooling, change in frequency, or form of stool.[43] IBS is believed to be multifactorial in origin and related to the hypersensitivity of the viscera leading to disproportionate pain with intestinal distension, dysregulation of gastrointestinal motility, and endocrine effects of hypothalamic pituitary axis.[44]

IBS is a diagnosis of exclusion. Other causes that may cause bowel dysfunction, such as Crohn's disease, diverticulitis, sprue, lactose allergy, and chronic appendicitis, must be ruled out. There is a strong association between CPP and IBS; 65% to 79% of patients with IBS have CPP and 60% of patients have associated dysmenorrhea.[45]

Dietary modification may be helpful to decrease symptomatology. For patients with diarrhea, loperamide, cholestyramine, and alosetron (for women) are most commonly recommended. A trial of rifaximin has been shown to provide symptom relief but is not yet approved by the FDA for IBS.[46] Constipation is generally treated with dietary and supplementary fiber, stool softener, or cathartics such as lactulose and polyethylene glycol. A 2007 Cochrane database reviewed the use of tegaserod, a 5-hydroxytryptamine^4 partial agonist and found patients were more likely to have modest relief than with placebo.[47] Tricyclic antidepressants, smooth muscle relaxants, and serotonin reuptake inhibitors have also been used with some success.[43]

Chronic proctalgia

Chronic proctalgia is defined as chronic or recurrent anorectal pain lasting for 20 minutes or longer, in the absence of other anorectal causes of pain such as hemorrhoids, fissures, and coccygodynia. Patients often describe a burning sensation, which may worsen with defecation or sitting and improve when supine. Symptoms are generally more common in women and are often associated with other bowel dysfunction, such as obstructed defecation. Proctalgia has an incidence of 2% to 5%.[48] First-line therapy for patients with chronic proctalgia and obstructed defecation is generally biofeedback with success rates as high as 65%.[49] For patients without defecatory symptoms, Botox may be used as well. Tricyclic antidepressants, sacral nerve stimulation, and pain medication are reserved for refractory cases.

Proctalgia fugax

Proctalgia fugax is sudden nocturnal cramping that occurs and spontaneously resolves without objective findings and has an incidence of 8% to 18%.[50,51] Episodes are localized to the anus or lower rectum and last for seconds to minutes. Complete cessation of pain occurs between episodes.[52] There is some association with high resting and squeeze pressures that may improve with biofeedback.[53] If pain is unilateral, entrapment of the pudendal nerve at the Alcock's canal should be considered.[54] First-line treatment includes topical diltiazem or nitroglycerin, injection of Botox, or strip myomectomy in severe cases in which internal anal sphincter is thickened.[49,55,56] Injection of the pudendal nerve and sphincterotomy have both been used with some success.[57,58] Sacral nerve modulation has also been effective.[59]

Musculoskeletal

Pelvic girdle pain

Pelvic girdle pain presents as posterior sacral or buttock pain of variable intensity.[60] It is generally associated with recent pregnancy or pain that started during pregnancy.[61] One to sixteen percent of women have pain lasting longer than 12 months postpartum.[62] Evaluation consists of musculoskeletal testing, including straight leg raise, provocative testing, palpation of sacroiliac ligament, resisted hip abduction, and adduction tests.[63] Treatment is generally multidisciplinary and includes an exercise program focusing on restoring pelvic stability. Occasionally intra-articular injections with steroids are given for sacroiliac joint pain.[64] Pain medications are generally avoided, except for antiinflammatory medications. For severe cases, radiofrequency thermocoagulation, cryoneurolysis under fluoroscopic guidance, and pulsed radiofrequency have been used with lasting improvement.[65,66]

Levator syndrome

Levator syndrome is generally attributed to muscle spasm of the pelvic floor musculature and consists of wide range of complex musculoskeletal disorders, including piriformis and puborectalis syndromes. Symptoms are generally a vague dull pressure or ache that may worsen with sitting or lying down. It is often associated with incomplete evacuation. It is more common in women, with an incidence of approximately 6%.[67] Diagnosis is made with palpation of muscles and associated tenderness. Digital massage is associated with improvement in symptoms in up to 68% of patients.[68] Lidocaine, methylprednisolone, and triamcinolone have also been injected with varied results.[69,70] Case reports also demonstrate improvement after injection of Botox.[71] Biofeedback has been used with approximately 30% of patients noting improvement.[72]

Coccygodynia

Coccygodynia is pain at or around the coccyx evoked by manipulation of the coccyx. It is typically associated with local trauma, prolonged sitting, or cycling. It may be exacerbated by sitting, bending, or arising, as well as during intercourse or defecation. Coccygodynia may be secondary to hypertonicity of the pelvic floor and decreased coccyx mobility. The cause may be unknown in up to 30% of cases. Diagnosis can be confirmed by relief of pain after injection of local anesthetic. Treatment options include antiinflammatory medications, rest, coccyx cushion, physical therapy, and massage. If the coccyx is unstable or hypermobile, local injection may be more useful compared with manual stretching.[73] Radiofrequency thermocoagulation, pulsed radiofrequency, cryoneurolysis, and sacral modulation have been promoted.[74] Coccygectomy should be assiduously avoided.

Pelvic floor prolapse

Pelvic prolapse may be noted in as many as 50% of multiparous women. The cause of pelvic prolapse is believed to be a multifactorial combination of aging, trauma, devascularization, changing collagen content, and lowered estrogen levels.[75] Pelvic floor prolapse in young premenopausal patients has been associated with decreased collagen content compared with normal controls.[76] Pop-Q examination and visualization are the gold standard for diagnosis; MRI defecography may be helpful in some situations. Organ prolapse may include the anterior compartment: cystocele, uterine prolapse, and enterocele. Rectocele may cause issues with obstructive defecation. Rectal prolapse can be associated with mucous discharge and incontinence. Surgical treatment has been the gold standard for most gynecologic, urologic, or gastrointestinal prolapse, although use of a pessary may relieve symptoms for anterior pelvic floor prolapse in some patients. The causes and treatment options for rectal prolapse are discussed elsewhere in this issue.

Infectious Causes

Gynecologic diseases, such as chlamydia, gonorrhea, syphilis, HIV-AIDS, trichomoniasis, vaginitis, and genital herpes, may cause pelvic pain.[77] Symptoms include bloody or malodorous vaginal discharge, urinary symptoms, dyspareunia, and cervical motion tenderness on examination. Objective findings may be minimal and reinfection without partner treatment is common. Treatment may be delayed if there is not a high level of suspicion. Chronic infections may contribute to infertility.

Chronic Pain Syndromes
___

A substantial number of patients with CPP do not demonstrate objective findings. These patients often undergo substantial workup and may have had transient improvements from treatment, but they continue to have recurrent pain. In these patients, Janicki[14] describes a chronic pain syndrome that involves the hypersensitization of nerve cells, increased role of the autonomic nervous system, and "windup" of the pain environment. Once patients experience this phenomenon, even minor pain stimulants can exacerbate or maintain the pain. Howard and colleagues[78] describe pain mapping of the visceral organs using a blunt probe laparoscopically under conscious sedation. Treatment involves injection at pressure points.

TREATMENT OPTIONS FOR PATIENTS WITHOUT DEFINED CAUSE

Patients in whom a specific cause for their pain cannot be identified often undergo a variety of treatments. Predictors of successful treatment include history of other pain syndromes, good family and social support systems, employment status, and beliefs about pain.[7] First-line treatment is generally scheduled NSAIDs to decrease pain and inflammation. Narcotics are not recommended, secondary to concerns for abuse and addiction potential as well as risks of constipation or antimotility side effects. Tricyclic antidepressants and neuropathic medications such as gabapentin lack good quality evidence to demonstrate efficacy, although they may be helpful for some patients.

Neuroablative techniques include radiofrequency thermocoagulation, pulsed radiofrequency, cooled radiofrequency, and cryoneurolysis. Neuroablative techniques are used primarily for neuralgias of the abdominal wall or pelvic floor and may destroy neural tissue directly or alter neuron conduction. Although most techniques have been used with success, side effects including neuroma formation and postprocedural neuritis have been documented.[79–81] Chemical neuroablation has also been used. Traditional techniques involve the use of alcohol, phenol, or hypertonic saline for patients refractory to other techniques.[82] Side effects include flaccid paralysis of injected and surrounding nerves. Botox is a strong neurotoxin that prevents release of acetylcholine at the neuromuscular junction. Analgesic effects last approximately 3 to 5 months longer than muscle relaxant effects.[83] Botox is increasingly used with some success for both pelvic floor muscle spasms and undifferentiated CPP.[84] A 2013 review of literature demonstrated relief in subjects with CPP secondary to pelvic floor muscle spasm; however, a lack of data on optimum dosage, technique, and duration of effect was noted.[85]

Laparoscopy has also been used as both a diagnostic and therapeutic tool. The most common causes of CPP discovered on laparoscopy include adhesions and endometriosis. Up to 58% of gynecologic laparoscopies are associated with pelvic pain, but more than half of patients will have a negative laparoscopy.[86–88] Adhesions are often thought to be a source of CPP; however, a prospective, randomized, clinical trial observed no benefit to surgical lysis of adhesions to treat CPP.[89] A second trial randomized subjects to either diagnostic laparoscopy alone or laparoscopic adhesiolysis. Both groups experienced a significant initial improvement in pain scores, but there was no difference between the groups at 1 year.[90] Only 45% of subjects treated with laparoscopic adhesiolysis experienced improvement in quality-of-life scores at the 2-year follow-up. Additionally, 55% of subjects were noted to have complete relapse of pain following adhesiolysis.[91]

In cases of severe pelvic pain, hysterectomy has been performed. Up to 10% of all hysterectomies are performed for CPP.[92] However, up to 40% of patients will have recurrent pelvic pain after hysterectomy. Risks factors for recurrence include lack of pelvic pathologic diagnosis, lack of commercial insurance, and age younger than 30.[93]

In one study, standard treatment was compared with integrated approach. Subjects in the standard treatment group underwent traditional treatment with root cause analysis and frequent laparoscopy. In the integrated approach, equal attention was devoted to somatic, physiologic, dietary, environmental, and physiotherapeutic factors. The groups were similar in baseline clinical characteristics and pain scores. Evaluation of pain scores at 1 year revealed the superiority of the integrated approach.[89]

CHALLENGES FACING DIAGNOSIS, TREATMENT, AND ELIMINATION OF CPP

CPP is a heterogenous group of disorders that cover a wide range of specialties. Because of the diversity in expertise, diagnosis, and treatment options, facilitating care for these patients can be difficult for the following reasons:

- The patient population is varied, which complicates research in terms of extrapolating findings or treatment success to a broader group of patients.
- There are minimal data from randomized controlled trials to direct treatment.
- Data available in one specialty may not be accessed by other specialties. Data in the gynecologic literature may not be read by gastroenterologists, urologists, or physiatrists, which limits incorporation of new findings.
- Data suggest that multidisciplinary treatment may benefit patients, but there is lack of funding and impetus to create and maintain such collaborative efforts.

REFERENCES

1. Reiter RC. Evidence-based management of chronic pelvic pain. Clin Obstet Gynecol 1998;41(2):422–35.
2. Apte G, Nelson P, Brismée JM, et al. Chronic female pelvic pain—part 1: clinical pathoanatomy and examination of the pelvic region. Pain Pract 2012;12(2): 88–110.
3. Mathias SD, Kuppermann M, Liberman RF, et al. Chronic pelvic pain: prevalence, health-related quality of life, and economic correlates. Obstet Gynecol 1996; 87(3):321–7.
4. Zondervan KT, Yudkin PL, Vessey MP, et al. The community prevalence of chronic pelvic pain in women and associated illness behaviour. Br J Gen Pract 2001; 51(468):541–7.
5. Grace VM, Zondervan KT. Chronic pelvic pain in New Zealand: prevalence, pain severity, diagnoses and use of the health services. Aust N Z J Public Health 2004; 28(4):369–75.
6. Garry R. Diagnosis of endometriosis and pelvic pain. Fertil Steril 2006;86:1307–9.
7. Reiter RC, Gambone JC. Demographic and historic variables in women with idiopathic chronic pelvic pain. Obstet Gynecol 1990;75(3 Pt 1):428–32.
8. Walling MK, Reiter RC, O'Hara MW, et al. Abuse history and chronic pain in women: I. Prevalences of sexual abuse and physical abuse. Obstet Gynecol 1994;84(2):193–9.
9. Collett BJ, Cordle CJ, Stewart CR, et al. A comparative study of women with chronic pelvic pain, chronic nonpelvic pain and those with no history of pain attending general practitioners. Br J Obstet Gynaecol 1998;105(1):87–92.
10. Ryder RM. Chronic pelvic pain. Am Fam Physician 1996;54:2225–32.

11. International Pelvic Pain Society history and physical form. Available at: http://www.pelvicpain.org/pdf/History_and_Physical_Form/IPPS-H&PformR-MSW.pdf. Accessed May 2013.
12. Steege JF. Office assessment of chronic pelvic pain. Clin Obstet Gynecol 1997; 40(3):554–63.
13. Gunter J. Chronic pelvic pain: an integrated approach to diagnosis and treatment. Obstet Gynecol Surv 2003;58(9):615–23.
14. Janicki TI. Chronic pelvic pain as a form of complex regional pain syndrome. Clin Obstet Gynecol 2003;46(4):797–803.
15. Dwarkasing RS, Schouten WR, Geeraedts TE, et al. Chronic anal and perianal pain resolved with MRI. AJR Am J Roentgenol 2013;200(5):1034–41.
16. Pearce C, Curtis M. A multidisciplinary approach to self-care in chronic pelvic pain. Br J Nurs 2007;16:82–5.
17. Nelson P, Apte G, Justiz R 3rd, et al. Chronic female pelvic pain—part 2: differential diagnosis and management. Pain Pract 2012;12(2):111–41.
18. Buttram VC Jr. The rationale for use of medical suppressive therapy prior to endoscopic surgery. Ann N Y Acad Sci 1994;734:445–9.
19. Scardapane A, Lorusso F, Bettocchi S, et al. Deep pelvic endometriosis: accuracy of pelvic MRI completed by MR colonography. Radiol Med 2013;118(2): 323–38.
20. Manganaro L, Vittori G, Vinci V, et al. Beyond laparoscopy: 3-T magnetic resonance imaging in the evaluation of posterior cul-de-sac obliteration. Magn Reson Imaging 2012;30(10):1432–8.
21. Reid S, Lu C, Casikar I, et al. Prediction of pouch of Douglas obliteration in women with suspected endometriosis using a new real-time dynamic transvaginal ultrasound technique: the sliding sign. Ultrasound Obstet Gynecol 2013; 41(6):685–91.
22. Macario S, Chassang M, Novellas S, et al. The value of pelvic MRI in the diagnosis of posterior cul-de-sac obliteration in cases of deep pelvic endometriosis. AJR Am J Roentgenol 2012;199(6):1410–5.
23. Hudelist G, Fritzer N, Staettner S, et al. Uterine sliding sign: a simple sonographic predictor for presence of deep infiltrating endometriosis of the rectum. Ultrasound Obstet Gynecol 2013;41(6):692–5.
24. Wayne PM, Kerr CE, Schnyer RN, et al. Japanese-style acupuncture for endometriosis-related pelvic pain in adolescents and young women: results of a randomized sham-controlled trial. J Pediatr Adolesc Gynecol 2008;21(5):247–57.
25. Highfield ES, Laufer MR, Schnyer RN, et al. Adolescent endometriosis-related pelvic pain treated with acupuncture: two case reports. J Altern Complement Med 2006;12(3):317–22.
26. Proctor ML, Farquhar CM, Sinclair OJ, et al. Surgical interruption of pelvic nerve pathways for primary dysmenorrhea. Cochrane Database Syst Rev 2002;(4):CD001896.
27. Liddle AD, Davies AH. Pelvic congestion syndrome: chronic pelvic pain caused by ovarian and internal iliac varices. Phlebology 2007;22:100–4.
28. Tu FF, Hahn D, Steege JF. Pelvic congestion syndrome-associated pelvic pain: a systematic review of diagnosis and management. Obstet Gynecol Surv 2010; 65(5):332–40.
29. Reed BD. Vulvodynia: diagnosis and management. Am Fam Physician 2006;73: 1231–8.
30. Smart OC, MacLean AB. Vulvodynia. Curr Opin Obstet Gynecol 2003;15(6): 497–500.

31. Krieger JN, Nyberg L Jr, Nickel JC. NIH consensus definition and classification of prostatitis. JAMA 1999;282(3):236–7.
32. Nickel JC, Alexander RB, Schaeffer AJ, et al, Chronic Prostatitis Collaborative Research Network Study Group. Leukocytes and bacteria in men with chronic prostatitis/chronic pelvic pain syndrome compared to asymptomatic controls. J Urol 2003;170(3):818–22.
33. Clemons JL, Arya LA, Myers DL. Diagnosing interstitial cystitis in women with chronic pelvic pain. Obstet Gynecol 2002;100:337–41.
34. Parson CL, Greenberger M, Gabal L, et al. The role of urinary potassium in the pathogenesis and diagnosis of interstitial cystitis. J Urol 1998;159:1862–6.
35. Sant GR, Hanno PM. Interstitial cystitis: current issues and controversies in diagnosis. Urology 2001;57(Suppl 6A):82–8.
36. Moldwin RM, Sant GR. Interstitial cystitis: a pathophysiology and treatment update. Clin Obstet Gynecol 2002;45:259–72, 62.
37. Mulholland SG, Hanno PM, Parsons CL. Pentosan polysulfate sodium for therapy of interstitial cystitis. Urology 1990;35:522–58.
38. Dawson TE, Jamison J. Intravesical treatments for painful bladder syndrome/interstitial cystitis. Cochrane Database Syst Rev 2007;(4):CD006113.
39. Kuo HC, Chancellor MB. Comparison of intravesical botulinum toxin type A injections plus hydrodistention with hydrodistention alone for the treatment of refractory interstitial cystitis/painful bladder syndrome. BJU Int 2009;104: 657–61.
40. Zabihi N, Mourtzinos A, Maher MG, et al. Short-term results of bilateral S2-S4 sacral neuromodulation for the treatment of refractory interstitial cystitis, painful bladder syndrome, and chronic pelvic pain. Int Urogynecol J Pelvic Floor Dysfunct 2008;19:553–7.
41. Gürel H, Gürel SA, Atilla MK. Urethral syndrome and associated risk factors related to obstetrics and gynecology. Eur J Obstet Gynecol Reprod Biol 1999; 83(1):5–7.
42. Costantini E, Zucchi A, Del Zingaro M, et al. Treatment of urethral syndrome: a prospective randomized study with Nd:YAG laser. Urol Int 2006;76(2):134–8.
43. Longstreth GF, Thompson WG, Chey WD, et al. Functional bowel disorders. Gastroenterology 2006;130:1480–91.
44. Shin JH, Howard FM. Management of chronic pelvic pain. Curr Pain Headache Rep 2011;15:377–85.
45. Hogston P. Irritable bowel syndrome as a cause of chronic pain in women attending a gynaecology clinic. Br Med J (Clin Res Ed) 1987;294(6577):934–5.
46. Pimental M, Lembo A, Chey W, et al. Rifaximin therapy for patients with irritable bowel syndrome without constipation. N Engl J Med 2011;364:22–32.
47. Evans BW, Clark WK, Moore DJ, et al. Tegaserod for the treatment of irritable bowel syndrome and chronic constipation. Cochrane Database Syst Rev 2007;(4):CD003960.
48. Rao SS, Paulson J, Mata M, et al. Clinical trial: effects of botulinum toxin on levator ani syndrome—a double-blind, placebo controlled study. Aliment Pharmacol Ther 2009;29:985–91.
49. Atkin GK, Suliman A, Vaizey CJ. Patient characteristics and treatment outcome in functional anorectal pain. Dis Colon Rectum 2011;54(7):870–5.
50. Baranowski AP. Chronic pelvic pain. Best Pract Res Clin Gastroenterol 2009;23: 593–610.
51. Mazza L, Formento E, Fonda G. Anorectal and perineal pain: new pathophysiological hypothesis. Tech Coloproctol 2004;8:77–83.

52. Rome III diagnostic criteria for functional gastrointestinal disorders. Available at: http://www.romecriteria.org/assets/pdf/19_RomeIII_apA_885–898.pdf. Accessed January 3, 2011.
53. Grimaud JC, Bouvier M, Naudy B, et al. Manometric and radiologic investigations and biofeedback treatment of chronic idiopathic anal pain. Dis Colon Rectum 1991;34:690–5.
54. Pisani R, Stubinski R, Datti R. Entrapment neuropathy of the internal pudendal nerve: report of two cases. Scand J Urol Nephrol 1997;31:407–10.
55. Lowenstein B, Cataldo PA. Treatment of proctalgia fugax with topical nitroglycerin: report of a case. Dis Colon Rectum 1998;41:667–8.
56. Katsinelos P, Kalomenopoulou M, Christodoulou K, et al. Treatment of proctalgia fugax with botulinum A toxin. Eur J Gastroenterol Hepatol 2001;13:1371–3.
57. Takano M. Proctalgia fugax: caused by pudendal neuropathy? Dis Colon Rectum 2005;48:114–20.
58. Gracia Solanas JA, Ramirez Rodriguez JM, Elia Guedea M, et al. Sequential treatment for proctalgia fugax. Mid-term follow-up. Rev Esp Enferm Dig 2005;97:491–6.
59. Falletto E, Masin A, Lolli P, et al. Is sacral nerve stimulation an effective treatment for chronic idiopathic anal pain? Dis Colon Rectum 2009;52:456–62.
60. Nilsson-Wikmar L, Holm K, Oijerstedt R, et al. Effect of three different physical therapy treatments on pain and activity in pregnant women with pelvic girdle pain: a randomized clinical trial with 3, 6, and 12 months follow-up postpartum. Spine 2005;30:850–6.
61. O'Sullivan PB, Beales DJ. Diagnosis and classification of pelvic girdle pain disorders – part 1: a mechanism based approach within a biopsychosocial framework. Man Ther 2007;12:86–97.
62. Ferreira CW, Alburquerque-Sendín F. Effectiveness of physical therapy for pregnancy-related low back and/or pelvic pain after delivery: a systematic review. Physiother Theory Pract 2013;29(6):419–31.
63. Mens JM, Vleeming A, Snijders CJ, et al. The active straight leg raising test and mobility of the pelvic joints. Eur Spine J 1999;8:468–73.
64. Bollow M, Braun J, Taupitz M, et al. CT-guided intraarticular corticosteroid injection into the sacroiliac joints in patients with spondyloarthropathy: indication and follow-up with contrast-enhanced MRI. J Comput Assist Tomogr 1996;20(4):512–21.
65. Cohen SP, Hurley RW, Buckenmaier CC 3rd, et al. Randomized placebo-controlled study evaluating lateral branch radiofrequency denervation for sacroiliac joint pain. Anesthesiology 2008;109:279–88.
66. Kapural L, Nageeb F, Kapural M, et al. Cooled radiofrequency system for the treatment of chronic pain from sacroiliitis: the first case-series. Pain Pract 2008; 8:348–54.
67. Drossman D, Li Z, Andruzzi E, et al. U.S. householder survey of functional gastrointestinal disorders: prevalence, sociodemography, and health impact. Dig Dis Sci 1993;38(9):1569–80.
68. Grant SR, Salvati EP, Rubin RJ. Levator syndrome: an analysis of 316 cases. Dis Colon Rectum 1975;18:161–3.
69. Nicosia JF, Abcarian H. Levator syndrome: a treatment that works. Dis Colon Rectum 1985;28:406–8.
70. Wald A. Functional anorectal and pelvic pain. Gastroenterol Clin North Am 2001; 30:243–51.
71. Thomson AJ, Jarvis SK, Lenart M, et al. The use of botulinum toxin type A (BOTOX) as treatment for intractable chronic pelvic pain associated with spasm of the levator ani muscles. BJOG 2005;112(2):247–9.

72. Gilliland R, Heymen J, Altomare D, et al. Biofeedback for intractable rectal pain. Dis Colon Rectum 1997;40(2):190–6.
73. Maigne JY, Chatellier G, Faou ML, et al. The treatment of chronic coccydynia with intrarectal manipulation: a randomized controlled study. Spine 2006;31:E621–7.
74. Patijn J, Janssen M, Hayek S, et al. Coccygodynia. Pain Pract 2010;10(6):554–9.
75. Tinelli A, Malvasi A, Rahimi S, et al. Age-related pelvic floor modifications and prolapse risk factors in postmenopausal women. Menopause 2010;17:204–12.
76. Soderberg MW, Falconer C, Bystrom B, et al. Young women with genital prolapse have a low collagen concentration. Acta Obstet Gynecol Scand 2004;83:1193–8.
77. Tarr ME, Gilliam ML. Sexually transmitted infections in adolescent women. Clin Obstet Gynecol 2008;51:306–18.
78. Howard FM, EL-Minawi AM, Sanchez RA. Conscious pain mapping by laparoscopy in women with chronic pelvic pain. Obstet gynecol 2000;96:934–9.
79. Rhame EE, Levey KA, Gharibo CG. Successful treatment of refractory pudendal neuralgia with pulsed radiofrequency. Pain Physician 2009;12:633–8.
80. Vallejo R, Benyamin RM, Kramer J, et al. Pulsed radiofrequency denervation for the treatment of sacroiliac joint syndrome. Pain Med 2006;7:429–34.
81. Mitra R, Zeighami A, Mackey S. Pulsed radiofrequency for the treatment of chronic ilioinguinal neuropathy. Hernia 2007;11:369–71.
82. Chen FP, Soong YK. The efficacy and complications of laparoscopic presacral neurectomy in pelvic pain. Obstet Gynecol 1997;90:974–7.
83. Tsui JK, Eisen A, Stoessl AJ, et al. Double- blind study of botulinum toxin in spasmodic torticollis. Lancet 1986;2:245–6.
84. Abbott JA, Jarvis SK, Lyons SD, et al. Botulinum toxin type A for chronic pain and pelvic floor spasm in women: a randomized controlled trial. Obstet Gynecol 2006; 108:915–23.
85. Bhide AA, Puccini F, Khullar V, et al. Botulinum neurotoxin type A injection of the pelvic floor muscle in pain due to spasticity: a review of the current literature. Int Urogynecol J 2013;24(9):1429–34.
86. Howard FM. The role of laparoscopy as a diagnostic tool in chronic pelvic pain. Baillieres Best Pract Res Clin Obstet Gynaecol 2000;14(3):467–94.
87. Peterson HB, Hulka JF, Phillips JM. American Association of Gynecologic Laparoscopists' 1988 membership survey on operative laparoscopy. J Reprod Med 1990;35(6):587–9.
88. Hulka JF, Peterson HB, Phillips JM, et al. Operative laparoscopy. American Association of Gynecologic Laparoscopists 1991 membership survey. J Reprod Med 1993;38(8):569–71.
89. Peters AA, van Dorst E, Jellis B, et al. A randomized clinical trial to compare two different approaches in women with chronic pelvic pain. Obstet Gynecol 1991; 77(5):740–4.
90. Swank DJ, Swank-Bordewijk SC, Hop WC, et al. Laparoscopic adhesiolysis in patients with chronic abdominal pain: a blinded randomised controlled multi-centre trial. Lancet 2003;361(9365):1247–51.
91. Dunker MS, Bemelman WA, Vijn A, et al. Long-term outcomes and quality of life after laparoscopic adhesiolysis for chronic abdominal pain. J Am Assoc Gynecol Laparosc 2004;11(1):36–41.
92. Carlson KJ, Nichols DH, Schiff I. Indications for hysterectomy. N Engl J Med 1993;328(12):856–60.
93. Hillis SD, Marchbanks PA, Peterson HB. The effectiveness of hysterectomy for chronic pelvic pain. Obstet Gynecol 1995;86(6):941–5.

Surgical Evaluation and Treatment of the Patient with Chronic Pelvic Pain

M. Brigid Holloran-Schwartz, MD

KEYWORDS

- Diagnostic laparoscopy and chronic pelvic pain
- Conscious laparoscopic pain mapping • Hysterectomy and chronic pain
- Presacral neurectomy • Laparoscopic uterine nerve ablation
- Adhesions and chronic pain

KEY POINTS

- Evaluation of the patient with chronic pelvic pain requires a detailed patient history, physical examination, ultrasonography, and pain diary.
- Nongynecologic sources of pelvic pain should be addressed concurrently. For example, constipation should be treated at the same time as cyclic dysmenorrhea.
- Diagnostic surgical evaluation should be offered to patients who have obvious abnormality on ultrasonography, in whom medical management has failed, or in whom the acuity of pain warrants an urgent diagnosis.
- Diagnostic laparoscopy and conscious laparoscopic pain mapping are useful in the surgical evaluation and treatment of chronic pelvic pain.
- Surgical treatments including excision of endometriosis, adhesiolysis, hysterectomy, and presacral neurectomy have been shown to provide relief to select patients. The possibility of persistent pain and new adhesion formation should be discussed with any patient considering surgery.

INTRODUCTION

Most gynecologists consider the definition of chronic pelvic pain to be pelvic pain of 6 months' duration. The subjective nature of pain makes studying pelvic pain with well-designed studies inherently difficult. Complicating matters, investigators of chronic pelvic pain often use variable definitions that include cyclic, intermittent, and noncyclic. In Practice Bulletin no. 51, the American College of Obstetricians and Gynecologists suggests one definition of chronic pelvic pain to be pain of 6 or more months' duration that localizes to the anatomic pelvis, anterior abdominal wall

This article originally appeared in Obstetrics and Gynecology Clinics, Volume 41, Issue 3, September 2014.
The author has nothing to disclose.
Saint Louis University School of Medicine, Department of Obstetrics, Gynecology and Women's Health, 6420 Clayton Road, Suite 230, St Louis, MO 63117, USA
E-mail address: holloran@slu.edu

at or below the umbilicus, the lumbosacral back, or the buttocks, and is of sufficient severity to cause functional disability or lead to medical care.[1] Approximately 15% to 20% of women aged 18 to 50 years have pelvic pain for longer than 1 year.[1] Despite this prevalence, there are many patients for whom the etiology is unclear.[2]

At the patient's initial consultation, medical and surgical options should be outlined (**Fig. 1**). Reviewing possible gynecologic, gastrointestinal, genitourinary, and musculoskeletal causes of pain will help the patient understand the importance of documenting alleviating and aggravating influences. Having the patient keep a pain diary for 3 months is helpful to further characterize the pain. Medical options, including nonsteroidal anti-inflammatory drugs, combined oral contraceptives, gonadotropin-releasing hormone agonists, and progesterone therapy may be offered as nonsurgical options, especially if there is a cyclical pattern.[3–8] If the patient suffers from predominantly gastrointestinal or genitourinary symptoms, referral should be made to these specialties to rule out other nongynecologic causes before diagnostic laparoscopy. If these patients return with persistent pain, especially after improvement in these systems, diagnostic laparoscopy may be offered. For the patient suffering from severe, disabling pain or the patient who declines or does not respond to medical therapy, a diagnostic laparoscopy may be offered. This article focuses on surgical interventions that may be offered for chronic pelvic pain, excluding endometriosis (addressed separately in the article by Yeung elsewhere in this issue).

DIAGNOSTIC SURGICAL PROCEDURES
Diagnostic Laparoscopy

The etiology of chronic pelvic pain is not always obvious after thorough history, physical examination, and imaging. Diagnostic laparoscopy can be offered in the absence of abnormality on physical examination or imaging, and has been increasingly used as

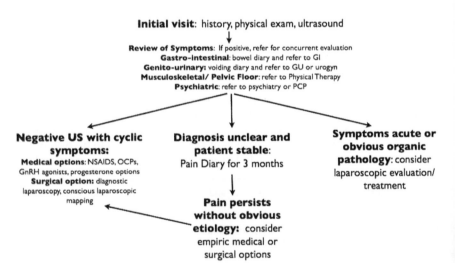

Fig. 1. Pathways of chronic pelvic pain management. GI, gastrointestinal; GnRH, gonadotropin-releasing hormone; GU, genitourinary; NSAIDs, nonsteroidal anti-inflammatory drugs; OCPs, oral contraceptive pills; PCP, primary care physician.

a diagnostic tool, accounting for upward of 40% of laparoscopic procedures.[2] Despite its frequent use, there are no clear guidelines as to when this should be offered.

Diagnostic laparoscopy may be helpful in the evaluation of visceral sources of pain such as endometriosis, adhesions, ovarian masses, pelvic inflammatory disease, and malignancy.[9] Counseling patients about the risks, benefits, and expectations before surgery is important. Pelvic ultrasonography should be done preoperatively to allow discussion of obvious possible abnormality such as ovarian cysts. The patient should be consented for possible peritoneal biopsies and adhesiolysis. The goal of a laparoscopy is ideally to establish a diagnosis and provide surgical treatment in a single step. As the risk of adhesions increases with the total number of abdominal and pelvic surgeries, every surgery needs to be considered carefully.[2]

A thorough diagnostic laparoscopy usually involves at least a camera port and an accessory port to manipulate organs and assist with exposure. Additional ports may be needed if peritoneal biopsies or adhesiolysis is needed. Peritoneal biopsies of abnormal peritoneum are ideal for establishing a diagnosis, especially if endometriosis is suspected.[2] The patient should be counseled preoperatively on the possibility of not being able to identify any abnormality.

Conscious Laparoscopic Pain Mapping

Conscious laparoscopic pain mapping has been advocated by some as a useful tool in the evaluation of chronic pain.[10] The reasoning is that there is often poor correlation of the patient's symptoms and the findings at laparoscopy, even in the presence of obvious abnormality such as adhesive disease and endometriosis.[11,12] Nociceptive signals may originate from more than 1 organ, and adding the patient's own feedback can provide useful information to direct treatment options.

The procedure involves establishing laparoscopic access and then waking the patient sufficiently to allow her to comprehend questioning and provide feedback. This approach usually involves using short-acting anesthetic agents such as fentanyl and midazolam. A blunt probe is used to establish a "control area"; the surgeon may than proceed with palpating sites where the pain is suspected, such as the ovary or appendix. Care is taken to minimize other discomforts related to the surgical procedure itself, so lidocaine is used liberally at the site of the uterine manipulator and skin incisions, while lidocaine jelly is used with Foley catheter placement.[13] Possible outcomes of pain mapping should be discussed preoperatively with patients, including a possible plan of action (ie, appendectomy if there is pain in the appendix). If additional, more extensive surgery is needed, general anesthesia can be introduced and the procedure completed during the same operative event.[13]

Limitations are seen in those of higher body mass index who may require significant Trendelenburg and increased torque with instrument manipulation at port sites. Patients with anxiety, agoraphobia, claustrophobia, or a low pain tolerance may not able to tolerate the procedure.[10,14]

Patient responses have been described by Palter[13,15] and Palter and Olive,[16] who categorized these into 3 groups:

1. Focal pain elicited is greater in one area than in adjacent areas
2. Pain is stimulated not at all or at universally low levels of the pelvis
3. High levels of pain are generated throughout most of the pelvic structures probed

Well-designed studies are inherently difficult to design, as the patients and surgeons cannot be blinded and patient selection makes randomization difficult. Small case series have found successful pain mapping in 70% to 100% of patients.[9,16] The lack of more recent studies suggests a limitation on this being used as a global tool for general gynecologists.[10] At present, there remain no substantial data to confirm the accuracy or improved clinical outcomes with laparoscopic pain mapping.[1]

FINDINGS POTENTIALLY AMENABLE TO SURGICAL TREATMENT

Previous published studies of laparoscopic findings for the patient with chronic pelvic pain suggest that endometriosis is diagnosed in 33%, adhesive disease in 24%, and no visible abnormality in 35%.[2] This finding may differ in various parts of the world, as demonstrated by a recent publication from of Hyderabad, where pelvic tuberculosis was the most common disorder followed by endometriosis, pelvic inflammatory disease, and adhesions.[17] At the time of laparoscopy, careful attention and biopsy of all abnormally appearing peritoneum is helpful to confirm a histologic diagnosis, particularly given all the different appearances endometriosis can have.[9] In a well-designed study, Walter and colleagues[18] demonstrated the importance of biopsy confirmation of abnormality. In his study, the visual appearance of endometriosis, when compared with histologic diagnosis, had a positive predictive value of 45%, negative predictive value of 99%, sensitivity of 97%, and specificity of 77%. These values varied by location of anatomic site. Histologic confirmation is critical, especially if the patient's pain persists or recurs at a later time after surgery. Included in this review is a discussion of possible causes of pelvic pain that may be diagnosed or treated with laparoscopy, with the exclusion of endometriosis, which again is addressed by Yeung's article elsewhere in this issue.

Laparoscopy and Pelvic Adhesions

The incidence of pelvic adhesive disease is unknown, and its role in the patient with chronic pelvic pain is controversial. Pelvic adhesions can generally result from any peritoneal irritation or inflammation, such as previous pelvic surgery, endometriosis, appendicitis, or pelvic inflammatory disease. One of these is present in the history of approximately 50% of women with pelvic adhesions, with the remaining 50% having no such previous history.[19] Stovall and colleagues[19] found the incidence of pelvic adhesions to be between 27% and 60% in women undergoing laparoscopy for pelvic pain. Nerve fibers have been identified in the adhesions of patients with and without chronic pain.[20] However, most women with pelvic adhesions are asymptomatic.[9] Furthermore, the extent or location of pelvic adhesions does not always correlate with the location or severity of the pain.[2]

It is hypothesized that adhesions may be a source of pain when they cause distortion of the normal anatomic relationships and/or when activities cause stretching of the peritoneum or organ serosa at the adhesion's attachment site.[20] It may be a band, of variable density and vascularity, or a cohesive connection of surfaces without an intervening band. Bowel adhesions are a proposed cause of chronic pelvic pain, and a known cause of partial and complete small bowel obstruction, that tend to have more acute presentations. Physical examination and preoperative imaging are not always useful predictors of the presence or location of pelvic adhesions. Diagnostic laparoscopy is the procedure of choice for diagnosing pelvic adhesive disease. The goal of adhesiolysis is to restore normal anatomy, but it must be recognized that new adhesions may form after any surgical procedure (**Figs. 2** and **3**).

Meticulous surgical technique is critical, including minimizing tissue trauma, achieving optimal hemostasis, and minimizing the risk of infection. Unfortunately, despite these efforts new adhesions can be generated with each surgical procedure.[21,22] Surgeons may consider using adhesion-prevention adjuncts, although there is no ideal agent. Several anti-inflammatory drugs such as dexamethasone have been

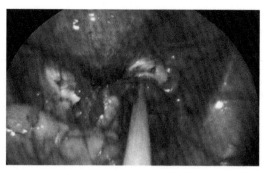

Fig. 2. An obliterated cul-de-sac in a patient with chronic pelvic pain and dense ovarian and bowel adhesions.

studied but have not proved to be effective.[23] In addition, there is insufficient evidence that peritoneal instillates such as normal saline or Ringer lactate, with or without heparin, prevent adhesions.[23] **Table 1** lists the advantages and disadvantages of the most effective adhesion-prevention barriers: Gore-Tex (Gore & Associates, Inc), Seprafilm (Genzyme), and Interceed (Ethicon Endo-Surgery).[21] One should avoid using oxidized regenerated cellulose (Interceed; Ethicon Endo-Surgery) in a patient for whom absolute hemostasis has not been achieved, as this may increase the risk of adhesions.[21]

The studies investigating laparoscopic adhesiolysis as a treatment for chronic pain are difficult to interpret collectively. Vrijland and colleagues[24] reviewed several observational studies with improvement ranging from 38% to 84%, but were limited by variable postoperative follow-up and pain-assessment tools. A randomized study assessing laparotomy alone versus laparotomy with adhesiolysis noted relief only for patients in whom dense bowel adhesions were noted.[25] Swank and colleagues[12] conducted a randomized controlled trial of diagnostic laparoscopy versus laparoscopic adhesiolysis in 100 participants (men and women) and found no difference in outcomes of pain or quality of life. At 1-year follow-up, 27% from each group continued to experience improved pain relief.

Laparoscopy and Ovarian Pathology

Ovarian cysts are thought to be an infrequent cause of chronic pelvic pain, accounting for only 3% of cases.[2] Most ovarian cysts are functional and asymptomatic, but can be a source of acute pain in the event of hemorrhage or torsion. If a functional ovarian cyst is suspected on ultrasonography in a stable patient, it generally can be followed with

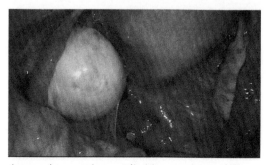

Fig. 3. Dense adhesions and an ovarian cyst limiting ovarian mobility.

Table 1
Advantages and disadvantages of adhesion prevention barriers

Adhesion Barrier	Advantages	Disadvantages
Polytetrafluoroethylene (Gore-Tex; W.L. Gore & Associates, Inc, Flagstaff, AZ)	Most effective adhesion barrier	Permanent material that needs to be sutured for security and later removed at subsequent surgery
Modified sodium hyaluronate/ carboxymethylcellulose (Seprafilm; Genzyme Corp, Boston, MA)	Effective at preventing adhesion formation in open surgery (myomectomies)	Lacking long-term studies. Not well studied laparoscopically
Oxidized regenerated cellulose (Interceed; Ethicon Endo-Surgery, Inc, Blue Ash, OH)	Effective at reducing pelvic adhesions during laparoscopy and laparotomy	May increase adhesion formation in the presence of blood

Data from Robertson D, Lefebvre G, Leyland N, et al. Adhesion prevention in gynaecological surgery. J Obstet Gynaecol Can 2010;32(6):598–608.

sonography and resolution documented after 1 to 2 cycles.[2] If recurrent, functional cyst formation is suspected as the source of intermittent cyclic pain, ovarian suppression with medical therapy, such as oral contraceptives, is usually successful.[2] The exception to this is ovarian endometriomas, which are most effectively treated with surgical cystectomy. Cystectomy is preferred over ovarian cyst drainage or cauterization of cyst lining, showing an improved reduction in pain and cyst recurrence (**Fig. 4**).[26]

Ovarian remnant syndrome is defined as the presence of ovarian tissue in a woman with a history of bilateral salpingo-oophorectomy that usually is the result of unintentional incomplete excision in the setting of severe adhesions, endometriosis, chronic pelvic inflammatory disease, or malignancy.[27] A premenopausal follicle-stimulating hormone value in a woman with a history of a bilateral salpingo-oophorectomy may help identify these patients. Various studies quote ovarian remnant syndrome as the

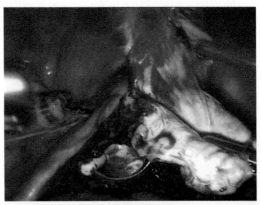

Fig. 4. Removal of ovarian cyst capsule using traction and countertraction, ligating small vessels.

cause of chronic pelvic pain in 18% to 26% of patients.[28,29] One study reported that in patients with chronic pelvic pain, a history of a bilateral salpingo-oophorectomy, and adnexal mass, ovarian remnant syndrome was identified in 76.5% of patients.[30] Management involves surgical excision through laparoscopy or laparotomy.[29,30]

Laparoscopy and Hernias

Hernias are found in only 1.6% to 6% of women with chronic pelvic pain.[31–33] Inguinal and femoral hernias may present with lateralizing chronic pelvic pain that may worsen with an upright position.[9] Sciatic hernias may radiate to the buttocks and posterior thigh.[34] A sciatic hernia is defined as a peritoneal sac with variable contents (fallopian tube or ovary) that protrudes through the greater or lesser sciatic foramen.[2] Inguinal, femoral, and sciatic hernias can be identified and repaired at laparoscopy.

Previous studies have described laparoscopic inguinal exploration and mesh placement in patients with chronic pelvic pain without a clinical hernia, hypothesizing that incarcerated fat in the inguinal canal may be a source of chronic pain.[35,36] Yong and colleagues[37] recently conducted a retrospective cohort study of empiric laparoscopic inguinal exploration and mesh placement in women with lateralizing chronic pelvic pain. Of 48 patients, 7 had an occult hernia they classified as a patent processus vaginalis, shown in **Fig. 5**.

Regardless of this finding, all 48 patients had inguinal exploration and mesh placement. Thirty-five percent had pain improvement regardless of the presence of an occult hernia. An additional 42% had initial improvement and later recurrence of pain (range of follow-up 73.2 ± 30.6 months). Patients with a positive Carnett test in the ipsilateral lower abdomen correlated with an improvement in pain. A positive Carnett test is defined as worsening in tenderness with abdominal wall flexion or contraction.[37] Additional studies are needed before this can be widely accepted as a treatment modality.

Laparoscopy and Pelvic Congestion Syndrome

Pelvic congestion syndrome is described as the presence of pelvic varices with subsequent venous stasis and congestion of the pelvic organs that results in chronic pelvic pain.[38] Laparoscopy has limited potential for the diagnosis of pelvic congestion syndrome, as the Trendelenburg position often results in the collapse of varicosities. Pelvic varicosities may be suspected if dilated veins (>8–10 mm in diameter) are seen in the reverse Trendelenburg position, but this has been shown to have a low sensitivity for diagnosis.[2,38] Venography, performed either transuterine or percutaneously, remains the gold standard for diagnosis of pelvic vascular congestion.[2,38]

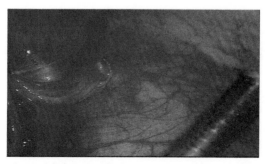

Fig. 5. A shallow peritoneal defect classified as a patent processus vaginalis or occult hernia.

Medical, surgical, and radiologic treatment options have been proposed for pelvic congestion syndrome. One randomized controlled trial by Soysal and colleagues[39] demonstrated improvement in symptoms with suppression of ovarian function with medroxyprogesterone acetate and goserelin. Hysterectomy, with and without bilateral salpingo-oophorectomy, has been shown to be effective in women in whom medical therapy has failed, but given the limited number of studies it should be used as a last resort.[40]

Radiographic embolotherapy has been shown to be as effective as hysterectomy in treating the symptoms of pelvic congestion syndrome.[41] Embolotherapy has the advantage of leaving no obvious scar, and can be performed on an outpatient basis. Several studies have documented the long-term effectiveness of this approach. Kim and colleagues[42] demonstrated efficacy in patients followed for 45 months. In addition, in a more recent study Laborda and colleagues[43] showed improvement in visual analog scores up to 5 years.

Laparoscopy and Endosalpingiosis

Endosalpingiosis is the presence of fallopian tube glandular epithelium in an ectopic location. It often resembles and is mistaken for endometriosis. Again this emphasizes the importance of excisional biopsies of abnormal peritoneum for tissue diagnosis in the management of the patient with chronic pain. The evidence supporting endosalpingiosis as a cause of chronic pelvic pain is primarily observational, based on a limited number of patients.[2] A recent study by Prentice and colleagues[44] found no significant relationship between endosalpingiosis, chronic pelvic pain, and infertility (**Fig. 6**).

PROCEDURES OFFERED FOR THE TREATMENT OF CHRONIC PELVIC PAIN
Hysterectomy

The role of hysterectomy in the treatment of idiopathic chronic pelvic pain is controversial. Approximately 12% of the 600,000 hysterectomies in the United States are done for reasons of chronic pelvic pain.[45] Before hysterectomy is considered, a multidisciplinary evaluation of any possible gastrointestinal, genitourinary, musculoskeletal, and/or psychiatric causes is necessary. When counseling patients considering hysterectomy for chronic pelvic pain, they should be informed that up to 40% of women will continue to have pain and 5% may have worsening symptoms.[46]

Lamvu[46] recently published a review on the role of hysterectomy in the treatment of chronic pelvic pain. She quoted a study by Stovall and colleagues[47] wherein patients who had failed other medical and surgical options underwent hysterectomy with a

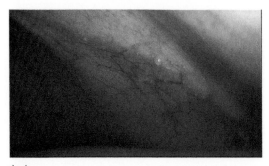

Fig. 6. Endosalpingiosis.

78% improvement rate. Of note, from this same study, 22% had persistence of pain even in the presence of histologic evidence of uterine disease.[47] Hillis and colleagues[48] found that in specific subsets of women, up to 40%, will continue to have pain. Specifically, women at increased risk for persistence were found to be younger than 30 years, uninsured, covered by Medicaid, had a history of pelvic inflammatory disease, and no identifiable abnormality at surgery. Lamvu[46] noted that these studies did not examine variables such as preexisting depression, anxiety, and history of abuse, which have been proved to be important in the modulation of long-term pain outcomes.

Hartmann and colleagues[49] looked at quality of life and sexual function after hysterectomy in patients with preoperative pain and depression over a 24-month period. Approximately 80% of patients were found to have improvement in pain, even in the presence of preexisting chronic pain, depression, or both after hysterectomy. Approximately 60% of patients reported improvement in pain with intercourse, although the frequency of intercourse remained unchanged.[49]

A 2006 retrospective cohort of 124 patients looked at patients with persistent chronic pain after hysterectomy and bilateral salpingo-oophorectomy. The most common histopathologic findings were adhesions (93%), adnexal remnants (32%), and endometriosis (18%).[28] Lamvu[46] concluded that all patients should have a thorough multidisciplinary evaluation before surgery to exclude other nonreproductive causes of pain before recommending hysterectomy with or without bilateral salpingo-oophorectomy. In addition, they should be counseled about the possible persistence of pain.

Laparoscopic Uterine Nerve Ablation

Laparoscopic uterine nerve ablation (LUNA) involves transection of the uterosacral ligaments at their insertion into the uterus with the purpose of interrupting the cervical sensory nerve fibers. It has been hypothesized that dividing these trunks may help women with dysmenorrhea.[50] A 2009 randomized controlled trial of 487 patients with chronic pelvic pain followed for 69 months, who had undergone laparoscopy with and without LUNA, found no difference in pain, dysmenorrhea, dyspareunia, or quality of life between the 2 arms.[50] Furthermore, a 2010 meta-analysis of randomized trials further analyzed available data and found no difference in improvement in pain between those who did or did not undergo LUNA.[51] At present, there is insufficient evidence to recommend LUNA (**Fig. 7**).

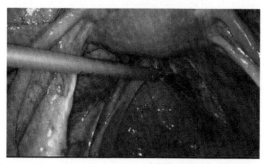

Fig. 7. The technique of laparoscopic uterine nerve ablation is performed by transecting both uterosacral ligaments at their attachment to the cervix. This photo shows transection of the right uterosacral ligament.

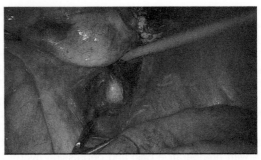

Fig. 8. Exposure of the presacral space for presacral neurectomy. The sacral promontory is noted at the tip of the laparoscopic grasper.

Presacral Neurectomy

Presacral neurectomy targets the superior hypogastric plexus (presacral nerves) that supply the cervix, uterus, and proximal fallopian tubes with afferent nociception. Surgical resection of this plexus has been shown to decrease dysmenorrhea unresponsive to other treatments.[1] It is significantly more effective than LUNA for the treatment of primary dysmenorrhea.[52] It is notable that central midline pelvic pain is much more responsive to presacral neurectomy than lateral pelvic pain, regardless of pathologic features.[1]

A recent 2012 retrospective analysis collected over 6 years demonstrated improvement in midline pain in 73% (22 of 30) of patients.[53]

Clinical trials in the early 1990s supported presacral neurectomy as an adjunct to conservative surgery for endometriosis, demonstrating additional midline pain relief associated with menses but not dyspareunia or nonmenstrual pain.[54,55] A more recent randomized controlled trial of 141 patients followed over 24 months demonstrated improvement in dysmenorrhea, dyspareunia, and quality of life in patients with endometriosis who underwent a concurrent presacral neurectomy at the time of conservative laparoscopic surgery over those who did not (**Fig. 8**).[56]

SUMMARY

It is important to characterize pelvic pain with a detailed patient history, physical examination, imaging, and a pain diary. Other possible nongynecologic causes must be addressed concurrently for optimal patient outcomes. Medical and surgical options should be outlined. Surgical therapy can be useful in patients with visceral sources of pain such as endometriosis, adhesions, ovarian disorder, hernias, pelvic inflammatory disease, and malignancy. In carefully selected patients, pelvic pain can be relieved with adhesiolysis, excision of endometriosis, hernia repair, hysterectomy, and presacral neurectomy. Before surgery the possibility of a negative laparoscopy, persistent postoperative pain, and new adhesion formation should be discussed.

REFERENCES

1. ACOG Practice Bulletin. Clinical management guidelines for obstetrician-gynecologists. No. 51, March 2004.
2. Howard FM. The role of laparoscopy in the chronic pelvic pain patient. Clin Obstet Gynecol 2003;46:749–66.

3. Owen PR. Prostaglandin synthetase inhibitions in the treatment of primary dysmenorrhea: outcome trials reviewed. Am J Obstet Gynecol 1984;148: 96–103.
4. Marjoribanks J, Proctor ML, Farquhar C. Nonsteroidal antiinflammatory drugs for primary dysmenorrhea [cochrane review]. In: Mary McLennan, Andrew Steele, Fah Che Leong, editors. The Cochrane library, Issue 4. Chichester (United Kingdom): John Wiley & Son, Ltd; 2003.
5. Proctor ML, Roberts H, Farquhar C. Combined oral contraceptive pill (OCP) as treatment for primary dysmenorrhea [cochrane review]. In: Mary McLennan, Andrew Steele, Fah Che Leong, editors. The Cochrane library, Issue 4. Chichester (United Kingdom): John Wiley & Son, Ltd; 2003.
6. Vercellini P, Aimi G, Panazza S, et al. A levonorgestrel-releasing intrauterine system for the treatment of dysmenorrhea associated with endometriosis. Fertil Steril 1999;72:505–8.
7. Telimaa S, Ronnberg L, Kauppila A. Placebo-controlled comparison of danazol and high-dose medroxyprogesterone acetate in the treatment of endometriosis after conservative surgery. Gynecol Endocrinol 1987;1:363–71.
8. Farquhar CM, Rogers V, Franks S, et al. A randomized controlled trial of medroxyprogesterone acetate and psychotherapy for the treatment of pelvic congestion. Br J Obstet Gynaecol 1989;96:1153–62.
9. Lamvu G, Tu F, As-Sanie S, et al. The role of laparoscopy in the diagnosis and treatment of conditions associated with chronic pelvic pain. Obstet Gynecol Clin North Am 2004;31:619–30.
10. Yunker A, Steege J. Practical guide to laparoscopic pain mapping. J Minim Invasive Gynecol 2010;17:8–11.
11. Fukaya T, Hoshiai H, Yajima A. Is pelvic endometriosis always associated with chronic pain? A retrospective study of 618 cases diagnosed by laparoscopy. Am J Obstet Gynecol 1993;169:719–22.
12. Swank DJ, Swank-Bordewijk SC, Hop WC, et al. Laparoscopic adhesiolysis in patients with chronic abdominal pain: a blinded randomized controlled multi-center trial. Lancet 2003;361:1247–51.
13. Palter S. Microlaparoscopy under local anesthesia and conscious pain mapping for the diagnosis and management of pelvic pain. Curr Opin Obstet Gynecol 1999;11:387–93.
14. Swanton A, Iyer L, Reginald PW. Diagnosis, treatment and follow up of women undergoing conscious pain mapping for chronic pelvic pain: a prospective cohort study. BJOG 2006;113:792–6.
15. Palter S. Office-based surgery and its role in the management of pelvic pain. In: Blackwell R, Olive D, editors. Chronic pelvic pain. New York: Springer; 1998. p. 167–82.
16. Palter S, Olive D. Office microlaparoscopy under local anesthesia for chronic pelvic pain. J Am Assoc Gynecol Laparosc 1996;3:359–64.
17. Baloch S, Khaskheli M, Malik A. Diagnostic laparoscopic findings in chronic pelvic pain. J Coll Physicians Surg Pak 2013;23(3):190–3.
18. Walter AJ, Hentz JG, Magtiboy PM, et al. Endometriosis: correlation between histologic and visual findings at laparoscopy. Am J Obstet Gynecol 2001;184: 1407–11.
19. Stovall TG, Elder RF, Ling FW. Predictors of pelvic adhesions. J Reprod Med 1989;34:345–8.
20. Hammoud A, Gago A, Diamond M. Adhesions in patients with chronic pelvic pain: a role for adhesiolysis. Fertil Steril 2004;82:1483–91.

21. Robertson D, Lefebvre G, Leyland N, et al. Adhesion prevention in gynaecological surgery. J Obstet Gynaecol Can 2010;32(6):598–608.
22. Neis KJ, Neis F. Chronic pelvic pain: cause, diagnosis and therapy from a gynaecologist's and an endoscopist's point of view. Gynecol Endocrinol 2009;25(11): 757–61.
23. Pfeifer S, Lobo R, Goldberg J, et al, Practice Committee of American Society for Reproductive Medicine in collaboration with Society of Reproductive Surgeons. Pathogenesis, consequences and control of peritoneal adhesions in gynecologic surgery: a committee opinion. Fertil Steril 2013;99(6):1550–5.
24. Vrijland WW, Jeekel J, Geldor HJ, et al. Abdominal adhesions: intestinal obstruction, pain, and infertility. Surg Endosc 2003;17(7):1017–22.
25. Peters AA, Trimbos-Kemper GC, Admiraal C, et al. A randomized clinical trial on the benefits of adhesiolysis in patients with intaperitoneal adhesions and chronic pelvic pain. BJOG 1992;99:59–62.
26. Yoshida S, Harada T, Iwabe T, et al. Laparoscopic surgery for the management of ovarian endometrioma. Gynecol Obstet Invest 2002;54(Suppl 1): 24–7.
27. Shemwell RW, Weed JC. Ovarian remnant syndrome. Obstet Gynecol 1970;36: 299–300.
28. Behera M, Vilos G, Hollett-Caines J, et al. Laparoscopic findings, histopathologic evaluation, and clinical outcomes in women with chronic pelvic pain after hysterectomy and bilateral salpingo-oophorectomy. J Minim Invasive Gynecol 2006;13: 431–5.
29. Abu-Rafeh B, Vilos GA, Misra M. Frequency and laparoscopic management of ovarian remnant syndrome. J Am Assoc Gynecol Laparosc 2003;10:33–7.
30. Senapati S, Advincula AP. Adnexal remnant syndrome: a new paradigm. J Am Assoc Gynecol Laparosc 2005;12:S7.
31. Banerjee S, Farrell RJ, Lembo T. Gastroenterological causes of pelvic pain. World J Urol 2001;19:166–72.
32. Carter JE. Combined hysteroscopic and laparoscopic findings in patients with chronic pelvic pain. J Am Assoc Gynecol Laparosc 1994;2:43–7.
33. Demco LA. Effect on negative laparoscopy rate in chronic pelvic pain patients using patient assisted laparoscopy. JSLS 1997;1:319–21.
34. Miklos JR, O'Reilly MJ, Saye WB. Sciatic hernia as a cause of chronic pelvic pain in women. Obstet Gynecol 1998;91:998–1001.
35. Metzger DA. Hernias in women: uncommon or unrecognized? Laparoscopy Today 2004;3(1):8–10.
36. Janicki TI, Onders R, Blood BJ, et al. Occult inguinal hernias in women with chronic pelvic pain. J Am Assoc Gynecol Laparosc 2001;8(Suppl 3):S28.
37. Yong P, Williams C, Allaire C. Laparoscopic inguinal exploration and mesh placement for chronic pelvic pain. JSLS 2013;17:74–81.
38. Liddle AD, Davies AH. Pelvic congestion syndrome: chronic pelvic pain caused by ovarian and internal iliac varices. Phlebology 2007;22(3):100–4.
39. Soysal ME, Soysal S, Vicdan K, et al. A randomised controlled trial of goserelin and medroxyprogesterone acetate in the treatment of pelvic congestion. Humanit Rep 2001;16:931–9.
40. Beard RW, Kennedy RG, Gangar KF, et al. Bilateral oophorectomy and hysterectomy in the treatment of intractable pelvic pain associated with pelvic congestion. Br J Obstet Gynaecol 1991;98:988–92.
41. Chung MH, Huh CY. Comparison of treatments for pelvic congestion syndrome. Tohoku J Exp Med 2003;201:131–8.

42. Kim HS, Malhotra AD, Rowe PC, et al. Embolotherapy for pelvic congestion syndrome: long-term results. J Vasc Interv Radiol 2006;17(2 Pt 1):289–97.
43. Laborda A, Medrano J, de Blas I, et al. Endovascular treatment of pelvic vascular congestion syndrome: visual analog score (VAS) long term follow up clinical evaluation in 202 patients. Cardiovasc Intervent Radiol 2013;36(4):1006–14. http://dx.doi.org/10.1007/s00270-013-0586-2.
44. Prentice L, Stewart A, Mohiuddin S, et al. What is endosalpingiosis? Fertil Steril 2012;98(4):942–7.
45. We JM, Wechter ME, Geller EJ, et al. Hysterectomy rates in the United States, 2003. Obstet Gynecol 2007;110:1091–5.
46. Lamvu G. Role of hysterectomy in the treatment of chronic pelvic pain. Obstet Gynecol 2011;117:1175–8.
47. Stovall TG, Ling FW, Crawford DA. Hysterectomy for chronic pelvic pain of presumed uterine etiology. Obstet Gynecol 2004;104:701–9.
48. Hillis SD, Marchbanks PA, Peterson HB. The effectiveness of hysterectomy for chronic pelvic pain. Obstet Gynecol 1995;86:941–5.
49. Hartmann KE, Ma C, Lamvu GM, et al. Quality of life and sexual function after hysterectomy in women with preoperative pain and depression. Obstet Gynecol 2004;104:701–9.
50. Daniels J, Gray R, Hills RK, et al. Laparoscopic uterine nerve ablation for alleviating chronic pelvic pain: a randomized controlled trial. JAMA 2009;302(9): 955–61.
51. Daniels JP, Middleton L, Xiong T, et al. Individual patient data meta-analysis of randomized evidence to assess the effectiveness of laparoscopic uterine nerve ablation in patients with chronic pelvic pain. Hum Reprod Update 2010;16(6): 568–76.
52. Chen FP, Chang SD, Chu KK, et al. Comparison of laparoscopic presacral neurectomy and laparoscopic uterine nerve ablation for primary dysmenorrhea. J Reprod Med 1996;41:463–6.
53. Kapetanakis V, Jacob K, Klauschie J, et al. Robotic presacral neurectomy - technique and results. Int J Med Robot 2012;8:73–6.
54. Canadiani GB, Fedele L, Vercillini P, et al. Presacral neurectomy for the treatment of pelvic pain associated with endometriosis: a controlled study. Am J Obstet Gynecol 1992;167:100–3.
55. Tjaden B, Schlaff WD, Kimball A, et al. The efficacy of presacral neurectomy for the relief of midline dysmenorrhea. Obstet Gynecol 1990;76:89–91.
56. Zullo F, Palomba S, Zupi E, et al. Long-term effectiveness of presacral neurectomy for the treatment of severe dysmenorrhea due to endometriosis. J Am Assoc Gynecol Laparosc 2004;11:23–8.

Complementary and Alternative Medications for Chronic Pelvic Pain

Fah Che Leong, MS, MD

KEYWORDS

- Complementary medicine • Alternative medicine • Chronic pelvic pain
- Interstitial cystitis • Endometriosis

KEY POINTS

- The use of complementary and alternative medicine is common and can account for as much as 11.2% of out-of-pocket expenditures for medical care.
- Patients seek information from peers as well as physicians with regard to alternative medical treatments.
- Rigorous controlled studies of the use of alternative medicine for pelvic pain are lacking.
- Some complementary medicine adjuncts such as dietary supplementation show some promise, but more studies are necessary.

INTRODUCTION

Chronic pelvic pain is a common condition that has significant clinical as well as economic impact. Medical and surgical management may be inadequate in either improving or eliminating the patient's pain, and many patients as well as practitioners have considered the use of complementary and alternative treatments. The causes for chronic pelvic pain can be structural or functional, and frequently can be both. There can be significant difficulty in finding the causes affecting the individual, and, when sufficiently frustrated, patients and physicians turn to alternatives. In 2007, 38.1 million adults made 354 million visits to alternative medicine practitioners and spent $34 billion for all medical conditions.[1] According to the US National Center for Complementary and Alternative Medicine (NCCAM) of the National Institutes of Health, complementary medicine costs are about 11.2% of the total out-of-pocket expenditures on health care. Chronic pelvic pain can affect 14.7% of women between the ages of 18 and 50 years, with an estimated direct cost of $881.5 million.[2] In an earlier study,

This article originally appeared in Obstetrics and Gynecology Clinics, Volume 41, Issue 3, September 2014.
Obstetrics Gynecology and Women's Health, Saint Louis University, 6420 Clayton Road, St Louis, MO 63117, USA
E-mail address: leongfc@slu.edu

Clinics Collections 4 (2014) 381–388
http://dx.doi.org/10.1016/j.ccol.2014.10.024
2352-7986/14/$ – see front matter © 2014 Elsevier Inc. All rights reserved.

12% of all hysterectomies and up to 40% of all laparoscopies were performed for chronic pelvic pain in women.[3] Although the focus of this article is pelvic pain in women, it can be difficult to differentiate pelvic pain from pain in other areas in the low back and low abdomen. Other common conditions include low back pain, arthritic pain, neuropathic pain, and conditions such as fibromyalgia, irritable bowel disease, chronic fatigue syndrome, vulvodynia, and rectal pain. Any patient may have more than one coexisting chronic pain condition. It is as difficult for the practitioner to tease out the nuances of the patient's complaints as it is for the patient to avoid self-diagnosis. At the time of writing, there were more than 5 million hits on a Google search for chronic pelvic pain, more than 4 million for treatment of chronic pelvic pain, and 1.4 million for alternative treatments for chronic pelvic pain. There were 234,000 hits from a search for a forum to discuss pelvic pain with other patients (https://www.google.com/#q=forum+pelvic+pain).

Complementary and alternative medicine (CAM) options that are most commonly sought are dietary supplements and herbs, acupuncture, mind/body medicine, and mind/body manipulative methods.

MANAGEMENT GOALS

The difficulty in treating patients with chronic pelvic pain is exacerbated by differences in expectations. Patients expect a cure, and cures are rare. Patients seek care with new providers out of frustration because of a lack of improvement or perceived degree of improvement. It is important to set realistic expectations for the treatment. Even with accurate diagnosis and effective treatment, cure (to the degree of never having the pain again) is rare.[4] Specific goals must be discussed, and this may be difficult if treatment involves more than one discipline. It is important for the treatment team to communicate with each other and with the patient. It is also important for the team to concentrate on the complementary portion of CAM instead of the alternative portion.

HERBAL AND DIETARY STRATEGIES
Dietary Changes

Up to 90% of patients with interstitial cystitis report sensitivities to foods and drink. Common irritants include coffee, tea, citrus, tomatoes, alcohol, and vitamin C. Patients can benefit from finding their own sensitivities and the use of a symptom diary is helpful. Patients are asked to diary their symptoms, menstrual cycle if indicated, emotional state, foods, and drinks over a month. They can also be provided with a list of possible dietary irritants, and be instructed on an elimination diet in which they ingest none of the possible irritants, adding them in stepwise to see the effect of the addition.[5] Although it is logical to presume that dietary changes affect urinary pain, they have also been studied in other areas of pelvic pain. Improvement of pain was reported by 75% of patients who were placed on a gluten-free diet and followed for 12 months.[6] In patients with endometriosis, the use of the antioxidant vitamins E and C improved the pain in 43% of patients, with a concomitant finding of a decrease in peritoneal fluid inflammatory markers.[7]

Phytotherapy (Herbal Medicine)

NCCAM began funding clinical trials in herbal medicine in 2002. Herbal medicine is widely used all over the world, and, in 2007, of the 40% of adults who used CAM, 17.7% used so-called natural products or herbal medications.[8]

Of the $34 billion spent on CAM, $14.8 billion was spent on natural products.[1]

Calcium Glycerophosphate

Seventy-five percent of patients surveyed rated the use of calcium glycerophosphate (Prelief; AKPharma) as helpful in patients with interstitial cystitis.[9] In an earlier study, patients were instructed to use it before meals for 4 weeks. A decrease in severity was noted in more than 40% of the respondents when used with pizza, coffee, acidic fruit, spicy foods, and tomato-based foods, and up to 30% with carbonated drinks, alcohol, and chocolate.[10]

CystoProtek (Meda Consumer Healthcare)

This is an oral supplement containing glucosamine, chondroitin, hyaluronate, quercetin, olive kernel extract, and rutin. In an uncontrolled study, 252 patients who had failed other treatments were studied for up to 12 months. The women experienced a 49% improvement, measured via a visual analog scale.[11]

Intravesical Instillations Not Approved by the US Food and Drug Administration

Many physicians already use combinations of varying contents including heparin, steroid, sodium bicarbonate, and local anesthetic as rescue instillations. There are several products available in Europe that are used for this purpose (dimethyl sulfoxide is the only product approved by the US Food and Drug Administration for this indication in the United States). Hyaluronic acid, available as an instillation agent with the brand name Cystistat (Mylan Pharma), when used in a small number of patients, showed decreases in nocturia (40%) and pain (30%).[12] Other studies have found similar results but used small numbers of patients.[13,14] However, in forum postings, patients have been advised by their peers to obtain these medications from Canada. Other such commercially branded instillations available in foreign markets include Gepan (Pohl-Boskamp; chondroitin sulfate 0.2%), Uracyst (Tribute Pharmaceuticals; chondroitin sulfate 2%), iAluril (Institut Biochemique SA; hyaluronic acid 1.6% and chondroitin sulfate 2%), Hyacyst (Syner-Med; hyaluronic acid solution), and Cystilieve (Medicines By Design Ltd; lidocaine and sodium bicarbonate).

Quercetin

Quercetin is a bioflavonoid found in red wine, green tea, and onions. It reduces inflammation via the inhibition of the production of cytokines interleukin (IL)-6, IL-8, and tumor necrosis factor. Many of the studies using quercetin are of men with pelvic pain attributed to chronic prostatitis.[15] A form of quercetin is available as Cysta-Q (Farr Labs) and has been used for interstitial cystitis. In an open-label study, 22 patients were given 1 capsule twice a day for 4 weeks. In these patients, pain and symptom indices improved.[16]

Marshmallow Root

Although there are no rigorous studies on the use of marshmallow root for pelvic pain, advice on its use is commonly found in Internet forums. It is thought to reduce pain and inflammation, and has been used for more than 2000 years.

Dextroamphetamine Sulfate

All the literature for the use of amphetamines for pelvic pain and interstitial cystitis come from the laboratory of Dr Jerome Check. All 9 citations listed are case reports but the premise that defects in the sympathetic nervous system contributes to pelvic pain is intriguing.[17–19] Complex regional pain syndrome has been thought to be sympathetically mediated,[20] and similarly patients with chronic pelvic pain without discernible anatomic problems are often thought to have neuropathic pain. However, controlled studies are lacking.

Pollen Extract

Pollen extract has been used for chronic pelvic pain for more than 40 years, but most of the literature has been in men. It is available as a dietary supplement under a variety of trade names, such as Cernilton, Prostat/Poltit, and Pollstimol. The main components, cernitin T60 and cernitin GBX have shown spasmolytic and antiinflammatory properties in animal and in-vitro studies. In a recent small study, 90% of the participants reported less pain and increased quality of life.[21] In a controlled study, 73% of the treatment arm showed improvement, compared with 36% in the control arm.[22]

Cannabinoids

Cannabinoid CB-1 receptors are found in the mouse urinary bladder and, as they are activated, bladder activity is modulated.[23] In a study in which bladder biopsies were taken from patients with painful bladder syndrome (PBS) and idiopathic detrusor overactivity (IDO), there was a significant increase of CB-1-immunoreactive suburothelial nerve fibers in PBS and IDO. Patients with chronic pain who were already on narcotics and were given vaporized cannabis showed an average of 27% decrease in pain without any increase in narcotic use.[24]

NONPHARMACOLOGIC STRATEGIES
Acupuncture

Acupuncture is among the oldest healing practices in the world. Thin needles are used to stimulate specific points in the body. The traditional Chinese medicine theory states that this regulates the flow of qi or vital energy that flows along meridians in the body. The most common use for acupuncture is for pain, with back pain being the most common indication. There is difficulty in creating studies with controls for acupuncture, and there may be a significant placebo effect in patients. In a study of men with chronic pelvic pain, acupuncture was controlled using sham acupuncture (needles placed 1 cm away from the acupuncture point). Seventy-three percent of the patients having acupuncture showed improvement, compared with 47% with sham acupuncture.[25] In an analysis of studies of acupuncture for endometriosis, only 1 of 24 studies met the investigators' criteria for a controlled study with adequate diagnostic studies and outcome measures. Auricular acupuncture reduced dysmenorrhea in 92% of patients.[26] Perhaps just as important is the patients' attitude toward the treatment. In a 2007 study, participants who expected acupuncture to relieve pain experienced significantly more pain relief.[27]

Hypnosis

Hypnosis has been used in a variety of pain conditions but studies for specific conditions are few. It has been studied for cancer pain, headaches, low back pain, fibromyalgia, sickle cell disease, and even temporomandibular joint syndrome. Some of the difficulty with extrapolating the results is lack of standardization for hypnosis, small studies, and variables including instructions for self-hypnosis. Many studies use imagery and relaxation techniques. There are some promising data, but better studies are needed.[28] In a study of men with chronic pelvic pain, 16 men were taught self-hypnosis. After 1 month, 47% reported moderate to marked improvement of symptoms, and, after 6 months, 36% continued to have that improvement. However, the investigators stated that the selected participants had moderate to high hypnotic ability, as identified with the Tellegen Absorption Scale, so those with low hypnotic ability were excluded.[29] The sessions were highly individualized so it is difficult to generalize the study to other populations.

Hyperbaric Oxygen

The premise for using hyperbaric oxygen therapy is that interstitial cystitis is perhaps caused by a relative ischemia leading to lower bladder vascular perfusion and pain. With this in mind, the investigators embarked on a pilot study of 6 patients. The treatment was well tolerated, and 4 of 6 patients rated themselves as improved.[30] The investigators then did a sham-controlled, double-blinded study with 21 total patients with only 3 of the 14 patients in the treatment arm improving.[31] An uncontrolled study from Japan showed improvement in 7 of 11 patients who were refractory to other treatments.[32]

Extracorporeal Shock Wave Lithotripsy

Extracorporeal shock wave lithotripsy (ESWL) was found incidentally to improve chronic pelvic pain in men during treatment of urolithiasis. The mechanism is unknown. In a randomized sham-controlled study, 60 patients were divided and treated once weekly for a month, and followed for 12 weeks after treatment was started. ESWL was administered to the perineum without anesthesia. All the patients in the treated arm showed a significant improvement in pain, quality of life, and voiding. There were no side effects noted.[33] In another randomized sham-controlled study with 40 patients, improvement in quality of life and chronic prostatitis symptom index scores were noted.[34] Whether these results are applicable to women is unknown.

Meditation

The most common mind-body therapy is meditation. Most patients use mind-body therapy in combination with traditional medicine and often in consultation with their physician (80% of patients had discussed this with their physician).[35] The philosophy of meditation has its roots in Buddhism. The 2 most common forms of meditation used in clinical relaxation are transcendental meditation (TM) and mindfulness. TM involves concentrating on a mantra (a repetition of a sound, word, or phrase), and mindfulness involves being aware of one's thoughts and letting go of those without emotional attachments.[36] A cross-sectional study of 13 highly trained Zen meditators showed that they had low sensitive to pain, and experienced analgesic effects during Zen meditation.[37] In a pilot study of women with chronic pelvic pain, the women who completed the study had significant improvement in pain scores, physical function, and mental health. However, only 12 of 22 enrolled subjects completed the study.

SUMMARY

Part of the allure of CAM is that many of them do not require prescription by a physician. Another part is the patient's dissatisfaction with current treatment. Even in the best of circumstances, patients with chronic pelvic pain are not cured, but are in good control. Some of what they choose are recommendations by peers, some from their physicians, and some from overpromises in advertisements. In a survey of the use of complementary medicine for interstitial cystitis, one of the most frequent recommenders (55%) were physicians or their office staff.[9] However, this study includes recommendations for dietary changes (avoidance of dietary irritants) and physical therapy, which are more mainstream and also found in American Urological Association guidelines. Research is limited, and studies with good results often are case studies or small uncontrolled series. In a survey of patients by the Interstitial Cystitis Association, the only alternative treatment rated helpful by a significant number of patients was calcium glycerophosphate (Prelief).[9] The therapies discussed are adjuncts and complementary rather than the primary treatments used by patients. Some of the current publications suggest that they may be helpful, but carefully controlled studies are needed.

REFERENCES

1. Nahin RL, Barnes PM, Stussman BJ, et al. Costs of complementary and alternative medicine (CAM) and frequency of visits to CAM practitioners. Hyattsville (MD): US Department of Health and Human Services, Centers for Disease Control and Prevention, National Center for Health Statistics, 2008. National health statistics reports. 2009; p. 1–14.
2. Mathias SD, Kuppermann M, Liberman RF, et al. Chronic pelvic pain: prevalence, health-related quality of life, and economic correlates. Obstet Gynecol 1996;87: 321–7.
3. Reiter RC. A profile of women with chronic pelvic pain. Clin Obstet Gynecol 1990; 33:130–6.
4. Abercrombie PD, Learman LA. Providing holistic care for women with chronic pelvic pain. J Obstet Gynecol Neonatal Nurs 2012;12:1–23.
5. Friedlander JI, Shorter B, Moldwin RM. Diet and its role in interstitial cystitis/bladder pain syndrome (IC/BPS) and comorbid conditions. BJU Int 2012;109:1584–91.
6. Marziali M, Venza M, Lazzaro S, et al. Gluten-free diet: a new strategy for management of painful endometriosis related symptoms? Minerva Chir 2012;67: 499–504.
7. Santanam N, Kavtaradze N, Murphy A, et al. Antioxidant supplementation reduces endometriosis-related pelvic pain in humans. Transl Res 2013;161:189–95.
8. Barnes PM, Bloom B, Nahin RL. Complementary and alternative medicine use among adults and children. Hyattsville (MD): US Department of Health and Human Services, Centers for Disease Control and Prevention, National Center for Health Statistics, 2008. National health statistics reports. 2008; p. 1–23.
9. O'Hare PG 3rd, Hoffmann AR, Allen P, et al. Interstitial cystitis patients' use and rating of complementary and alternative medicine therapies. Int Urogynecol J 2013;24:977–82.
10. Bologna RA, Gomelsky A, Lukban JC, et al. The efficacy of calcium glycerophosphate in the prevention of food-related flares in interstitial cystitis. Urology 2001; 57:119–20.
11. Theoharides TC, Kempuraj D, Vakali S, et al. Treatment of refractory interstitial cystitis/painful bladder syndrome with CystoProtek–an oral multi-agent natural supplement. Can J Urol 2008;15:4410–4.
12. Kallestrup EB, Jorgensen SS, Nordling J, et al. Treatment of interstitial cystitis with Cystistat: a hyaluronic acid product. Scand J Urol Nephrol 2005;39:143–7.
13. Figueiredo AB, Palma P, Riccetto C, et al. Clinical and urodynamic experience with intravesical hyaluronic acid in painful bladder syndrome associated with interstitial cystitis. Actas Urol Esp 2011;35:184–7 [in Spanish].
14. Van Agt S, Gobet F, Sibert L, et al. Treatment of interstitial cystitis by intravesical instillation of hyaluronic acid: a prospective study on 31 patients. Prog Urol 2011; 21:218–25 [in French].
15. Shoskes DA, Nickel JC. Quercetin for chronic prostatitis/chronic pelvic pain syndrome. Urol Clin North Am 2011;38:279–84.
16. Katske F, Shoskes DA, Sender M, et al. Treatment of interstitial cystitis with a quercetin supplement. Tech Urol 2001;7:44–6.

17. Check JH, Cohen G, Cohen R, et al. Sympathomimetic amines effectively control pain for interstitial cystitis that had not responded to other therapies. Clin Exp Obstet Gynecol 2013;40:227–8.
18. Check JH, Cohen R. Chronic pelvic pain–traditional and novel therapies: part II medical therapy. Clin Exp Obstet Gynecol 2011;38:113–8.
19. Check JH, Wilson C, Cohen R. Sympathetic nervous system disorder of women that leads to pelvic pain and symptoms of interstitial cystitis may be the cause of severe backache and be very responsive to medical therapy rather than surgery despite the presence of herniated discs. Clin Exp Obstet Gynecol 2011;38:175–6.
20. Mazzola TJ, Poddar SK, Hill JC. Complex regional pain syndrome I in the upper extremity. Curr Sports Med Rep 2004;3:261–6.
21. Cai T, Luciani LG, Caola I, et al. Effects of pollen extract in association with vitamins (DEPROX 500®) for pain relief in patients affected by chronic prostatitis/chronic pelvic pain syndrome: results from a pilot study. Urologia 2013; 80(Suppl 22):5–10.
22. Elist J. Effects of pollen extract preparation Prostat/Poltit on lower urinary tract symptoms in patients with chronic nonbacterial prostatitis/chronic pelvic pain syndrome: a randomized, double-blind, placebo-controlled study. Urology 2006;67:60–3.
23. Walczak JS, Price TJ, Cervero F. Cannabinoid CB1 receptors are expressed in the mouse urinary bladder and their activation modulates afferent bladder activity. Neuroscience 2009;159:1154–63.
24. Abrams DI, Couey P, Shade SB, et al. Cannabinoid-opioid interaction in chronic pain. Clin Pharmacol Ther 2011;90:844–51.
25. Lee SH, Lee BC. Use of acupuncture as a treatment method for chronic prostatitis/chronic pelvic pain syndromes. Curr Urol Rep 2011;12:288–96.
26. Zhu X, Hamilton KD, McNicol ED. Acupuncture for pain in endometriosis. Cochrane Database Syst Rev 2011;(9):CD007864.
27. Linde K, Witt CM, Streng A, et al. The impact of patient expectations on outcomes in four randomized controlled trials of acupuncture in patients with chronic pain. Pain 2007;128:264–71.
28. Elkins G, Jensen MP, Patterson DR. Hypnotherapy for the management of chronic pain. Int J Clin Exp Hypn 2007;55:275–87.
29. Anderson RU, Nagy TF, Orenberg E. Feasibility trial of medical hypnosis and cognitive therapy for men with refractory chronic prostatitis/chronic pelvic pain syndrome. UroToday Int J 2011;4:2–12.
30. van Ophoven A, Rossbach G, Oberpenning F, et al. Hyperbaric oxygen for the treatment of interstitial cystitis: long-term results of a prospective pilot study. Eur Urol 2004;46:108–13.
31. van Ophoven A, Rossbach G, Pajonk F, et al. Safety and efficacy of hyperbaric oxygen therapy for the treatment of interstitial cystitis: a randomized, sham controlled, double-blind trial. J Urol 2006;176:1442–6.
32. Tanaka T, Nitta Y, Morimoto K, et al. Hyperbaric oxygen therapy for painful bladder syndrome/interstitial cystitis resistant to conventional treatments: long-term results of a case series in Japan. BMC Urol 2011;11:11.
33. Zimmermann R, Cumpanas A, Miclea F, et al. Extracorporeal shock wave therapy for the treatment of chronic pelvic pain syndrome in males: a randomised, double-blind, placebo-controlled study. Eur Urol 2009;56:418–24.
34. Vahdatpour B, Alizadeh F, Moayednia A, et al. Efficacy of extracorporeal shock wave therapy for the treatment of chronic pelvic pain syndrome: a randomized, controlled trial. ISRN Urol 2013;2013:972601.

35. Wolsko PM, Eisenberg DM, Davis RB, et al. Use of mind-body medical therapies. J Gen Intern Med 2004;19:43–50.
36. Teixeira ME. Meditation as an intervention for chronic pain: an integrative review. Holist Nurs Pract 2008;22:225–34.
37. Grant JA, Rainville P. Pain sensitivity and analgesic effects of mindful states in Zen meditators: a cross-sectional study. Psychosom Med 2009;71:106–14.

Opioid Use and Depression in Chronic Pelvic Pain

Andrew Steele, MD

KEYWORDS

- Chronic pelvic pain • Addiction • Opioid • Narcotic • Depression

KEY POINTS

- Opioid prescribing is a national epidemic, associated with high rates of diversion of prescription therapeutics.
- Opioid therapy should rarely be initiated for patients with chronic pelvic pain, even in the setting of a referring practice or emergency department.
- Screening tools can help predict and detect opioid addiction and diversion.
- Women on chronic opioid therapy for chronic noncancer pain should be weaned off their medication before attempted conception.
- Women with chronic pain should be screened for depression and treatment or referral provided when positive.

INTRODUCTION

Prescription medication abuse has become a national epidemic. In 2011, more than 238 million narcotic analgesic prescriptions were written, with more attributable deaths than heroin and cocaine combined.[1] According to data from the 2010 National Survey on Drug Use and Health,[2] the nonmedical misuse of prescription psychotherapeutics, including opioids, was the second leading type of illicit drug abuse, behind marijuana. Further data from the Survey found that almost one-third of people aged 12 and over who initiated illicit drug use for the first time began by using a prescription drug nonmedically. In addition, review articles on the use of opioids for chronic pain have found limited data supporting their long-term use in a variety of pain conditions.[3]

Women's health care providers are confronted with several chronic pain syndromes ranging from irritable bowel syndrome, interstitial cystitis and endometriosis, to musculoskeletal pain, vestibulitis, and pelvalgia. Often patients present to the consultant already having received long-term narcotic prescriptions, initiated from other providers. Volkow and McLellan[4] found that the main prescribers of opioids are primary care

This article originally appeared in Obstetrics and Gynecology Clinics, Volume 41, Issue 3, September 2014.
The author has nothing to disclose.
Obstetrics, Gynecology and Women's Health, Surgery, Saint Louis University, 6420 Clayton Road, St Louis, MO 63117, USA
E-mail address: steeleac@slu.edu

providers, followed by dentists and orthopedic surgeons, with the main prescribers for patients aged 10 to 19 being dentists. Emergency room visits also led to significant opioid prescribing. In one large insurance database, it was found that more than 400,000 narcotic prescriptions were written in 2009 through emergency departments for plan enrollees aged 18 to 64. More startling was that 10% of these patients who received narcotic prescriptions did so despite identifiable risk factors for opioid misuse.[5]

Primary care providers have reported unease at chronic opioid prescribing, while simultaneously noting the difficulty of referral to pain management centers.[6] In the author's practice, the patient's access to medication management by trained pain specialists is often limited by insurance considerations as well as the procedural focus (ie, injection therapy) of many pain management physicians.

THE PAIN EXPERIENCE

The experience of pain varies from patient to patient and is a factor of the patient's underlying coping skills, mental health, support, and potential secondary gain.[7] Furthermore, chronic pain and the medications used to treat pain lead to other complications, such as sleeplessness, job performance issues, and relationship issues (**Fig. 1**).

The perception of pain carries 2 components best summed in the legal term, "pain and suffering." The pain component, or sensory-discriminative component, is quantifiable and amenable to therapy. Suffering, or the affective-motivational component, is more difficult to quantify and treat with therapies targeted at the disease process.[7] Thus, one aspect of the physician-patient educational component is that therapy may, "fix your pain but not your suffering." It is important that alternative options for pain control are discussed with the patient. Physicians should be aware of resources in his or her community. Establishing collegial relationships with local counselors, acupuncturists, and pain management specialists allows the obstetrician/gynecologist (OB/GYN) to develop a multidisciplinary approach to the patient with chronic pelvic pain (CPP).

NARCOTIC ACTIONS

Nociceptive (pain) signals are transmitted to the superficial dorsal horn of the brain via sodium-dependent depolarization predominantly via A-δ and C fibers.[8] Opioids have

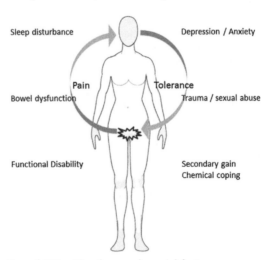

Fig. 1. The interaction of CPP with other psychosocial factors.

their primary effect on mu receptors. These receptors are located in the cortex, thalamus, and periaqueductal gray matter as well as the spinal cord. Two types of mu receptors have been proposed. Mu1 receptors have a high affinity for morphine and its derivatives and are dominant receptors in supraspinal analgesia as well as the development of physical tolerance. Mu2 receptors have a lower affinity to morphine and are implicated in narcotic side effects, such as respiratory depression and constipation.[9] Mu receptors are also involved in the reward response associated with opioid use via increasing dopaminergic release. Medications with the most rapid onset of action tend to cause the most euphoria, and that euphoric reward is the first effect lost with developing tolerance. Thus, patients need increasing doses to achieve the same euphoric reward response. Side effects of opioid medications are generally dose-dependent and include constipation, meiosis, sedation, and respiratory depression.[10]

TOLERANCE, DEPENDENCE, AND ADDICTION

Tolerance, physical dependence, and addiction are not synonymous terms, although all 3 may lead to aberrant medication-taking behaviors (AMTB). Over time, patients on chronic narcotics may develop tolerance to the medication requiring escalating dosages. Patients demonstrating AMTBs because of inadequate analgesia have what is termed pseudo-addiction. Physical dependence represents physiologic adaptation with signs and symptoms of withdrawal if the opioid is abruptly stopped and is an effect of tolerance. Both tolerance and dependence may be anticipated with chronic narcotic use. Addiction manifests with AMTBs representing impaired control over opioid use and a preoccupation with obtaining opioids. In cases of addiction, patients will also continue opioid use despite evidence of harm from the medications, such as, declining function in relationships or work, intoxication, or persistent oversedation.[11] Medication diversion is another concern with narcotic prescribing. Approximately 76% of opioids used for nonmedical purposes were originally prescribed to someone else.[12]

DETECTING "AT-RISK" PATIENTS

Screening tools exist to help determine those patients at higher risk for opioid misuse. A prior history of personal or family history of substance abuse is major risk factor for opioid misuse. Smoking is a significant risk factor for opioid misuse, because up to 95% of patients treated for another substance abuse disorder also smoke.[13] Questionnaires provide a means of assessing for potential opioid misuse. The SOAPP (Screener and Opioid Assessment for Patients with Pain) is a 24-question validated survey in which patients answer questions in domains, such as lifestyle, physician-patient relationship, antisocial behaviors, medication-use behaviors, psychiatric disorders, and psychosocial difficulties.[14,15] An abbreviated, 14-question version has also been reported.[13] Another potentially useful questionnaire is the Opioid Risk Tool (ORT). Both elevated as well as low scores on the ORT have been associated with a high and low likelihood of demonstrating later AMTBs, respectively.[16] Although questionnaires are safe and easy to administer, a recent review has shown variable utility in the identification of at-risk patients, with studies showing a mixed picture with overall weak associations between positive screens and future medication misuse.[17]

AMTB

Aberrant drug-related behaviors can be markers of prescription medication abuse or diversion (**Fig. 2**). These behaviors may include patients receiving narcotics from

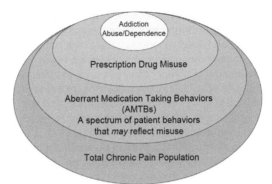

Fig. 2. The spectrum of opioid tolerance and abuse disorders. (*From* Alford D. Chronic pain and opioid risk management. Chief Resident Immersion Training (CRIT) Program in Addiction Medicine, Boston University. 2010. Available at: http://www.bumc.bu.edu/care/files/2010/09/11.-ALFORD-Chronic-Pain-and-Opioid-Risk-Management.pdf. Accessed February 15, 2014; with permission.)

multiple providers simultaneously; requesting specific, short-acting medications; or relating allergies to nonnarcotic pain medications. These behaviors often serve as "yellow flags" or "red flags" to the clinician.[18] It is important to remember that all patients with AMTBs are not addicted to opioids, nor even misusing them. Rather, there is a spectrum of use in which concern needs to be raised when AMBTs are demonstrated (**Box 1**).

Studies have found significant gender differences in AMBTs. Simoni-Wastila and colleagues[19,20] have noted that women have significantly higher rates of nonmedical use of prescription opioids compared with men, noting that women are 48% more likely than men to use any abusable prescription drug, when controlled for demographics, health and economic status, and diagnosis.[20] Women are also more likely to supplement their nonmedical use with other prescription drugs, such as anxiolytics or sedatives.[21,22]

However, aberrant and drug-seeking behaviors have another, more subtle effect. The patient who calls frequently for refills, or calls after hours or on weekends, also places tremendous strain on a doctor's office personnel, staff, or colleagues. This

---

Box 1
Aberrant drug-seeking behaviors

Warning signs of addiction

  Multiple lost or stolen prescriptions

  Failure to comply with monitoring (random drug screens)

  Current use of alcohol or illicit drugs

  Multiple prescriptions from different physicians or pharmacies

  Forging, selling, or stealing prescriptions

Possible misuse, logistically burdensome

  Calls after hours/weekends for refills

  Requesting narcotic adjustment or changes by phone

  Narcotic hoarding/overutilization

practice, in turn, harms the physician-patient relationship and may ultimately lead to severing of care in a patient who legitimately needs assistance. Strategies to minimize AMTBs and limit adverse narcotic events will benefit both the patient and the provider.

OPIOID MANAGEMENT STRATEGIES

There is scant evidence supporting the role of opioid therapy in chronic pain, and risks to the patient from narcotics are not insignificant.[23] As such, providers should be hesitant to initiate any narcotic therapy for CPP, even in the initial evaluation phase while tests are pending. In patients presenting with CPP, simple screening questions may help identify patients at risk for opioid misuse.

Several strategies exist to help minimize AMBTs and decrease the likelihood of abuse or redirection (**Boxes 2** and **3**). Patient contracts are widely used for patients seeking long-term opioid prescriptions. Often, patients will require a separate visit to undergo screening and to review and initiate the contract; remember that the opioid need itself can represent a disease state that needs the same attention as the gynecologic condition. Contracts spell out policies and expectations but must be used in conjunction with a clear overall strategy for narcotic use. Simply listing the AMBTs that will cause the patient to be disengaged from the practice is inadequate. Instead, expectations for periodic reassessment of the efficacy of the pain management, practice policies regarding refills, and exit strategies for discontinuing these medications should be spelled out at initiation of the therapy. Some suggestions are listed in **Box 2**.

PERIODIC REASSESSMENT

Periodic reassessment in the office is a valuable method for ensuring adequate analgesia and limiting abuse. Several tools are available for clinical use.

Pill Counts

Pill counts aid in assessing overuse, underuse as well as diversion. Pill counts may be especially useful for the patient who calls before the scheduled renewal complaining of intolerance or ineffectiveness of a current medication and requesting a prescription change. In general, these patients are asked to schedule a visit to discuss the need for medication adjustment, to assess for new conditions that would lead to a deterioration in their pain control, and to undergo pill counting of the unused medication. In patients being managed on fentanyl patches, the used patches should be returned because a small amount of fentanyl could be still be extracted.

Box 2
PEG physician-administered pain score

1. What number best describes your pain on average in the past week? (0 No pain to 10 pain as bad as you can imagine)

2. What number best describes how, during the past week, pain has interfered with your enjoyment of life? (0 Does not interfere to 10 completely interferes)

3. What number best describes how, during the past week, pain has interfered with your general activity? (0 Does not interfere to 10 completely interferes)

Adapted from Krebs EE, Lorenz KA, Bair MJ, et al. Development and initial validation of the PEG, a three-item scale assessing pain intensity and interference. J Gen Intern Med 2009;24(6):733–8.

Box 3
Strategies to prevent abuse and redirection of prescribed opioids

Strategies to prevent abuse and redirection

   Patient contracts

   Single provider and pharmacy for all opioid prescriptions

   Urine drug testing

   Regular validated questionnaires

   Pill counts

Strategies to prevent abuse and minimize practice impact

   Concurrent use of complementary and alternative therapies

      Acupuncture

      NSAIDs

      Stress management

      Counseling

   Regularly scheduled follow-up visits specifically addressing pain management

   Communication of office practice expectations

      No after-hours refill requests

      No medication dose/frequency adjustment by phone

      No phone replacement of lost/stolen prescriptions

Urine Drug Testing

Urine drug testing may be accomplished in an office-based practice.[24] Urine drug testing may sometimes detect unrecognized abuse or misuse even in "model" patients. Katz and Fanciullo[25] reported findings that 21% of chronic pain patients had positive urine drug screens despite demonstrating no ABMTs. A negative urine drug screen in a patient on chronic opioid therapy may represent unintentional underutilization, diversion, or disingenuous specimen substitution. Although commonly recommended in discussions of opioid prescribing, the practice raises many questions. Medical urine drug testing is not a forensic process. At the same time, the practitioner must use judgment in evaluating results. For instance, will the specimen collection be supervised? Will temperature or creatinine be checked to discourage substitution? What are the limitations, such as cross-reactivity, of the specific urine drug test and laboratory you will be using?[26]

Patient Questionnaires

As with other decisions in medicine, the ongoing benefits of chronic opioid therapy should be weighed against the risks of its use. The "4 A's" of the therapy should be periodically assessed and include evaluating *Analgesia*, *Activities* of daily living, *Adverse* events, and *Aberrant* drug-taking behaviors.[27] One way to assess the ongoing utility of the therapy, as well as the development of tolerance or addiction, is with questionnaires. These questionnaires can be either patient-administered or physician-administered. The Current Opioid Misuse Measure is a patient self-administered, validated questionnaire. The 17-point list has a negative sensitivity of 77% but a specificity of only 66%, suggesting that not all screen positives will be misusing medications.[28] Another physician-administered questionnaire is the PEG (pain, enjoyment, general activity) Scale.[29] Patients rate the following on a 0 to 10 scale with 10 being most severe or disruptive (see **Box 2**).

It should be noted that these questionnaires differ from previously mentioned screening strategies for detecting possible abuse; instead, they represent methods of assessing the effectiveness and negative impact of the ongoing opioid treatment.

EXIT STRATEGIES

Exit strategies should be addressed early in the relationship as part of the informed consent process. The patient should be made aware of the possibility that medication therapy will be discontinued or modulated if the risks of medication use to the patient outweigh the benefits. This discussion should be kept separate from threats to disengage the patient from care. Even when exiting from opioid prescribing, the OB/GYN should focus on ongoing treatments for the disease process or processes.[18] Referral should be considered for more specialized care at tertiary referral centers as well as for addiction evaluation and treatment if needed.

OPIOIDS AND PREGNANCY

One special population confronting the obstetrician is the pregnant patient presenting on chronic opioid therapy. Although some concern existed in animal studies, until recently standard texts in the field reported no definite association between the development of congenital anomalies in women with the use of morphine derivatives, including codeine, oxycodone, or hydromorphone.[30] More recent large studies, however, have called the safety of opioids in pregnancy into question. Broussard and colleagues,[31] using the Birth Defects Prevention Database, found statistically significant increases in the following anomalies in mothers using opioids in the peri-conceptual period (1-month preconception) and first trimester. These anomalies included conoventricular septal defects (odds ratio [OR], 2.7; 95% confidence interval [CI], 1.1–6.3), atrioventricular septal defects (OR, 2.0; 95% CI, 1.2–3.6), hypoplastic left heart syndrome (OR, 2.4; 95% CI, 1.4–4.1), spina bifida (OR, 2.0; 95% CI, 1.3–3.2), and gastroschisis (OR, 1.8; 95% CI, 1.1–2.9).[31] The Swedish Medical Register presented data on more than 7000 infants born to mothers who reported the use of opioids during early pregnancy. In that study, the only anomaly reaching statistical significance was pes equinovarus in women taking tramadol.[32] Studies using databases on the effects of opioid medications during pregnancy are often confounded by polysubstance use in subjects, as well as the retrospective nature of the data collection. Nonetheless, women requiring chronic opioid therapy should be encouraged to wean off their medication before attempted conception. In those women who present already on chronic narcotic therapy, referral to maternal fetal medicine and pain management specialists may be indicated.

ABUSE, DEPRESSION, AND CHRONIC PAIN

The relationship between women suffering from CPP and prior traumatic events has been well established.[33–35] Up to 50% of women with CPP in a referral population had a history of prior sexual or physical abuse. In that series, Meltzer-Brody and colleagues[36] found that 1 in 3 women also demonstrated evidence of posttraumatic stress disorder. The association between domestic physical and sexual abuse in dysfunctional households may make the contribution of either component difficult to determine[33,37,38]; however, women with CPP have been clearly found to have a higher incidence of early (under age 15) sexual abuse as well as severe childhood sexual abuse.[33,39]

Depression is much more common in women with CPP. Walker and colleagues[35] found that women with CPP had a higher incidence of several psychiatric conditions, including major depression, substance abuse, adult sexual dysfunction, and somatization.[35] This higher incidence of psychiatric conditions was the case despite similar degrees of intra-abdominal pathologic abnormality. The underlying associations between chronic pain and depression are complex. The 2 conditions may coexist because underlying adverse life experiences predispose women to both conditions. Depression may occur because the underlying pain condition leads to vegetative changes in function manifesting as depression. Finally, the strong association may exist because women with depression have a greater sensitization to noxious stimuli and diminished neuroendocrine coping mechanisms. In most cases, it may be difficult to tell which condition predisposed a given patient to the other.[40] Research has suggested that the loss of norepinephrine and serotonin in the periaqueductal gray matter can occur with ongoing painful stimuli. This area of the brain is thought to be responsible for the modulation of pain, so that loss of modulatory function here leads to an increase in attention to and emotional association with pain.[41] Thus, from the standpoint of neuropathology, there may not be a distinction that can be made between cause and consequence.

Women presenting with CPP should be specifically questioned about a past history of sexual abuse or trauma, especially in childhood. Screening for posttraumatic stress disorder should also be undertaken.[36] Several simple screening tools exist for the clinician's use. The main key is that this is done early in the therapeutic relationship. Waiting to delve into these issues until the patient has undergone a series of negative tests may send a message to the patient that the psychosocial issues are secondary or untreatable. Screening questions may be introduced by discussing the holistic understanding of the patient to include medical, spiritual, and mental facets.

There is limited evidence to support the use of antidepressants in women specifically for CPP.[42] In women with CPP and associated depression, treatment of their depression may be initiated during the evaluation of their pain. Tricyclic antidepressants, such as amitriptyline or nortriptyline, and serotonin-norepinephrine reuptake inhibitors, such as duloxetine, are commonly used antidepressants in patients with other chronic, non-pelvic pain syndromes.[43] When initiating antidepressants, the clinician should "start low and go slow."[43] Care should be taken to evaluate for suicidal ideation. A review of potential medication interactions should be completed based on the specific medication prescribed. Clinicians unfamiliar with treating depression should consider referral. In addition, nonmedical therapy, including psychologic evaluation and counseling, should be offered.

SUMMARY

OB/GYN physicians frequently deal with chronic pain patients. Whenever possible, initiating narcotics in patients with CPP should be avoided, even when the physician is covering a patient with chronic pain in the emergency department. When patients present already on narcotics, the patient may have already been formally or informally disengaged from the referring practice, leaving the OB/GYN in the unenviable position of needing to deal with the condition as well as the opioid requirements that other physicians have established. When the OB/GYN becomes the primary prescriber, establishing boundaries and goals is important. In those cases, screening for addiction risks and completing a pain contract should be considered, along with developing a plan for periodic reassessments.

REFERENCES

1. Manchikanti L, Helm S 2nd, Fellows B, et al. Opioid epidemic in the United States. Pain Physician 2012;15(Suppl 3):ES9–38.
2. Substance Abuse and Mental Health Services Administration. Results from the 2010 National Survey on Drug Use and Health: Summary of National Findings. NSDUH Series H-41, HHS Publication No. (SMA) 11-4658. Rockville (MD): Substance Abuse and Mental Health Services Administration; 2011. Available at: www.samhsa.gov/data/NSDUH/2k10NSDUH/2k10Results.pdf.
3. Von Korff M, Kolodny A, Deyo RA, et al. Long-term opioid therapy reconsidered. Ann Intern Med 2011;155(5):325–8.
4. Volkow ND, McLellan TA. Curtailing diversion and abuse of opioid analgesics without jeopardizing pain treatment. JAMA 2011;305(13):1346–7.
5. Logan J, Liu Y, Paulozzi L, et al. Opioid prescribing in emergency departments: the prevalence of potentially inappropriate prescribing and misuse. Med Care 2013;51(8):646–53.
6. Barry DT, Irwin KS, Jones ES, et al. Opioids, chronic pain, and addiction in primary care. J Pain 2010;11(12):1442–50.
7. Savage SR, Kirsh KL, Passik SD. Challenges in using opioids to treat pain in persons with substance use disorders. Addict Sci Clin Pract 2008;4(2):4–25.
8. Giordano J. The neurobiology of nociceptive and anti-nociceptive systems. Pain Physician 2005;8(3):277–90.
9. Koneru A, Satyanarayana S, Rizwan S. Endogenous opioids: their physiological role and receptors. Global Journal Pharmacology 2009;3(3):149–53.
10. Yaksh T, Wallace MS. Opioids, analgesia, and pain management. In: Brunton LL, Chabner BA, Knollmann BC, editors. Goodman & Gilman's the pharmacological basis of therapeutics. 12th edition. New York: McGraw-Hill Medical. Available at: http://accessmedicine.mhmedical.com/content.aspx?bookid=374&Sectionid=41266224. Accessed May 30, 2014.
11. Miller SC, Frankowski D. Prescription opioid use disorder: a complex clinical challenge. Current Psychiatry 2012;11(8):15–22. Available at: http://www.currentpsychiatry.com/index.php?id=22661&tx_ttnews(tt_news)=176994.
12. U.S. Department of Health and Human Services. Substance Abuse and Mental Health Services Administration. Office of Applied Studies. Results from the 2009 national survey on drug use and health: volume I. Available at: http://www.samhsa.gov/data/NSDUH/2k9NSDUH/2k9Results.htm. Accessed June 20, 2012.
13. Akbik H, Butler SF, Budman SH, et al. Validation and clinical application of the Screener and Opioid Assessment for Patients with Pain (SOAPP). J Pain Symptom Manage 2006;32(3):287–93.
14. Butler SF, Fernandez K, Benoit C, et al. Validation of the Revised Screener and Opioid Assessment for Patients with Pain (SOAPP-R). J Pain 2008;9(4):360–72.
15. Butler SF, Budman SH, Fernandez K, et al. Screener and opioid assessment measure for patients with chronic pain. Pain 2004;112(1–2):65–75.
16. Webster LR, Webster RM. Predicting aberrant behaviors in opioid treated patients: preliminary validation of the Opioid Risk Tool. Pain Med 2005;6(6):432–42.
17. Chou R, Fanciullo GJ, Fine PG, et al. Opioids for chronic noncancer pain: prediction and identification of aberrant drug-related behaviors: a review of the evidence for an American Pain Society and American Academy of Pain Medicine clinical practice guideline. Pain 2009;10(2):131–46.
18. Alford D. Chronic pain and opioid risk management. Chief Resident Immersion Training (CRIT) Program in Addiction Medicine, Boston University 2010. Available

at: http://www.bumc.bu.edu/care/files/2010/09/11.-ALFORD-Chronic-Pain-and-Opioid-Risk-Management.pdf. Accessed February 15, 2014.

19. Simoni-Wastila L, Ritter G, Strickler G. Gender and other factors associated with the nonmedical use of abusable prescription drugs. Subst Use Misuse 2004; 39(1):1–23.

20. Simoni-Wastila L. The use of abusable prescription drugs: the role of gender. J Womens Health Gend Based Med 2000;9(3):289–97.

21. Back SE, Payne RA, Waldrop AE, et al. Prescription opioid aberrant behaviors: a pilot study of gender differences. Clin J Pain 2009;25(6):477–84.

22. Tetrault JM, Desai RA, Becker WC, et al. Gender and non-medical use of prescription opioids: results from a national US survey. Addiction 2008;103(2): 258–68.

23. Manchikanti L, Abdi S, Atluri S, et al. American Society of Interventional Pain Physicians (ASIPP) Guidelines for responsible opioid prescribing in chronic non-cancer pain: Part I – Evidence assessment. Pain Physician 2012;15(Suppl 3): S1–65.

24. Christo PJ, Manchikanti L, Ruan X, et al. Urine drug testing in chronic pain. Pain Physician 2011;14(2):123–43.

25. Katz N, Fanciullo GJ. Role of urine toxicology testing in the management of chronic opioid therapy. Clin J Pain 2002;18(Suppl 4):S76–82.

26. Starrels JL, Becker WC, Alford DP, et al. Systematic review: treatment agreements and urine drug testing to reduce opioid misuse in patients with chronic pain. Ann Intern Med 2010;152(11):712–20.

27. Passik SD. Issues in long-term opioid therapy: unmet needs, risks, and solutions. Mayo Clin Proc 2009;84(7):593–601.

28. Current Opioid Misuse Measure. Available at: http://nationalpaincentre. mcmaster.ca/documents/comm_sample_watermarked.pdf. Accessed February 15, 2014.

29. Krebs EE, Lorenz KA, Bair MJ, et al. Development and initial validation of the PEG, a three-item scale assessing pain intensity and interference. J Gen Intern Med 2009;24(6):733–8.

30. Reuvers M, Schaefer C. Analgesics and anti-inflammatory drugs. In: Briggs, Freeman, Yaffe, editors. Drugs during pregnancy and lactation. 9th edition. Amsterdam: Elsevier; 2007. p. 33–7 Ebook.

31. Broussard CS, Rasmussen SA, Reefhuis J, et al. National Birth Defects Prevention Study. Maternal treatment with opioid analgesics and risk for birth defects. Am J Obstet Gynecol 2011;204(4):314.e1–11.

32. Kallen B, Borg N, Reis M. The use of central nervous system active drugs during pregnancy. Pharmaceuticals 2013;6:1221–86.

33. Lampe A, Solder E, Ennemoser A, et al. Chronic pelvic pain and previous sexual abuse. Obstet Gynecol 2000;96:929–33.

34. Golding JM, Wilsnack SC, Learman LA. Prevalence of sexual assault history among women with common gynecologic symptoms. Am J Obstet Gynecol 1998;179:1013–9.

35. Walker EA, Katon W, Harrop-Griffiths J, et al. Relationship of chronic pelvic pain to psychiatric diagnoses and childhood sexual abuse. Am J Psychiatry 1988;145: 75–80.

36. Meltzer-Brody S, Leserman J, Zolnoun D, et al. Trauma and posttraumatic stress disorder in women with chronic pelvic pain. Obstet Gynecol 2007;4(109):902–8.

37. Rapkin AJ, Kames LD, Darke LL, et al. History of physical and sexual abuse in women with chronic pelvic pain. Obstet Gynecol 1990;76(1):92–6.

38. Drossman DA, Leserman J, Nachman G, et al. Sexual and physical abuse in women with functional or organic gastrointestinal disorders. Ann Intern Med 1990;113(11):828–33.
39. Walker EA, Katon WJ, Hansom J, et al. Medical and psychiatric symptoms in women with childhood sexual abuse. Psychosom Med 1992;54(6):658–64.
40. Ghally A, Chien P. Chronic pelvic pain: clinical dilemma or clinician's nightmare. Sex Transm Infect 2000;76:419–25.
41. Bair MJ, Robinson RL, Eckert GJ, et al. Impact of pain on depression treatment response in primary care. Psychosom Med 2004;66:17–22.
42. Cheong YC, Smotra G, Williams AC. Non-surgical interventions for the management of chronic pelvic pain. Cochrane Database Syst Rev 2014;(3):CD008797.
43. Schultz E, Malone DA. A practical approach to prescribing antidepressants. Cleve Clin J Med 2013;80(10):625–31.

Pain, Perceptions, and Perceived Conflicts

Improving the Patient's Experience

Patricia Kunz Howard, PhD, RN, CEN, CPEN, NE-BC, FAEN, FAAN[a],*,
Penne Allison, RN, BSN, MSOM, NE-BC[b], Matthew Proud, BSN, RN, CEN[c],
Jennifer Forman, RN, BSN[d]

KEYWORDS

- Pain • Perceptions • Patient • Experience • Clinical outcomes • Management

KEY POINTS

- Provider attitudes about pain management may influence the patient's feelings about their care in the emergency department.
- There is support that patients' perceptions of their care, and specifically management of their pain, impacts their clinical outcomes.
- Pain education and innovative approaches to nurse-driven protocols are essential to ensure the most optimal provision of care and clinical outcomes.

INTRODUCTION

Pain is the number 1 reason patients 15 years of age and older seek care in an emergency department (ED).[1] ED visits for nontraumatic abdominal pain increased 31% from 1999 to 2008.[1] Patients' experiences with pain management in the ED may be impacted most by delays in crowded emergency departments. Provider attitudes about pain management may influence patients' feelings about their care in the ED. Innovative strategies for pain management need to be considered to meet patients' expectations about their pain.

This article originally appeared in Nursing Clinics of North America, Volume 49, Issue 1, March 2014.
[a] Emergency Services, University of Kentucky Chandler Medical Center, 1000 South Limestone Street A.00.403, Lexington, KY 40536, USA; [b] Emergency Services, UK Healthcare, 1000 South Limestone Street A.00.402, Lexington, KY 40536, USA; [c] Emergency Services, University of Kentucky Chandler Medical Center, 1000 South Limestone Street A.00.404, Lexington, KY 40536, USA; [d] Critical Care Services, UK Healthcare Good Samaritan Hospital, 310 South Limestone Street, Lexington, KY 40508, USA
* Corresponding author.
E-mail address: pkhoward@uky.edu

BACKGROUND

A review of the literature provides substantive evidence that pain management in the ED does not meet patients' expectations of care related to their pain.[2] In a multicenter study, the researchers illustrated that pain management did not meet patients' expectations for pain relief. These investigators identified a lack of ED research related to pain.[2]

Optimal clinical outcomes are facilitated by adequate pain control. There is support that patients' perceptions of their care, and specifically management of their pain, impacts their clinical outcomes.[3] Patients' perceptions of their illness and functional abilities improved when their pain was reduced. These investigators also suggested that further study may be warranted to examine the relationship between the patient's pain and mental well-being.

Emergency care is episodic, and pain management in the ED may be complicated by long waits, health care professionals' concerns for misuse/abuse, and, more recently, regulatory limitations in some states.[2,4] In 2012, regulations were promulgated in Kentucky that limit the amount of narcotics prescribed in an episodic care setting to a 48-hour supply. This legislation was directed at prescription abuse and "pill mills," yet may have some unintended negative consequences for patients who have limited access to care.[5]

Poor patient satisfaction has been associated with ineffective pain management.[6] A review of qualitative data from patient satisfaction surveys highlighted a poor likelihood to recommend when the patient scored pain control as poor. The voice of the patient showcases how important helpful pain strategies are to perceptions of care.

A limiting factor for effective pain management may be clinical staff attitudes about pain and pain management. An innovative approach to address this was developed from less than desirable patient satisfaction scores directly attributable to pain control. A team of interprofessional stakeholders (ED nursing leadership, ED attending physicians, ED pharmacists, ED registered nurses, pain nurse, ED nursing staff development) was assembled to develop strategies for improvement. It was determined that a multifaceted approach would be used to improve pain management and, indirectly, patient satisfaction scores. The stakeholders' overarching goals were to increase awareness and importance of treating pain by all those who care for ED patients, and reeducate all staff on pain management with an end goal of a comprehensive holistic approach to ED pain management. Pain champions were appointed and included nursing, physician, and pharmacy representation. These interprofessional champions were charged with engaging and educating the staff to improve pain care. Nursing champions attended the "Pain Resource Nurse" (PRN)[7] course to increase their personal knowledge to better educate their peers. Pain champions were critical to the success of the initiative.

An investigation into pain, perceptions, and perceived conflicts of ED staff was developed to gain an understanding about staff-managed pain in an academic medical center. Approval from the medical institutional review board was received for this study; the study objectives can be found in **Box 1**. The study design used a prospective pretest/posttest with a 5-point Likert-type scale that was adapted from the attitudes survey from the PRN course.[7] Letters were sent to emergency nurses and emergency medicine residents requesting voluntary participation in this study. A link to the confidential Internet-based survey was included in the study letter sent via department e-mail (**Table 1**). A review of the baseline survey results revealed areas of knowledge deficit and misperceptions about pain management techniques. Pain champions from the stakeholder team developed "Operation Pain." This project

---

Box 1
Study objectives

Determine the impact of education on ED staff perception related to pain management.

Describe 2 methods to measure staff knowledge of pain management.

Investigate effects of pain management education on patient satisfaction scores related to pain.

Determine which pain management strategies are more commonly used by staff.

---

was developed to promote effective pain measures for every patient every time. There were several educational aspects of Operation Pain: brief themed pain management techniques during the preshift huddles for a week (**Box 2**), a banner in the ED, and language on the white board in each patient room "tell us if you have pain." The pain champions coordinated a 4-hour interprofessional education offering that was mandatory for all clinical staff. Content for the education was modeled from some aspects of the PRN course.[7] Weekly pain pearls were e-mailed to nursing staff by the pain champions who also worked collaboratively with staff development to verify pain management competencies for clinical staff need while leading by example in the clinical arena. After completion of the 4-hour education session and verification of competency, the postsurvey link was sent to staff. The original study protocol was amended to add 6 survey questions about pain management strategies (**Fig. 1**).

Table 1
Attitudes survey

Attitudes Survey	Strongly Disagree	Disagree	Neutral	Agree	Strongly Agree
Older people can bore you to death talking about pain.	1	2	3	4	5
I like to be known as a person who doesn't complain about pain.	1	2	3	4	5
Older women complain about pain more than older men.	1	2	3	4	5
Men are supposed to be brave and not let anybody know if they have pain.	1	2	3	4	5
Some patients exaggerate their pain as a way of getting attention.	1	2	3	4	5
Patients are often embarrassed to tell their nurse that they're hurting.	1	2	3	4	5
Learning to live with pain builds character.	1	2	3	4	5
Life is painful. There is no getting around that.	1	2	3	4	5
By suffering pain in this life, we are purifying ourselves for life to come.	1	2	3	4	5
If patients can still get around or do things, I have to wonder if they are in that much pain.	1	2	3	4	5

Box 2
Operation pain

Daily Huddle Focus:

Monday: ABCs of Pain Assessment

- A – ask regularly
- B – believe patient's report of pain
- C – choose treatment options based on assessment
- D – deliver interventions in a timely way
- E – evaluate treatment effectiveness by reassessment

Tuesday: Set a Realistic Pain Goal

- Achievable
- Mutually acceptable
- Each and every patient

Wednesday: Complete Pain Assessments

- Onset
- Location
- Duration
- Quality
- Intensity
- Type of pain
- Special considerations

Thursday: Use Nonpharmacologic Pain Measures

- 5-minute hand massage
- Distraction
- Heat
- Ice
- Relaxation techniques

Friday: Assess Your Patients' Pain

- Are they getting the right medication
- The right time frame
- The right dose for their type of pain
- Follow-up with your physician

Saturday: Reassess Pain Interventions: Don't Forget to Document What You've Done

- Within 30 minutes of parenteral drug administration
- Within 1 hour of oral medication administration
- With each report of new pain
- With unrelieved pain
- With each report of changes in pain
- Before, during, and after procedures
- Whenever pain is suspected

Sunday: Look for Nonverbal Pain Cues

- Facial expressions
- Verbalizations, vocalizations
- Mental status changes
- Body movements
- Changes in interpersonal interactions
- Changes in activity

DISCUSSION

Seventy-six ED nurses and residents responded to the baseline survey. Thirty-six ED nurses completed the postsurvey. It was unclear why the residents did not complete the postsurvey, although survey fatigue was considered. The mean pretest and post-test scores showed little change for attitudes and were not statistically significant but did trend more positively after the education (**Fig. 2**). Staff reported that they perceived pain differently and had a greater focus on pain interventions after the education. Most significant was the change in patient satisfaction scores related to pain control. Before Operation Pain was implemented, the "how well my pain was managed" mean score was 67.3 (seventh percentile). The quarter following the education and pain champion activities, the "how well my pain was managed" mean score increased to 80.3 (73rd percentile).

Staff responses about pain management strategies were not measured at baseline. The opportunity to learn staff practices regarding pain management (**Fig. 3**) supported a tendency to start with suboptimal management pain control practices, as identified

Pain Question			Yes	No
I am an advocate for pain				
I always assess patient's levels on admission				
I routinely re-assess patient's pain after an intervention				
I always assess patient's pain level at/prior to discharge				
I ensure that patient's pain is improved prior to discharge or transfer				
Strategy:	Distraction	Basic Measures ice, elevation	NSAIDS	Narcotics
The first pain management technique I use with patients with a pain score less than 4 is:				
The first pain management technique I use with patients with a pain score greater than 4 is:				
The follow-up pain management technique I use with patients with a pain score greater than 4 is:				

Fig. 1. Postsurvey pain management strategies.

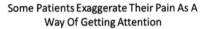

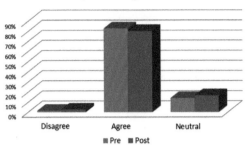

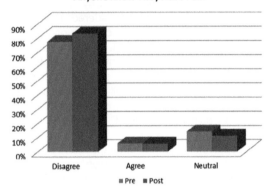

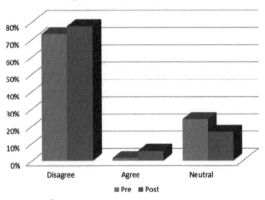

Fig. 2. Attitudes survey results.

in the Pain and Emergency Medicine Initiative (PEMI) study.[2] Validating these practices led to additional education being provided by the pain champions on the advanced nursing protocols, with more substantive pain management modalities. Advanced nursing protocols are nurse-driven order sets approved by the ED medical staff. The nurse can choose to implement these protocols based on clinical assessment. This is most effective when the ED is crowded, delays are likely, and the patient is experiencing moderate to severe pain.

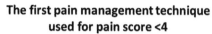

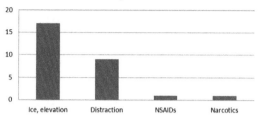

The first pain management technique used for pain score <4

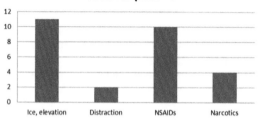

The first pain management technique used for pain >4

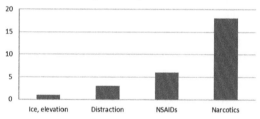

Follow-up pain management techniques for pain score >4

Fig. 3. Pain management survey results.

The strengths associated with this study were a potential Hawthorne effect and a meaningful change in patients' pain control as measured in the change in patient satisfaction scores. The increased emphasis on effective pain control has resulted in more staff focus on pain management strategies, both nonpharmacologic and pharmacologic measures for all ages. ED clinical staff are committed to ensuring that pain is assessed early, with frequent reassessments postintervention. Limitations of this investigation include disparity between the pretest and posttest sample sizes, as well as lack of homogeneity between the subjects in each sample. These inequities make it difficult to be certain this could be generalized to other EDs.

SUMMARY

According to Saint Augustine, "The greatest evil is physical pain." This is reflected in patients' perceptions of their pain. Pain education and innovative approaches to nurse-driven protocols are essential to ensure the most optimal provision of care and clinical outcomes. ED welcome brochures include information about pain control and the "Universal Pain Tool" in 8 languages. ED staff attitudes have changed over time, and the increased advocacy has benefited their patients. Emergency nurses participating in Operation Pain placed a higher priority on pain management for their patients.

Pain control remains a priority for the ED. Staff perform purposeful rounding to consistently assess pain levels. Pain assessment and interventions are monitored through reports from the electronic medical record on a monthly basis. It is an expectation that 80% of all patients with a pain score greater than 4 will have an intervention completed and documented with reassessment noted. Metrics related to pain interventions are included in the ED dashboard and shared with staff. Patient satisfaction data related to "how well pain was controlled" is disseminated in the weekly note sent to ED nursing and medical staff. Pain is the reason most patients come to the ED, it is nursing's accountability to ensure they receive the appropriate intervention.

REFERENCES

1. Bhuiya F, Pitts S, McCraig L. Emergency department visits for chest pain and abdominal pain: United States, 1999–2008. NCHS Data Brief. Hyattsville (MD): National Center for Health Statistics; 2010. p. 43.
2. Todd K, Ducharme J, Choiniere M, et al. Pain in the emergency department: results of the pain and emergency medicine initiative (PEMI) multicenter study. J Pain 2007;8:460–6.
3. Moss-Morris R, Humphrey K, Johnson M, et al. Patient's perceptions of their pain condition across a multidisciplinary pain management program: do they change and if so does it matter? Clin J Pain 2007;23:558–64.
4. Bergman C. Emergency nurses' perceived barriers to demonstrating caring when managing adult patients' pain. J Emerg Nurs 2012;38:218–25.
5. Commonwealth of Kentucky Legislative Review Commission. KRS Chapter 218A. Available at: http://www.kbml.ky.gov/NR/rdonlyres/DFFF4843-1343-4468-9574-C9BE26CE48CF/0/HouseBill1.pdf. Accessed September 15, 2013.
6. DuPree E, Martin L, Anderson R, et al. Improving patient satisfaction with pain management using six sigma tools. Jt Comm J Qual Patient Saf 2009;35:343–50.
7. Dahl J, Gordon D, Palce J, editors. Pain resource nurse program curriculum and planning guide. Madison (WI): The Resource Center of the Alliance of State Pain Initiatives; 2008.

Cognitive-Behavioral Therapy for Comorbid Insomnia and Chronic Pain

Patrick H. Finan, PhD*, Luis F. Buenaver, PhD,
Virginia T. Runko, PhD, Michael T. Smith, PhD

KEYWORDS

- Insomnia • Chronic pain • Comorbid • Cognitive-behavioral therapy for insomnia

KEY POINTS

- Cognitive-behavioral therapy for insomnia (CBT-I) for comorbid insomnia and chronic pain demonstrates clinically meaningful improvements in sleep symptoms, particularly sleep continuity.
- CBT-I for comorbid insomnia and chronic pain does not consistently improve pain severity, but appears to reduce pain interference and disability in several studies.
- Hybrid interventions that target both pain and insomnia have demonstrated feasibility in small pilot samples, but further conclusions must be deferred until a larger trial is reported.
- More comprehensive and dynamic pain assessment strategies may reveal effects for CBT-I and hybrid interventions not captured through single-occasion pain severity measures.

INTRODUCTION

Most patients with chronic pain report poor sleep quality. Insomnia, the most prevalent form of sleep disturbance in chronic pain, may directly contribute to poor long-term outcomes by affecting multiple dimensions of chronic pain pathophysiology and psychosocial functioning. Sleep loss impairs immune function,[1,2] emotion regulation,[3,4] and cognitive function,[5,6] and heightens pain sensitivity.[7] These processes are considered both vulnerabilities to and consequences of chronic pain.[8-11] As such, there is a growing interest in the development and evaluation of sleep-related interventions among patients with chronic pain and in individuals at risk for developing chronic pain.

This article originally appeared in Sleep Medicine Clinics, Volume 9, Issue 2, June 2014.
Department of Psychiatry and Behavioral Sciences, Johns Hopkins University School of Medicine, Baltimore, MD, USA
* Corresponding author.
E-mail address: pfinan1@jhu.edu

Treating sleep disturbance in patients with chronic pain is of interest for several reasons. First, a recent systematic review indicates that psychological and pharmacologic strategies for chronic pain management show only modest effects in reducing pain and pain-related disability.[12] Targeting additional symptom clusters that may actively contribute to chronic pain severity and persistence, such as sleep disturbance, may be necessary to improve pain-management outcomes. Furthermore, and perhaps somewhat surprisingly, recent prospective studies using rigorous statistical methodologies have suggested that in some idiopathic pain conditions, such as temporomandibular joint disorder,[13] sleep disturbance might in fact be a more robust predictor of subsequent pain than vice versa. A recent laboratory study demonstrated that extension of sleep among individuals with mild chronic sleep loss was associated with reduced pain sensitivity.[14] Thus, it is reasonable to hypothesize that interventions that target sleep in patients with chronic pain may produce improvements in pain symptoms as insomnia dissipates.

Cognitive-behavioral therapy for insomnia (CBT-I) is the standard of care for treating chronic primary insomnia. The efficacy of CBT-I in primary insomnia is comparable with that of modern sedative hypnotics, with the advantages of long-term sustainability of treatment effects[15,16] and a favorable side-effect profile.[17] CBT-I is standardized, and can be implemented in a wide range of outpatient settings and formats.[18–21] In the past decade, CBT-I has increasingly been investigated for the treatment of insomnia occurring in the context of medical and psychiatric comorbidities, with promising results.[22] Most of these studies limited their primary outcomes to sleep parameters. A handful of researchers, however, have recently begun to study the effects of CBT-I on sleep and pain-related outcomes. The theoretical frameworks and some of the coping skills taught in CBT-I overlap with the skills taught in cognitive-behavioral therapy for pain (CBT-P), but the 2 treatments also retain many distinct pain-related and sleep-related components. There is a potential for skills taught in CBT-I to improve pain-related outcomes despite a primary focus on insomnia. In addition, it is reasonable to hypothesize that the components of CBT-I and CBT-P may be blended into a hybrid intervention format that works synergistically on sleep and pain symptoms. Both of these possibilities have been tested in preliminary randomized controlled trials (RCTs), which are the focus of this article. The objectives of this review are to: (1) summarize the findings of this first wave of published clinical trials; (2) discuss the limitations; and (3) identify promising directions for the next wave of studies.

CBT-I FOR COMORBID INSOMNIA AND CHRONIC PAIN

CBT-I is most commonly practiced as a multicomponent treatment that uses a variety of behavioral interventions and cognitive restructuring approaches. It is a short-term intervention that is typically conducted over 4 to 8 individual or group sessions. The most commonly used therapeutic elements include: (1) general sleep education; (2) the application of operant and classical conditioning principles via stimulus control instructions; (3) the replacement of sleep-interfering behaviors with sleep-promoting behaviors through sleep-hygiene education and behavior-change counseling; (4) relaxation training (eg, deep breathing, guided imagery); (5) the alteration of circadian regularity and alignment; (6) the manipulation of homeostatic sleep drive to consolidate sleep via sleep restriction[23]; and (7) the use of cognitive therapy techniques to modify maladaptive sleep-related cognitions. Much of the therapy is data driven, relying on the patient's self-monitoring of daily sleeping patterns, including time in bed (TIB), sleep onset latency (SOL), wake after sleep onset (WASO), and total sleep time (TST).

Currie and Colleagues

Primary findings

The first RCT of CBT-I for patients with comorbid insomnia and chronic pain (N = 60) compared seven 2-hour CBT-I group sessions held weekly with a self-monitoring/wait-list control.[24] The components of therapy followed traditional CBT-I guidelines (**Table 1**), with one notable modification: the contribution of pain to sleep problems was specifically addressed through guided readings and group discussion. The investigators found that patients in the CBT-I condition demonstrated significant improvements in daily diary–measured SOL, sleep efficiency (SE), WASO, and sleep quality. These effects were maintained at the 3-month follow-up assessment. Actigraphic measures of nocturnal physical activity were also significantly reduced in the CBT-I condition. Of note, however, pain severity ratings did not significantly improve.

Analysis

This study[24] established that CBT-I may produce clinically significant changes in self-reported and actigraphy-measured sleep for patients with insomnia and comorbid chronic pain. The use of a wait-list control condition, however, significantly tempers the strength of this conclusion, because of the strong expectation for minimal improvement created by randomization to a wait list. That pain was not significantly reduced in the CBT-I group raises the possibility that clinical improvements in sleep do not directly lead to reductions in pain severity. However, methodological constraints may limit this interpretation. First, participants were selected on the basis of having insomnia symptoms that developed secondary to chronic pain, and information about their pain status before the development of insomnia was not available. Because it is not possible to determine if and to what extent the development of insomnia symptoms altered pre-existing pain symptoms in this sample, one cannot conclude that the lack of pain changes following treatment of insomnia necessarily indicate that CBT-I is inefficacious for pain symptoms. Rather, it could be that the pain symptoms, by virtue of having preceded the development of insomnia symptoms, were not being maintained by insomnia and therefore were not influenced by improvements in insomnia symptoms. This possibility could be evaluated in future studies by assessing time-contingent dependencies between insomnia and pain symptoms through daily diaries before and after treatment. A second limitation is that pain severity was the only pain-related outcome measured, and was considered a secondary outcome; a wider range of pain-related outcomes that measure the multidimensional nature of pain (eg, pain interference, pain catastrophizing) would be necessary to adequately evaluate the broader influence of CBT-I on pain-related outcomes. Third, although groups did not significantly differ from pretreatment to posttreatment on changes in pain, the means trended in this direction. The between-groups effect size (Cohen's d[25]) of CBT-I versus Control on pain was 0.51 at posttreatment and 0.64 at the 3-month follow-up. These values are considered medium effect sizes.[25] As a point of comparison, a recent meta-analysis of the effect of CBT-P shows small to medium effect sizes on pain severity, disability, and catastrophizing at posttreatment, with even smaller effects at follow-up.[12,26] That reductions in pain severity were observed (though not to the point of statistical significance) by Currie and colleagues[24] at 3 months for the CBT-I group might be considered clinically relevant, and raises the issue of whether longer-term follow-up periods are needed to realize the full effect of CBT-I on pain and pain-related outcomes.

Rybarczyk and Colleagues

Primary findings

Expanding on the study by Currie and colleagues,[24] Rybarczyk and colleagues[27] compared CBT-I (n = 23) with a stress-management and wellness control (n = 28)

Table 1
Comparison of CBT-I and hybrid clinical trials for comorbid insomnia and chronic pain

Authors,[Ref.] Year	Treatment Type	Study Sample	PSG Exclusion Criteria	Active Treatment Components	Treatment Duration	Treatment Format	Pain Measures	Sleep Measures	Significant CBT-Related Improvements in Pain?	Significant CBT-Related Improvements in Sleep?
Currie et al,[24] 2000	CBT-I vs wait-list control	Chronic nonmalignant pain + insomnia N = 60	PSG not administered	GSE; SCT; SRT; SHE; RT; CT Pain coping education	7 weekly sessions; 2 h/session	Group; 5–7 patients/ group	MPI	Daily diary; actigraphy; PSQI	No	Yes 1. Diary SOL, SE, WASO 2. Sleep quality 3. Nocturnal activity
Rybarczyk et al,[27] 2005; Vitiello et al,[28] 2009	CBT-I vs stress management control	Osteoarthritis + insomnia N = 51	AHI <15 PLMI <30	SCT; SRT; SHE; RT; CT	8 weekly sessions; 2 h/session	Group; 5 patients/ group	MPQ; SF-36 Bodily Pain	Daily Diary	Yes 1. SF-36 Bodily Pain	Yes 1. Diary SOL; SE; WASO
Edinger et al,[31] 2005	CBT-I vs sleep-hygiene control vs usual care	Fibromyalgia + insomnia N = 47	AHI <15 PLMI <15	GSE; SCT; SRT	6 weekly sessions; 45–60 min in week 1, 15–30 min in weeks 2–6	Individual	MPQ; BPI	Daily diary; actigraphy; ISQ	No	Yes 1. Diary SOL; SE; TWT 2. Actigraphy SOL and SOL variability; TST variability 3. Insomnia Severity
Jungquist et al,[35] 2010; Jungquist et al,[38]	CBT-I vs contact control	Chronic nonmalignant pain + insomnia N = 28	AHI <10 PLM not specified	SCT; SRT; SHE; CT	8 weekly sessions; 30–60 min/ session	Individual	Daily diary; MPQ; MPI; PDI	Daily diary; ISI; ESS	Yes 1. Pain interference (MPI)	Yes 1. Diary SOL; SE; WASO; awakenings 2. Insomnia

Studies in Which a Hybrid CBT-I/-P Was the Active Treatment

Authors,[Ref.] Year	Treatment Types	Study Population	Active Treatment Components	Treatment Duration	Treatment Format	Pain Measures	Sleep Measures	Significant Hybrid Treatment-Related Improvements in Pain?	Significant Hybrid Treatment-Related Improvements in Sleep?
Pigeon et al,[40] 2012	Hybrid CBT-I/-P vs CBT-I vs CBT-P vs wait-list control	Chronic nonmalignant pain + insomnia N = 21 AHI <10 PLMI not specified	GSE; SCT; SRT; SHE; RT; sleep-related CT; sleep-related relapse prevention; pain education; pain-related CT; activity pacing; problem solving; communication skills training; pain-related relapse prevention	10 weekly sessions; session time not reported	Individual	MPI; PDI	Daily diary; ISI; ESS	No	Yes 1. Insomnia Severity[a]
Tang et al,[41] 2012	Hybrid CBT-I/-P vs symptom monitoring control	Chronic nonmalignant pain + insomnia N = 20 PSG not administered	GSE; SCT; SRT; CT; pain education; behavioral activation; pain-related CT	4 weekly sessions; 2 h/session	Individual	Daily diary; BPI; CISP; PSPS	Daily diary; actigraphy; ISI; DBAS; PSAS; APSQ	Yes 1. Pain Interference (BPI)	Yes 1. Insomnia Severity (ISI) 2. Diary SOL; SE; WASO; TST

(continued on next page)

Table 1
(continued)

Studies in Which a Hybrid CBT-I/-P Was the Active Treatment

Authors,[Ref.] Year	Treatment Types	Study Population		Active Treatment Components	Treatment Duration	Treatment Format	Pain Measures	Sleep Measures	Significant Hybrid Treatment-Related Improvements in Pain?	Significant Hybrid Treatment-Related Improvements in Sleep?
Vitiello et al,[42] 2013	Hybrid CBT-I/P vs CBT-P vs Education	Chronic osteoarthritis and insomnia	PSG not administered	SHE; SCT; SRT; pain education; behavioral activation; relaxation; activity pacing; imagery; pain-related CT	6 weekly session; 90 min/session	Groups; 5–12/group	Graded Chronic Pain Scale; arthritis symtpoms	ISI; Actigraphy SE	No	Yes 1. ISI 2. SE

Abbreviations: APSQ, Anxiety and Preoccupation about Sleep Questionnaire; BPI, Brief Pain Inventory; CBT, cognitive-behavioral therapy; CBT-I, cognitive-behavioral therapy for insomnia; CBT-P, cognitive-behavioral therapy for pain; CISP, Catastrophizing in Pain Scale; CT, cognitive therapy; DBAS, Dysfunctional Beliefs About Sleep Scale; ESS, Epworth Sleepiness Scale; GSE, general sleep education; ISI, Insomnia Severity Index; ISQ, Insomnia Symptom Questionnaire; MPI, Multidimensional Pain Inventory; MPQ, McGill Pain Questionnaire; PDI, Pain Disability Index; PSAS, Presleep Arousal Scale; PSPS, Pain Self-Perception Scale; PSQI, Pittsburgh Sleep Quality Index; RT, relaxation training; SCT, stimulus control therapy; SE, sleep efficiency; SF-36, 36-item Short-Form Survey; SHE, sleep-hygiene education; SII, Sleep Impairment Index; SOL, sleep onset latency; SRT, sleep restriction therapy; TST, total sleep time; TWT, total wake time; WASO, wake after sleep onset.

[a] The hybrid group evidenced a larger effect size than CBT-I, but was not significantly different after adjusting for multiple comparisons.

in a subsample of patients with comorbid insomnia and osteoarthritis (OA). The CBT-I intervention (see **Table 1**) did not specifically address pain interference with sleep, and the OA patients participated in group sessions along with patients with other nonpainful medical conditions. The focus here is on the data for the OA/pain subsample only. Results indicated that, relative to the stress-management control, CBT-I significantly improved daily diary–reported SE, WASO, and SOL.[28] Pain on the McGill Pain Questionnaire (MPQ[29]), which measures both sensory and affective components of pain, was not significantly reduced by the CBT-I intervention. However, a follow-up analysis[28] revealed that CBT-I patients reported significantly less pain on the SF-36 Bodily Pain scale[30] at posttreatment, and tended to maintain those benefits at 1-year follow-up (P = .08).

Analysis

By including an active control condition, this study[27] permitted a more rigorous test of CBT-I against a stress management control with similar cognitive demand and expectancy characteristics. Overall, the findings from this study confirmed the efficacy of CBT-I for self-reported sleep-related outcomes in patients with comorbid chronic pain and insomnia. Findings on pain-related measures were equivocal, perhaps owing to differences in measurement. The MPQ assesses sensory and affective characteristics of the pain experience, whereas the SF-36 is a measure that includes items measuring both pain severity and interference in function.[30] Similar to the study by Currie and colleagues,[24] this study was primarily focused on sleep-related outcomes, and lacked a comprehensive pain-assessment strategy. Nonetheless, the superiority of CBT-I over an active control on primary sleep outcomes offers compelling support for its efficacy in treating sleep among patients with insomnia and comorbid chronic pain.

Edinger and Colleagues

Primary findings

Similar CBT-I benefits were observed in a small RCT involving patients with comorbid fibromyalgia and insomnia.[31] Clinically significant improvements in daily diary SE and TST were observed in 43% (6 of 14) of CBT-I patients compared with 7% (1 of 15) in a control condition receiving only sleep-hygiene education, and in 0 of 7 in a usual-care condition. Objective actigraphic measures of sleep yielded comparable results, including shorter mean SOL and lower variability across days in both SOL and TST, suggesting that sleep became more reliable following CBT-I, an underappreciated but common outcome associated with CBT-I. Across most sleep outcomes, treatment gains were maintained at 6-month follow-up. Significant differences between the CBT-I and control groups were not observed for pain outcomes (ie, severity and sensory/affective pain), although means trended in that direction and effect sizes between the CBT-I and usual-care groups at postintervention were medium to large (Cohen d 0.51 and 1.74 for pain severity[32] and sensory/affective pain,[29] respectively). Of interest, patients in the sleep-hygiene group scored significantly differently to usual-care controls on both pain severity and sensory/affective pain measures. Subgroup analyses indicated that the association of sleep-hygiene treatment and pain-related improvements was driven by a portion of patients in the sleep-hygiene group who self-initiated the behavioral strategy of standardizing their sleep times and achieved a 25% or greater reduction in TIB variability. This subgroup showed a significantly greater reduction in self-reported sensory/affective pain than usual-care controls.

Analysis

Overall, the results of this study[31] suggest that CBT-I may be an effective intervention for patients with fibromyalgia, as it provided favorable results on both subjective and objective sleep criteria. However, as with prior studies in other chronic nonmalignant pain populations, the results were equivocal with respect to the efficacy of CBT-I for reducing pain and pain-related symptoms. Fibromyalgia pain may be substantively different from pain associated with osteoarthritis and other types of degenerative musculoskeletal disorders, so it is difficult to compare general pain measures across studies. Future efforts with this population could expand outcome measures to include fibromyalgia-specific measures, such as a body map or the Fibromyalgia Impact Questionnaire.[33] Furthermore, because nonrestorative sleep is such a prevalent complaint among patients with fibromyalgia,[34] it would be important to know if CBT-I improvements in SOL, SE, and TST are associated with improvements in the perception of restorative sleep.

Jungquist and Colleagues

Primary findings
Another RCT[35] of patients with chronic nonmalignant back and/or neck pain and comorbid insomnia found that, relative to a contact control (n = 9), CBT-I (n = 19) produced significant posttreatment improvements in daily diary–reported SOL, SE, WASO, number of awakenings, insomnia severity, and pain interference measured with the Multidimensional Pain Inventory.[36] CBT-I did not significantly improve posttreatment daily diary–reported pain severity or pain disability measured with the Pain Disability Index.[37] Although TST was not significantly enhanced at posttreatment, which is commonly the case among interventions that include sleep restriction, clinically and statistically significant gains in TST (23 minutes) were observed at 6-month follow-up.[38] In addition, posttreatment reductions in pain interference were maintained at both 3-month and 6-month follow-up periods, providing preliminary evidence for the sustainability of CBT-I effects on a key functional pain-related outcome.

Analysis
The multimodal (ie, diary and single-occasion measurement), multidimensional (ie, severity vs disability and interference) assessment of pain is a particular strength of this study,[35] and an important advancement in the literature. Whereas the self-reported perception of pain severity was essentially unaltered by CBT-I, the extent to which pain reportedly interfered with daily functioning was significantly reduced. One implication of this finding is that CBT-I may be more efficacious for improving the ability to cope with pain rather than perceptions of pain severity/intensity itself. It seems that, despite minimal changes in the severity of pain, patients are less inclined to perceive pain-related functional limitations following CBT-I. Although the reason for this distinction at present is unclear, the authors speculate that as the perception of pain interference declines, patients may be less likely to experience disability and impairment of social functioning.[39] In turn, this may promote an increase in healthy pain-coping behaviors. Such effects may not translate into pain severity changes in the short term, and the failure of CBT-I to produce short-term changes in pain severity, despite changes in pain interference, is consistent with effects observed in trials of CBT-P, in which pain coping is directly targeted.[26] Thus, longer-term follow-ups in the range of 1 to 2 years may be warranted for these effects to be fully manifested. Such a study would be reasonable given the durability of CBT-I over these longer-term periods, and the general intractability of many chronic pain conditions.

HYBRID CBT-I FOR COMORBID INSOMNIA AND CHRONIC PAIN

If the inconsistency in pain severity changes across CBT-I trials in patients with comorbid insomnia and chronic pain is due to a narrow treatment focus on sleep behaviors and cognitions, it is possible that a hybrid intervention targeting both sleep and pain may produce more favorable results. Given the similarity in theoretical grounding of cognitive and behavioral skills taught in both CBT-I and CBT-P, it is reasonable to hypothesize that a hybrid of the two may be feasibly delivered and more efficiently treat symptoms of both insomnia and pain. Two preliminary pilot studies have examined the effects of a hybrid intervention of CBT-I/CBT-P on pain and insomnia symptoms.

Pigeon and Colleagues

Primary findings

A 10-week hybrid intervention was delivered to patients with chronic noncancer pain and comorbid insomnia.[40] The efficacy of the hybrid intervention (n = 6) was compared with CBT-P alone (n = 5), CBT-I alone (n = 6), and a wait-list control (n = 4) at postintervention, but no follow-up time points. The hybrid intervention contained all components of both the CBT-I and CBT-P conditions (see **Table 1** for complete treatment components). The pain treatment components in both the CBT-P and hybrid conditions included pain psychophysiology education, relaxation training, pacing, pain-specific cognitive therapy, activity planning, problem solving, communication skills, pain flare-up planning, and relapse prevention.[40] The timing and sequence of specific intervention components was not explicitly described. Results indicated that the largest effect for pain severity was observed in the CBT-P group, whereas the CBT-I and hybrid groups did not show improvements in pain severity (**Table 2**). CBT-P also produced the largest reduction in pain disability, but modest reductions on pain disability were also observed for CBT-I and the hybrid intervention (between-group Cohen d = 0.28 and

Table 2
Between-group effect size estimates for CBT-I and hybrid interventions on key outcomes after intervention

Authors,[Ref.] Year	Diary SOL	Diary SE	Diary WASO	Diary TST	Pain Severity	Functional Pain Measure
Studies in which CBT-I was the active treatment						
Currie et al,[24] 2000	0.76	1.02	0.94	0.40	0.51	—
Rybarczyk et al,[27] 2005; Vitiello et al,[28] 2009	0.36	0.75	0.89	0.03	0.53	—
Edinger et al,[31] 2005[a]	0.08	0.73	1.51	0.01	0.17	—
Jungquist et al,[35] 2010; Jungquist et al,[38] 2012	2.28	1.95	1.69	1.12	0.81	0.67 (MPI) 1.06 (PDI)
Studies in which hybrid CBT-I/-P was the active treatment						
Pigeon et al,[40] 2012[b]	—	1.48	—	0.66	0.37	0.39 (PDI)
Tang et al,[41] 2012	1.84	1.94	2.10	0.73	0.05	1.34 (BPI)
Vitiello et al,[42] 2013[c]	—	2.64[d]	—		0.10	—

Values are Cohen's d effect-size estimates derived from between-group (treatment vs control) comparisons at posttreatment time points.
Abbreviations: BPI, Brief Pain Inventory, Pain Interference Subscale; MPI, Multidimensional Pain Inventory, Pain Interference Subscale; PDI, Pain Disability Index.
[a] Study included multiple control groups; effect size derived from CBT-I/usual care comparison.
[b] Study included multiple control groups; effect size derived from hybrid/wait-list control comparison.
[c] Study included multiple control groups; effect size derived from hybrid/education control comparison.
[d] Actigraphy was the only modality used to assess SE in this study.

0.35, respectively). With respect to insomnia severity, however, the largest effect was observed for the hybrid treatment, followed by CBT-I, and a smaller, nonsignificant effect for CBT-P. The hybrid and CBT-I interventions evidenced similar gains in diary-measured sleep continuity, including approximately 50-minute increases in TST from baseline, and mean SE higher than 90% (from baseline mean <70%) at postintervention, both clinically significant (but not statistically significant) marks.

Analysis

In sum, the findings of this study establish the feasibility of a hybrid insomnia/pain intervention. Across outcomes of both sleep and pain, the hybrid intervention was comparable with CBT-I. Of interest, the hybrid intervention was not efficacious for pain severity and was not significantly different to control for pain disability, despite a modest reduction. The small sample size, however, precludes any firm conclusions. One interesting aspect of this study is the use of a CBT-P arm, which demonstrated benefits for chronic pain symptoms but failed to alleviate insomnia symptoms. As with the studies reviewed earlier, the findings of Pigeon and colleagues[40] should be cautiously interpreted until a larger study is conducted.

Tang and Colleagues

Primary findings

One other pilot study[41] investigated the effects of a 4-week hybrid intervention (n = 10; see **Table 1** for treatment component details) in comparison with a symptom-monitoring control group (n = 10) in patients with chronic heterogeneous, nonmalignant pain and comorbid insomnia. The sleep interventions included stimulus control and sleep-restriction therapies. The pain treatment components in the hybrid intervention included pain education, behavioral activation, and cognitive therapy focused on reducing pain catastrophizing, safety-seeking behavior, and increasing positive reappraisal and growth strategies. Sessions lasted 2 hours, but the sequencing of individual components was not explicitly described. Significant improvements at postintervention were observed for the hybrid intervention relative to the control in insomnia severity, diary-reported SOL, WASO, SE, and TST (see **Table 2** for between-group effect sizes), in addition to actigraphically assessed SOL, WASO, TST, and TIB. The hybrid intervention was associated with significant postintervention improvements in pain interference but not pain severity. Primary diary and actigraphy measures were not obtained on follow-up, but 1-month and 6-month follow-up data were available for retrospective questionnaire data, which included insomnia severity, pain severity, and interference. Significant pre-post gains in insomnia severity and pain interference were maintained at 1-month and 6-month follow-up.

Vitiello and Colleagues

Primary findings

Vitiello and colleagues[42] reported results from the largest RCT of CBT for comorbid insomnia and chronic pain, with 367 older adults randomized to receive a hybrid CBT-I/P, CBT-P, or an education control. The hybrid intervention resulted in significantly greater reductions in self-reported insomnia severity than either CBT-P or the education control, and these effects were maintained at 9 month follow-up. The only objective sleep outcome reported—actigraphically-measured SE—improved in both CBT-I/P and CBT-P, and declined in the education control group. Neither CBT-I/P nor CBT-P significantly improved in pain severity. Secondary analyses on all primary outcomes in a subgroup of patients with heightened baseline pain did not reveal a substantively different pattern of results.

Analysis

The primary strengths of the Vitiello and colleagues[42] were its large sample size, rigorous design, and excellent retention of participants at 9-month follow-up. The findings support those of Pigeon et al. and Tang et al. in 2 respects. First, all three studies suggest CBT-I/P is efficacious in reducing insomnia severity. Second, all three studies suggest CBT-I/P is not efficacious in reducing pain severity. Together, the data from the studies of Tang and colleagues[41] and Pigeon and colleagues[40] confirm the feasibility of a hybrid intervention. Furthermore, they demonstrate that brief (ie, 4 sessions) and longer (ie, 10 sessions) hybrid intervention formats produce comparable results on sleep outcomes. There was overlap in the content of hybrid interventions in both of these studies (see **Table 1** for comparisons). Relative to the study by Pigeon and colleagues,[40] Tang and colleagues'[41] intervention notably omitted relaxation and relapse prevention modules for both insomnia and pain. Pigeon and colleagues reported "pain-specific cognitive therapy" as a therapeutic module, but did not provide additional details about the content of the cognitive therapy. By contrast, Tang and colleagues reported incorporating specific modules on positive reappraisal and growth, in addition to cognitive therapy to reduce pain catastrophizing. It is notable that within the intervention of Pigeon and colleagues,[40] the hybrid condition included twice as many components in the same number of sessions as both the CBT-I and CBT-P comparison conditions. Although speculative, it is possible that the absence of hybrid intervention effects on pain severity in this study was due to patient difficulty in managing the demands of simultaneously learning a large number of pain-coping skills and sleep-habit changes. Although Vitiello and colleagues spread their hybrid modules over more sessions, they too failed to find pain reduction following CBT-I/P. It would be interesting to see in future studies whether reducing the number of skills taught improves pain-related outcomes in hybrid interventions (although Pigeon and colleagues[40] noted that patients and therapists anecdotally remarked that the number of sessions could actually be reduced and still accommodate the material). Future hybrid interventions may be better evaluated by measuring process and adherence measures in addition to discrete outcomes. For example, it would be useful to know whether patients adhered to sleep and pain home practice assignments differently in the hybrid intervention when compared with the CBT-I and CBT-P interventions.

INTEGRATED ANALYSIS AND FUTURE DIRECTIONS

The available evidence consistently indicates that cognitive-behavioral interventions targeting sleep in patients with chronic pain, including both stand-alone CBT-I and hybrid CBT-I/CBT-P interventions, are efficacious for a range of outcomes derived from sleep diaries and actigraphy, including sleep duration, continuity, and perceived quality. Furthermore, CBT-I and hybrid interventions may improve pain-related outcomes, with greater effects on pain interference and disability relative to pain severity. The 2 preliminary hybrid interventions incorporating elements of both pain and sleep seem to primarily benefit sleep, with modest effects on pain interference and disability. Despite the promise of these initial findings, they are limited by several factors that must be addressed in future research.

Sample Size

Small sample sizes in the treatment and control conditions of all of the RCTs to date threaten the reliability and validity of the data. Increasing the sample size is the most straightforward way to improve reliability and validity in the outcome data available from existing trials.

Optimization of Sleep Outcome Measurement

A more complex issue than sample size is how to optimize outcome measurement. All RCTs reviewed used daily diaries to assess primary sleep outcomes, and 5 studies[24,31,35,41,42] additionally used actigraphic measurements. In general, the diary procedures are minimally described across studies, and only very limited data pertaining to participant adherence are available across studies. In several studies, it is not clear whether the diaries were paper/pencil or electronic, the latter of which can be objectively verified with time stamps and, therefore, may produce more reliable data. Thus, it is unclear whether diary entries were reliably made within specified windows, and how much retrospective bias may have interfered with self-report estimations. Furthermore, no empirically validated methods are available to guide the analysis of actigraphy data for patients with comorbid insomnia and chronic pain. It is plausible, for example, that patients with certain chronic pain disorders may evidence greater WASO on actigraphy by virtue of heightened motor activity related to the pain source (eg, leg movements due to knee osteoarthritis). This pattern was observed in the study by Jungquist and colleagues,[38] in which actigraphy-assessed WASO was significantly greater than daily diary–assessed WASO. By contrast, Edinger and colleagues[31] did not report any systematic differences between diary-based and actigraphy-based outcomes. Future research should examine the validity of actigraphy as an outcome measure by determining whether actigraphically assessed sleep parameters are different in patients with certain types of chronic pain. As ambulatory polysomnography (PSG) becomes increasingly available and affordable, the reliability and validity of actigraphy data may be readily compared with those of PSG.

Optimization of Pain Outcome Measurement

Though interpreted with caution because of small sample sizes, the available data suggest that pain severity may not be robustly altered by CBT-I and hybrid CBT-I/CBT-P, and therefore may be a poor primary end point, at least when measured within 6 months. Other more functionally relevant outcomes, such as pain interference, seem to be more strongly influenced by CBT-I and hybrid interventions.[35,41] The minimal effects on pain severity contrast with those in the experimental literature because they suggest that changes in sleep do not precipitate changes in pain. However, an alternative explanation is that the pain assessments in clinical trials to date have not been sufficiently broad to capture the true variance or complexities underpinning the association of insomnia with chronic pain. For example, in future studies it may prove important to incorporate a broader range of diary-based pain-related outcomes and to evaluate time-variant contingencies in pain, sleep, functional disability, mood, and stress from day to day.[43,44] Such an assessment strategy would yield potentially important information about the psychosocial antecedents and sequelae of changes in pain and sleep from one day to the next, and whether such contingent daily associations change following treatment. In addition, it may be useful to investigate individual differences in response to quantitative sensory testing (QST). QST includes a range of nociceptive stimuli (eg, thermal, pressure, electrodermal) that evoke a variable range of pain responses in individuals with and without chronic pain.[8] Experimental studies have demonstrated that response to QST, including pain threshold[45–48] and endogenous pain inhibition,[49] are altered by sleep deprivation. The evaluation of changes in QST responses throughout treatment may shed light on the ability of CBT-I to effect change on neurobiologically mediated processes that may contribute to the maintenance of chronic pain, such as central sensitization[50,51] and endogenous pain inhibition.[52] The mechanisms by which such changes may take place are not clear at present, although sleep has been identified as a potential source of variance in these endogenous pain modulatory processes.[49,53] In addition, physical function and psychosocial factors are associated with dysfunctional endogenous pain modulation.[50,54] If CBT-I and hybrid interventions are shown to reliably improve sleep and functional pain-related outcomes, it is reasonable to postulate that such effects may be associated with improved endogenous pain modulation, which might be hypothesized to precede changes in clinical pain reporting. The potential for such changes to affect clinical pain severity might be best determined over long-term follow-up (eg, 1–3 years), and therefore may not be reflected in the results of the studies reviewed here.

Examination of Demographic Moderators

Many of the studies reviewed were not large enough to investigate or explore the possibility that key moderators known to influence pain sensitivity and sleep, such as sex, age, and ethnicity,[55–60] may have obscured the effects. Although the Vitiello and colleagues study was powered to explore such effects, they did not report them in their initial publication. Future studies should examine these moderation models. It is possible, for example, that demographic subgroups vary in the magnitude or time course of response to CBT-I and/or a hybrid intervention.

Evaluation of Secondary Sleep-Related Phenomena

Another potentially important issue that creates complexity within this literature is the possibility that other sleep-related phenomena, such as central or obstructive apneas and periodic limb movements (PLMs), may influence some of the pain-related outcomes. Although all studies reviewed here attempted to identify many of these intrinsic sleep disorders for the purpose of exclusion through self-report (eg, Structured Interview for Sleep Disorders), 3 studies[24,41,42] did not use polysomnography to rule out sleep disorders other than insomnia, and the remaining studies varied in the thresholds used to exclude subjects based on apnea-hypopnea index (AHI; number of apneas and hypopneas per hour of sleep) and PLM index (number of PLMs per hour of sleep) (see **Table 1**). It is likely that severe cases of sleep apnea and PLM disorder were excluded from the studies, but it is possible that variability among individuals with mild apnea (eg, AHI 5–15) and PLMs (eg, PLM index <15) may have influenced results. None of the studies reviewed attempted to control or assess the effect of these indices on outcomes. However, emerging data suggest, for example, that sleep-related hypoxemia may actually reduce pain sensitivity in patients with chronic pain.[61,62] Other data suggest that nocturnal hypoxemia may increase pain sensitivity, especially in healthy subjects.[63] Thus, future studies should covary continuous measures of hypoxemia and other relevant nocturnal phenomena to partial out any potential influence on primary outcomes.

Process-Oriented Evaluation of Hybrid Intervention Components

Theoretically, hybrid interventions may offer advantages over CBT-I for pain outcomes by incorporating strategies to behaviorally manage both sleep and pain.[64] Future hybrid studies may yet bear this out, as the effect sizes of CBT-I on pain severity are comparable with the effects of CBT-P on pain severity. However, at present it seems that findings in the experimental[7,14,45,48,49,65] and longitudinal literature[13,53,66,67] that support a causal association between sleep and pain severity may not easily translate into the treatment context in this first wave of studies. That said, it may simply be the case that a more systematic refinement of hybrid treatment protocols may be needed to yield treatment gains. Issues related to the sequencing of pain-related and sleep-related treatment components may be critical and have yet to be investigated. It may additionally be necessary to evaluate which sleep and pain components are the most compatible, and whether specific pairings of sleep and pain components enhances or detracts from outcomes. It is possible that flooding patients with too many skills over too short a period of time may have contributed to the relatively disappointing preliminary findings, particularly with respect to the study by Pigeon and colleagues.[40] Tang and colleagues'[41] intervention incorporated fewer treatment components, but needs to be tested against CBT-I and CBT-P with long-term follow-up to understand its true promise.

Larger-scale investigations of CBT-I in patients with comorbid insomnia and chronic pain are currently under way. An ongoing RCT in the authors' laboratory is comparing the effects of CBT-I with those of an active placebo (behavioral desensitization) on clinical pain and QST in patients with knee osteoarthritis and comorbid insomnia.

SUMMARY

Insomnia and chronic pain harbor a high rate of comorbidity, and have been regarded as reciprocally related conditions. Four RCTs have investigated the efficacy of CBT-I and 2 RCTs have investigated the efficacy of hybrid CBT-I/CBT-P interventions in reducing insomnia and pain symptoms. In general, these interventions demonstrate clinically meaningful improvements in sleep symptoms. Improvements in pain-related outcomes have been observed in functional domains, such as pain interference and disability, with limited evidence supporting the short-term efficacy of CBT-I or hybrid interventions for pain severity. Hybrid interventions are feasible, and one large-scale RCT now supports the findings of 2 pilot studies, suggesting that hybrid interventions, as currently designed, improve sleep, but not pain severity. Future clinical trials should consider using more comprehensive pain assessments with longer-term follow-up assessment of at least 1 year or more. Measurement strategies that permit the analysis of time-variant contingencies in sleep, pain, and associated psychosocial variables may also be particularly informative. Larger-scale investigations are needed to clarify the limited efficacy data from the small pilot RCTs on hybrid interventions. Future studies aimed at developing hybrid interventions should be designed to investigate issues related to the sequencing of pain and sleep components, and should address the trade-off between the number of new skills patients are expected to master and the quality and mastery of critical components. Hybrid approaches that combine sleep and pain intervention components continue to hold promise for improving the treatment of chronic pain among patients with comorbid insomnia.

REFERENCES

1. Irwin M, McClintick J, Costlow C, et al. Partial night sleep deprivation reduces natural killer and cellular immune responses in humans. FASEB J 1996;10(5): 643–53.
2. Mullington JM, Haack M, Toth M, et al. Cardiovascular, inflammatory and metabolic consequences of sleep deprivation. Prog Cardiovasc Dis 2009;51(4):294.
3. Yoo SS, Gujar N, Hu P, et al. The human emotional brain without sleep: a prefrontal amygdala disconnect. Curr Biol 2007;17(20):R877–8.
4. Zohar D, Tzischinsky O, Epstein R, et al. The effects of sleep loss on medical residents' emotional reactions to work events: a cognitive-energy model. Sleep 2005;28(1):47–54.
5. Durmer JS, Dinges DF. Neurocognitive consequences of sleep deprivation. Semin Neurol 2005;25(1):117–29.

6. Thomas M, Sing H, Belenky G, et al. Neural basis of alertness and cognitive performance impairments during sleepiness. I. Effects of 24 h of sleep deprivation on waking human regional brain activity. J Sleep Res 2000;9(4):335–52.

7. Lautenbacher S, Kundermann B, Krieg JC. Sleep deprivation and pain perception. Sleep Med Rev 2006;10(5):357–69.

8. Edwards RR, Sarlani E, Wesselmann U, et al. Quantitative assessment of experimental pain perception: multiple domains of clinical relevance. Pain 2005;114(3): 315–9.

9. Lumley MA, Cohen JL, Borszcz GS, et al. Pain and emotion: a biopsychosocial review of recent research. J Clin Psychol 2011;67(9):942–68.

10. Marchand F, Perretti M, McMahon SB. Role of the immune system in chronic pain. Nat Rev Neurosci 2005;6(7):521–32.

11. Weiner DK, Rudy TE, Morrow L, et al. The relationship between pain, neuropsychological performance, and physical function in community-dwelling older adults with chronic low back pain. Pain Med 2006;7(1):60–70.

12. Williams AC, Eccleston C, Morley S. Psychological therapies for the management of chronic pain (excluding headache) in adults. Cochrane Database Syst Rev 2012;(11):CD007407.

13. Quartana PJ, Wickwire EM, Klick B, et al. Naturalistic changes in insomnia symptoms and pain in temporomandibular joint disorder: a cross-lagged panel analysis. Pain 2010;149(2):325–31.

14. Roehrs TA, Harris E, Randall S, et al. Pain sensitivity and recovery from mild chronic sleep loss. Sleep 2012;35(12):1667–72.

15. Morin CM, Colecchi C, Stone J, et al. Behavioral and pharmacological therapies for late-life insomnia. JAMA 1999;281(11):991–9.

16. Morin CM, Valleres A, Guay B, et al. Cognitive behavioral therapy, singly and combined with medication, for persistent insomnia. JAMA 2009;301(19): 2005–15.

17. Sivertsen B, Krokstad S, Overland S, et al. The epidemiology of insomnia: associations with physical and mental health. The HUNT-2 study. J Psychosom Res 2009;67(2):109–16.

18. Bastien CH, Morin CM, Ouellet MC, et al. Cognitive-behavioral therapy for insomnia: comparison of individual therapy, group therapy, and telephone consultations. J Consult Clin Psychol 2004;72(4):653.

19. Edinger JD, Sampson WS. A primary care "friendly" cognitive behavioral insomnia therapy. Sleep 2003;26(2):177–84.

20. Backhaus J, Hohagen F, Voderholzer U, et al. Long-term effectiveness of a short-term cognitive-behavioral group treatment for primary insomnia. Eur Arch Psychiatry Clin Neurosci 2001;251(1):35–41.

21. Manber R, Edinger JD, Gress JL, et al. Cognitive behavioral therapy for insomnia enhances depression outcome in patients with comorbid major depressive disorder and insomnia. Sleep 2008;31(4):489.

22. Smith MT, Huang MI, Manber R. Cognitive behavior therapy for chronic insomnia occurring within the context of medical and psychiatric disorders. Clin Psychol Rev 2005;25(5):559–92.

23. Spielman AJ, Saskin P, Thorpy MJ. Treatment of chronic insomnia by restriction of time in bed. Sleep 1987;10(1):45–56.

24. Currie SR, Wilson KG, Pontefract AJ, et al. Cognitive-behavioral treatment of insomnia secondary to chronic pain. J Consult Clin Psychol 2000;68(3):407.

25. Cohen J. Statistical power analysis for the behavioral sciences. 2nd edition. Hillsdale (NJ): Erlbaum; 1988.

26. Morley S, Eccleston C, Williams A. Systematic review and meta-analysis of randomized controlled trials of cognitive behaviour therapy and behaviour therapy for chronic pain in adults, excluding headache. Pain 1999;80(1):1–13.
27. Rybarczyk B, Stepanski E, Fogg L, et al. A placebo-controlled test of cognitive-behavioral therapy for comorbid insomnia in older adults. J Consult Clin Psychol 2005;73(6):1164.
28. Vitiello MV, Rybarczyk B, Von Korff M, et al. Cognitive behavioral therapy for insomnia improves sleep and decreases pain in older adults with co-morbid insomnia and osteoarthritis. J Clin Sleep Med 2009;5(4):355.
29. Melzack R. The short-form McGill pain questionnaire. Pain 1987;30(2):191–7.
30. Ware JE, Kosinski M, Keller S. SF-36 physical and mental health summary scales: a user's manual. Health Assessment Lab; 1994.
31. Edinger JD, Wohlgemuth WK, Krystal AD, et al. Behavioral insomnia therapy for fibromyalgia patients: a randomized clinical trial. Arch Intern Med 2005;165(21):2527.
32. Cleeland CS, Ryan KM. Pain assessment: global use of the Brief Pain Inventory. Ann Acad Med Singapore 1994;23(2):129.
33. Burckhardt CS, Clark SR, Bennett RM. The fibromyalgia impact questionnaire: development and validation. J Rheumatol 1991;18(5):728–33.
34. Roizenblatt S, Neto NS, Tufik S. Sleep disorders and fibromyalgia. Curr Pain Headache Rep 2011;15(5):347–57.
35. Jungquist CR, O'Brien C, Matteson-Rusby S, et al. The efficacy of cognitive-behavioral therapy for insomnia in patients with chronic pain. Sleep Med 2010;11(3):302–9.
36. Kerns RD, Turk DC, Rudy TE. The West Haven-Yale Multidimensional Pain Inventory (WHYMPI). Pain 1985;23(4):345–56.
37. Chibnall JT, Tait RC. The Pain Disability Index: factor structure and normative data. Arch Phys Med Rehabil 1994;75(10):1082.
38. Jungquist CR, Tra Y, Smith MT, et al. The durability of cognitive behavioral therapy for insomnia in patients with chronic pain. Sleep Disord 2012;2012:679648.
39. Wittink H, Turk DC, Carr DB, et al. Comparison of the redundancy, reliability, and responsiveness to change among SF-36, Oswestry Disability Index, and Multidimensional Pain Inventory. Clin J Pain 2004;20(3):133–42.
40. Pigeon WR, Moynihan J, Matteson-Rusby S, et al. Comparative effectiveness of CBT interventions for co-morbid chronic pain & insomnia: a pilot study. Behav Res Ther 2012;50:685–9.
41. Tang NK, Goodchild CE, Salkovskis PM. Hybrid cognitive-behaviour therapy for individuals with insomnia and chronic pain: a pilot randomised controlled trial. Behav Res Ther 2012;50:814–21.
42. Vitiello MV, McCurry SM, Shortreed SM, et al. Cognitive-behavioral treatment for comorbid insomnia and osteoarthritis pian in primary care: The Lifestyles Randomized Controlled Trial. Journal of the American Geriatrics Society 2013;61:947–56.
43. Davis MC, Zautra AJ, Smith BW. Chronic pain, stress, and the dynamics of affective differentiation. J Pers 2004;72(6):1133–59.
44. Zautra AJ, Affleck GG, Tennen H, et al. Dynamic approaches to emotions and stress in everyday life: Bolger and Zuckerman reloaded with positive as well as negative affects. J Pers 2005;73(6):1511–38.
45. Kundermann B, Spernal J, Huber MT, et al. Sleep deprivation affects thermal pain thresholds but not somatosensory thresholds in healthy volunteers. Psychosom Med 2004;66(6):932–7.

46. Lentz MJ, Landis CA, Rothermel J, et al. Effects of selective slow wave sleep disruption on musculoskeletal pain and fatigue in middle aged women. J Rheumatol 1999;26(7):1586.

47. Onen SH, Alloui A, Gross A, et al. The effects of total sleep deprivation, selective sleep interruption and sleep recovery on pain tolerance thresholds in healthy subjects. J Sleep Res 2001;10(1):35–42.

48. Roehrs T, Hyde M, Blaisdell B, et al. Sleep loss and REM sleep loss are hyperalgesic. Sleep 2006;29(2):145.

49. Smith MT, Edwards RR, McCann UD, et al. The effects of sleep deprivation on pain inhibition and spontaneous pain in women. Sleep 2007;30(4):494–505.

50. Edwards RR, Smith MT, Stonerock G, et al. Pain-related catastrophizing in healthy women is associated with greater temporal summation of and reduced habituation to thermal pain. Clin J Pain 2006;22(8):730–7.

51. Girbes EL, Nijs J, Torres-Cueco R, et al. Pain treatment for patients with osteoarthritis and central sensitization. Phys Ther 2013;93:842–51.

52. Yarnitsky D. Conditioned pain modulation (the diffuse noxious inhibitory control-like effect): its relevance for acute and chronic pain states. Curr Opin Anaesthesiol 2010;23(5):611–5.

53. Edwards RR, Grace E, Peterson S, et al. Sleep continuity and architecture: associations with pain-inhibitory processes in patients with temporomandibular joint disorder. Eur J Pain 2009;13(10):1043–7.

54. Edwards RR, Ness TJ, Weigent DA, et al. Individual differences in diffuse noxious inhibitory controls (DNIC): association with clinical variables. Pain 2003;106(3):427–37.

55. Durrence HH, Lichstein KL. The sleep of African Americans: a comparative review. Behav Sleep Med 2006;4(1):29–44.

56. Foley D, Ancoli-Israel S, Britz P, et al. Sleep disturbances and chronic disease in older adults: results of the 2003 National Sleep Foundation Sleep in America Survey. J Psychosom Res 2004;56(5):497–502.

57. Mogil JS. Sex differences in pain and pain inhibition: multiple explanations of a controversial phenomenon. Nat Rev Neurosci 2012;13(12):859–66.

58. Ohayon MM, Carskadon MA, Guilleminault C, et al. Meta-analysis of quantitative sleep parameters from childhood to old age in healthy individuals: developing normative sleep values across the human lifespan. Sleep 2004;27(7):1255–73.

59. Song Y, Ancoli-Israel S, Lewis CE, et al. The association of race/ethnicity with objectively measured sleep characteristics in older men. Behav Sleep Med 2011;10(1):54–69.

60. Zhang B, Wing Y. Sex differences in insomnia: a meta-analysis. Sleep 2006;29(1):85.

61. Lovati C, Zardoni M, D'Amico D, et al. Possible relationships between headache—allodynia and nocturnal sleep breathing. Neurol Sci 2011;32(1):145–8.

62. Smith MT, Wickwire EM, Grace EG, et al. Sleep disorders and their association with laboratory pain sensitivity in temporomandibular joint disorder. Sleep 2009;32(6):779.

63. Onen S, Onen F, Albrand G, et al. Pain tolerance and obstructive sleep apnea in the elderly. J Am Med Dir Assoc 2010;11(9):612–6.

64. Tang NK. Cognitive-behavioral therapy for sleep abnormalities of chronic pain patients. Curr Rheumatol Rep 2009;11(6):451–60.

65. Irwin MR, Olmstead R, Carrillo C, et al. Sleep loss exacerbates fatigue, depression, and pain in rheumatoid arthritis. Sleep 2012;35(4):537.

66. Lewandowski AS, Palermo TM, De la Motte S, et al. Temporal daily associations between pain and sleep in adolescents with chronic pain versus healthy adolescents. Pain 2010;151(1):220.
67. Tang NK, Goodchild CE, Sanborn AN, et al. Deciphering the temporal link between pain and sleep in a heterogeneous chronic pain patient sample: a multilevel daily process study. Sleep 2012;35(5):675.

Co-occurring Depression and Pain in Multiple Sclerosis

Kevin N. Alschuler, PhD*, Dawn M. Ehde, PhD, Mark P. Jensen, PhD

KEYWORDS

- Depression • Pain • Multiple sclerosis

KEY POINTS

- Depression and pain are highly prevalent among individuals with multiple sclerosis (MS), often co-occur, and likely make each other worse.
- Both depression and pain impact quality of life, medical utilization, and the effectiveness of interventions.
- Although there are effective interventions for depression and pain, no interventions have yet been developed that target comorbid pain and depression in individuals with MS.

INTRODUCTION

A classic element of multiple sclerosis (MS) is the presence of multiple symptoms that impact functioning. In prior reviews,[1,2] the authors have commented on the significance of individual problems, specifically pain and depression, reporting on prevalence rates and outlining recommendations for the treatment of each one individually. The reality, however, is that these problems often co-occur and likely have bidirectional effects, with each amplifying the other. The purpose of this article is to summarize the theory and existing literature on the comorbidity of pain and depression and describe how their presence impacts individuals with MS. Additionally, the article discusses how existing treatments for pain and depression could be adapted to address shared mechanisms and overcome barriers to treatment utilization.

This article originally appeared in Physical Medicine and Rehabilitation Clinics of North America, Volume 24, Issue 4, November 2013.

Sources of support: The contents of this article were developed under grants from: (1) the Institutes of Health, National Institute of Child Health and Human Development, National Center for Medical Rehabilitation Research (grant number R01HD057916); (2) the National Multiple Sclerosis Society (grant number MB 0008); and (3) the Department of Education (grant number H133B080025). The article does not necessarily represent the policy of the Department of Education, and you should not assume endorsement by the federal government.

Department of Rehabilitation Medicine, University of Washington School of Medicine, Box 358815, 1536 North 115th Street, Seattle, WA 98133, USA

* Corresponding author. Department of Rehabilitation Medicine, UW Medicine Multiple Sclerosis Center, University of Washington School of Medicine, Box 358815, 1536 North 115th Street, Seattle, WA 98133.

E-mail address: kalschul@uw.edu

Clinics Collections 4 (2014) 427–438
http://dx.doi.org/10.1016/j.ccol.2014.10.028

PREVALENCE OF PAIN, DEPRESSION, AND THEIR COMORBIDITY

Several prior studies have reported that pain and depression are both common in individuals with MS. For example, 50% of the people with MS in clinical samples are reported to experience chronic pain at any one point in time.[3] In a community sample of people with MS and pain, 75% reported experiencing some pain and 40% reported an average pain severity of 3 or greater on a scale of 0 to 10,[4] which is understood to be pain of at least moderate intensity in people with MS.[5] In another community sample of people with MS and pain, 25% described their pain as severe.[6]

The 12-month prevalence of major depressive disorder in people with MS is about twice that of the general population (15.7% vs 7.4%, respectively).[7] The lifetime prevalence of depressive disorders in MS is 2 to 3 times that of the general population.[2,8] Many people with MS, as high as 50% at any one time, experience depressive symptoms that may not always reflect a clinical diagnosis of a mood disorder but are nonetheless clinically significant.[9–12]

Although many studies described the associations between pain and depressive symptoms in individuals with MS, few have reported on the prevalence of their co-occurrence.[3,6,13,14] A recent study using varying criteria to identify depression and pain in a community sample of people with MS reported that pain and depression co-occurred in 6% to 19% of the sample, depending on which criteria for pain and depression were used.[4] Pain was experienced by 86% to 100% of people meeting depression criteria, and pain of moderate severity was experienced by 67% to 77% of people meeting depression criteria. In contrast, 11% to 34% of people experiencing *any* pain met depression criteria and 15% to 37% of people experiencing pain of at least moderate severity met criteria for clinical depression. In a prior study of a community sample of people with MS, 53% of the people with pain reported having clinically significant levels of depressive symptoms.[6]

AMPLIFYING EFFECTS OF PAIN AND DEPRESSION ON ONE ANOTHER

Prior MS research has reported high associations between pain and depression, such that higher pain is associated with worse depressive symptoms.[3,6,13,14] This finding suggests the possibility that the presence of one condition amplifies the presence or severity of the other. Indeed, cross-sectional studies in MS[4] and longitudinal studies in the general population[15–17] have shown that chronic pain is a risk factor for subsequent depression; similarly, depression is a risk factor for chronic pain. At the same time, a substantial percentage of individuals with MS have only pain or depression,[4] suggesting that there may be both overlapping and unique aspects of the two conditions.[16]

When looking at studies in this area in individuals who do not have MS, the evidence is mixed regarding whether pain has a larger impact on depression than depression has on pain. For example, an earlier review of 191 studies examining the association between pain and depression in a large variety of patient and nonpatient samples reported consistent support for the *consequence* hypothesis (depression is influenced by the presence or severity of chronic pain) and inconsistent support for the *antecedent* hypothesis (depression precedes pain).[18] A recent longitudinal study of 95 adolescents diagnosed with chronic pain or depression reported evidence for a bidirectional association between depression and pain, although the impact of pain on depression was stronger than the impact of depression on pain.[19] In contrast, a study of 500 primary care patients with chronic musculoskeletal pain demonstrated that the two had an equally adverse impact on the other.[16] In their sample, change in severity of either depression or pain predicted a change in severity of the other symptom over time. Longitudinal research tracking pain and depression in people with MS would illuminate the nature and consequences of their relationships over time.

In the research literature outside of MS, researchers have suggested several reasons why pain and depression co-occur and why the presence of either pain or depression makes the other more likely.[15,16,18] In terms of pathophysiology, prior reviews of depression and pain have noted that central nociceptive and affective pathways overlap,[15,18] which supports the understanding that chronic pain is modulated centrally.[20] The experience of depressive symptoms and pain also share underlying neurotransmitters, with both norepinephrine and serotonin implicated in mood disorders and in the processing of pain. Beyond pathophysiology, there are potential psychological and behavioral reasons that pain and depression may amplify one another. For example, depressive symptoms have been found to impact the evaluative and affective aspects of pain and pain-related disability.[21,22] Pain often impacts the extent to which individuals engage in physical activity, which can limit an individual's participation in activities that were previously valued or enjoyed and, thus, puts the individual at risk for low mood.[23] Although it is highly likely that these same mechanisms play a role in individuals with MS, additional research is needed to understand the importance of these mechanisms and to understand whether additional, unique factors may also be implicated in the MS population.

OVERLAPPING IMPACT OF PAIN AND DEPRESSION ON FUNCTIONING AND QUALITY OF LIFE

Depression and chronic pain have a significant negative impact on individuals living with MS.[24] Major depression is associated with poorer neuropsychological functioning, lower quality of life, increased time lost from work, social disruption, and poorer health. Chronic pain in MS has been associated with poorer health-related quality of life, including greater interference with daily activities, energy/vitality, mental health, and social functioning.[3,6] Depression and pain have been linked to higher risk for unemployment[25]; both are also thought to affect fatigue negatively, another common and often disabling symptom of MS. For example, people with MS and clinically significant depressive symptoms are 6.2 times more likely to have disabling fatigue than nondepressed controls with MS.[26] Studies in MS have highlighted that higher levels of depressive symptoms and pain are associated with lower quality of life independent of other confounding symptoms.[27–31] Furthermore, research in other medical populations has shown that pain and depression have a reciprocal and additive adverse impact on quality of life and disability.[16,32]

Depression and pain may also impact the ability of a person with MS to self-manage their condition and its effects on daily life. Depression is thought to affect self-management through its adverse effects on energy, motivation, concentration, self-efficacy, and interpersonal interactions.[33] For example, a meta-analysis found that people with depression and chronic medical illness had a 3-fold higher rate of nonadherence to self-care regimens compared with nondepressed controls.[34] Consistent with these findings, depression has been associated with a decreased ability to manage MS symptoms, including adherence to disease-modifying medications.[35–37] Individuals with MS and chronic pain are also more likely to be inactive[13] and to report lower self-efficacy for managing their MS, including pain.[38] The extent to which comorbid pain and depression conjointly influence individuals' MS self-management is an area worthy of further exploration.

IMPACT ON TREATMENT UTILIZATION AND EFFECTIVENESS

Depression and pain likely influence health care utilization and treatment effectiveness. For example, in a recent study, the authors described how the rates of pain treatment utilization of patients with MS were higher among the subset of patients who were also depressed.[39] Individuals with comorbid pain and depression were found to have made more visits to medical providers for pain intervention, tried more pain treatments, and trended toward making more emergency department visits for pain intervention relative to individuals with pain alone. This finding is consistent with research in other medical populations that has shown that pain and depression are associated with higher rates of health care utilization.[40,41] In other medical conditions, pain and depression are also thought to reduce the effectiveness of treatments for the other condition (see Bair and colleagues[15,42] for a review of this literature). In other words, the presence of pain may interfere with depression treatment and vice versa. Such relationships have not been studied in people with MS, pain, and depression, however. Further, this prior research has suggested that the presence of pain distracts providers from detecting the presence of depression and subsequently results in the undertreatment of depression in pain populations.[15] Whether pain is a contributing factor to the underidentification and treatment of depression among patients with MS[11,43] is unknown.

INTERVENTIONS FOR COMORBID PAIN AND DEPRESSION

Descriptions of pharmacologic and cognitive-behavioral interventions for depression[2] and pain[1] have been provided in prior articles. However, the authors are unaware of research on combined treatments for depression and pain in MS, despite their co-occurrence and presumed bidirectional impact on each other. Effective treatment of depression has been shown to have a secondary effect of improving pain in primary care patients.[42] Research in other medical populations also points to the potential for successful treatment of comorbid pain and depression through antidepressant therapy, cognitive-behavioral therapy (CBT), and self-hypnosis training, although results have been far from definitive to this point.[15]

Antidepressants are commonly prescribed to patients with MS with neuropathic pain to address not only pain but also depression and sleep. However, little is known about the efficacy of antidepressants for treating neuropathic pain in MS.[13] Tricyclic antidepressants have some evidence for their efficacy in treating chronic pain in other neuropathic pain disorders,[44] although they are typically prescribed at doses lower than those needed for depression treatment. Side effects of tricyclic antidepressants can also be a deterrent to their use for pain and depression. There is also evidence that the serotonin-norepinephrine reuptake inhibitors duloxetine and venlafaxine are effective in the treatment of neuropathic pain in a range of conditions, although their efficacy in MS pain has not been studied.[13] Only a few antidepressants have been evaluated for their benefits in treating depression in MS via randomized controlled trials for depression,[45,46] and no studies were found reporting the benefits of treating depression with antidepressants on pain.

Among the available psychological treatments for depression and pain, CBT has the most evidence supporting its efficacy in individuals with MS. In a series of randomized controlled trials, Mohr and colleagues[35,46–49] demonstrated that CBT, delivered both in person and by telephone, is efficacious in reducing depression as well as fatigue, disability, and quality of life.[50] CBT for chronic pain has been less extensively studied in MS populations, although preliminary evidence in MS[51] and a substantial body of evidence in other painful conditions[52] support its use for chronic pain in MS. However, although CBT for depression and pain share many ingredients (such as relaxation training, cognitive restructuring, behavioral activation), treatments targeting both have not been developed or tested, to the authors' knowledge.

One of the treatments for pain with the longest history, hypnosis, had not been tested in controlled trials until recently. However, research has established its efficacy for several chronic pain conditions.[53,54] Even more recently, controlled trials of hypnosis in individuals with MS and chronic pain have demonstrated its efficacy for reducing pain intensity and pain interference.[55,56] In addition, preliminary research suggests that hypnotic interventions may also be effective for reducing depressive symptoms.[57-59] Although research is needed to confirm that hypnosis and hypnotic interventions are as effective in individuals with MS and depression as they are in individuals who present with pain or depression as a primary problem, there is no a priori reason to hypothesize the benefits would not generalize to an MS population.

UTILIZATION OF AND ACCESS TO INTERVENTIONS FOR COMORBID PAIN AND DEPRESSION

Outside of the development of treatments targeting the pain-depression comorbidity, a pressing issue is the ability of patients to access and appropriately use the interventions that are currently available. Specifically, prior research has shown that although effective treatments for pain and depression are available, these two conditions remain underidentified and undertreated in MS populations.[3,6,43,60] An estimated two-thirds of people with MS and major depression are untreated.[35,61,62] Similarly, although psychosocial interventions specifically targeting MS and depression have been found to be effective,[35] both real and perceived barriers impact the follow-through with depression treatment referrals.[63] The MS literature also reflects poor utilization of screening information to improve treatment referrals, even when screening is systematically implemented.[11] Pain is also inadequately treated; treatments that patients identify as most helpful are not necessarily the most frequently used, and non-pharmacologic pain management strategies are used at very low rates despite their potential to reduce pain and associated suffering.[55] (Ehde DM, Osborne TL, Hanley MA, et al. Use and perceived effectiveness of treatments for pain associated with multiple sclerosis. submitted for publication) These studies highlight the need to implement and evaluate new systems of care for pain and depression to address the undertreatment of depression and pain in people with MS.

INNOVATIVE APPROACHES TO THE MANAGEMENT OF COMORBID DEPRESSION AND PAIN

In other medical populations whereby depression and/or chronic pain are common, the collaborative care model has been found to be an effective systems-based approach to managing chronic comorbid conditions. This model emphasizes implementing systemic changes complete with self-management support, clinical information systems, delivery system redesign, decision support, health care organization, and community resources.[64,65] Health professionals are not simply colocated; they use established principles of chronic care management and interdisciplinary collaborative care teams in which professionals with complementary skills work closely together to care for a population of patients with complex medical conditions. Specialists and primary medical providers actively collaborate in providing integrated care, usually assisted by a care manager who guides patients collaboratively through various decisions about and aspects of care. The specialists, such as psychiatrists or pain specialists, supervise the care managers. The specialists are also available to consult primary medical providers on patients who are clinically challenging or who need additional specialty services and to see patients themselves when required. Collaborative care also typically features a stepped-care approach in which interventions are titrated based on the response to treatment. Collaborative care emphasizes measurement-based care, including screening and ongoing measurement and monitoring of treatment outcomes. Thus, the severity of problems such as depression and pain are repeatedly measured, and the treatment is systematically intensified or modified to ensure that the targeted improvements are achieved.

Collaborative care has repeatedly proven to be an effective model for maximizing access to, and efficacy of, medical treatment of chronic conditions. Collaborative care has improved depression outcomes and quality of care in patients with co-occurring chronic conditions, such as diabetes, coronary heart disease, and osteoarthritis.[60,66–72] A meta-analysis of 37 randomized controlled trials showed that collaborative care is more effective than standard care in improving short-term and long-term (up to 5 years) depression outcomes in primary care settings.[67] Recent trials have successfully tested collaborative care for patients with chronic pain (with or without depression) and produced useful benefits over usual care in improving pain, depression, and functional outcomes.[60,73–77]

The collaborative care approach is consistent with many of the conclusions of a 2002 MS stakeholder consensus conference on the identification and treatment of depression in MS.[43] Their recommendations for improving depression care in patients with MS included standardization of depression treatment, individualized care based on patient preferences, treatment to remission, and integrated biopsychosocial treatments that include options for both pharmacologic and psychosocial care.[43] Although they did not mention collaborative care in their published statement, their recommendations are consistent with a collaborative care model of depression care. Despite these recommendations made 10 years ago, collaborative care is not yet standard practice in MS care. In fact, the authors are aware of only one small, nonrandomized study that used the collaborative care model to treat depression in MS.[78] Results showed that at 6 months after baseline, fewer (33.3%) patients who received care management met diagnostic criteria for major depression relative to historical controls who received standard care (55.2%, $P = .15$). Although preliminary, this study supports the need for further evaluation of a collaborative care intervention, including by tailoring the intervention to match the needs of people with MS.

Given the tremendous barriers to receiving adequate behavioral health services,[79] an additional direction for future intervention development and research is the use of technology to deliver pain and depression care. Although not previously studied in people with MS, literature from other patient populations suggests that only one-third of patients with depression receive any psychotherapy.[80] Of these, 25% attend only one session and only 50% attend 4 or more sessions.[81,82] The barriers for people with MS may be even greater, spanning across limited transportation, inability to drive, and other motivational (eg, fatigue), cognitive, social, and financial problems that interfere with their ability to attend regularly scheduled in-person appointments. Telehealth and other forms of technology hold promise for overcoming some of these barriers to care in MS.

Evidence is building for the feasibility and efficacy of telehealth interventions in MS care. Various telehealth technologies have been used to treat MS-related fatigue,[83,84] to deliver MS self-management support,[85] and to monitor MS symptoms remotely.[86] It has also been used to treat depression and pain. In a series of randomized controlled trials, Mohr and colleagues[35,47,87] demonstrated that telephone-delivered CBT is efficacious in treating depression in MS. In the authors' clinical trials of behavioral interventions for pain, they have found telephone-delivered CBT to also be a feasible and effective treatment of reducing chronic pain and its negative impact on functioning in people with MS.[88] Neither of these lines of research specifically targeted both depression and pain, however. Telephone-based care overcomes some of the associated barriers as well as the potential stigma associated with seeking mental health care. Whether telehealth interventions will be adopted in real-world (eg, clinic) settings remains to be seen.

FUTURE DIRECTIONS FOR RESEARCH AND CLINICAL INTERVENTIONS

Research on the co-occurrence of pain and depression in MS is truly in its infancy. Recent research has yielded sufficient evidence to suggest that depression and pain are among the most common symptoms experienced by people with MS,[1,2] greater depression severity and greater pain severity are positively associated with each other, and clinical levels of depression and pain often co-occur.[3] Little research has been conducted on the effects of the pain-depression comorbidity on quality of life, treatment utilization, and clinical outcomes.

In recent research on depression and pain in non-MS populations, researchers have improved our understanding of depression, pain, and their impact on quality of life by examining longitudinal outcome trajectories using newer methods of data analysis (such as latent growth mixture modeling) to identify subsets of individuals with similar symptom trajectories.[89–91] As opposed to cross-sectional analyses that identify differential outcomes at a single time point or usual longitudinal analyses that rely on comparisons of group means or change scores over time, these longitudinal analyses provide information on distinct patterns that present over time for any given variable. These methods not only identify and describe subgroups of individuals with similar trajectories over time but can also identify baseline variables that are predictive of subgroup membership. Longitudinal research with this type of analysis would greatly improve our understanding of pain, depression, their comorbidity, and their impact on quality of life.

The authors' recent study, which found that the rates of pain treatment utilization of patients with MS were higher among those who were also depressed,[39] suggests that the impact of comorbid pain and depression on treatment utilization is an important area for future research. Furthermore, research from other settings suggesting that depression influences pain outcomes and pain influences depression outcomes[15,16] indicates that it would be worthwhile to explore the impact of pain and/or depression on treatment response in these conditions. Research is also needed on how comorbid pain and depression influence other important MS treatment outcomes, such as the adherence to disease-modifying therapies or rehabilitation interventions.

Clinically, there are many effective pharmacologic and psychological interventions for depression and pain,[1,2] but the authors are unaware of any research on the treatment of the pain-depression comorbidity in MS. There are good reasons, however, to think that existing treatments could be adapted to effectively treat this comorbidity. For example, duloxetine and venlafaxine have been shown to effectively treat depression and pain simultaneously in patients with fibromyalgia,[92] another population with highly comorbid pain and depression. Similarly, CBT is one of the most commonly used psychological interventions for depression and for pain, with standard protocols using similar components for both conditions, suggesting that it could be relatively easy to merge the two into a single, effective intervention. Finally, as noted earlier, hypnosis is effective in the treatment of pain and depression,[53–59] suggesting that a protocol could be developed to have an effect on the comorbidity.

Taken together, the available research on depression and pain in MS provides the impetus for further research in this area. By better understanding the patients who present with both pain and depression, clinicians can improve their tailoring of interventions for patients.[93] Consistent with the current trend in the mental health literature, transdiagnostic interventions could be effective in treating these comorbid problems that have so many shared elements.[94] Research expanding our understanding of and treatments for comorbid pain and depression will ultimately reduce their morbidity and improve outcomes for individuals with MS.

REFERENCES

1. Ehde DM, Osborne TL, Jensen MP. Chronic pain in persons with multiple sclerosis. Phys Med Rehabil Clin N Am 2005;16(2):503–12.
2. Ehde DM, Bombardier CH. Depression in persons with multiple sclerosis. Phys Med Rehabil Clin N Am 2005;16(2):437–48, ix.
3. O'Connor AB, Schwid SR, Herrmann DN, et al. Pain associated with multiple sclerosis: systematic review and proposed classification. Pain 2008;137(1): 96–111.
4. Alschuler KN, Ehde DM, Jensen MP. The co-occurrence of pain and depression in adults with multiple sclerosis. Rehabil Psychol 2013;58(2):217–21.
5. Alschuler KN, Jensen MP, Ehde DM. Defining mild, moderate, and severe pain in persons with multiple sclerosis. Pain Med 2012;13(10):1358–65.
6. Ehde DM, Gibbons LE, Chwastiak L, et al. Chronic pain in a large community sample of persons with multiple sclerosis. Mult Scler 2003;9(6):605–11.
7. Patten SB, Beck CA, Williams JV, et al. Major depression in multiple sclerosis: a population-based perspective. Neurology 2003;61(11):1524–7.
8. Patten SB, Metz LM, Reimer MA. Biopsychosocial correlates of lifetime major depression in a multiple sclerosis population. Mult Scler 2000;6(2):115–20.
9. Patten SB, Metz LM. Depression in multiple sclerosis. Psychother Psychosom 1997;66(6):286–92.
10. Sadovnick AD, Remick RA, Allen J, et al. Depression and multiple sclerosis. Neurology 1996;46(3):628–32.
11. Mohr DC, Hart SL, Julian L, et al. Screening for depression among patients with multiple sclerosis: two questions may be enough. Mult Scler 2007;13(2): 215–9.
12. Chwastiak L, Ehde DM, Gibbons LE, et al. Depressive symptoms and severity of illness in multiple sclerosis: epidemiologic study of a large community sample. Am J Psychiatry 2002;159(11):1862–8.
13. Ehde DM, Kratz AL, Robinson JP, et al. Chronic pain. In: Finlayson M, editor. Multiple sclerosis rehabilitation: from impairment to participation. London: Taylor & Francis; 2013. p. 199–226.
14. Arnett PA, Barwick FH, Beeney JE. Depression in multiple sclerosis: review and theoretical proposal. J Int Neuropsychol Soc 2008;14(5):691–724.
15. Bair MJ, Robinson RL, Katon W, et al. Depression and pain comorbidity: a literature review. Arch Intern Med 2003;163(20):2433–45.
16. Kroenke K, Wu J, Bair MJ, et al. Reciprocal relationship between pain and depression: a 12-month longitudinal analysis in primary care. J Pain 2011; 12(9):964–73.
17. Husted JA, Tom BD, Farewell VT, et al. Longitudinal study of the bidirectional association between pain and depressive symptoms in patients with psoriatic arthritis. Arthritis Care Res (Hoboken) 2012;64(5):758–65.

18. Fishbain DA, Cutler R, Rosomoff HL, et al. Chronic pain-associated depression: antecedent or consequence of chronic pain? A review. Clin J Pain 1997;13(2):116–37.
19. Lewandowski Holley A, Law EF, Zhou C, et al. Reciprocal longitudinal associations between pain and depressive symptoms in adolescents. Eur J Pain 2013; 17(7):1058–67.
20. Melzack R. Pain and the neuromatrix in the brain. J Dent Educ 2001;65(12): 1378–82.
21. Geisser ME, Gaskin ME, Robinson ME, et al. The relationship of depression and somatic focus to experimental and clinical pain in chronic pain patients. Psychol Health 1993;8(6):405–15.
22. Alschuler KN, Theisen-Goodvich ME, Haig AJ, et al. A comparison of the relationship between depression, perceived disability, and physical performance in persons with chronic pain. Eur J Pain 2008;12(6):757–64.
23. Fordyce WE. Behavioral methods for chronic pain and illness. St Louis (MO): Mosby; 1976.
24. Zwibel HL, Smrtka J. Improving quality of life in multiple sclerosis: an unmet need. Am J Manag Care 2011;17(Suppl 5 improving):S139–45.
25. Honarmand K, Akbar N, Kou N, et al. Predicting employment status in multiple sclerosis patients: the utility of the MS functional composite. J Neurol 2011; 258(2):244–9.
26. Chwastiak LA, Gibbons LE, Ehde DM, et al. Fatigue and psychiatric illness in a large community sample of persons with multiple sclerosis. J Psychosom Res 2005;59(5):291–8.
27. Göksel Karatepe A, Kaya T, Günaydn R, et al. Quality of life in patients with multiple sclerosis: the impact of depression, fatigue, and disability. Int J Rehabil Res 2011;34(4):290–8.
28. Kargarfard M, Eetemadifar M, Mehrabi M, et al. Fatigue, depression, and health-related quality of life in patients with multiple sclerosis in Isfahan, Iran. Eur J Neurol 2012;19(3):431–7.
29. Solaro C, Uccelli MM. Management of pain in multiple sclerosis: a pharmacological approach. Nat Rev Neurol 2011;7(9):519–27.
30. Brochet B, Deloire MS, Ouallet JC, et al. Pain and quality of life in the early stages after multiple sclerosis diagnosis: a 2-year longitudinal study. Clin J Pain 2009; 25(3):211–7.
31. Newland PK, Naismith RT, Ullione M. The impact of pain and other symptoms on quality of life in women with relapsing-remitting multiple sclerosis. J Neurosci Nurs 2009;41(6):322–8.
32. Arnow BA, Blasey CM, Lee J, et al. Relationships among depression, chronic pain, chronic disabling pain, and medical costs. Psychiatr Serv 2009;60(3):344–50.
33. Katon WJ. Clinical and health services relationships between major depression, depressive symptoms, and general medical illness. Biol Psychiatry 2003;54(3): 216–26.
34. DiMatteo MR, Lepper HS, Croghan TW. Depression is a risk factor for noncompliance with medical treatment: meta-analysis of the effects of anxiety and depression on patient adherence. Arch Intern Med 2000;160(14):2101–7.
35. Mohr DC, Likosky W, Bertagnolli A, et al. Telephone-administered cognitive-behavioral therapy for the treatment of depressive symptoms in multiple sclerosis. J Consult Clin Psychol 2000;68(2):356–61.
36. Mohr DC, Goodkin DE, Likosky W, et al. Treatment of depression improves adherence to interferon beta-1b therapy for multiple sclerosis. Arch Neurol 1997;54(5): 531–3.

37. Tarrants M, Oleen-Burkey M, Castelli-Haley J, et al. The impact of comorbid depression on adherence to therapy for multiple sclerosis. Mult Scler Int 2011; 2011:271321.
38. Osborne TL, Jensen MP, Ehde DM, et al. Psychosocial factors associated with pain intensity, pain-related interference, and psychological functioning in persons with multiple sclerosis and pain. Pain 2007;127(1–2):52–62.
39. Alschuler KN, Jensen MP, Ehde DM. The association of depression with pain-related treatment utilization in patients with multiple sclerosis. Pain Med 2012; 13(12):1648–57.
40. Katon W, Berg AO, Robins AJ, et al. Depression–medical utilization and somatization. West J Med 1986;144(5):564–8.
41. Rowan PJ, Davidson K, Campbell JA, et al. Depressive symptoms predict medical care utilization in a population-based sample. Psychol Med 2002;32(5):903–8.
42. Bair MJ, Robinson RL, Eckert GJ, et al. Impact of pain on depression treatment response in primary care. Psychosom Med 2004;66(1):17–22.
43. Goldman Consensus Group. The Goldman consensus statement on depression in multiple sclerosis. Mult Scler 2005;11(3):328–37.
44. Saarto T, Wiffen PJ. Antidepressants for neuropathic pain: a Cochrane review. J Neurol Neurosurg Psychiatry 2010;81(12):1372–3.
45. Ehde DM, Kraft GH, Chwastiak L, et al. Efficacy of paroxetine in treating major depressive disorder in persons with multiple sclerosis. Gen Hosp Psychiatry 2008;30(1):40–8.
46. Mohr DC, Boudewyn AC, Goodkin DE, et al. Comparative outcomes for individual cognitive-behavior therapy, supportive-expressive group psychotherapy, and sertraline for the treatment of depression in multiple sclerosis. J Consult Clin Psychol 2001;69(6):942–9.
47. Mohr DC, Hart SL, Julian L, et al. Telephone-administered psychotherapy for depression. Arch Gen Psychiatry 2005;62(9):1007–14.
48. Mohr DC, Hart SL, Goldberg A. Effects of treatment for depression on fatigue in multiple sclerosis. Psychosom Med 2003;65(4):542–7.
49. Mohr DC, Hart S, Vella L. Reduction in disability in a randomized controlled trial of telephone-administered cognitive-behavioral therapy. Health Psychol 2007;26(5): 554–63.
50. Cosio D, Jin L, Siddique J, et al. The effect of telephone-administered cognitive-behavioral therapy on quality of life among patients with multiple sclerosis. Ann Behav Med 2011;41(2):227–34.
51. Ehde DM, Jensen MP. Feasibility of a cognitive restructuring intervention for treatment of chronic pain in persons with disabilities. Rehabil Psychol 2004;49(3):254–8.
52. Eccleston C, Williams AC, Morley S. Psychological therapies for the management of chronic pain (excluding headache) in adults. Cochrane Database Syst Rev 2009;(2):CD007407.
53. Patterson DR, Jensen M. Hypnosis and clinical pain. Psychol Bull 2003;29: 495–521.
54. Jensen MP. Hypnosis for chronic pain management: a new hope. Pain 2009; 146(3):235–7.
55. Jensen MP, Ehde DM, Gertz KJ, et al. Effects of self-hypnosis training and cognitive restructuring on daily pain intensity and catastrophizing in individuals with multiple sclerosis and chronic pain. Int J Clin Exp Hypn 2011;59(1):45–63.
56. Jensen MP, Barber J, Romano JM, et al. A comparison of self-hypnosis versus progressive muscle relaxation in patients with multiple sclerosis and chronic pain. Int J Clin Exp Hypn 2009;57(2):198–221.

57. Alladin A. Cognitive hypnotherapy for major depressive disorder. Am J Clin Hypn 2012;54(4):275–93.

58. Alladin A. Evidence-based hypnotherapy for depression. Int J Clin Exp Hypn 2010;58(2):165–85.

59. Alladin A, Alibhai A. Cognitive hypnotherapy for depression: an empirical investigation. Int J Clin Exp Hypn 2007;55(2):147–66.

60. Lin EH, Katon W, Von Korff M, et al. Effect of improving depression care on pain and functional outcomes among older adults with arthritis: a randomized controlled trial. JAMA 2003;290(18):2428–9.

61. Feinstein A. An examination of suicidal intent in patients with multiple sclerosis. Neurology 2002;59(5):674–8.

62. Mohr DC, Hart SL, Fonareva I, et al. Treatment of depression for patients with multiple sclerosis in neurology clinics. Mult Scler 2006;12(2):204–8.

63. Mohr DC, Hart SL, Howard I, et al. Barriers to psychotherapy among depressed and nondepressed primary care patients. Ann Behav Med 2006;32(3):254–8.

64. Bodenheimer T, Wagner EH, Grumbach K. Improving primary care for patients with chronic illness: the chronic care model, part 2. JAMA 2002;288(15): 1909–14.

65. Bodenheimer T, Wagner EH, Grumbach K. Improving primary care for patients with chronic illness. JAMA 2002;288(14):1775–9.

66. Gilbody S, Bower P, Fletcher J, et al. Collaborative care for depression: a cumulative meta-analysis and review of longer-term outcomes. Arch Intern Med 2006; 166(21):2314–21.

67. Katon WJ, Von Korff M, Lin EH, et al. The Pathways Study: a randomized trial of collaborative care in patients with diabetes and depression. Arch Gen Psychiatry 2004;61(10):1042–9.

68. Katon WJ, Lin EH, Von Korff M, et al. Collaborative care for patients with depression and chronic illnesses. N Engl J Med 2011;363(27):2611–20.

69. Rollman BL, Belnap BH, LeMenager MS, et al. Telephone-delivered collaborative care for treating post-CABG depression: a randomized controlled trial. JAMA 2009;302(19):2095–103.

70. Roy-Byrne P, Craske MG, Sullivan G, et al. Delivery of evidence-based treatment for multiple anxiety disorders in primary care: a randomized controlled trial. JAMA 2010;303(19):1921–8.

71. Roy-Byrne PP, Craske MG, Stein MB, et al. A randomized effectiveness trial of cognitive-behavioral therapy and medication for primary care panic disorder. Arch Gen Psychiatry 2005;62(3):290–8.

72. Zatzick D, Roy-Byrne P, Russo J, et al. A randomized effectiveness trial of stepped collaborative care for acutely injured trauma survivors. Arch Gen Psychiatry 2004;61(5):498–506.

73. Kroenke K, Bair MJ, Damush TM, et al. Optimized antidepressant therapy and pain self-management in primary care patients with depression and musculoskeletal pain: a randomized controlled trial. JAMA 2009;301(20):2099–110.

74. Dobscha SK, Corson K, Perrin NA, et al. Collaborative care for chronic pain in primary care: a cluster randomized trial. JAMA 2009;301(12):1242–52.

75. Kroenke K, Theobald D, Wu J, et al. Effect of telecare management on pain and depression in patients with cancer: a randomized trial. JAMA 2010;304(2): 163–71.

76. Ahles TA, Wasson JH, Seville JL, et al. A controlled trial of methods for managing pain in primary care patients with or without co-occurring psychosocial problems. Ann Fam Med 2006;4(4):341–50.

77. Chelminski PR, Ives TJ, Felix KM, et al. A primary care, multi-disciplinary disease management program for opioid-treated patients with chronic non-cancer pain and a high burden of psychiatric comorbidity. BMC Health Serv Res 2005;5(1):3.

78. Patten SB, Newman S, Becker M, et al. Disease management for depression in an MS clinic. Int J Psychiatry Med 2007;37(4):459–73.

79. Simon GE, Von Korff M, Rutter CM, et al. Treatment process and outcomes for managed care patients receiving new antidepressant prescriptions from psychiatrists and primary care physicians. Arch Gen Psychiatry 2001;58(4):395–401.

80. Katon W, von Korff M, Lin E, et al. Adequacy and duration of antidepressant treatment in primary care. Med Care 1992;30(1):67–76.

81. Young AS, Klap R, Sherbourne CD, et al. The quality of care for depressive and anxiety disorders in the United States. Arch Gen Psychiatry 2001;58(1):55–61.

82. Horvitz-Lennon M, Normand SL, Frank RG, et al. "Usual care" for major depression in the 1990s: characteristics and expert-estimated outcomes. Am J Psychiatry 2003;160(4):720–6.

83. Moss-Morris R, McCrone P, Yardley L, et al. A pilot randomised controlled trial of an Internet-based cognitive behavioural therapy self-management programme (MS Invigor8) for multiple sclerosis fatigue. Behav Res Ther 2012;50(6):415–21.

84. Finlayson M, Preissner K, Cho C, et al. Randomized trial of a teleconference-delivered fatigue management program for people with multiple sclerosis. Mult Scler 2011;17(9):1130–40.

85. Miller DM, Moore SM, Fox RJ, et al. Web-based self-management for patients with multiple sclerosis: a practical, randomized trial. Telemed J E Health 2011; 17(1):5–13.

86. Zissman K, Lejbkowicz I, Miller A. Telemedicine for multiple sclerosis patients: assessment using health value compass. Mult Scler 2012;18(4):472–80.

87. Mohr DC, Vella L, Hart S, et al. The effect of telephone-administered psychotherapy on symptoms of depression and attrition: a meta-analysis. Clin Psychol (New York) 2008;15(3):243–53.

88. Ehde DM. Efficacy of telephone-delivered cognitive behavioral therapy for chronic pain. National Institutes of Health, National Institute of Child Health and Human Development, National Center for Medical Rehabilitation Research Grant; 2008-2013.

89. Dunn LB, Cooper BA, Neuhaus J, et al. Identification of distinct depressive symptom trajectories in women following surgery for breast cancer. Health Psychol 2011;30(6):683–92.

90. Miaskowski C, Cooper B, Paul SM, et al. Identification of patient subgroups and risk factors for persistent breast pain following breast cancer surgery. J Pain 2012;13(12):1172–87.

91. Bonanno GA, Kennedy P, Galatzer-Levy IR, et al. Trajectories of resilience, depression, and anxiety following spinal cord injury. Rehabil Psychol 2012; 57(3):236–47.

92. Bellato E, Marini E, Castoldi F, et al. Fibromyalgia syndrome: etiology, pathogenesis, diagnosis, and treatment. Pain Res Treat 2012;2012:426130.

93. Thieme K, Turk DC, Flor H. Responder criteria for operant and cognitive-behavioral treatment of fibromyalgia syndrome. Arthritis Rheum 2007;57(5): 830–6.

94. Craske MG. Transdiagnostic treatment for anxiety and depression. Depress Anxiety 2012;29(9):749–53.

Myofascial Pain Syndrome Treatments

Joanne Borg-Stein, MD*, Mary Alexis Iaccarino, MD

KEYWORDS

- Myofascial pain syndrome • Regional muscle pain • Treatment
- Myofascial trigger points • Pharmacotherapy

KEY POINTS

- Myofascial pain syndrome is a painful condition arising from myofascial trigger points.
- Treatment of myofascial pain syndrome consists of pharmacologic and nonpharmacologic interventions.
- Exercise and education are the mainstay treatments for all patients.
- Medications, physical modalities, dry needling, and trigger point injection are adjunct therapies that are appropriate in some patient subsets to treat myofascial pain and associated symptoms.

INTRODUCTION

Myofascial pain syndrome (MPS) is a painful condition of myofascial trigger points (MTrPs) in the skeletal muscle.[1] It can occur alone or in combination with other pain generators. MTrPs are focal areas of taut bands found in skeletal muscle that are hypersensitive to palpation. When manual pressure is applied over an MTrP, it produces a distinct local and referred pain that is consistent with the patient's presenting pain symptoms.[2] MPS is often grouped with other pain syndromes; however, it is distinct from diagnoses such as fibromyalgia in that it is focal, does not require multiple pain generators, and involves a taut band in skeletal muscle.[3]

EPIDEMIOLOGY

The prevalence of myofascial pain varies in the general population. In internal medicine and orthopedics clinics, the estimated prevalence is 21% to 30%. In a nationwide German study of more than 300 physicians experienced in treating patients with pain, 46% of patients had active MTrPs.[4] In other specialty pain clinics, estimates as high as 85% to 90% have been reported.[5] Unlike other chronic pain

This article originally appeared in Physical Medicine and Rehabilitation Clinics of North America, Volume 25, Issue 2, May 2014.
Department of Physical Medicine and Rehabilitation, Harvard Medical School, 300 First Avenue, Boston, MA 02129, USA
* Corresponding author.
E-mail address: jborgstein@partners.org

disorders, which are more prevalent in women, men and women are equally affected by MPS. However, studies in nationalized health care systems have found women to be more limited by musculoskeletal pain, with higher pain scores and more frequent absence from work.[6]

CLINICAL PRESENTATION

For a detailed review of clinical presentation, the reader is referred to the article on MPS diagnosis elsewhere in this issue by Dr Gerwin. Topics relevant to determining appropriate treatment of myofascial pain are discussed here.

MPS can be of insidious onset or occur as a result of trauma or injury. Patients complain of varying degrees of pain from mild to severe, characterized as deep and aching. Pain is focal and can have discrete referral patterns, which can help identify the muscle that contains the causative MTrP.[1] Patients may report associated autonomic dysfunction. Diaphoresis, lacrimation, flushing, dermatographia, pilomotor activity, and temperature change are common in MPS.[7] Cervical myofascial pain has been associated with vestibular symptoms, such as dizziness, blurred vision, and tinnitus.[8] Hyperesthesia, numbness, tingling, and twitching may occur if nearby nerves are irritated by the MTrPs. Decreased work tolerance, muscle fatigue, weakness, and other functional complaints may be present, and over time, mood and sleep disturbance can develop.[9–11] Eliciting associated symptoms and assessing their degree of impact on the patient is helpful in guiding treatment strategies.

Physical examination aids diagnosis and may guide treatment, particularly if local trigger point therapy is being considered. A thorough medical, neurologic, and musculoskeletal examination should be performed. Myofascial pain can be caused by postural stress, muscle imbalance, and repetitive overuse. Therefore biomechanics, joint function, and posture should be evaluated to assess their contribution.[12] Myofascial pain is associated with restricted range of motion. Muscles around the restricted area should be palpated for active MTrPs. To identify MTrPs, the examiner applies gentle pressure perpendicular to the muscle fibers. A taut band should be palpable, and direct pressure should produce significant pain, which reproduces the patient's local and referred symptoms.[12]

Laboratory studies may be useful to exclude systemic diagnoses, particularly when the clinical presentation is not definitive. In MPS, blood counts, chemistry and liver panel, erythrocyte sedimentation rate, and C-reactive protein levels are normal. A thyroid panel may be used to exclude thyroid disease as a cause of muscle pain. Radiography and advanced imaging may show concurrent osteoarthritis, diskogenic disease, neural irritation, and other mechanical changes. The relevance of these findings must be determined in individual cases based on the clinical scenario.

DIFFERENTIAL DIAGNOSIS

MPS and other muscle pain diagnoses can have overlapping and related symptoms. MTrPs occur insidiously or secondary to mechanical dysfunction and other disease states. Determining both primary and secondary causes of myofascial pain helps formulate a treatment plan. The following are questions that may aid clinicians in identifying contributing factors.

- Is there regional myofascial pain with trigger points present?
- Is myofascial pain the primary pain generator or are there other coexisting or underlying structural diagnoses?

- Is there a nutritional, metabolic, psychological, visceral, or inflammatory disorder contributing to the myofascial pain?
- Is there widespread pain that does not resemble the pattern associated with regional myofascial pain?

Table 1 provides a list of common differential diagnoses for myofascial pain. This list is not exhaustive. For a list of differential diagnoses by region of pain, please refer to the article on diagnosis of MPS elsewhere in this issue.

In difficult-to-treat cases with refractory pain symptoms, consider MPS when other diagnoses have been exhausted. In the literature, MPS has had uncommon presentations. It has been implicated in patients with chronic unilateral shoulder pain, lateral epicondylalgia, and chronic tension-type headache.[13–15] It has been found concurrently in the affected limb in patients with complex regional pain syndrome.[16] In a review of pelvic pain, symptoms of dysuria, dyspareunia, dyschezia, constipation, and

Table 1 Differential diagnosis for MPS	
Joint disorders	Zygapophyseal joint disorders Osteoarthritis Loss of normal joint motion
Inflammatory disorders	Polymyositis Polymyalgia rheumatica Rheumatoid arthritis
Neurologic disorders	Radiculopathy Entrapment neuropathy Metabolic myopathy
Regional soft tissue disorders	Bursitis Epicondylitis Tendonitis Cumulative trauma
Diskogenic disorders	Degenerative disk disease Annular tears Disk protrusion or herniation
Visceral referred pain	Gastrointestinal Cardiac Pulmonary Renal
Mechanical stress	Postural dysfunction Scoliosis Leg length discrepancy
Nutritional, metabolic, and endocrine disorders	Vitamin deficiency (B_1, B_{12}, D, calcium, folic acid, iron, magnesium) Alcoholic and toxic myopathy Hypothyroidism
Psychological disorders	Depression Anxiety Disordered sleep
Infectious disease	Viral illness Chronic hepatitis Bacterial or viral myositis
Widespread chronic pain	Fibromyalgia

From Borg-Stein J. Treatment of fibromyalgia, myofascial pain, and related disorders. Phys Med Rehabil Clin N Am 2006;17(2):491–510, viii; with permission.

testicular pain can be presenting symptoms of pelvic floor myofascial pain.[17] In a study of patients with suspected carpal tunnel syndrome, approximately one-third were found to have infraspinatus trigger points and normal nerve conduction studies, suggesting that MPS may mimic or be concurrent with carpal tunnel syndrome.[18] Postoperative myofascial pain after thoracotomy and mastectomy has also been described.[19–22]

TREATMENT OF MPS

Treatment of MPS targets MTrPs and aims to correct the structural and mechanical imbalance that prompted MTrP formation. Treatment should also address sympathetic dysfunction, identify emotional stressors, and treat late complications. The following is a discussion of therapeutic interventions for MPS. Education, pharmacotherapy, local needle therapy, and exercise serve to reduce pain and associated symptoms. Most often a combination of therapies is used simultaneously or in sequence and appropriate initial therapy is patient and provider dependent.

EDUCATION

- Based on the patient's symptoms and pain characteristics, a firm diagnosis of MPS should be made.
- Build rapport with the patient by approaching them with an attitude of empathy and understanding. Validate their concerns and reassure them that their symptoms are real and not psychogenic.
- In difficult-to-treat or refractory cases of pain, the patient may have had other diagnoses. The patient should be educated on the symptoms of MPS, and explanation should be provided as to why other diagnoses are less likely.
- Unnecessary tests should be avoided.
- Probable mechanisms of pain should be discussed in simple terms, emphasizing that the muscle pain associated with MPS is not dangerous and does not cause tissue damage.
- Inquire about associated symptoms.
- Determine what is most aggravating to the patient: intolerance to pain, loss of function, lack of sleep, or fear of underlying structural or catastrophic disease. Associated symptoms vary from patient to patient but help guide individual management.
- Educate the patient on each proposed modality of treatment: pharmacotherapy, manual modalities such as osteopathy or manual release, and injection.
- Recognize and address underlying psychosocial factors, such as depression, anxiety, stress at home or work, and poor coping skills.
- Educate the patient that psychological factors exacerbate pain. A few patients may require referral to mental health providers.
- Educate patients on the importance of restful sleep, cardiovascular fitness, and body mechanics to overall lifestyle.
- Promote behavioral modification through education, including cognitive behavioral techniques.

PHARMACOLOGIC MANAGEMENT

The pathophysiology of MPS is not completely understood. However, it is believed that there are local muscle, peripheral nerve, and central nervous system components. Therefore, medications that target each of these areas may be effective in treating

MPS. For each medication, it is important to consider mechanism of action and side effect profile, which is discussed in the addendum, in the context of individual patients. The adage of starting at a low dose and slowly increasing is important to patient tolerance and compliance. The side effect profile of medications is outlined in the article on side effects of commonly prescribed analgesic medications elsewhere in this issue.

Nonsteroidal Antiinflammatory Drugs

There is a paucity of literature on the use of oral nonsteroidal antiinflammatory drugs (NSAIDs) for MPS. Several studies show effectiveness for chronic pain and fibromyalgia in combination with other medications such as diazepam, alprazolam, cyclobenzaprine, and amitriptyline, but little is known on the efficacy of oral NSAIDs in MPS.[23–26] Topical NSAIDs have been shown to be useful in MPS. In general, they have fewer systemic side effects than oral NSAIDs but are often more expensive.[27] A study of diclofenac patch use in patients with upper trapezius myofascial pain found a significant reduction in pain based on visual analog scale, neck range of motion, and cervical disability index.[28] Despite limited evidence, NSAIDs are often part of MPS treatment because they are readily available and many patients are comfortable using them without physician input. Until further evidence is offered, providers should inquire about frequency of patient use, advise on the common side effects, monitor use in patients who find it helpful, and encourage discontinued use for those who find it ineffective.

Muscle Relaxants

Muscle relaxants are a group of drugs with varying pharmacology that act on the central nervous system to disrupt nociceptive pain.[29]

Cyclobenzaprine targets muscle relaxation without affecting muscle function. Its mechanism of action is not known, but its structure is similar to that of a tricyclic antidepressant. It is often used for both pain relief and sleep, because it has a sedating effect. In 41 patients with myofascial jaw pain, cyclobenzaprine was slightly better than clonazepam or placebo in pain relief but not more effective at improving sleep.[30] A Cochrane review in 2009[31] found that because of insufficient studies, there is not enough evidence to support its use in MPS. However, cyclobenzaprine is commonly prescribed for musculoskeletal pain and is well tolerated. In MPS, prescribing this medication at night can provide analgesia and promote sleep.

Tizanidine, an α_2-adrenergic agonist, acts centrally at the level of the spinal cord to inhibit spinal polysynaptic pathways and reduce the release of substance P.[32] Studies in animal models show that, in the thalamus, it reduces the release of neurotransmitters in ascending pathways involved in central sensitization.[33,34] In a prospective study of 29 women with MPS treated with tizanidine for 5 weeks,[35] pain, sleep, and disability all significantly improved. Tizanidine has a sedating effect and can cause hypotension, therefore dosing at night may limit noticeable side effects and aid sleep. This medication is also used for spasticity, with doses titrated up to 36 mg daily. In MPS, available studies have used lower doses of tizanidine with success.[36,37]

Benzodiazepines

Clonazepam and diazepam are benzodiazepine derivatives with multiple applications as anxiolytics, anticonvulsants, and muscle relaxants and are used in the treatment of MPS.[38] Most studies of MPS treatment with benzodiazepines were performed in a subset of patients with orofacial and temporomandibular pain.[26] In 2000, an open trial of clonazepam in patients with MPS from a multidisciplinary pain facility found a significant reduction in visual analog scale pain scores. However, of 46 participants, about 20% dropped out of the study because of intolerable side effects before reaching an effective dose.[39] The success of benzodiazepines on MPS may be targeting not only pain but also commonly associated symptoms, including muscle tension, anxiety, restless leg syndrome, and sleep disturbance. However, disadvantages to their use include a potent side effect profile, including ataxia, weakness, cognitive impairment, memory dysfunction, fatigue, depression, and adverse withdrawal symptoms.[29,40]

Serotonin and Norepinephrine Selective Reuptake Inhibitors and Tricyclic Antidepressants

There is an increasing role for antidepressants in the treatment of chronic pain, including tricyclic antidepressants, selective serotonin reuptake inhibitors (SSRIs), and serotonin norepinephrine reuptake inhibitors (SNRIs). Trials examining chronic tension headache and myofascial pain found amitriptyline to be effective for many patients.[41,42] A systematic review by Annaswamy and colleagues[43] supported the use of amitriptyline in some MPS conditions. Fewer studies have assessed the efficacy of nortriptyline.

An increasing body of evidence exists for the use of SSRIs and SNRIs in the treatment of fibromyalgia and other pain disorders.[44–46] There is little research on their use in regional muscle pain, such as MPS. However, these agents, particularly SNRIs, are used to treat regional myofascial pain. The rationale for their use stems from the fact that regional and widespread muscle pain have some overlap in signs and symptoms and approach to treatment. Thus, extrapolating from the chronic pain literature, SSRIs and SNRIs may be beneficial adjuvant pharmacotherapy. Should patients show signs and symptoms of mood disturbance in combination with MPS, antidepressant therapy may be warranted along with referral to a mental health professional.[47]

Tramadol

Tramadol is a weak opioid agonist and inhibits reuptake of serotonin and norepinephrine in the dorsal horns of the spinal cord. There are no published studies to support the use of tramadol in myofascial pain. However, several studies support its use in chronic widespread pain, chronic low back pain, and osteoarthritis, which are commonly associated with regional MPS.[48–51]

Lidocaine Patch

The lidocaine patch is a transdermal application of a local anesthetic with effective local penetration and limited systemic absorption. It has been proposed as an alternative treatment to needle injection of local anesthetics in patients with hypersensitivity associated with MPS. In a randomized control study, the lidocaine patch was effective in treatment of MPS. It did not generate as great a pain reduction score as needle infiltration, but patients were satisfied with its analgesic effect, and its use was associated with less discomfort than needle infiltration.[52]

Over-the-Counter Agents

There are a surplus of over-the-counter or nonprescription topical agents that are recommended for joint and muscle pain. Many of these products, such as Biofreeze, Salonpas, Icyhot, Tiger Balm, and others, use the active ingredient methyl salicylate or menthol to create a cool or warm sensation that dulls pain. Although published evidence for their use in myofascial pain is limited, some patients find that these medications have an analgesic effect. They can be used in combination with oral medications, although they should not be mixed or coadministered with other topical agents. In general, they are well tolerated and have minimal side effects.

NONPHARMACOLOGIC MANAGEMENT
Exercise for Myofascial Pain

Exercise is one of the most important aspects of rehabilitation and management of musculoskeletal pain. It helps to improve flexibility, increase functional status, optimize mood, and reduce pain.

Initiating a stretching exercise program is fundamental in MPS treatment. Stretching lengthens the tight bands of skeletal muscle that have become shortened and are causing pain. Stretching improves joint range of motion, leading to decreased pain, increased mobility, and restoration of normal activity. After optimal muscle length is restored and pain is reduced, adding strengthening to the exercise program can help establish new movement patterns and increase muscle endurance.[1] This goal can be achieved with the assistance of physical therapy to strengthen weak muscle groups, correct posture, and provide feedback so as not to overuse dominant muscle groups. For example, overuse of the upper trapezius and levator scapulae for shoulder motion can be corrected by stretching of the overactive muscles, and strengthening of scapular stabilizers, such as latissimus dorsi, rhomboids, and the lower trapezius. Patients should be encouraged to maintain an active lifestyle and incorporate a cardiovascular and aerobic fitness program into their routine. Educating patients on manual techniques, exercises, and stretches that relieve pain empowers patients to self-manage symptoms and effectively move from formal physical therapy to a home exercise program.[53] As pain relief improves, patients can resume normal activity, which improves function and prevents recurrence of MTrPs.

For some patients, the pain associated with MPS may preclude an effective exercise program, and other treatments, such as trigger point injection (TPI), may be required first. However, exercise should be incorporated into the treatment plan for all patients with MPS. Clinical experience suggests that leaving a muscle in a shortened position aggravates MTrPs and prevents resolution of symptoms.[2]

Postural, Mechanical, and Ergonomic Modifications

In occupational health and ergonomics research, there is evidence that repetitive loads in undesirable positions cause muscle pain and predispose workers to injury.[54–57] Theoretically, the overused or poorly conditioned muscle develops microtrauma and myofascial shortening, placing the muscle at risk of MTrP formation. Based on this theory, it is standard clinical practice to recommend correction of postural and ergonomic abnormalities.[58] Incorporating postural training for workers[59] and patients with temporomandibular joint pain has led to improvement in pain symptoms.[60] However, there are limited long-term efficacy data to support postural change as an effective treatment of myofascial pain. Nevertheless, in occupation-related injury or a situation in which a specific repetitive or strenuous task cannot be avoided, ergonomic modifications to correct abnormal postures are encouraged.

Stress Reduction

There are many types of interventions to reduce stress in MPS, including cognitive behavioral therapy (CBT), mediation and relaxation training, and biofeedback (**Table 2**). It is theorized that autonomic innervation to muscles may provide a link between stress and muscle pain. Thus, strategies to reduce emotional and physical stress may aid in treatment of MPS. McNulty and colleagues[61] found a higher increase

Table 2	
Stress reduction interventions	
CBT	A psychotherapy technique that facilitates behavior change by altering patients' beliefs or thought patterns
Meditation	Encompasses a variety of practice all with the similar goal of facilitating a sense of personal well-being or relaxation
Biofeedback	Any technique or device that increases awareness of physiologic changes in the body to improve emotions or change behavior

in needle electromyographic activity in trapezius MTrPs than in other areas of the muscle during psychological stress. A small study of patients with myofascial jaw pain found stress reduction intervention to be as effective as transcutaneous electrical nerve stimulation (TENS).[62] A randomized control trial of 3 months of CBT in chronic temporomandibular joint pain found improvements in pain, function, and activity after 1 year.[63] Stress reduction methods have also been shown to treat chronic pain, such as fibromyalgia.[64–66] Extrapolating from the fibromyalgia literature and incorporating the few studies on regional myofascial pain, stress reduction techniques and behavioral medicine may be useful adjunct therapies. However, further research would help to validate this intervention in the treatment of MPS.

Acupuncture

Acupuncture has been shown to be effective in treating myofascial pain.[67–72] In 2 Cochrane systematic reviews, acupuncture showed short-term benefit in mechanical neck pain and chronic low back pain when compared with sham acupuncture or no treatment.[67,68] Birch and Jamison[69] found that acupuncture alone over painful areas in the neck had better outcomes than NSAID treatment combined with acupuncture over nonpainful areas.

There are still several clinical questions about acupuncture that are unanswered, including number of needles used, duration of effect, and the mechanism by which it produces an antinociceptive effect. There is a close relationship between acupuncture points and trigger points, making the distinction between treatment with dry needling of MTrPs and local acupuncture more difficult to differentiate.[73] Overall, there is some evidence for the use of acupuncture as an adjunctive therapy for MPS, but further research is needed to determine treatment course and specific needling procedure.

Massage, Electrotherapy, and Ultrasonography

Massage is often sought as an alternative therapy for MPS. Anecdotal evidence and small clinic studies report it as an effective treatment; however, large vigorous trials are lacking. Two studies have found that combined with stretching, massage is helpful in reducing pain intensity and number of MTrPs.[74,75]

Several electrotherapies have been investigated for pain reduction of MTrPs, including TENS, electrical muscle stimulation (EMS), frequency-modulated neural stimulation (FREMS), and electrical twitch-obtaining intramuscular stimulation (ETOIMS). Compared with EMS or placebo, TENS has been found to be superior in pain reduction.[76–78] However, its effects seem limited to immediately after treatment, with 1 study finding no reduction in symptoms at 1 and 3 months after treatment.[78] In comparison, FREMS is shown to be as effective as TENS for myofascial pain, and its effect persisted at 3 months, whereas the TENS group did not.[79] ETOIMS, an emerging electrotherapy technique, acts on deep motor end plates to produce a muscle twitch. It has been used in MPS, but there are few studies and limited evidence on pain reduction.[80–82]

Ultrasound applies mechanical and thermal energy to tissue, and is believed to increase circulation, improve metabolism, and increase tissue pliability. Several studies have found that ultrasound alone, or in combination with exercise, improves pain in MPS.[75,83–85] Ay and colleagues[85] conducted a blinded randomized controlled trial, in which ultrasound was found to improve pain and number of MTrPs better than sham ultrasound. This study also found ultrasound alone to be as effective as ultrasound with diclofenac. Other studies of heat and antiinflammatory use with ultrasound have reported positive effect on pain in MPS.[86,87] In conclusion, ultrasound can be an effective adjunct therapy for MPS, and some patients may benefit from the addition of heat or antiinflammatory medication with ultrasound.

NEEDLING THERAPY

The regional pain associated with MPS stems from tight bands in the muscle called MTrPs. Dry needling and TPI are treatments that directly target MTrPs. Ordinarily, stretching and exercise are the foundation for pain reduction in MPS, but in the case of persistent MTrPs, providers can offer needling therapy.[88] Dry needling or TPI are most effective when they are accompanied by manual release of MTrPs and stretching that patients can perform themselves or with physical therapy.[89]

When needle therapy is necessary, it can be performed weekly over a series of several visits. At each visit, the amount of improvement and location of trigger points should be evaluated and compared with previous visits. When needling is used in combination with other therapies, some patients may find significant relief after only a few visits, whereas others may have recalcitrant areas that require more treatment. In general, TPI is performed as a series of injections. Patients need to be educated that there may be local soreness after injection, which should resolve, and that several treatments may be needed before results are noticeable.[3]

The hallmark of needling therapy is the production of a local twitch response in the targeted muscle. It is theorized that the needle mechanically disrupts and stops the dysfunctional activity of the motor end plate of the skeletal muscle motor neuron. Hong[90] described a fast-in–fast-out needling technique, which may be beneficial in eliciting maximal number of local twitch responses. In this technique, the needle penetrates the taut muscle band, is withdrawn to the superficial tissue, and then redirected to another area without coming out of the skin. Anesthetic can be injected when a twitch response is felt.

Dry needling is a low-risk intervention that is minimally invasive and inexpensive but requires training to achieve competence.[91,92] A prospective double-blind randomized controlled trial of 39 patients with MPS in an outpatient clinic found dry needling of MTrPs significantly reduced pain compared with sham dry needling.[93] A recent meta-analysis of dry needling in MPS found 3 studies in which dry needling improved pain in the cervicothoracic region both immediately and 4 weeks after treatment.[94]

Dry needling can be performed either superficially or deep. The technique of superficial dry needling is believed to deactivate MTrPs by stimulation of cutaneous A δ fibers without producing a muscle twitch response.[95] Conversely, deep dry needling targets muscular afferents and has been shown to produce greater pain reduction.[96] In a systematic review by Annaswamy and colleagues,[43] deep dry needling was found to be more effective than superficial dry needling for relief of pain from MTrPs. However, if there is a risk for damaging deep structures such as the lung or vasculature, the superficial method is preferred and is still efficacious. A preinjection block can be performed in the region or muscle of interest to allow more thorough and extensive needling with less patient discomfort. Preinjection blocks are also believed to block central sensitization and decrease any neurogenic component of the trigger point.[97]

TPI targets MTrPs by needle stimulation and treatment with anesthetics, steroids, or botulinum toxin. Shorter-acting and lower concentration anesthetic such as 0.25% lidocaine has shown to be less myotoxic than long-acting anesthetics like bupivacaine and less painful to inject than higher concentrations such as 1% lidocaine.[98,99] Although inflammation does play a role in MPS, the role of steroids in TPI is limited. A study of 45 patients with headache and MPS[100] found that steroid injection plus lidocaine produced a greater reduction of postinjection sensitivity than dry needling or lidocaine alone, but was no better at improving overall pain or cervical range of motion at 12 weeks.

Multiple systematic reviews, randomized controlled trials, and a Cochrane review have found no substantial evidence that injection provides more effective pain relief than dry needling alone.[85,100,101] Despite its limited evidence, anesthetic injection is still used in clinical practice. Because needling of MTrPs can cause local pain, the immediate antinociceptive effect of lidocaine and reduced latent soreness can improve the treatment experience overall. A single blinded randomized controlled trial of 29 patients with cervical MTrPs found TPI to be better than dry needling,[100] and Hong and colleagues[102] found that injection with lidocaine produced less postinjection soreness than dry needling alone. In addition, third-party payers in the United States reimburse for TPI but do not cover dry needling. Dry needling is an out-of-pocket expense for many patients, giving some preference to TPI. In the absence of significant adverse effect and recognizing the patient's cost burden, TPI may prove a useful treatment strategy. However, more research is needed to show the benefits of injection over dry needling.

Overall, there is no conclusive evidence that 1 needling technique is more effective than another. In their systemic literature review, Cummings and White concluded "because no technique is better than any other, we recommend that the method safest and most comfortable for the patient should be used."[101] Moreover, these techniques are based on the ability to accurately palpate and identify trigger points and discern them from other pain generators. In 1997, Gerwin[103] established that, with specialized training, interrater reliability in trigger point identification is good, but without training, localizing MTrPs and discerning twitch response during treatment is poor. Thus, using the technique that is most comfortable for the patient and with which the examiner is most proficient is likely to yield the best results.

Botulinum Toxin Injection

Botulinum toxin type A is a neurotoxic substance that is believed to act both centrally and peripherally to decrease pain. At the neuromuscular junction, it blocks the release of acetylcholine to prevent muscle hyperactivity and spasm. Its action at the neuromuscular junction allows it to target MTrPs, reducing local ischemia within muscles, and freeing entrapped nerve endings.[104] It has antinociceptive properties, preventing release of pain neurotransmitters at primary sensory neurons.[105] It also may act centrally, at the spinal and supraspinal levels,[106] and in the somatic and autonomic nervous system.[104] Botulinum toxin has an off-label use in myofascial pain and chronic musculoskeletal pain. Its multiple sites of action may prove beneficial not only to release tight MTrPs but also to disrupt nociceptive pain and treat associated autonomic symptoms.

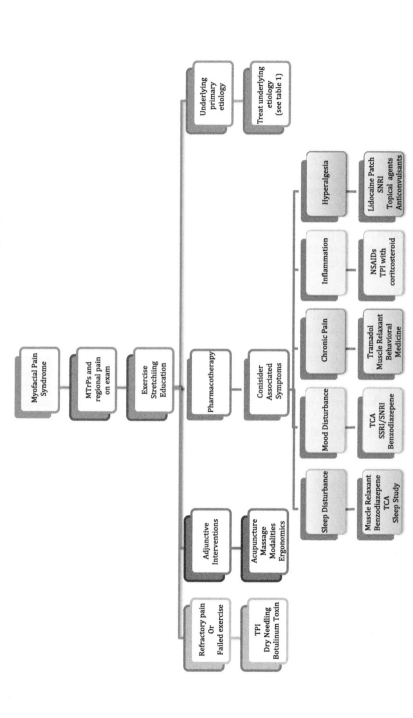

Fig. 1. MPS treatment summary. NSAIDs, nonsteroidal antiinflammatory drugs; SNRI, serotonin norepinephrine reuptake inhibitor; SSRI, selective serotonin reuptake inhibitor; TCA, tricyclic antidepressant; TPI, trigger point injection.

Studies on the efficacy of botulinum toxin in MPS are mixed. A 2012 Cochrane review[107] of botulinum toxin in MPS of the body (excluding the head and neck), evaluated 4 studies, including 233 patients, and found insufficient evidence for its use. Similarly, Ferrante and colleagues[108] conducted a randomized controlled trial of botulinum toxin for neck and shoulder pain and found it no better than placebo. Wheeler and colleagues[109] had similar results in the treatment of refractory cervicothoracic myofascial pain. However, other studies of MPS have found botulinum toxin to be beneficial.[110–114] In a multicenter randomized placebo-controlled trial of 145 patients with back and shoulder myofascial pain, Gobel and colleagues[115] found significant improvement in pain with botulinum toxin injection. Still other literature endorses that botulinum toxin may be best used in refractory cases of pain, taking advantage of its antinociceptive and muscular effects.[116]

Variations in study outcomes make the use of botulinum toxin difficult to endorse over other conservative, proven interventions. In a recent review by Gerwin,[117] the potential pitfalls of botulinum toxin studies were explored and an explanation offered for results variability. These pitfalls include a robust response to placebo, confounding variable in the control groups, incomplete treatments, and inappropriate periods between treatment and reassessment. More studies are required to better understand the role of botulinum toxin treatment in MPS.

SUMMARY

MPS is common in musculoskeletal practice, either as a primary or secondary pain disorder. As well as causing local muscle pain and limiting function, it can be associated with sympathetic dysfunction, emotional stressors, postural malalignment, and sleep disturbance. It is critically important to take a multifaceted approach to treatment (**Fig. 1**). Patient education and engagement in active training and exercise are necessary for functional restoration. Pharmacotherapy and needling therapy can be added to address primary complaints and comorbid symptoms. With a variety of tools available for treatment, MPS continues to be one of the most challenging yet rewarding musculoskeletal pain conditions to treat.

REFERENCES

1. Simons D, Travell J, Simons L. Myofascial Pain and Dysfunction: The Trigger Point Manual, Vol. 1. Upper Half of Body. Baltimore (MD): Williams & Wilkins; 1999.
2. Borg-Stein J, Simons DG. Focused review: myofascial pain. Arch Phys Med Rehabil 2002;83(3 Suppl 1):S40–7, S48–9.
3. Borg-Stein J. Treatment of fibromyalgia, myofascial pain, and related disorders. Phys Med Rehabil Clin N Am 2006;17(2):491–510, viii.
4. Fleckenstein J, Zaps D, Ruger LJ, et al. Discrepancy between prevalence and perceived effectiveness of treatment methods in myofascial pain syndrome: results of a cross-sectional, nationwide survey. BMC Musculoskelet Disord 2010; 11:32.
5. Gerwin RD. Classification, epidemiology, and natural history of myofascial pain syndrome. Curr Pain Headache Rep 2001;5(5):412–20.
6. Rollman GB, Lautenbacher S. Sex differences in musculoskeletal pain. Clin J Pain 2001;17(1):20–4.
7. Fricton JR, Kroening R, Haley D, et al. Myofascial pain syndrome of the head and neck: a review of clinical characteristics of 164 patients. Oral Surg Oral Med Oral Pathol 1985;60(6):615–23.

8. Krabak BJ, Borg-Stein J, Oas JA. Chronic cervical myofascial pain syndrome: improvement in dizziness and pain with a multidisciplinary rehabilitation program. A pilot study. J Back Musculoskelet Rehabil 2000;15(2):83–7.

9. Altindag O, Gur A, Altindag A. The relationship between clinical parameters and depression level in patients with myofascial pain syndrome. Pain Med 2008;9(2): 161–5.

10. Dohrenwend BP, Raphael KG, Marbach JJ, et al. Why is depression comorbid with chronic myofascial face pain? A family study test of alternative hypotheses. Pain 1999;83(2):183–92.

11. Schwartz RA, Greene CS, Laskin DM. Personality characteristics of patients with myofascial pain-dysfunction (MPD) syndrome unresponsive to conventional therapy. J Dent Res 1979;58(5):1435–9.

12. Hong C. Muscle pain syndromes. In: Braddom R, editor. Physical medicine and rehabilitation. Philadelphia: WB Saunders; 2011. p. 971–1002.

13. Bron C, Dommerholt J, Stegenga B, et al. High prevalence of shoulder girdle muscles with myofascial trigger points in patients with shoulder pain. BMC Musculoskelet Disord 2011;12:139.

14. Couppe C, Torelli P, Fuglsang-Frederiksen A, et al. Myofascial trigger points are very prevalent in patients with chronic tension-type headache: a double-blinded controlled study. Clin J Pain 2007;23(1):23–7.

15. Fernandez-Carnero J, Fernandez-de-Las-Penas C, de la Llave-Rincon AI, et al. Prevalence of and referred pain from myofascial trigger points in the forearm muscles in patients with lateral epicondylalgia. Clin J Pain 2007;23(4):353–60.

16. Rashiq S, Galer BS. Proximal myofascial dysfunction in complex regional pain syndrome: a retrospective prevalence study. Clin J Pain 1999;15(2):151–3.

17. Itza F, Zarza D, Serra L, et al. Myofascial pain syndrome in the pelvic floor: a common urological condition. Actas Urol Esp 2010;34(4):318–26.

18. Qerama E, Kasch H, Fuglsang-Frederiksen A. Occurrence of myofascial pain in patients with possible carpal tunnel syndrome–a single-blinded study. Eur J Pain 2009;13(6):588–91.

19. Diaz JH, Gould HJ 3rd. Management of post-thoracotomy pseudoangina and myofascial pain with botulinum toxin. Anesthesiology 1999;91(3):877–9.

20. Fernandez-Lao C, Cantarero-Villanueva I, Fernandez-de-Las-Penas C, et al. Development of active myofascial trigger points in neck and shoulder musculature is similar after lumpectomy or mastectomy surgery for breast cancer. J Bodyw Mov Ther 2012;16(2):183–90.

21. Hamada H, Moriwaki K, Shiroyama K, et al. Myofascial pain in patients with post-thoracotomy pain syndrome. Reg Anesth Pain Med 2000;25(3):302–5.

22. Karmakar MK, Ho AM. Postthoracotomy pain syndrome. Thorac Surg Clin 2004; 14(3):345–52.

23. Goldenberg DL, Felson DT, Dinerman H. A randomized, controlled trial of amitriptyline and naproxen in the treatment of patients with fibromyalgia. Arthritis Rheum 1986;29(11):1371–7.

24. Fossaluzza V, De Vita S. Combined therapy with cyclobenzaprine and ibuprofen in primary fibromyalgia syndrome. Int J Clin Pharmacol Res 1992; 12(2):99–102.

25. Russell IJ, Fletcher EM, Michalek JE, et al. Treatment of primary fibrositis/fibromyalgia syndrome with ibuprofen and alprazolam. A double-blind, placebo-controlled study. Arthritis Rheum 1991;34(5):552–60.

26. Singer E, Dionne R. A controlled evaluation of ibuprofen and diazepam for chronic orofacial muscle pain. J Orofac Pain 1997;11(2):139–46.

27. Castelnuovo E, Cross P, Mt-Isa S, et al. Cost-effectiveness of advising the use of topical or oral ibuprofen for knee pain; the TOIB study [ISRCTN: 79353052]. Rheumatology (Oxford) 2008;47(7):1077–81.
28. Hsieh LF, Hong CZ, Chern SH, et al. Efficacy and side effects of diclofenac patch in treatment of patients with myofascial pain syndrome of the upper trapezius. J Pain Symptom Manage 2010;39(1):116–25.
29. Frontera W, DeLisa J, Gans B, et al. Delisa's physical medicine and rehabilitation principles and practice. Philadelphia: Lippincott Williams & Wilkins; 2010.
30. Herman CR, Schiffman EL, Look JO, et al. The effectiveness of adding pharmacologic treatment with clonazepam or cyclobenzaprine to patient education and self-care for the treatment of jaw pain upon awakening: a randomized clinical trial. J Orofac Pain 2002;16(1):64–70.
31. Leite FM, Atallah AN, El Dib R, et al. Cyclobenzaprine for the treatment of myofascial pain in adults. Cochrane Database Syst Rev 2009;(3):CD006830.
32. Ono H, Mishima A, Ono S, et al. Inhibitory effects of clonidine and tizanidine on release of substance P from slices of rat spinal cord and antagonism by alpha-adrenergic receptor antagonists. Neuropharmacology 1991;30(6):585–9.
33. Hirata K, Koyama N, Minami T. The effects of clonidine and tizanidine on responses of nociceptive neurons in nucleus ventralis posterolateralis of the cat thalamus. Anesth Analg 1995;81(2):259–64.
34. Davies J. Selective depression of synaptic transmission of spinal neurones in the cat by a new centrally acting muscle relaxant, 5-chloro-4-(2-imidazolin-2-yl-amino)-2, 1, 3-benzothiodazole (DS103-282). Br J Pharmacol 1982;76(3):473–81.
35. Malanga GA, Gwynn MW, Smith R, et al. Tizanidine is effective in the treatment of myofascial pain syndrome. Pain Physician 2002;5(4):422–32.
36. Berry H, Hutchinson DR. A multicentre placebo-controlled study in general practice to evaluate the efficacy and safety of tizanidine in acute low-back pain. J Int Med Res 1988;16(2):75–82.
37. Berry H, Hutchinson DR. Tizanidine and ibuprofen in acute low-back pain: results of a double-blind multicentre study in general practice. J Int Med Res 1988;16(2):83–91.
38. Manfredini D, Landi N, Tognini F, et al. Muscle relaxants in the treatment of myofascial face pain. A literature review. Minerva Stomatol 2004;53(6):305–13.
39. Fishbain DA, Cutler RB, Rosomoff HL, et al. Clonazepam open clinical treatment trial for myofascial syndrome associated chronic pain. Pain Med 2000;1(4):332–9.
40. Harkins S, Linford J, Cohen J, et al. Administration of clonazepam in the treatment of TMD and associated myofascial pain: a double-blind pilot study. J Craniomandib Disord 1991;5(3):179–86.
41. Bendtsen L, Jensen R. Amitriptyline reduces myofascial tenderness in patients with chronic tension-type headache. Cephalalgia 2000;20(6):603–10.
42. Plesh O, Curtis D, Levine J, et al. Amitriptyline treatment of chronic pain in patients with temporomandibular disorders. J Oral Rehabil 2000;27(10):834–41.
43. Annaswamy TM, De Luigi AJ, O'Neill BJ, et al. Emerging concepts in the treatment of myofascial pain: a review of medications, modalities, and needle-based interventions. PM R 2011;3(10):940–61.
44. Arnold LM, Lu Y, Crofford LJ, et al. A double-blind, multicenter trial comparing duloxetine with placebo in the treatment of fibromyalgia patients with or without major depressive disorder. Arthritis Rheum 2004;50(9):2974–84.

45. Offenbaecher M, Ackenheil M. Current trends in neuropathic pain treatments with special reference to fibromyalgia. CNS Spectr 2005;10(4): 285–97.
46. Sayar K, Aksu G, Ak I, et al. Venlafaxine treatment of fibromyalgia. Ann Pharmacother 2003;37(11):1561–5.
47. Khatun S, Huq MZ, Islam MA, et al. Clinical outcomes of management of myofacial pain dysfunction syndrome. Mymensingh Med J 2012;21(2):281–5.
48. Rosenberg MT. The role of tramadol ER in the treatment of chronic pain. Int J Clin Pract 2009;63(10):1531–43.
49. Kean WF, Bouchard S, Roderich Gossen E. Women with pain due to osteoarthritis: the efficacy and safety of a once-daily formulation of tramadol. Pain Med 2009;10(6):1001–11.
50. Schnitzer TJ, Gray WL, Paster RZ, et al. Efficacy of tramadol in treatment of chronic low back pain. J Rheumatol 2000;27(3):772–8.
51. Wilder-Smith CH, Hill L, Spargo K, et al. Treatment of severe pain from osteoarthritis with slow-release tramadol or dihydrocodeine in combination with NSAID's: a randomised study comparing analgesia, antinociception and gastrointestinal effects. Pain 2001;91(1–2):23–31.
52. Affaitati G, Fabrizio A, Savini A, et al. A randomized, controlled study comparing a lidocaine patch, a placebo patch, and anesthetic injection for treatment of trigger points in patients with myofascial pain syndrome: evaluation of pain and somatic pain thresholds. Clin Ther 2009;31(4):705–20.
53. Lin SY, Neoh CA, Huang YT, et al. Educational program for myofascial pain syndrome. J Altern Complement Med 2010;16(6):633–40.
54. Treaster D, Marras WS, Burr D, et al. Myofascial trigger point development from visual and postural stressors during computer work. J Electromyogr Kinesiol 2006;16(2):115–24.
55. Edwards RH. Hypotheses of peripheral and central mechanisms underlying occupational muscle pain and injury. Eur J Appl Physiol Occup Physiol 1988; 57(3):275–81.
56. Madeleine P. On functional motor adaptations: from the quantification of motor strategies to the prevention of musculoskeletal disorders in the neck-shoulder region. Acta Physiol (Oxf) 2010;199(Suppl 679):1–46.
57. Hoyle JA, Marras WS, Sheedy JE, et al. Effects of postural and visual stressors on myofascial trigger point development and motor unit rotation during computer work. J Electromyogr Kinesiol 2011;21(1):41–8.
58. Bhatnager V, Drury CG, Schiro SG. Posture, postural discomfort, and performance. Hum Factors 1985;27(2):189–99.
59. Rota E, Evangelista A, Ciccone G, et al. Effectiveness of an educational and physical program in reducing accompanying symptoms in subjects with head and neck pain: a workplace controlled trial. J Headache Pain 2011;12(3): 339–45.
60. Komiyama O, Kawara M, Arai M, et al. Posture correction as part of behavioural therapy in treatment of myofascial pain with limited opening. J Oral Rehabil 1999;26(5):428–35.
61. McNulty WH, Gevirtz RN, Hubbard DR, et al. Needle electromyographic evaluation of trigger point response to a psychological stressor. Psychophysiology 1994;31(3):313–6.
62. Crockett DJ, Foreman ME, Alden L, et al. A comparison of treatment modes in the management of myofascial pain dysfunction syndrome. Biofeedback Self Regul 1986;11(4):279–91.

63. Turner JA, Mancl L, Aaron LA. Short- and long-term efficacy of brief cognitive-behavioral therapy for patients with chronic temporomandibular disorder pain: a randomized, controlled trial. Pain 2006;121(3):181–94.

64. Ferraccioli G, Ghirelli L, Scita F, et al. EMG-biofeedback training in fibromyalgia syndrome. J Rheumatol 1987;14(4):820–5.

65. Grossman P, Tiefenthaler-Gilmer U, Raysz A, et al. Mindfulness training as an intervention for fibromyalgia: evidence of postintervention and 3-year follow-up benefits in well-being. Psychother Psychosom 2007;76(4):226–33.

66. Kaplan KH, Goldenberg DL, Galvin-Nadeau M. The impact of a meditation-based stress reduction program on fibromyalgia. Gen Hosp Psychiatry 1993; 15(5):284–9.

67. Furlan AD, van Tulder M, Cherkin D, et al. Acupuncture and dry-needling for low back pain: an updated systematic review within the framework of the Cochrane Collaboration. Spine (Phila Pa 1976) 2005;30(8):944–63.

68. Peloso P, Gross A, Haines T, et al. Medicinal and injection therapies for mechanical neck disorders. Cochrane Database Syst Rev 2007;(3):CD000319.

69. Birch S, Jamison RN. Controlled trial of Japanese acupuncture for chronic myofascial neck pain: assessment of specific and nonspecific effects of treatment. Clin J Pain 1998;14(3):248–55.

70. Irnich D, Behrens N, Molzen H, et al. Randomised trial of acupuncture compared with conventional massage and "sham" laser acupuncture for treatment of chronic neck pain. BMJ 2001;322(7302):1574–8.

71. Ga H, Choi JH, Park CH, et al. Acupuncture needling versus lidocaine injection of trigger points in myofascial pain syndrome in elderly patients–a randomised trial. Acupunct Med 2007;25(4):130–6.

72. Zhang JF, Wu YC, Mi YQ. Observation on therapeutic effect of acupuncture at pain points for treatment of myofascial pain syndrome. Zhongguo Zhen Jiu 2009;29(9):717–20.

73. Melzack R, Stillwell DM, Fox EJ. Trigger points and acupuncture points for pain: correlations and implications. Pain 1977;3(1):3–23.

74. Trampas A, Kitsios A, Sykaras E, et al. Clinical massage and modified proprioceptive neuromuscular facilitation stretching in males with latent myofascial trigger points. Phys Ther Sport 2010;11(3):91–8.

75. Gam AN, Warming S, Larsen LH, et al. Treatment of myofascial trigger-points with ultrasound combined with massage and exercise–a randomised controlled trial. Pain 1998;77(1):73–9.

76. Ardic F, Sarhus M, Topuz O. Comparison of two different techniques of electrotherapy on myofascial pain. J Back Musculoskelet Rehabil 2002;16(1):11–6.

77. Graff-Radford SB, Reeves JL, Baker RL, et al. Effects of transcutaneous electrical nerve stimulation on myofascial pain and trigger point sensitivity. Pain 1989; 37(1):1–5.

78. Smania N, Corato E, Fiaschi A, et al. Repetitive magnetic stimulation: a novel therapeutic approach for myofascial pain syndrome. J Neurol 2005;252(3):307–14.

79. Farina S, Casarotto M, Benelle M, et al. A randomized controlled study on the effect of two different treatments (FREMS AND TENS) in myofascial pain syndrome. Eura Medicophys 2004;40(4):293–301.

80. Chu J, Schwartz I. eToims twitch relief method in chronic refractory myofascial pain (CRMP). Electromyogr Clin Neurophysiol 2008;48(6–7):311–20.

81. Chu J, Takehara I, Li TC, et al. Electrical twitch obtaining intramuscular stimulation (ETOIMS) for myofascial pain syndrome in a football player. Br J Sports Med 2004;38(5):E25.

82. Chu J, Yuen KF, Wang BH, et al. Electrical twitch-obtaining intramuscular stimulation in lower back pain: a pilot study. Am J Phys Med Rehabil 2004;83(2): 104–11.
83. Majlesi J, Unalan H. High-power pain threshold ultrasound technique in the treatment of active myofascial trigger points: a randomized, double-blind, case-control study. Arch Phys Med Rehabil 2004;85(5):833–6.
84. Srbely JZ, Dickey JP. Randomized controlled study of the antinociceptive effect of ultrasound on trigger point sensitivity: novel applications in myofascial therapy? Clin Rehabil 2007;21(5):411–7.
85. Ay S, Evcik D, Tur BS. Comparison of injection methods in myofascial pain syndrome: a randomized controlled trial. Clin Rheumatol 2010;29(1): 19–23.
86. Draper DO, Mahaffey C, Kaiser D, et al. Thermal ultrasound decreases tissue stiffness of trigger points in upper trapezius muscles. Physiother Theory Pract 2010;26(3):167–72.
87. Shin SM, Choi JK. Effect of indomethacin phonophoresis on the relief of temporomandibular joint pain. Cranio 1997;15(4):345–8.
88. Graff-Radford SB, Reeves JL, Jaeger B. Management of chronic head and neck pain: effectiveness of altering factors perpetuating myofascial pain. Headache 1987;27(4):186–90.
89. Edwards J, Knowles N. Superficial dry needling and active stretching in the treatment of myofascial pain–a randomised controlled trial. Acupunct Med 2003;21(3):80–6.
90. Hong CZ. Considerations and recommendations regarding myofascial trigger point injection. J Muscoskel Pain 1994;2(1):29–54.
91. Kalichman L, Vulfsons S. Dry needling in the management of musculoskeletal pain. J Am Board Fam Med 2010;23(5):640–6.
92. Tsai CT, Hsieh LF, Kuan TS, et al. Remote effects of dry needling on the irritability of the myofascial trigger point in the upper trapezius muscle. Am J Phys Med Rehabil 2010;89(2):133–40.
93. Tekin L, Akarsu S, Durmus O, et al. The effect of dry needling in the treatment of myofascial pain syndrome: a randomized double-blinded placebo-controlled trial. Clin Rheumatol 2013;32(3):309–15.
94. Kietrys DM, Palombaro KM, Azzaretto E, et al. Effectiveness of dry needling for upper quarter myofascial pain: a systematic review and meta-analysis. J Orthop Sports Phys Ther 2013;43(9):620–34.
95. Baldry P, Yunus M, Inanici F. Myofascial pain and fibromyalgia syndrome: a clinical guide to diagnosis and management. Edinburgh (United Kingdom): Churchill Livingstone; 2001.
96. Ceccherelli F, Rigoni MT, Gagliardi G, et al. Comparison of superficial and deep acupuncture in the treatment of lumbar myofascial pain: a double-blind randomized controlled study. Clin J Pain 2002;18(3):149–53.
97. Lennard T. Trigger point injections. In: Lennard T, editor. Pain procedures in clinical practice. Philadelphia: Elsevier; 2011. p. 89.
98. Iwama H, Akama Y. The superiority of water-diluted 0.25% to neat 1% lidocaine for trigger-point injections in myofascial pain syndrome: a prospective, randomized, double-blinded trial. Anesth Analg 2000;91(2):408–9.
99. Iwama H, Ohmori S, Kaneko T, et al. Water-diluted local anesthetic for trigger-point injection in chronic myofascial pain syndrome: evaluation of types of local anesthetic and concentrations in water. Reg Anesth Pain Med 2001;26(4): 333–6.

100. Venancio Rde A, Alencar FG, Zamperini C. Different substances and dry-needling injections in patients with myofascial pain and headaches. Cranio 2008;26(2):96–103.
101. Cummings TM, White AR. Needling therapies in the management of myofascial trigger point pain: a systematic review. Arch Phys Med Rehabil 2001;82(7): 986–92.
102. Hong CZ. Lidocaine injection versus dry needling to myofascial trigger point. The importance of the local twitch response. Am J Phys Med Rehabil 1994; 73(4):256–63.
103. Gerwin RD, Shannon S, Hong CZ, et al. Interrater reliability in myofascial trigger point examination. Pain 1997;69(1–2):65–73.
104. Casale R, Tugnoli V. Botulinum toxin for pain. Drugs R D 2008;9(1):11–27.
105. Aoki KR. Review of a proposed mechanism for the antinociceptive action of botulinum toxin type A. Neurotoxicology 2005;26(5):785–93.
106. Gobel H, Heinze A, Heinze-Kuhn K, et al. Botulinum toxin A for the treatment of headache disorders and pericranial pain syndromes. Nervenarzt 2001;72(4): 261–74.
107. Soares A, Andriolo RB, Atallah AN, et al. Botulinum toxin for myofascial pain syndromes in adults. Cochrane Database Syst Rev 2012;(4):CD007533.
108. Ferrante FM, Bearn L, Rothrock R, et al. Evidence against trigger point injection technique for the treatment of cervicothoracic myofascial pain with botulinum toxin type A. Anesthesiology 2005;103(2):377–83.
109. Wheeler AH, Goolkasian P, Gretz SS. A randomized, double-blind, prospective pilot study of botulinum toxin injection for refractory, unilateral, cervicothoracic, paraspinal, myofascial pain syndrome. Spine (Phila Pa 1976) 1998;23(15): 1662–6 [discussion: 1667].
110. Porta M. A comparative trial of botulinum toxin type A and methylprednisolone for the treatment of myofascial pain syndrome and pain from chronic muscle spasm. Pain 2000;85(1–2):101–5.
111. Fishman LM, Konnoth C, Rozner B. Botulinum neurotoxin type B and physical therapy in the treatment of piriformis syndrome: a dose-finding study. Am J Phys Med Rehabil 2004;83(1):42–50 [quiz: 51–3].
112. Lang AM. Botulinum toxin type B in piriformis syndrome. Am J Phys Med Rehabil 2004;83(3):198–202.
113. Fishman LM, Anderson C, Rosner B. BOTOX and physical therapy in the treatment of piriformis syndrome. Am J Phys Med Rehabil 2002;81(12):936–42.
114. Qerama E, Fuglsang-Frederiksen A, Kasch H, et al. A double-blind, controlled study of botulinum toxin A in chronic myofascial pain. Neurology 2006;67(2): 241–5.
115. Gobel H, Heinze A, Reichel G, et al. Efficacy and safety of a single botulinum type A toxin complex treatment (Dysport) for the relief of upper back myofascial pain syndrome: results from a randomized double-blind placebo-controlled multicentre study. Pain 2006;125(1–2):82–8.
116. Kamanli A, Kaya A, Ardicoglu O, et al. Comparison of lidocaine injection, botulinum toxin injection, and dry needling to trigger points in myofascial pain syndrome. Rheumatol Int 2005;25(8):604–11.
117. Gerwin R. Botulinum toxin treatment of myofascial pain: a critical review of the literature. Curr Pain Headache Rep 2012;16(5):413–22.

Autoinflammatory Disorders, Pain, and Neural Regulation of Inflammation

Michael C. Chen, PhD*, Matthew H. Meckfessel, PhD

KEYWORDS

- Autoinflammatory disorders • Neural crosstalk • IL-1β • Inflammasome • Pain
- Neuromodulation

KEY POINTS

- Current dermatologic disorders with predominant inflammatory components, such as rosacea and acne, possess hallmark features of autoinflammatory disorders.
- The contribution of interleukin-1 beta (IL-1β) in mediating pain through underlying neural pathways is underappreciated in the context of autoinflammatory disorders, and needs to be further explored.
- Disorders marked by increases in IL-1β in the absence of adaptive immune activation, in conjunction with inexplicable pain and inflammation, may be considered diagnostic criteria for classifying autoinflammatory disorders.
- Further exploration into the causative link between inflammation and the nervous system may lead to new therapeutic modalities for autoinflammatory disorders, such as neuromodulation.

INTRODUCTION

Autoinflammatory disorders are a newly described class of disorders marked predominantly by dysregulation of the innate immune system.[1] This heterogeneous class of disorders is clinically distinct from autoimmune disorders.[1-3] Autoinflammatory disorders are currently recognized as "clinical disorders marked by abnormally increased inflammation, mediated predominantly by the cells and molecules of the innate immune system, with a significant host predisposition."[1] Increased levels of interleukin-1 beta (IL-1β) cause abnormal inflammatory responses and are central to these disorders. Infection has yet to be found during episodic flares and does not

This article originally appeared in Dermatologic Clinics, Volume 31, Issue 3, July 2013.
Funding Sources/Support: Galderma Laboratories, L.P., Fort Worth, TX.
Conflict of Interest: None.
Galderma Laboratories, LP, 14501 North Freeway, Fort Worth, TX 76177, USA
* Corresponding author.
E-mail address: michael.chen@galderma.com

Clinics Collections 4 (2014) 457–469
http://dx.doi.org/10.1016/j.ccol.2014.10.030
2352-7986/14/$ – see front matter

seem to be a precipitating factor in the disorders. High-titer antibodies and antigen-specific autoreactive T cells are also absent.

A large number of disorders are now recognized as autoinflammatory and the number continues to grow. Affected systems are diverse and include skin, joints, and the nervous system.[1] The hereditary periodic fever (HPF) syndromes were among the first to be labeled as autoinflammatory.[2] Gout, type 2 diabetes, obesity-induced insulin resistance, Blau syndrome, and others are now classified as autoinflammatory.[1,4] Some autoinflammatory disorders, including pyogenic arthritis-pyoderma gangrenosum-acne (PAPA) syndrome and Blau syndrome, affect the skin.[5,6] Other dermatologic disorders with an inflammatory component, such as rosacea or acne, may potential be autoinflammatory disorders.

Many of the autoinflammatory disorders have a strong pain component that is overlooked. Episodic flares in the HPF syndromes and gout can cause debilitating pain. Cytokines, including IL-1β, and other inflammatory mediators are known to play important roles in neuronal perception of pain.[7] Thus abnormal innate immune responses may abnormally affect neuronal perception of pain. The nervous system plays an important role in regulating inflammation and inflammatory pain.[8] Neural-inflammation crosstalk may be disrupted in autoinflammatory disorders and contribute to the symptoms. Although crosstalk between inflammation and perception of pain is known to occur, it has not been highlighted in autoinflammatory disorders. Highlighting the inflammatory/neural crosstalk may allow a richer understanding of autoinflammatory disorders and potentially help to broaden the current disorder classification. This article provides an overview of current autoinflammatory disorders and how inexplicable inflammation and pain may factor into classifying new autoinflammatory disorders.

THE INFLAMMASOME

Identification of the inflammasome and its physiologic role helped to elucidate autoinflammatory disorders as being caused by dysregulation of the innate immune system. The inflammasome is a complex of proteins composed of a sensor protein, the adapter protein apoptosis-associated speck-like protein with CARD domain (ASC), and caspase-1.[9] Four sensor proteins have been identified: NLRP1, NLRP3, NLRC4, and AIM2.[10] Binding of stimuli to the sensor protein promotes assembly of the complex and activation of caspase-1. The NLRP1, NLRC4, and AIM2 inflammasomes are activated by specific microbial stimuli, whereas NLRP3 can be activated by a broad range of microbial and sterile stimuli.[4,9] Once activated, the inflammasome processes proIL-1β into its active form. IL-1β is a potent regulator of inflammatory responses. Activation of IL-1β in response to inflammatory stimuli is a 2-step process.[11] The first step involves increased production of proIL-1β. Basal expression of proIL-1β is low and is induced by nuclear factor (NF)-κB.[11] Activation of NF-κB occurs through pathogen-associated molecular patterns (PAMPs) that stimulate phagocytic cells or through primary cytokines.[12] The second step is activation of inflammasomes.

The NLRP3 inflammasome is the most studied inflammasome. Microbial activation can occur through bacteria, fungi, and viruses.[13–15] Unlike other inflammasomes, the NLRP3 inflammasome can be activated in sterile environments by nonmicrobial stimuli; extracellular ATP, monosodium crystals, calcium pyrophosphate dehydrate crystals, cholesterol crystals, and oligomers of islet amyloid polypeptide are all capable of activating NLRP3 inflammasomes.[16–19] Several of these nonmicrobial activators are also involved in the pathogenesis of other diseases with a strong inflammatory component such as gout and type 2 diabetes. Thus a broad range of stimuli or genetic defects can cause dysregulation of the innate immune system and induce an autoinflammatory response. In the established HPF syndromes and the emerging autoinflammatory disorders, dysregulation of the innate immune system, specifically the inflammasome, is at the epicenter and abnormal inflammasome activity results in increased IL-1β levels.

INFLAMMASOME AUTOACTIVATION DISORDERS

Familial Mediterranean fever (FMF) is an HPF disorder. Patients with FMF experience episodic bouts of fever and serosal inflammation lasting up to 3 days and occurring every 10 days to once a year.[20] During attacks, patients also experience debilitating muscle and joint pain.[21] Defects in the *MEFV* gene encoding for pyrin have been found to cause FMF.[22] Pyrin is a regulator of capsase-1 activation. The defective pyrin protein causes an overactive inflammasome, which leads to increased levels of IL-1β.[23]

Mutations in the *PSTPIP1* (proline-serine-threonine-phosphatase interacting protein 1) gene have been identified as the cause of PAPA syndrome.[24] PAPA syndrome is an autosomal dominant hereditary syndrome that has some clinical similarities to FMF. Sterile arthritis of the knees, elbows, and ankles develops in early childhood in patients with PAPA.[25] Symptoms also include cystic acne and pyoderma gangrenosum, which last into adulthood and may cause debilitating pain.[5] Infection has yet to be found in cultures from skin lesions or joint fluids.[5,24] PSTPIP1 interacts with pyrin to regulate inflammasome activity.[26] Mutations result in hyperphosphorylation of PSTPIP1 disrupting regulation of the NLRP3 inflammasome, which causes increased production of IL-1β.

The cryopyrin-associated periodic syndromes (CAPSs) are a group of 3 syndromes that are also HPF syndromes: familial cold autoinflammatory syndrome (FCAS), Muckle-Wells syndrome (MWS), and neonatal-onset multisystem inflammatory disease (NOMID). FCAS is the least severe and is characterized by cold-induced fever and rashes.[11] MWS is more severe and is accompanied by hearing loss and arthritis. NOMID is the most severe and is characterized by chronic fever, hives, hearing loss, overgrowth of the epiphyses of the long bones, chronic meningitis, cerebral atrophy, and delayed atrophy.[27] All 3 are caused by inherited or de novo mutations in the *NLRP3/CIAS1* gene (previously called cryopyrin).[28,29] The encoded NLRP3 protein is defective in regulation and is constitutively active.[30] Subjects afflicted with any of the CAPSs have increased levels of IL-1β. Biologic therapies for the CAPSs target IL-1β and are effective in managing the disorders.[31,32] Although CAPS is caused by defects in *NLRP3*, the causes of increased levels of IL-1β and the origin of the IL-1β remain unknown. It is also unknown why CAPSs only affect certain organs and not others. Mouse models of CAPS have been developed which will help to address these questions.[33,34]

METABOLITE AUTOINFLAMMATORY DISEASES

Gout is an autoinflammatory disorder marked by severe swelling and pain of the joints. Attacks are recurring and acute, and, if left untreated, can progress into chronic tophaceous gout.[35] Gout is caused by an accumulation of monosodium urate (MSU) crystals. However, MSU crystals are not the sole causative agent in gout.[36] One study investigated what effect MSU crystals or free fatty acids (FFAs) had on human peripheral blood mononuclear cells (PBMCs) and murine macrophages in vitro.[37] Neither produced IL-1β when exposed to MSU crystals or FFAs alone. When PBMCs or murine macrophages were simultaneously exposed to both, large amounts of IL-1β were produced. Thus accumulation of MSU crystals and FFAs activate the NLRP3 inflammasome, resulting in increased levels of IL-1β.[17] This finding is consistent with the clinical manifestation of gout frequently occurring during night. Released IL-1β then binds IL-1 receptors on macrophages, which leads to additional production of proinflammatory cytokines and chemokines.[38]

Mevalonate kinase deficiency (MKD; formerly called hyperimmunoglobulinemia D syndrome [HIDS]) is an HPF syndrome caused by a recessively inherited defect in the mevalonate kinase gene.[39] Mevalonate kinase is the second enzyme in the meval-onate pathway of cholesterol synthesis. Deficiencies result in reduced levels of down-stream metabolites. Episodic attacks last longer than those associated with FMF. Symptoms can include abdominal pain, headache, cervical lymphadenopathy, arthritis, and diarrhea.[40] Dysregulation of the inflammasome in HIDS has also been identified.[41] Experiments that inhibited mevalonate kinase by alendronate in human PBMCs treated with lipopolysaccharide (LPS) resulted in a 20-fold increase in NLRP3 expression and increased levels of secreted IL-1β. When treated with alendr-onate or LPS alone, NLRP3 expression was only increased approximately 2.5-fold. Basal levels of NLRP3 in PBMCs isolated from 2 subjects with MKD were also increased. When these PBMCs were stimulated with just LPS, levels of IL-1β increased. Thus a functioning mevalonate kinase gene and downstream metabolites are necessary for proper inflammasome regulation. Similar to gout, it also seems that multiple stimuli are required to elicit an autoinflammatory response in MKD.

Type 2 diabetes is now recognized as an autoinflammatory disease.[36] High levels of glucose stimulate beta cells to produce IL-1β, indicating a direct role for IL-1β in the disease.[42] Glucose, FFAs, and leptin all induce production of IL-1β from human is-lets.[43–45] Adipocyte differentiation and insulin resistance are controlled by caspase-1 activation and production of IL-1β.[46] Inhibition of IL-1β improves insulin sensitivity. Taken together, these results highlight the central role of IL-1β in type 2 diabetes and confirm its classification as autoinflammatory.

NF-κB DISEASES

Tumor necrosis factor (TNF) receptor–associated periodic syndrome (TRAPS) was the first disorder to be recognized as autoinflammatory.[47] TRAPS is a dominantly inherited disorder characterized by episodic periods of fever, abdominal pain, migratory erythema, myalgia, and periorbital edema.[48] Molecular cloning identified a missense mutation in the TNFRSF1A gene, which encodes for a TNF receptor.[47] Mutations result in increased activity of NF-κB and, ultimately, increased production of IL-1β.

Blau syndrome is an autosomal dominant hereditary disease with a childhood onset.[6] Symptoms include iritis, skin rash, granulomatous arthritis, and periarticular synovial cysts. Blau syndrome is caused by mutations in the NOD2 gene.[49–51] NOD2 is a cytosolic protein that recognizes muramyl dipeptide (MDP), the minimal active peptidoglycan motif common to bacteria.[52,53] On MDP recognition, NOD2 ac-tivates and interacts with RIP2 activating NF-κB. Mutations in NOD2 cause excessive activation and signaling of NF-κB, resulting in increased IL-1β levels.[51]

AUTOINFLAMMATORY DISORDERS DOWNSTREAM OF IL-1β

Deficiency of the IL-1 receptor agonist (DIRA) is a recently described autoinflammatory disorder.[54,55] Symptoms present within 2.5 weeks of birth and include fetal distress, pustular rash, joint swelling, oral mucosal lesions, pain with movement, and cutaneous pustulosis.[54] The pathogenesis of DIRA is caused by deletion or truncation of the IL1RN gene.[55,56] Patients with DIRA fail to produce a functioning IL-1 receptor agonist (IL1RA), which plays a crucial role in modulating the effects of IL-1β at the receptor level. Other autoinflammatory disorders can be traced to mutations or changes to stimuli upstream of IL-1β production or activation, but DIRA is unique because the disorder is caused by defects downstream of IL-1β.

AUTOINFLAMMATORY PAIN

There are 3 types of recognized pain: nociceptive, neuropathic, and inflammatory.[57] Nociceptive pain is the result of noxious stimuli activating sensory neurons. Nociceptors respond to temperature, chemical, and mechanical stimuli. Neuropathic pain arises from damage or dysfunction to the nervous system. Normal sensory cells generate action potentials from the end of the nerve at the receptive field. Damaged nerve cells can generate pathologic ectopic discharges from the site of injury, and healthy nerve fibers near damaged nerves can also spontaneously generate pain.[58,59] Ectopic and spontaneous pain are examples of neuropathic pain. Inflammatory pain results from damaged tissue, cancer cells, and other inflamed tissues, which release inflammatory mediators known as an inflammatory soup that modulates nociceptors to perceive pain.[57] Posttranslational modification to nociceptors alters their response, making them more sensitive to pain. Peripheral nociceptors are normally dormant in the absence of stimuli. When activated, they produce an acute response that provides a warning of eminent danger and plays an essential function in an organism's survival.

In particular, IL-1β hypersensitizes nociceptors and proinflammatory cytokines play an important role in hyperalgesia and inflammatory pain.[60–62] Part of this response is alterations of periphery nociceptors that reduce their threshold and increase their sensitivity.[63] The goal of hyperalgesia is to heighten pain awareness to prevent further injury to the afflicted area. Dysregulation of IL-1β can result in increased nociceptor sensitization and eventually neuropathic pain.[64] Attacks and increased levels of IL-1β are episodic in the HPF syndromes; associated pain is acute and does not progress into neuropathic pain. Other autoinflammatory disorders that are not episodic may have associated chronic pain.

The symptoms of gout are extremely painful. Gout initially presents as acute flares, but can progress into a chronic state. Activation of IL-1β produces increased levels of inflammatory mediators and chemokines, which create an influx of neutrophils into the joint. In addition to the direct role that IL-1β has in modulating pain, neutrophils may also have hyperalgesic properties.[65] Chemokines are also important in modulating pain.[66] Thus IL-1β may not only increase pain in gout but also amplify it. Treatment of gout with anakinra, a recombinant IL-1 receptor antagonist, or canakinumab, an anti–IL-1β monoclonal antibody, improves symptoms of acute and chronic tophaceous gout.[67–69] Blocking or inhibiting the effects of IL-1β in treating gout reinforces the central role IL-1β has in autoinflammation as well as pain.

Given the important role that IL-1β plays in pain modulation, subjects with type 2 diabetes frequently experience peripheral neuropathic pain.[70] However, only 3% to 25% of subjects experience peripheral neuropathic pain.[71] Why only a small portion of subjects with type 2 diabetes experience peripheral neuropathic pain is unclear. Clinical trials with anakinra in subjects with type 2 diabetes showed improvements in beta-cell function and inflammation.[72,73] Current pain management therapies for type 2 diabetes do not target IL-1β function. Treatments include lipoic acid, tricyclic antidepressants, gabapentin, pregabalin, duloxetine, and oxycodone.[71] Because of the central role IL-1β plays in pain, IL-1β antagonists and blockers could be potential therapeutic agents for pain relief as well as for helping to manage symptoms in subjects with type 2 diabetes.

The link between autoinflammation and pain is further underscored in animal models. One study screened *N*-ethyl-*N*-nitrosourea (ENU)–mutated mice to identify a mouse model for pain.[74] This line showed abnormal nociceptor responses and was hypersensitive to pain. The line also showed symptoms of autoinflammation. These mice showed normal behavior and were otherwise healthy. A mutation in the *PSTPIP2* gene, the same gene implicated in PAPA syndrome, was identified as the causative factor. A successful screen for a pain model in mice yielded a mutation known to cause an autoinflammatory disorder. The identification of this mouse model highlights the importance of pain in autoinflammatory disorder and how the two are interconnected.

POTENTIAL AUTOINFLAMMATORY DISORDERS

All of the disorders discussed thus far have 2 commonalities: unprovoked inflammation and pain. Dysregulation of the innate immune system is the causative agent in these diseases. However, the underlying cause of many disorders has yet to be identified. Are other disorders with seemingly inexplicable inflammation and a pain component autoinflammatory?

INTERSTITIAL CYSTITIS

Interstitial cystitis (IC) is a chronic inflammatory disorder affecting the bladder. IC is characterized by pelvic or perineal pain, urinary urgency and frequency, and nocturia.[75] IC is also marked with a strong pain component and is frequently called painful bladder syndrome. In the absence of a causative factor in IC, management is difficult. Current strategies to manage the symptoms of IC include behavior modification, pentosan polysulfate sodium, amitriptyline, hydroxyzine, and dimethyl sulfoxide.[76] IC is clinically distinct from other bladder and urinary disorders even though symptoms overlap. The cause of IC is not well understood. No diagnostic exists for IC and diagnostic tests are used to rule out other diseases.[77] Markers of inflammation have been identified in subjects with IC. Infiltration of mast cells into the bladder was identified in histologic analysis.[78] Urine samples collected over 24 hours in subjects with IC were increased in antiproliferative factor, epidermal growth factor, insulin growth factor–binding protein 3, and IL-6 compared with healthy subjects.[79] Urine and serum levels of nerve growth factor are also increased in subjects with IC.[80] However, urine markers do not always correlate with biopsy findings.[81] No direct evidence indicates that IC is an autoimmune disease, and there is no evidence of infection.[82,83] Does that indicate that IC is an autoinflammatory disease? Immunohistochemical analysis of tissue from the urothelial layer of the bladder showed the presence of NLRP3.[84] This finding suggests that the inflammasome may play a role in mediating bladder inflammation. The presence of mast cells may also indicate that IC is an autoinflammatory disorder. Mast cells are the source of IL-1β in urticarial rash in CAPS disorders.[85] Given the chronic inflammation, absence of an autoimmune response or infection, infiltrated mast cells, and the presence of NLRP3 in urothelial tissue from the bladder, it is plausible that dysregulation of the NLRP3 inflammasome and increased IL-1β may play a role in the cause of IC. Future studies in patients with IC should address this possibility.

ROSACEA

Rosacea is a chronic disease of the face characterized by flushing, persistent erythema, telangiectasia, papules, and pustules. Rosacea flares are frequently triggered by external stimuli such as ultraviolet (UV) light or temperature changes. The molecular and cellular mechanisms underlying rosacea have yet to be identified. Clinical and histopathologic analyses indicate that rosacea is the result of inflammatory processes.[86] Dysregulation of the innate immune system and an abnormal response to innocuous stimuli have been proposed as underlying causes of rosacea.[87] UV light, a rosacea trigger, is known to induce IL-1β and TNF-α in human skin.[88] UV light also activates inflammasomes in keratinocytes.[89] Biopsies taken from patients with rosacea revealed an increase in mast cells.[90] As discussed earlier, mast cells are a source of IL-1β production. Subjects with rosacea can also experience pain with changes in temperature that are normally perceived as benign.[91] Abnormal signaling by the transient receptor potential (TRP) channels TRPA1 and TRPV1 are thought to play a role in temperature pain. These receptors are located on periphery neurons and may release neurotransmitters that could increase inflammation. An abnormal response to stimuli, infiltration of mast cells, and the presence of pain indicate that rosacea has commonalities with other autoinflammatory disorders.

SUMMARY

Autoinflammatory disorders constitute a large and growing class of disorders (summarized in **Table 1**). Disorders that are seemingly unrelated, such as FMF, type 2 diabetes, and gout, are all similar because of dysregulation of the innate immune system, specifically IL-1β. Although the inflammatory components of these disorders are well recognized, the neural components underlying pain and regulation are not. Crosstalk between the neural networks and inflammatory machinery allows additional levels of regulation to fine tune inflammatory responses. Inflammation modulates pain responses to help protect the organism against further harm, whereas neurotransmitters inhibit inflammatory mediators to ease inflammation. This interplay is highlighted in the mouse model identified from a screen for a pain model that also had autoinflammatory disease. Further emphasizing the link between inflammation and the nervous system is that therapeutic neuromodulation of IC provides symptomatic relief of inflammatory symptoms.[92] Perhaps neuromodulation could also be a therapeutic option for other autoinflammatory disorders. The neural regulation of the inflammatory component in autoinflammatory disorders warrants further investigation. It is conceivable that

Table 1	
Autoinflammatory disorders discussed in this review and their causes	
Inflammasome Autoactivation Disorders Metabolite Disorders	
FMF	*MEFV*
PAPA	*PSTPIP1*
CAPS	*NLRP3*
NF-kB Disorders	
Blau syndrome	*NOD2*
TRAPS	*TNFRSF1A*
Metabolite Disorders	
Gout	MSU crystals and FFAs
MKD	Melavonate kinase
Type 2 diabetes	Glucose, FFAs, leptin
Potential Autoinflammatory Disorders	
Rosacea	Unknown
IC	Unknown

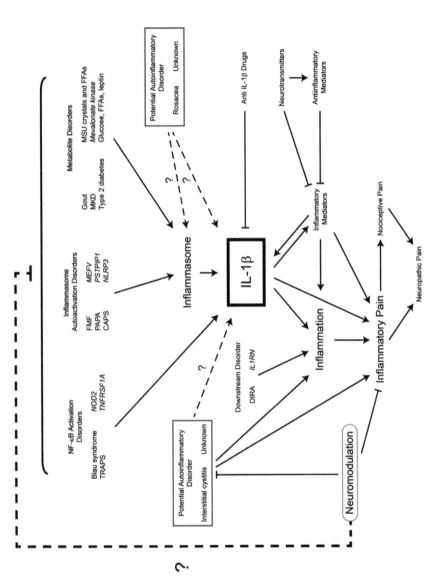

Fig. 1. Overview of known autoinflammatory disorders, potential autoinflammatory disorders, and their interplay with pain. Known and possible therapeutic options are also shown.

mutations or deficiencies in the nervous system could elicit unwarranted inflammatory responses. Perhaps neural dysfunction is the causative agent in disorders with an inflammatory component that have not had the underlying mechanisms identified.

Fig. 1 provides an overview of autoinflammatory disorders discussed in this article and their interplay with neural pathways. Other disorders with unexplained inflammation and pain may be autoinflammatory disorders. IC and rosacea each are marked by inflammation and pain. Thus, in the absence of an autoimmune component, these two diseases may be autoinflammatory. Other diseases that fit these criteria may also be classified as autoinflammatory as their causes become better understood, such as psoriasis or Behçet Disease. Taken together, the body of evidence supports a larger role for neural networks in pain and inflammatory regulation in autoinflammatory disorders than is currently appreciated.

REFERENCES

1. Kastner DL, Aksentijevich I, Goldbach-Mansky R. Autoinflammatory disease reloaded: a clinical perspective. Cell 2010;140(6):784–90.
2. Brydges S, Kastner DL. The systemic autoinflammatory diseases: inborn errors of the innate immune system. Curr Top Microbiol Immunol 2006;305: 127–60.
3. Kambe N, Satoh T, Tanizaki H, et al. Enhanced NF-kappaB activation with an in-flammasome activator correlates with activity of autoinflammatory disease associated with NLRP3 mutations outside of exon 3: comment on the article by Jeru et al. Arthritis Rheum 2010;62(10):3123–4 [author reply: 3124–5].
4. Menu P, Vince JE. The NLRP3 inflammasome in health and disease: the good, the bad and the ugly. Clin Exp Immunol 2011;166(1):1–15.
5. Smith EJ, Allantaz F, Bennett L, et al. Clinical, molecular, and genetic character-istics of PAPA syndrome: a review. Curr Genomics 2010;11(7):519–27.
6. Pastores GM, Michels VV, Stickler GB, et al. Autosomal dominant granulomatous arthritis, uveitis, skin rash, and synovial cysts. J Pediatr 1990;117(3):403–8.
7. Basbaum AI, Bautista DM, Scherrer G, et al. Cellular and molecular mechanisms of pain. Cell 2009;139(2):267–84.
8. Kavoussi B, Ross BE. The neuroimmune basis of anti-inflammatory acupuncture. Integr Cancer Ther 2007;6(3):251–7.
9. Gross O, Thomas CJ, Guarda G, et al. The inflammasome: an integrated view. Immunol Rev 2011;243(1):136–51.
10. Franchi L, Eigenbrod T, Munoz-Planillo R, et al. The inflammasome: a caspase-1-activation platform that regulates immune responses and disease pathogenesis. Nat Immunol 2009;10(3):241–7.
11. Ozkurede VU, Franchi L. Immunology in clinic review series; focus on autoinflam-matory diseases: role of inflammasomes in autoinflammatory syndromes. Clin Exp Immunol 2012;167(3):382–90.
12. Bauernfeind FG, Horvath G, Stutz A, et al. Cutting edge: NF-kappaB activating pattern recognition and cytokine receptors license NLRP3 inflammasome activa-tion by regulating NLRP3 expression. J Immunol 2009;183(2):787–91.
13. Franchi L, Munoz-Planillo R, Reimer T, et al. Inflammasomes as microbial sensors. Eur J Immunol 2010;40(3):611–5.
14. Joly S, Sutterwala FS. Fungal pathogen recognition by the NLRP3 inflammasome. Virulence 2010;1(4):276–80.
15. Rathinam VA, Fitzgerald KA. Inflammasomes and anti-viral immunity. J Clin Immu-nol 2010;30(5):632–7.

16. Ferrari D, Pizzirani C, Adinolfi E, et al. The P2X7 receptor: a key player in IL-1 processing and release. J Immunol 2006;176(7):3877–83.

17. Martinon F, Petrilli V, Mayor A, et al. Gout-associated uric acid crystals activate the NALP3 inflammasome. Nature 2006;440(7081):237–41.

18. Duewell P, Kono H, Rayner KJ, et al. NLRP3 inflammasomes are required for atherogenesis and activated by cholesterol crystals. Nature 2010;464(7293): 1357–61.

19. Masters SL, Dunne A, Subramanian SL, et al. Activation of the NLRP3 inflammasome by islet amyloid polypeptide provides a mechanism for enhanced IL-1beta in type 2 diabetes. Nat Immunol 2010;11(10):897–904.

20. Sohar E, Gafni J, Pras M, et al. Familial Mediterranean fever. A survey of 470 cases and review of the literature. Am J Med 1967;43(2):227–53.

21. Feng J, Zhang Z, Li W, et al. Missense mutations in the MEFV gene are associated with fibromyalgia syndrome and correlate with elevated IL-1beta plasma levels. PLoS One 2009;4(12):e8480.

22. Ancient missense mutations in a new member of the RoRet gene family are likely to cause familial Mediterranean fever. The International FMF Consortium. Cell 1997;90(4):797–807.

23. Yildirim K, Uzkeser H, Keles M, et al. Relationship between serum interleukin-1beta levels and acute phase response proteins in patients with familial Mediterranean fever. Biochem Med (Zagreb) 2012;22(1):109–13.

24. Nesterovitch AB, Hoffman MD, Simon M, et al. Mutations in the PSTPIP1 gene and aberrant splicing variants in patients with pyoderma gangrenosum. Clin Exp Dermatol 2011;36(8):889–95.

25. Contassot E, Beer HD, French LE. Interleukin-1, inflammasomes, autoinflammation and the skin. Swiss Med Wkly 2012;142:w13590.

26. Shoham NG, Centola M, Mansfield E, et al. Pyrin binds the PSTPIP1/CD2BP1 protein, defining familial Mediterranean fever and PAPA syndrome as disorders in the same pathway. Proc Natl Acad Sci U S A 2003;100(23):13501–6.

27. Prieur AM. A recently recognised chronic inflammatory disease of early onset characterised by the triad of rash, central nervous system involvement and arthropathy. Clin Exp Rheumatol 2001;19(1):103–6.

28. Hoffman HM, Mueller JL, Broide DH, et al. Mutation of a new gene encoding a putative pyrin-like protein causes familial cold autoinflammatory syndrome and Muckle-Wells syndrome. Nat Genet 2001;29(3):301–5.

29. Feldmann J, Prieur AM, Quartier P, et al. Chronic infantile neurological cutaneous and articular syndrome is caused by mutations in CIAS1, a gene highly expressed in polymorphonuclear cells and chondrocytes. Am J Hum Genet 2002; 71(1):198–203.

30. Agostini L, Martinon F, Burns K, et al. NALP3 forms an IL-1beta-processing inflammasome with increased activity in Muckle-Wells autoinflammatory disorder. Immunity 2004;20(3):319–25.

31. Hoffman HM, Throne ML, Amar NJ, et al. Efficacy and safety of rilonacept (interleukin-1 Trap) in patients with cryopyrin-associated periodic syndromes: results from two sequential placebo-controlled studies. Arthritis Rheum 2008;58(8):2443–52.

32. Lachmann HJ, Kone-Paut I, Kuemmerle-Deschner JB, et al. Use of canakinumab in the cryopyrin-associated periodic syndrome. N Engl J Med 2009;360(23):2416–25.

33. Brydges SD, Mueller JL, McGeough MD, et al. Inflammasome-mediated disease animal models reveal roles for innate but not adaptive immunity. Immunity 2009; 30(6):875–87.

34. Meng G, Zhang F, Fuss I, et al. A mutation in the Nlrp3 gene causing inflamma-some hyperactivation potentiates Th17 cell-dominant immune responses. Immunity 2009;30(6):860–74.
35. Dalbeth N, Haskard DO. Mechanisms of inflammation in gout. Rheumatology (Oxford) 2005;44(9):1090–6.
36. Dinarello CA. Blocking interleukin-1beta in acute and chronic autoinflammatory diseases. J Intern Med 2011;269(1):16–28.
37. Joosten LA, Netea MG, Mylona E, et al. Engagement of fatty acids with Toll-like receptor 2 drives interleukin-1beta production via the ASC/caspase 1 pathway in monosodium urate monohydrate crystal-induced gouty arthritis. Arthritis Rheum 2010;62(11):3237–48.
38. Kingsbury SR, Conaghan PG, McDermott MF. The role of the NLRP3 inflamma-some in gout. J Inflamm Res 2011;4:39–49.
39. Simon A, Cuisset L, Vincent MF, et al. Molecular analysis of the mevalonate kinase gene in a cohort of patients with the hyper-igd and periodic fever syndrome: its application as a diagnostic tool. Ann Intern Med 2001;135(5):338–43.
40. Goldfinger S. The inherited autoinflammatory syndrome: a decade of discovery. Trans Am Clin Climatol Assoc 2009;120:413–8.
41. Pontillo A, Paoluzzi E, Crovella S. The inhibition of mevalonate pathway induces upregulation of NALP3 expression: new insight in the pathogenesis of mevalo-nate kinase deficiency. Eur J Hum Genet 2010;18(7):844–7.
42. Maedler K, Sergeev P, Ris F, et al. Glucose-induced beta cell production of IL-1beta contributes to glucotoxicity in human pancreatic islets. J Clin Invest 2002;110(6):851–60.
43. Boni-Schnetzler M, Thorne J, Parnaud G, et al. Increased interleukin (IL)-1beta messenger ribonucleic acid expression in beta -cells of individuals with type 2 diabetes and regulation of IL-1beta in human islets by glucose and autostimula-tion. J Clin Endocrinol Metab 2008;93(10):4065–74.
44. Boni-Schnetzler M, Boller S, Debray S, et al. Free fatty acids induce a proinflam-matory response in islets via the abundantly expressed interleukin-1 receptor I. Endocrinology 2009;150(12):5218–29.
45. Maedler K, Sergeev P, Ehses JA, et al. Leptin modulates beta cell expression of IL-1 receptor antagonist and release of IL-1beta in human islets. Proc Natl Acad Sci U S A 2004;101(21):8138–43.
46. Stienstra R, Joosten LA, Koenen T, et al. The inflammasome-mediated caspase-1 activation controls adipocyte differentiation and insulin sensitivity. Cell Metab 2010;12(6):593–605.
47. McDermott MF, Aksentijevich I, Galon J, et al. Germline mutations in the extracel-lular domains of the 55 kDa TNF receptor, TNFR1, define a family of dominantly inherited autoinflammatory syndromes. Cell 1999;97(1):133–44.
48. Turner MD, Chaudhry A, Nedjai B. Tumour necrosis factor receptor trafficking dysfunction opens the TRAPS door to pro-inflammatory cytokine secretion. Biosci Rep 2012;32(2):105–12.
49. Tromp G, Kuivaniemi H, Raphael S, et al. Genetic linkage of familial granuloma-tous inflammatory arthritis, skin rash, and uveitis to chromosome 16. Am J Hum Genet 1996;59(5):1097–107.
50. Miceli-Richard C, Lesage S, Rybojad M, et al. CARD15 mutations in Blau syn-drome. Nat Genet 2001;29(1):19–20.
51. van Duist MM, Albrecht M, Podswiadek M, et al. A new CARD15 mutation in Blau syndrome. Eur J Hum Genet 2005;13(6):742–7.

52. Girardin SE, Boneca IG, Viala J, et al. Nod2 is a general sensor of peptidoglycan through muramyl dipeptide (MDP) detection. J Biol Chem 2003;278(11):8869–72.
53. Inohara N, Ogura Y, Fontalba A, et al. Host recognition of bacterial muramyl dipeptide mediated through NOD2. Implications for Crohn's disease. J Biol Chem 2003;278(8):5509–12.
54. Aksentijevich I, Masters SL, Ferguson PJ, et al. An autoinflammatory disease with deficiency of the interleukin-1-receptor antagonist. N Engl J Med 2009;360(23): 2426–37.
55. Reddy S, Jia S, Geoffrey R, et al. An autoinflammatory disease due to homozygous deletion of the IL1RN locus. N Engl J Med 2009;360(23):2438–44.
56. Jesus AA, Osman M, Silva CA, et al. A novel mutation of IL1RN in the deficiency of interleukin-1 receptor antagonist syndrome: description of two unrelated cases from Brazil. Arthritis Rheum 2011;63(12):4007–17.
57. Scholz J, Woolf CJ. Can we conquer pain? Nat Neurosci 2002;5(Suppl):1062–7.
58. Janig W, Grossmann L, Gorodetskaya N. Mechano- and thermosensitivity of regenerating cutaneous afferent nerve fibers. Exp Brain Res 2009;196(1):101–14.
59. Wu G, Ringkamp M, Hartke TV, et al. Early onset of spontaneous activity in uninjured C-fiber nociceptors after injury to neighboring nerve fibers. J Neurosci 2001;21(8):RC140.
60. Binshtok AM, Wang H, Zimmermann K, et al. Nociceptors are interleukin-1beta sensors. J Neurosci 2008;28(52):14062–73.
61. Watkins LR, Maier SF. Beyond neurons: evidence that immune and glial cells contribute to pathological pain states. Physiol Rev 2002;82(4):981–1011.
62. Milligan ED, Twining C, Chacur M, et al. Spinal glia and proinflammatory cytokines mediate mirror-image neuropathic pain in rats. J Neurosci 2003;23(3):1026–40.
63. Hucho T, Levine JD. Signaling pathways in sensitization: toward a nociceptor cell biology. Neuron 2007;55(3):365–76.
64. Ren K, Torres R. Role of interleukin-1beta during pain and inflammation. Brain Res Rev 2009;60(1):57–64.
65. Cunha TM, Verri WA Jr. Neutrophils: are they hyperalgesic or anti-hyperalgesic? J Leukoc Biol 2006;80(4):727–8 [author reply: 729–30].
66. Kiguchi N, Kobayashi Y, Kishioka S. Chemokines and cytokines in neuroinflammation leading to neuropathic pain. Curr Opin Pharmacol 2012;12(1):55–61.
67. So A, De Smedt T, Revaz S, et al. A pilot study of IL-1 inhibition by anakinra in acute gout. Arthritis Res Ther 2007;9(2):R28.
68. McGonagle D, Tan AL, Shankaranarayana S, et al. Management of treatment resistant inflammation of acute on chronic tophaceous gout with anakinra. Ann Rheum Dis 2007;66(12):1683–4.
69. So A, De Meulemeester M, Pikhlak A, et al. Canakinumab for the treatment of acute flares in difficult-to-treat gouty arthritis: results of a multicenter, phase II, dose-ranging study. Arthritis Rheum 2010;62(10):3064–76.
70. Boulton AJ, Malik RA, Arezzo JC, et al. Diabetic somatic neuropathies. Diabetes Care 2004;27(6):1458–86.
71. Tesfaye S, Boulton AJ, Dyck PJ, et al. Diabetic neuropathies: update on definitions, diagnostic criteria, estimation of severity, and treatments. Diabetes Care 2010;33(10):2285–93.
72. Larsen CM, Faulenbach M, Vaag A, et al. Interleukin-1-receptor antagonist in type 2 diabetes mellitus. N Engl J Med 2007;356(15):1517–26.
73. Larsen CM, Faulenbach M, Vaag A, et al. Sustained effects of interleukin-1 receptor antagonist treatment in type 2 diabetes. Diabetes Care 2009;32(9):1663–8.

74. Chen TC, Wu JJ, Chang WP, et al. Spontaneous inflammatory pain model from a mouse line with N-ethyl-N-nitrosourea mutagenesis. J Biomed Sci 2012;19:55.
75. Marshall K. Interstitial cystitis: understanding the syndrome. Altern Med Rev 2003;8(4):426–37.
76. Lau TC, Bengtson JM. Management strategies for painful bladder syndrome. Rev Obstet Gynecol 2010;3(2):42–8.
77. Moutzouris DA, Falagas ME. Interstitial cystitis: an unsolved enigma. Clin J Am Soc Nephrol 2009;4(11):1844–57.
78. Sant GR, Kempuraj D, Marchand JE, et al. The mast cell in interstitial cystitis: role in pathophysiology and pathogenesis. Urology 2007;69(Suppl 4):34–40.
79. Erickson DR, Xie SX, Bhavanandan VP, et al. A comparison of multiple urine markers for interstitial cystitis. J Urol 2002;167(6):2461–9.
80. Liu HT, Kuo HC. Increased urine and serum nerve growth factor levels in interstitial cystitis suggest chronic inflammation is involved in the pathogenesis of disease. PLoS One 2012;7(9):e44687.
81. Erickson DR, Tomaszewski JE, Kunselman AR, et al. Urine markers do not predict biopsy findings or presence of bladder ulcers in interstitial cystitis/painful bladder syndrome. J Urol 2008;179(5):1850–6.
82. van de Merwe JP. Interstitial cystitis and systemic autoimmune diseases. Nat Clin Pract Urol 2007;4(9):484–91.
83. Grover S, Srivastava A, Lee R, et al. Role of inflammation in bladder function and interstitial cystitis. Ther Adv Urol 2011;3(1):19–33.
84. Kummer JA, Broekhuizen R, Everett H, et al. Inflammasome components NALP 1 and 3 show distinct but separate expression profiles in human tissues suggesting a site-specific role in the inflammatory response. J Histochem Cytochem 2007; 55(5):443–52.
85. Nakamura Y, Kambe N, Saito M, et al. Mast cells mediate neutrophil recruitment and vascular leakage through the NLRP3 inflammasome in histamine-independent urticaria. J Exp Med 2009;206(5):1037–46.
86. Gerber PA, Buhren BA, Steinhoff M, et al. Rosacea: the cytokine and chemokine network. J Investig Dermatol Symp Proc 2011;15(1):40–7.
87. Yamasaki K, Gallo RL. The molecular pathology of rosacea. J Dermatol Sci 2009; 55(2):77–81.
88. Brink N, Szamel M, Young AR, et al. Comparative quantification of IL-1beta, IL-10, IL-10r, TNFalpha and IL-7 mRNA levels in UV-irradiated human skin in vivo. Inflamm Res 2000;49(6):290–6.
89. Faustin B, Reed JC. Sunburned skin activates inflammasomes. Trends Cell Biol 2008;18(1):4–8.
90. Schwab VD, Sulk M, Seeliger S, et al. Neurovascular and neuroimmune aspects in the pathophysiology of rosacea. J Investig Dermatol Symp Proc 2011;15(1): 53–62.
91. Aubdool AA, Brain SD. Neurovascular aspects of skin neurogenic inflammation. J Investig Dermatol Symp Proc 2011;15(1):33–9.
92. Peters KM. Neuromodulation for the treatment of refractory interstitial cystitis. Rev Urol 2002;4(Suppl 1):S36–43.

Acute Pain Management in Older Adults in the Emergency Department

Ula Hwang, MD, MPH[a,b,c],*, Timothy F. Platts-Mills, MD[d,e]

KEYWORDS

- Pain • Geriatrics • Emergency medicine • Pain assessment • Analgesics

KEY POINTS

- Effective treatment of acute pain in older patients is a common challenge faced by emergency providers.
- Because older adults are at increased risk for adverse events associated with systemic analgesics, pain treatment must proceed cautiously.
- Essential elements to quality acute pain care include an early initial assessment for the presence of pain, selection of an analgesic based on patient-specific risks and preferences, and frequent reassessments and retreatments as needed.

INTRODUCTION

Acute pain is a common reason for emergency department (ED) visits among older adults.[1] Effective treatment of acute pain is important for the relief of suffering and because unrelieved acute pain is associated with poorer outcomes during hospitalization, including persistent pain, longer hospital lengths of stay, missed or shortened physical therapy sessions, delays to ambulation, and delirium.[2–7] Despite the frequency with which this problem is encountered and the importance of effective pain treatment, disparities in pain care continue to exist for older adults when compared with younger adults as evidenced by high rates of pain at the end of the ED visit and lower rates of

This article originally appeared in Clinics in Geriatric Medicine, Volume 29, Issue 1, February 2013.

Disclosure: See last page of article.

[a] Department of Emergency Medicine, Mount Sinai School of Medicine, New York, NY, USA; [b] Brookdale Department of Geriatrics and Palliative Medicine, Mount Sinai School of Medicine, New York, NY, USA; [c] Geriatric Research, Education and Clinical Center, James J. Peters Veterans Affairs Medical Center, Bronx, NY, USA; [d] Department of Emergency Medicine, University of North Carolina Chapel Hill, Chapel Hill, NC, USA; [e] Department of Anesthesiology, University of North Carolina Chapel Hill, Chapel Hill, NC, USA

* Corresponding author. Department of Emergency Medicine, One Gustave L. Levy Place, Box 1620, New York, NY 10029.

E-mail address: ula.hwang@mountsinai.org

Clinics Collections 4 (2014) 471–484

http://dx.doi.org/10.1016/j.ccol.2014.10.031

2352-7986/14/$ – see front matter Published by Elsevier Inc.

treatment for older versus younger adults.[1,8-16] Although increased attention to this issue has resulted in some improvement in pain care documentation and use of analgesic in older adults,[17,18] older adults with acute pain are up to 20% less likely to receive treatment[1] than younger patients and still often leave the ED with pain.

The optimal management of acute pain in older adults requires an iterative process of treatment and assessment. This is true for all individuals with acute pain, but particularly so for older adults because of the increased risk of adverse events. Thus, reassessment of pain is as important as providing initial treatment, and failure to reassess pain is a common cause of under-treatment of pain in older adults.[19] Adverse events associated with analgesic treatment in older adults include over-sedation, respiratory depression, acute kidney injury, and gastrointestinal bleeding. Older adults are at increased risk for these events for several reasons: Polypharmacy increases risk for drug–drug interactions; physiologic changes and higher rates of chronic medical problems decrease drug metabolism and clearance; and higher rates of pretreatment functional impairments (physical and cognitive) lower the threshold at which patients may experience symptoms such as loss of balance. Thus, systemic analgesics must be used with caution in older adults.

Goals of Acute Pain Care Management

Goals of care should include early initial assessment of pain, selection of an analgesic based on patient-specific risks and preferences, and effective reduction in pain. Because of the increased risk of adverse drug events, the maxim "start low and go slow" is recommended when dosing analgesics for older adults. Careful titration with frequent reassessment allows for optimal and safe acute pain care in older adults.[20]

Pain Assessment

Older adults are less likely to have documented pain assessments in the ED,[13] despite studies that demonstrate that documentation of pain scores improves analgesic administration patterns in the ED.[21] Potential barriers to assessing and treating pain include patient limitations in the ability to report pain symptoms owing to cognitive and functional impairments and provider limitations in knowledge as well as misconceptions about the value of treating pain in older patients.[22,23] The need for titration of analgesic dosing requires frequent assessment and reassessment of pain in older adults. Thus, the assessment of pain is critical for the safe and effective treatment of acute pain.

Pain scores

Numerous pain assessment methods have been described and studied in older adults.[24] For patients who are cognitively intact, the verbal Numeric Rating Scale is the easiest, most commonly administered method of assessing pain, and preferred by patients.[25,26] The Verbal Descriptor Scale may serve as a more sensitive and reliable instrument for measuring pain in older adults than the Numeric Rating Scale,[26] but the marginal benefit of using a descriptor scale rather than a Numeric Rating Scale in cognitively intact older adults is unclear. For the Numeric Rating Scale and Verbal Descriptor Scale, see **Fig. 1**.

The assessment of pain in older adults with cognitive impairment generally combines information from multiple sources: Patient self-report, searches for potential

NRS: 0 1 2 3 4 5 6 7 8 9 10 [0, no pain; 10, worst pain ever experienced]

VDS[29]: no pain, mild pain, moderate pain, severe pain, extreme pain, most intense pain imaginable

Fig. 1. Numerical rating and verbal descriptor scales for pain.

causes of pain, observations of the patient's facial expressions and behaviors, surrogate reports, and a trial of analgesic therapy.[27,28] These tools include the Abbey Pain Scale (Abbey),[29] Assessment of Discomfort in Dementia protocol,[30] Checklist of Nonverbal Pain Indicators,[31] Noncommunicative Patient's Pain Assessment Instrument,[32] Pain Assessment Checklist for Seniors with Limited Ability to Communicate (PACSLAC[33] and PACSLAC-D-Revised[34]), Pain Assessment in Advanced Dementia,[35] the Critical Care Pain Observation Tool (CPOT),[36] and the Algoplus (**Fig. 2**).[37] Advantages and disadvantages of each of these are provided in **Table 1** based on a modified summary by Bjoro and colleagues.[38] Unfortunately, no single pain scale has been identified to be superior for assessing pain in older adults with limited communication ability, nor have any been developed or validated specifically for the ED setting. Choice of preferred pain assessment may ultimately be determined by feasibility and ease of quickly administering and assessing pain levels in the busy ED environment. More important than which scale is used is that an effort should be made to assess pain in all cognitively impaired patients and treat it when present.

Treatment

Patient goals of pain care

Incorporating patient preferences and goals of care for treatment and pain relief are also priorities of quality geriatric patient care.[39,40] Pain control in older adults almost always involves a balance between pain relief and the risk of unwanted side effects. An open discussion with the patient about their goals and expectations for pain relief can help the provider to understand the manner and degree to which the pain causes problems for the patient and what they perceive to be their risks of various side effects. A shared decision-making effort may result in greater satisfaction with the analgesic choice and improved pain reduction.[41] Among patients with acute severe pain, most patients desire that pain be treated in the ED, would like to be treated early on, and are agreeable to having a nurse administering medication before physician evaluation, but prefer pain control without sedation.[42] Because physician prescribed treatment of pain in the ED is often slow and worsened by ED crowding,[43,44] these preferences support the use of protocols for nurse-administered analgesia. However, nurse-administered analgesia in older adults should initiate treatment with a lower starting dose than for younger patients. A titrated approach will aid providers and patients in finding an appropriate balance between pain control and risk of side effects such as sedation.

Analgesic Options

No guidelines currently exist regarding acute analgesic treatment and dosing for older adults. Evidence-based guidelines in pain treatment for older adults have primarily

Score each grouped item YES / NO for *presence* or *absence*	YES / NO
1. Facial expressions: frowning, grimacing, wincing, clenching teeth, unexpressive	
2. Look: inattentive, blank stare, distant or imploring, teary-eyed, closed eyes	
3. Complaints: "ow-ouch", "that hurts", groaning, screaming	
4. Body position: Withdrawn, guarded, refuses to move, frozen posture	
5. Atypical behaviors: agitations, aggressivity, grabbing onto something or someone	

TOTAL YES   /5

Fig. 2. Algoplus pain scale: Acute pain behavior scale for older persons with inability to communicate verbally. (*Adapted from* Rat P, Jouve E, Pickering G, et al. Validation of an acute pain-behavior scale for older persons with inability to communicate verbally: algoplus. Eur J Pain 2011;15(2):198.e191–10; with permission.)

Table 1
Comparison of pain scales for patients with cognitive impairment or limited ability to communicate

Pain Scale	Objectives/Metrics of Scale	Validation Sample	Advantages (in the ED)	Disadvantages
Abbey Pain Scale[29]	Six questions based on observation of vocalization, facial expression, body language, behavioral, and physiologic and physical changes.	Nursing home resident with end- or late-stage dementia	<1 minute to complete	—
Assessment of Discomfort in Dementia Protocol[30]	Multiple checklist observations (physical symptoms, behavioral changes, sleep changes), use of nonpharmacologic comfort measures, appropriate use of pharmacologic interventions, coordination with physicians, and documentation of care protocols.	Long-term care patients	—	Pain care protocol that focuses on both assessment of discomfort, treatment of this, and use of psychotropic medication; not ED based.
Checklist of nonverbal pain indicators[31]	Summed score of 6 nonverbal indicators (vocalizations, grimaces, bracing, rubbing, restlessness, verbal complaint) observed at rest and with movement.	Cognitively impaired and intact patients with hip fracture during transfer from bed to chair	More appropriate for pain assessment in acute care and procedural pain situations[38]	—
Noncommunicative Patient's Pain Assessment Instrument (NOPPAIN): Nursing Assistant-Administered Pain Assessment Instrument for Use in Dementia[32]	During the performance of daily care activities (laying, turning, transferring from bed; sitting, dressing, feeding, talking, bathing) scaled intensity observations of pain responses with verbal and visualized cues.	Nursing home residents	—	Less than 5 minutes to complete, observation of tasks generally not completed in the ED (bathing, dressing, etc.)

PACSLAC: Pain Assessment Checklist for Seniors with Limited Ability to Communicate[33] PACSLAC-D-Revised[34]	Observation checklist of 60 facial expressions, activity/body movement, social/personality/mood indicators, and physiologic/eating/sleeping/vocal behaviors; Abbreviated version of PACSLAC scale reduced to 24 observed items.	Patients/nursing home resident with dementia and limited ability to communicate	Seems easy to use and preferred by nurses[38]	—
PAINAD: Pain Assessment In Advanced Dementia Scale[35]	Observation of 5 items (and scaled ratings) of breathing, negative vocalizations, facial expression, body language, consolability.	Dementia special care unit	—	Requires >5 minutes observation period
CPOT: Critical-care pain observation tool[36]	Observation of 4 items (facial expression, body movements, muscle tension and compliance with ventilator or vocalization).	Adult cardiac surgical patients in the intensive care unit	<1 minute observation period	—
Algoplus[37]	Observation for presence (yes/no) of 5 items (facial expressions, look, complaints, body position, atypical behaviors).	Cross section of patients ≥65 years in EDs, acute settings, rehabilitation units, long-term care facilities	Less than 1 minute observation period, specifically designed to assess acute pain in elders with inability to communicate verbally (ICV)	—

focused on treatment of chronic or persistent pain with medication recommendations divided into short- (<6 weeks) and long-term (>6 weeks) periods.[45] For older adults with acute moderate to severe pain (pain ≥4–10 on a 0–10 scale), opioids remain the standard of care. There is insufficient evidence at present to support guidelines further characterizing which patients with acute pain are most likely to benefit from opioids versus alternative therapies including nonsteroidal anti-inflammatory drugs (NSAIDs), acetaminophen, or regional anesthesia. For a summary of analgesic options for use in the ED setting, please see **Table 2**.

Non-opioids
Acetaminophen Acetaminophen is perhaps the safest analgesic in older ED patients because of the absence of gastrointestinal, renal, and cardiovascular risks with appropriate dosing.[45] Effective for musculoskeletal pain, acetaminophen is recommend by the American Geriatric Society as a first-line agent for mild ongoing and persistent pain, with increased dosing if pain relief is not satisfactory (up to 4 mg/24 hours) before moving onto a stronger alternative.[45] Risks of hepatic toxicity with acetaminophen are minimal and have primarily been observed with long-term use.[46] Unfortunately, acetaminophen may not be as effective as NSAIDs for pain secondary to inflammatory

Table 2 Common analgesic options for use in older adults: dosing, and considerations		
Analgesic	**Recommended Starting Dose**	**Considerations**
Acetaminophen (Tylenol)	325–500 mg every 4 h or 500–1,000 mg every 6 h	Recommended as first-line pharmacotherapy for pain. One of the safest analgesic profiles. Use limited by maximal daily dose of 4 g.
Ibuprofen	200 mg 3 times a day	If prescribing for prolonged periods, consider adding proton pump inhibitor to reduce gastric side effects.
Naproxen sodium	220 mg twice a day	If prescribing for prolonged periods, consider adding proton pump inhibitor to reduce gastric side effects.
Hydrocodone	2.5–5 mg every 4–6 h	Usually prescribed as a combination drug (with acetaminophen or ibuprofen) which will limit its maximal dosing.
Oxycodone	2.5–5 mg every 4–6 h	Usually prescribed as a combination drug (with acetaminophen or ibuprofen), which will limit its maximal dosing.
Morphine	Immediate release: 2.5–10 mg every 4 h Sustained release: 15 mg every 8–24 h	No maximal ceiling dose.
Hydromorphone (Dilaudid)	1–2 mg every 3–4 h	Effective for breakthrough pain (acute on chronic pain).
Tramadol (Ultram)	12.5–2.5 mg every 4–6 h	Drowsiness, constipation are still common side effects (though not as extreme as with other opioids), lowers seizure threshold.

Data from American Geriatrics Society Panel on the Pharmacologic Management of Persistent Pain in Older Persons. Pharmacologic management of persistent pain in older persons. J Am Geriatr Soc 2009;57:1331–46.

conditions,[47] and the analgesic benefit of acetaminophen is its ceiling dose that limits its effectiveness in treating severe pain.

NSAIDs All commonly used NSAIDs are on Beers list of inappropriate medications for older adults. Beers criteria[48] are a list of medications considered inappropriate for use in older adults in the nursing home, community, outpatient, and acute care settings. Initially developed in the early 1990s to assist in geriatric medication prescribing, the most recent update of Beers criteria have been compiled and reviewed by an interdisciplinary panel of experts in geriatric care, clinical pharmacology, and psychopharmacology has developed guidelines and criteria for appropriate medication use in older adults. Even short-term use of NSAIDS has been considered unacceptable in older adults with diabetes, impaired kidney function, or taking medications that may impair kidney function (diuretics, angiotensin-converting enzyme inhibitors) or metformin.[49] Both renal and gastrointestinal toxicity from NSAIDs are dose and time dependent.[50,51] The patient's risk factors for toxicities and adverse drug reactions (including renal insufficiency, congestive heart failure, hypertension, or concomitant medications such as warfarin use) and recent history of NSAID exposure should be reviewed before administering or prescribing NSAIDs.

Despite these concerns, ibuprofen and ketorolac are commonly used in the treatment of acute pain in older ED patients. Ketorolac (including its parenteral form) should not be used to treat pain secondary to its high potential for adverse gastrointestinal and renal toxicity. "Key issues in the selection of NSAID therapy are pain amelioration, cardiovascular risk, nephrotoxicity, drug interactions, and gastrointestinal toxicity."[45] Other NSAIDs, however, that may be considered for use are ibuprofen and naproxen sodium, and may be used judiciously in the acute setting for older patients who do not have contraindications to their use (decreased renal function, gastropathy, cardiovascular disease, congestive heart failure). When NSAIDs are administered, patients should be informed of the risks and warning signs of adverse effects (eg, decreased urine output, abdominal pain, nausea)[40] and initially started on lowest doses available. Gastric acid suppression with a proton pump inhibitor may also be considered if NSAIDs will be prescribed for prolonged periods ($\geq$4 weeks) at discharge.[52]

Opioids Opioids are recommended for the treatment of moderate to severe persistent pain in older adults by the American Geriatric Society.[45] Secondary to higher fat to lean body mass ratios, older adults should have starting doses 25% to 50% lower than those used in young adults.[53] Opioids commonly used in the ED include oxycodone, morphine, and hydromorphone.[54] Oxycodone is a preferred oral agent because it has a short half-life and little to no toxic metabolites. Morphine can be used with caution, with reduced dosing in patients with renal insufficiency. Tramadol (Ultram) is an atypical opioid analgesic that, although not classified as an opioid, has weak centrally acting opioid activity. For these reasons, some patients may not find it as potent as other opioids, but concurrently it has milder respiratory, abuse potential, and constipation side effects. It may be considered as another option for individuals with moderate pain who cannot tolerate NSAID side effects but are wary about taking opioids.[55] It is metabolized by the liver via the cytochrome P450 isoenzyme and then excreted by the kidney, so cautious dosing is recommended in patients with limited liver and renal function. Doses of warfarin may also need to reduced with concomitant use. Because of neurotoxic metabolites and the presence of safer alternatives,[48] meperidine is listed as inappropriate in older adults by the Beers criteria[48] and should be avoided. Codeine should be used with caution in older adults because it has been found to have greater central nervous system side effects and be associated with increased risk of falls and hip fractures.[56,57]

Common side effects of opioid therapy include nausea/vomiting, dizziness, constipation, and somnolence. Opioid use has also been associated with an increased risk for falls and fall-related injuries in older adults.[58] Thus, the post-ED visit use of opioids in older adults ought to consider the patient's risk of falls including prior history of falls, visual impairment, need for frequent toileting, or limited ability to walk or transfer.[59] A recent study in an adult veteran population found that higher doses of opioids were associated with increased risk of overdose death.[60]

Specific opioids have been associated with specific risks. Cardiovascular effects (QT prolongation and Torsades de pointes) are more commonly seen with methadone than other opioids.[61] A review of more than 5 million Medicare/Medicaid dual enrollees found that of the opioid medications, rates of injury-related ED visits were highest for patients who had recently filled prescriptions for methadone, propoxyphene, and fentanyl.[62]

When compared with hydrocodone, codeine carries an increased cardiovascular event risk after 180 days, and oxycodone and codeine had higher all-cause mortality at 30 days.[63] In another study by the same investigators, it was found that coxibs and opioids carried greater risks for cardiovascular events (when compared with NSAIDs) and opioids had increased risks for fracture, adverse events resulting in hospitalizations, and mortality.[64] Although potentially important for decisions regarding long-term pain management, these results are based on analyses of observational data and, despite appropriate methods for adjustment, may still be confounded by indication (ie, patients with a greater risk of death being more likely to receive opioids). As a result, it remains unclear how these results should inform acute pain treatment in older adults.[65]

Nonpharmacologic strategies

Regional anesthesia Femoral nerve blocks are a feasible and effective option for acute pain owing to hip fractures. Usually, this involves administration of a long-acting local anesthetic (eg, bupivacaine) under ultrasound guidance.[66] Regional anesthesia may provide excellent pain relief without exposing the patient to side effects from systemic analgesics. A combination of regional and systemic anesthesia may also be appropriate. Unfortunately, the use of regional anesthesia is limited primarily to injuries to the face, hands, and lower legs (**Fig. 3**).

Alternate non-pharmacologic therapies

The feasibility and effectiveness of using other types of non-pharmacologic therapies including complementary alternative therapies such as acupuncture, aromatherapy, biofeedback training, and physical modalities such as heat, cold, massage, positioning, and exercise have not been studied in the ED setting. These may, however, be considered by patients as self-management strategies for use once discharged from the ED. Cognitive–behavioral therapy has been demonstrated to be effective in the treatment of chronic pain in older adults.[67–70] Whether cognitive–behavioral therapy can improve outcomes for older adults with acute pain is unknown, but patients with acute severe pain at high risk for persistent pain are, in theory, likely to benefit from early exposure to coping strategies and methods of controlling negative cognitions associated with a new pain condition.

Reassessment

The complexity and risks of managing acute pain in older adults requires frequent reassessment of pain and response to analgesic treatment. Patients should be reassessed with 15 to 20 minutes after a dose of intravenous opioids and within 20 to 30 minutes of administration of oral analgesics. Consistent with the management of

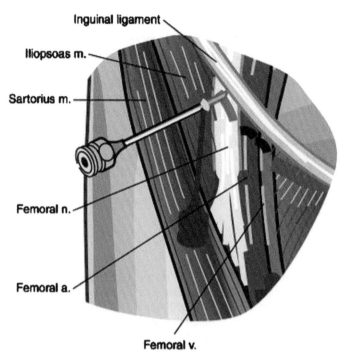

Fig. 3. Femoral nerve block. (*Adapted from* Waldman SD. Atlas of interventional pain management. 2nd edition. Philadelphia: Saunders; 2004. p. 453; with permission.)

diabetic ketoacidosis in the ED setting, where frequent measurements of patient glucose levels are necessary to appropriately manage hyperglycemia, effective management of acute pain in older adults similarly requires frequent reassessments of pain and often requires retreatment.

Geriatric ED Pain Care Quality Indicators

Quality indicators are operational metrics used to determine whether or not care is delivered well or poorly. They set a minimum standard for the care expected from clinicians. Following the Assessing Care of Vulnerable Elders quality indicator approach,[71] a task force convened by the Society for Academic Emergency Medicine and the American College of Emergency Physicians developed the following indicators to measure the quality of geriatric pain care received in the ED setting[72]:

1. Formal assessment for the presence of acute pain should be documented within 1 hour of ED arrival.
2. If a patient remains in the ED for longer than 6 hours, a second pain assessment should be documented.
3. If a patient receives pain treatment, a pain reassessment should be documented before discharge from the ED.
4. If a patient has moderate to severe pain, pain treatment should be initiated (or a reason documented why it was not initiated).
5. Meperidine (Demerol) should not be used to treat pain in older adults.
6. If a patient is prescribed opioid analgesics upon discharge from the ED, a bowel regimen should also be provided.

SUMMARY

Acute pain management in older adults is an increasingly common challenge faced by emergency clinicians. Because of the negative consequences of pain on the health and function of older adults, quality pain care is an important priority in this population. The high frequency of analgesic side effects in older adults, however, requires a cautious approach. Rigorous assessment, treatment, and reassessment of pain are the cornerstone of optimal acute pain care in older adults. Acetaminophen, NSAIDs, opioids, and non-pharmacologic options such as regional anesthesia each have a role to play in acute pain management. Understanding the limitations, contraindications, and risks of these medications are necessary in selecting the appropriate analgesic for both ED and early outpatient treatment in older patients. Communication about risks and close outpatient follow-up with a primary physician is essential to optimize the safe and effective treatment of pain in older adults.

DISCLOSURE

Ula Hwang is supported by a K23 (AG031218) and R21 (AG040734) from the National Institute on Aging to study pain care for older adults in the ED setting. Dr Platts-Mills is supported by Award Number KL2 TR000084 and UL1 TR000083 from the National Center for Research Resources through the North Carolina Translational and Clinical Science Institute. The content is solely the responsibility of the authors and does not necessarily represent the official views of the National Center for Research Resources, the National Institutes of Health, or the North Carolina Translational and Clinical Science Institute.

REFERENCES

1. Platts-Mills TF, Esserman DA, Brown DL, et al. Older US emergency department patients are less likely to receive pain medication than younger patients: results from a national survey. Ann Emerg Med 2012;60(2):199–206.
2. Desbiens N, Mueller-Rizner N, Connors A, et al. Pain in the oldest-old during hospitalization and up to one year later. J Am Geriatr Soc 1997;45:1167–72.
3. Dworkin R. Which individuals with acute pain are most likely to develop a chronic pain syndrome? Pain Forum 1997;6:127–36.
4. Katz J, Jackson M, Kavanaugh B, et al. Acute pain after thoracic surgery predicts long-term post-thoracotomy pain. Clin J Pain 1996;12:50–6.
5. Morrison RS, Magaziner J, McLaughlin MA, et al. The impact of post-operative pain on outcomes following hip fracture. Pain 2003;103(3):303–11.
6. Duggleby W, Lander J. Cognitive status and postoperative pain: older adults. J Pain Symptom Manage 1994;9:19–27.
7. Lynch E, Lazor M, Gelis J, et al. The impact of postoperative pain on the development of postoperative delirium. Anesth Analg 1998;86:781–5.
8. Terrell KT, Hui SL, Castelluccio P, et al. Analgesic prescribing for patients who are discharged from an emergency department. Pain Med 2010;11:1072–7.
9. Jones J, Johnson K, McNinch M. Age as a risk factor for inadequate emergency department analgesia. Am J Emerg Med 1996;14:157–60.
10. Heins J, Heins A, Grammas M, et al. Disparities in analgesia and opioid prescribing practices for patients with musculoskeletal pain in the emergency department. J Emerg Nurs 2006;32:219–24.

11. Heins A, Grammas M, Heins JK, et al. Determinants of variation in analgesic and opioid prescribing practice in an emergency department. J Opioid Manag 2006; 2:335–40.

12. Hwang U, Richardson LD, Harris B, et al. The quality of emergency department pain care for older adult patients. J Am Geriatr Soc 2010;58:2122–8.

13. Iyer RG. Pain documentation and predictors of analgesic prescribing for elderly patients during emergency department visits. J Pain Symptom Manage 2010;41: 367–73.

14. Arendts G, Fry M. Factors associated with delay to opiate analgesia in emergency departments. J Pain 2006;7:682–6.

15. Platts-Mills TF, Esserman DA, Brown L, et al. Older US emergency department patients are less likely to receive pain medication than younger patients: results from a national survey. Ann Emerg Med 2012;60:199–206.

16. Mills AM, Edwards JM, Shofer FS, et al. Analgesia for older adults with abdominal or back pain in emergency department. West J Emerg Med 2011;12:43–50.

17. Herr K, Titler M. Acute pain assessment and pharmacological management practices for the older adult with a hip fracture: review of ED trends. J Emerg Nurs 2009;35:312–20.

18. Cinar O, Ernst R, Fosnocht D, et al. Geriatric patients may not experience increased risk of oligoanalgesia in the emergency department. Ann Emerg Med 2012;60:207–11.

19. Wells N, Pasero C, McCaffery M. Improving the quality of care through pain assessment and management. patient safety and quality: an evidence-based handbook for nurses. Rockville (MD): Agency for Healthcare Research and Quality; 2008.

20. Fine PG. Treatment guidelines for the pharmacological management of pain in older persons. Pain Med 2012;13(Suppl 2):s57–66.

21. Silka PA, Roth MM, Moreno G, et al. Pain scores improve analgesic administration patterns for trauma patients in the emergency department. Acad Emerg Med 2004;11:264–70.

22. Duignan M, Dunn V. Barriers to pain management in emergency departments. Emerg Nurse 2008;15(9):30–4.

23. Rupp T, Delaney K. Inadequate analgesia in emergency medicine. Ann Emerg Med 2004;43:494–503.

24. Hwang U, Jagoda A. Geriatric emergency analgesia. In: Thomas S, editor. Emergency department analgesia. Cambridge (UK): Cambridge University Press; 2008. p. 42–51.

25. Ware LJ, Epps CD, Herr K, et al. Evaluation of the revised faces pain scale, verbal descriptor scale, numeric rating scale, and Iowa pain thermometer in older minority adults. Pain Manag Nurs 2006;7(3):117–25.

26. Herr K, Spratt K, Mobiliy P, et al. Pain intensity assessment in older adults: use of experimental pain to compare psychometric properties and usability of selected pain scales with younger adults. Clin J Pain 2004;20:207–19.

27. Herr K, Coyne PJ, Key T, et al. Pain assessment in the nonverbal patient: position statement with clinical practice recommendations. Pain Manag Nurs 2006;7(2): 44–52.

28. Herr K, Bjoro K, Decker S. Tools for assessment of pain in nonverbal older adults with dementia: a state-of-the-science review. J Pain Symptom Manage 2006; 31(2):170–92.

29. Abbey J, Piller N, De Belllis A, et al. The Abbey pain scale: a 1-minute numerical indicator for people with end-stage dementia. Int J Palliat Nurs 2004;10(1):6–13.

30. Kovach CR, Weissman DE, Griffie J, et al. Assessment and treatment of discomfort for people with late-stage dementia. J Pain Symptom Manage 1999;18(6): 412–9.
31. Feldt KS. The Checklist of nonverbal pain indicators (CNPI). Pain Manag Nurs 2000;1:13–21.
32. Snow AL, Weber JB, O'Malley KJ, et al. NOPPAIN: a nursing assistant-administered pain assessment instrument for use in dementia. Dement Geriatr Cogn Disord 2004;17(3):240–6.
33. Fuchs-Lacelle S, Hadjistavropoulos T. Development and preliminary validation of the pain assessment checklist for seniors with limited ability to communicate (PACSLAC). Pain Manag Nurs 2004;5(1):37–49.
34. Zwakhalen SM, Hamers JP, Berger MP. Improving the clinical usefulness of a behavioural pain scale for older people with dementia. J Adv Nurs 2007;58: 493–502.
35. Warden V, Hurley AC, Volicer L. Development and psychometric evaluation of the pain assessment in advanced dementia (PAINAD) scale. J Am Med Dir Assoc 2003;4(1):9–15.
36. Gelinas C, Fillion L, Puntillo KA, et al. Validation of the critical-care pain observation tool in adult patients. Am J Crit Care 2006;15(4):420–7.
37. Rat P, Jouve E, Pickering G, et al. Validation of an acute pain-behavior scale for older persons with inability to communicate verbally: algoplus. Eur J Pain 2011; 15(2). 198.e191–10.
38. Bjoro M, Herr K. Chapter 5-assessment of pain in the nonverbal and/or cognitively impaired older adults. In: Smith H, editor. Current therapy in pain. Philadelphia: Saunders Elsevier; 2009. p. 24–37.
39. Isaacs CG, Kistler C, Hunold KM, et al. Shared decision making in the selection of outpatient analgesics for older emergency department patients. Chicago: Society of Academic Emergency Medicine; 2012.
40. Bowling CB, O'Hare AM. Managing older adults with CKD: individualized versus disease-based approaches. Am J Kidney Dis 2012;59:293–302.
41. Isaacs CG, Kistler C, Hunold KM, et al. Shared decision making in the selection of outpatient analgesics for older emergency department patients. J Am Geriatr Soc, in press.
42. Beel TL, Mitchiner JC, Frederiksen SM, et al. Patient preferences regarding pain medication in the ED. Am J Emerg Med 2000;18:376–80.
43. Hwang U, Richardson LD, Sonuyi TO, et al. The effect of emergency department crowding on the management of pain in older adults with hip fracture. J Am Geriatr Soc 2006;54:270–5.
44. Pines JM, Hollander JE. Emergency department crowding is associated with poor care for patients with severe pain. Ann Emerg Med 2008;51:1–5.
45. American Geriatrics Society Panel on the Pharmacological Management of Persistent Pain in Older Persons. Pharmacological management of persistent pain in older persons. J Am Geriatr Soc 2009;57:1331–46.
46. Watkins PB, Kaplowitz N, Slattery JT, et al. Aminotransferase elevations in healthy adults receiving 4 grams of acetaminophen daily: a randomized controlled trial. JAMA 2006;296:87–93.
47. Weinecke T, Gotzsche PC. Paracetamol versus nonsteroidal anti-inflammatory drugs for rheumatoid arthritis. Cochrane Database Syst Rev 2004;(1):CD003789.
48. American Geriatrics Society 2012 Beers criteria update expert panel. American Geriatrics Society updated Beers Criteria for potentially inappropriate medication use in older adults. J Am Geriatr Soc 2012;60(4):616–31.

49. Platts-Mills TF, Richmond NL, Hunold KM, et al. Life-threatening hyperkalemia following two days of ibuprofen. Am J Emerg Med, in press.
50. Whelton A, Stout RL, Spilman PS, et al. Renal effects of ibuprofen, piroxicam, and sulindac in patients with asymptomatic renal failure. A prospective, randomized, crossover comparison. Ann Intern Med 1990;112(8):568–76.
51. Rainsford KD. Profile and mechanisms of gastrointestinal and other side effects of nonsteroidal anti-inflammatory drugs (NSAIDs). Am J Med 1999;107(6A): 27S–35S.
52. Rostom A, Dube C, Wells G, et al. Prevention of NSAID-induced gastrodudenal ulcers. Cochrane Database Syst Rev 2002;(4):CD0022960.
53. Abrahm JL. Advances in pain management for older adult patients. Clin Geriatr Med 2000;16:269–311.
54. Chang AK, Bijur PE, Baccelieri A, et al. Efficacy and safety profile of a single dose of hydromorphone compared with morphine in older adults with acute, severe pain: a prospective, randomized, double-blind clinical trial. Am J Geriatr Pharmacother 2009;7:1–10.
55. Barkin R, Barkin S, Barkin D. Perception, assessment, treatment, and management of pain in the elderly. Clin Geriatr Med 2005;21:465–90.
56. Shorr RI, Griffin MR, Daughterty JR, et al. Opioid analgesics and the risk of hip fracture in the elderly: codeine and propoxyphene. J Gerontol 1992;47: M111–5.
57. Turturro MA, Paris PM, Yealy DM, et al. Hydrocodone versus codeine in acute musculoskeletal pain. Ann Emerg Med 1991;20(10):1100–3.
58. Huang AR, Mallet L, Rochefort CM, et al. Medication-related falls in the elderly: causative factors and preventive strategies. Drugs Aging 2012;29:359–76.
59. Vassallo M, Stockdale R, Sharma JC, et al. A comparative study of the use of four fall risk assessment tools on acute medical wards. J Am Geriatr Soc 2005;53: 1034–8.
60. Bohnert AS, Valenstein M, Bair MJ, et al. Association between opioid prescribing patterns and opioid overdose-related deaths. JAMA 2011;305:1315–21.
61. Chan BK, Tam LK, Wat CY, et al. Opioids in chronic non-cancer pain. Expert Opin Pharmacother 2011;12:705–20.
62. Blackwell SA, Montgomery MA, Waldo D, et al. National study of medications associated with injury in elderly Medicare/Medicaid dual enrollees. J Am Pharm Assoc 2003;49(6):751–9.
63. Solomon DH, Rassen JA, Glynn RJ, et al. The comparative safety of opioids for nonmalignant pain in older adults. Arch Intern Med 2010;170:1979–86.
64. Solomon DH, Rassen JA, Glynn RJ, et al. The comparative safety of analgesics in older adults with arthritis. Arch Intern Med 2010;170:1968–76.
65. Hwang U, Morrison RS, Richardson LD, et al. A painful setback: misinterpretation of analgesic safety in older adults may inadvertently worsen pain care. Arch Intern Med 2011;171(12):1127.
66. Beaudoin FL, Nagdev A, Merchant RC, et al. Ultrasound-guided femoral nerve blocks in elderly patients with hip fractures. Am J Emerg Med 2010;28(1):76–81.
67. Abbasi M, Dehghani M, Keefe FJ, et al. Spouse-assisted training in pain coping skills and the outcome of multidisciplinary pain management for chronic low back pain treatment: a 1-year randomized controlled trial. Eur J Pain 2012;16(7): 1033–43.
68. Keefe FJ, Blumenthal J, Baucom D, et al. Effects of spouse-assisted coping skills training and exercise training in patients with osteoarthritic knee pain: a randomized controlled study. Pain 2004;110(3):539–49.

69. Morley S, Eccleston C, Williams A. Systematic review and meta-analysis of randomized controlled trials of cognitive behaviour therapy and behaviour therapy for chronic pain in adults, excluding headache. Pain 1999;80(1–2):1–13.
70. Waters SJ, Woodward JT, Keefe FJ. Cognitive-behavioral therapy for pain in older adults. In: Gibson SJ, Weiner DK, editors. Pain in older persons, progress in pain research and management, vol. 35. Seattle (WA): IASP Press; 2005. p. 239–61.
71. Wenger N, Shekelle P. Assessing care of vulnerable elders: ACOVE project overview. Ann Intern Med 2001;135(8 Part 2):642–6.
72. Terrell KT, Hustey FM, Hwang U, et al. Quality indicators for geriatric emergency care. Acad Emerg Med 2009;16:441–50.

Printed and bound by CPI Group (UK) Ltd, Croydon, CR0 4YY

03/10/2024

01040497-0012